Treatment of Pediatric Neurologic Disorders

Harvey S. Singer
Eric H. Kossoff
Adam L. Hartman
Thomas O. Crawford

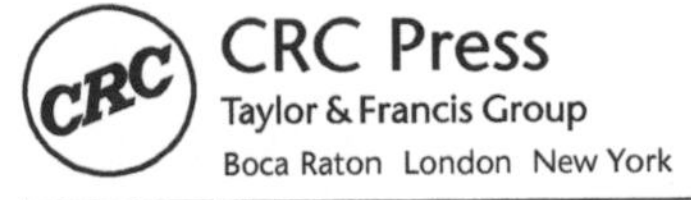

CRC Press is an imprint of the
Taylor & Francis Group, an **informa** business

CRC Press
Taylor & Francis Group
6000 Broken Sound Parkway NW, Suite 300
Boca Raton, FL 33487-2742

First issued in paperback 2019

ISBN-13: 978-0-8247-2693-5 (hbk)
ISBN-13: 978-0-367-39301-4 (pbk)

A CIP record for this book is available from the British Library.

Library of Congress Cataloging-in-Publication Data available on application

Visit the Taylor & Francis Web site at
http://www.taylorandfrancis.com

and the CRC Press Web site at
http://www.crcpress.com

Contents

Preface

The decision to pursue the challenge of producing a high quality text on treating disorders in child neurology was undertaken after much deliberation. In part, our ultimate motivation was based on both the need for such a book and a desire to include the expertise of individuals who have had a role in the child neurology program at the Johns Hopkins Hospital. It is, therefore, with great pleasure that we note that multiple chapters have been written by individuals, both faculty members and residents, with current or past ties to the program. The four editors, two senior faculty, one junior faculty, and a senior child neurology resident, have produced a text that we hope will be broadly acceptable to readers at all levels of experience. Lastly, we are proud to include a brief description of the history of the child neurology program at the Johns Hopkins University. We dedicate this book to the past leaders of the program, with special recognition to the first Director of the training program, Dr. John M. Freeman.

Harvey S. Singer
Eric H. Kossoff
Adam L. Hartman
Thomas O. Crawford
Division of Child Neurology
Johns Hopkins University School of Medicine,
Baltimore, Maryland

HISTORY OF CHILD NEUROLOGY AT JOHNS HOPKINS HOSPITAL

The Department of Neurology and its accompanying division of Child Neurology were formally established at Johns Hopkins in 1969. Before this time, there already existed a distinguished history of individuals with expertise in pediatric neurology, including such luminaries as William Osler, Frank Ford, and David Clark.

William Osler was Chief of Medicine at the Johns Hopkins Hospital from 1889 to 1905. His contributions to internal medicine and neurology are legendary, but his research and case presentations on pediatric topics are often overlooked. His bibliography contains publications on cerebral palsy, chorea, tics, muscular dystrophy, epilepsy, meningitis, and childhood migraine.

Frank Ford was one of the earliest child neurologists in the United States. Ford was born and schooled in Baltimore and ultimately rose to be head of neurology at Johns Hopkins, a position he held from 1932 to 1958. Based in part on his observations at the Harriet Lane Home Outpatient Clinic and interest in neuroanatomy and pathology, he was coauthor of a book entitled *Birth Injuries of the Nervous System*. Included in the section written by Ford was a description of developmental neurobiology, with an emphasis on perinatal birth injury. His second text on pediatric neurology, first published in 1937, was an encyclopedic 950 pages entitled *Diseases of the Nervous System in Infancy, Childhood and Adolescence*.

David Clark received his medical degree from the University of Chicago and trained in medicine and neurology at Johns Hopkins. As one of Frank Ford's students, he became an energetic, outstanding clinician and teacher, well known for his case analyses and virtuoso performances in case conferences. Clark left Hopkins in 1965 to become the chairman of the Department of Neurology at the University of Kentucky.

In the 1950s there were seven neurology faculty members within the neurology division of the Department of Medicine, three in pediatric neurology (Frank Ford, David Clark, and John Menkes). John Menkes left in 1966 to head child neurology in Los Angeles.

Although the concept of establishing a separate Department of Neurology had been frequently discussed, the decision to create the department was not finalized until Vernon Mouncastle, who held a strong belief in the "science of the brain and behavior," convinced the then Director of Medicine A. McGee Harvey of the benefits. Based, in part, on a recommendation by Robert Cooke, Chair of the Department of Pediatrics, Guy McKhann was selected as the first Neurology Department Chairman.

McKhann attended the Yale Medical School, trained in pediatrics at Yale and Hopkins, received neurology training at Boston Children's Hospital under the mentorship of Phillip Dodge, and spent several years studying cerebral metabolism at the NIH. In January 1969, he was the first chair of the newly created department and its sole child neurologist. It is said that he impressed the Hopkins pediatricians during his first month when he was asked to consult on a child with the acute onset of ataxia and opsoclonus. For reasons unclear to them, he requested a chest x-ray looking for a neuroblastoma. Although they were mystified at first, when the neuroblastoma was removed and the child improved, the future of child neurology was ensured.

One of Guy McKhann's earliest faculty appointments was a chief of pediatric neurology; he wisely chose John Freeman. Freeman completed his pediatric training at Hopkins where David Clark had served as his mentor and role model. This was followed by a child neurology fellowship at the Columbia Neurological Institute, under the mentorship of Dr. Sidney Carter. Freeman was initially recruited by McKhann to join him at Stanford, but after enjoying sunny California for only 3 years, he repacked and returned to the East coast. It is notable that three of the four initial neurology residents, Gary Goldstein, William Logan, and Mark Molliver, were all pediatric neurology trainees. Apparently, the Osler medical residents were not informed that they were being supervised by mere pediatricians. The goal from the outset was to train academic neurologists who would advance the field, as well as train others.

In starting the child neurology program, Freeman's initial goal was to reverse the segregation policy that had been in place during his residency. He established an integrated clinic that wall open to all—black, white, rich or poor—and staffed it with residents and medical students under his supervision. Freeman also organized a combined service for pediatric neurology and neurosurgery patients. Clearly, the patients received better and more consistent care than if they had been on only a surgical service. Unfortunately, in later years because of house staff shortages, billing, and other issues, this unique concept had to be abandoned. The goal of the pediatric neurology training program was identical to that of adult neurology, i.e., to train the future academic leaders of the field. In this regard, Freeman achieved success. During his tenure as Director of Child Neurology from 1969 to 1990, he trained 44 individuals in child neurology. Thirty-one of the 44 entered academic neurology and most went on to run their own training programs—wonderful legacy! His philosophy was to attract the best and the brightest and instill in than the joys of academia. As one of his pupils, I can personally attest to his strong character, teaching and motivational skills, academic achievements, but most importantly to his ability to be a friend and long-term counselor.

This book is a testimony to the quality and quantity of an impressive group of residents trained over the years at Johns Hopkins.

Harvey S. Singer, M.D.
Haller Professor of Pediatric Neurology
Director, Child Neurology
Johns Hopkins University School of Medicine

Contributors

Anthony M. Avellino Division of Pediatric Neurosurgery, Children's Hospital and Regional Medical Center, University of Washington School of Medicine, Seattle, Washington, U.S.A.

James F. Bale Division of Neurology, Department of Pediatrics, The University of Utah School of Medicine, Salt Lake City, U.S.A.

Shannon Barnett Department of Psychiatry, The Johns Hopkins Hospital, Baltimore, Maryland, U.S.A.

Anita L. Belman Department of Neurology, School of Medicine, State University of New York (SUNY) at Stony Brook, Stony Brook, New York, U.S.A.

Ann M. Bergin Childrens Hospital, Department of Neurology, Boston, Massachusetts, U.S.A.

Genila M. Bibat Neurogenetics Unit, Kennedy Krieger Institute, Johns Hopkins Medical Institutions, Baltimore, Maryland, U.S.A.

Ian Butler The University of Texas Medical School at Houston, Houston, Texas, U.S.A.

Benjamin S. Carson, Sr. Department of Neurological Surgery, Johns Hopkins Medical Institutions, Baltimore, Maryland, U.S.A.

Ronald D. Cohn Johns Hopkins Hospital, Children's Center, McKusick-Nathans Institute of Genetic Medicine, Baltimore, Maryland, U.S.A.

Anne M. Comi Johns Hopkins Hospital, Baltimore, Maryland, U.S.A.

Joan A. Conry George Washington University School of Medicine, Children's National Medical Center, Washington, D.C., U.S.A.

Helen E. Courvoisie Division of Child and Adolescent Psychiatry, Department of Psychiatry and Behavioral Sciences, The Johns Hopkins Medical Institutions, Baltimore, Maryland, U.S.A.

Thomas O. Crawford Johns Hopkins Hospital, Baltimore, Maryland, U.S.A.

Dana D. Cummings Kennedy Krieger Institute, Baltimore, Maryland, U.S.A.

Nancy P. Dalos All Children's Hospital, Clearwater, Florida, U.S.A.

Cecilia T. Davoli Kennedy Krieger Institute, Baltimore, Maryland, U.S.A.

Martha Bridge Denckla Johns Hopkins University School of Medicine, Kennedy Krieger Institute, Baltimore, Maryland, U.S.A.

Leon S. Dure, IV Division of Pediatric Neurology, Department of Pediatrics, The University of Alabama at Birmingham, Birmingham, Alabama, U.S.A.

Linda M. Famiglio Geisinger Health System, Danville, Pennsylvania, U.S.A.

Paul Grahan Fisher The Beirne Family Director of Neuro-Oncology at Packard Children's Hospital, Stanford University, Stanford, California, U.S.A.

John M. Freeman Pediatrics and Neurology, Johns Hopkins Hospital, Baltimore, Maryland, U.S.A.

Natan Gadoth Department of Neurology, Meir General Hospital, Kfar Saba, Israel

William Davis Gaillard Department of Neurology, Children's National Medical Center, Washington, D.C., U.S.A.

Philippe H. Gailloud Division of Interventional Neuroradiology, Johns Hopkins University School of Medicine, Baltimore, Maryland, U.S.A.

Donald L. Gilbert Cincinnati Children's Hospital Medical Center, Movement Disorders Clinics, Cincinnati, Ohio, U.S.A.

Fiona Goodwin Department of Pediatric Neurology, Child Health, University of Southampton and Southampton University Hospitals, Southampton, U.K.

Marco A. Grados The Johns Hopkins Hospital, Department of Psychiatry, Division of Child and Adolescent Psychiatry, Baltimore, Maryland, U.S.A.

Robert M. Gray Kennedy Krieger Institute, Department of Neuropsychology, Baltimore, Maryland, U.S.A.

Carolyn Elizabeth Hart Mecklenburg Neurological Associates, Charlotte, North Carolina, U.S.A.

Adam L. Hartman Johns Hopkins Hospital, Baltimore, Maryland, U.S.A.

Susan J. Hayflick Molecular and Medical Genetics, Pediatrics and Neurology, Oregon Health & Science University, Portland, Oregon, U.S.A.

J. Michael Hemphill Department of Neurology, Medical College of Georgia, Savannah Neurology, Savannah, Georgia, U.S.A.

Alec Hoon Johns Hopkins University School of Medicine, Kennedy Krieger Institute, Baltimore, Maryland, U.S.A.

Judy Huang Department of Neurosurgery, Johns Hopkins University School of Medicine, Baltimore, Maryland, U.S.A.

Rebecca N. Ichord Department of Neurology, Children's Hospital of Philadelphia, Philadelphia, Pennsylvania, U.S.A.

H.A. Jinnah Department of Neurology, Johns Hopkins University, Baltimore, Maryland, U.S.A.

Michael V. Johnston Department of Neurology and Developmental Medicine, Kennedy Krieger Institute, Johns Hopkins University School of Medicine, Baltimore, Maryland, U.S.A.

Charlotte Jones Joan C. Edwards School of Medicine, Marshall University, Huntington, West Virginia, U.S.A.

Lori C. Jordan Department of Neurology, Johns Hopkins University School of Medicine, Baltimore, Maryland, U.S.A.

Raymond S. Kandt Johnson Neurological Clinic, High Point, North Carolina, U.S.A.

Richard Kaplan Southern California Permanente Medical Group, San Diego, California, U.S.A.

Colin Kennedy Department of Pediatric Neurology, Child Health, University of Southampton and Southampton University Hospitals, Southampton, U.K.

Douglas Kerr Department of Neurology, Johns Hopkins University School of Medicine, Baltimore, Maryland, U.S.A.

Julie Newman Kingery Division of Child and Adolescent Psychiatry, Johns Hopkins University School of Medicine, Baltimore, Maryland, U.S.A.

Stephen L. Kinsman Departement of Pediatrics, University of Maryland School of Medicine, Baltimore, Maryland, U.S.A.

Eric H. Kossoff The Johns Hopkins Hospital, Baltimore, Maryland, U.S.A.

Chitra Krishnan Department of Neurology, Johns Hopkins University School of Medicine, Baltimore, Maryland, U.S.A.

William R. Leahy Neurological Medicine, Greenbelt, Maryland, U.S.A.

Benjamin H. Lee Departments of Anesthesiology, Critical Care Medicine, and Pediatrics, The John Hopkins Hospital, Baltimore, Maryland, U.S.A.

Maureen A. Lefton-Greif Johns Hopkins University School of Medicine, Baltimore, Maryland, U.S.A.

David Lieberman Johns Hopkins Hospital, Departments of Pediatric Neurology and Pediatric Infectious Disease, Baltimore, Maryland, U.S.A.

E. Mark Mahone Department of Neuropsychology, Kennedy Krieger Institute, Baltimore, Maryland, U.S.A.

Pedro Mancias The University of Texas Medical School at Houston, Houston, Texas, U.S.A.

Bernard L. Maria Medical University of South Carolina, Charleston, South Carolina, U.S.A.

Julia McMillan Johns Hopkins Hospital, Departments of Pediatric Neurology and Pediatric Infectious Disease, Baltimore, Maryland, U.S.A.

Lonnie J. Miner Division of Neurology, Department of Pediatrics, The University of Utah School of Medicine, Salt Lake City, U.S.A.

Xue Ming UMDNJ-New Jersey Medical School, Newark, New Jersey, U.S.A.

Jonathan W. Mink University of Rochester, Departments of Neurology, Neurobiology & Anatomy, and Pediatrics, Rochester, New York, U.S.A.

Leslie A. Morrison Department of Neurology, University of New Mexico, Albuquerque, New Mexico, U.S.A.

Hugo W. Moser Kennedy Krieger Institute, Johns Hopkins University, Baltimore, Maryland, U.S.A.

Stewart Mostofsky Kennedy Krieger Institute, Baltimore, Maryland, U.S.A.

Richard T. Moxley, III Department of Neurology, University of Rochester Medical Center, Rochester, New York, U.S.A.

Edwin C. Myer VCU Health System, Department of Neurology, Richmond, Virginia, U.S.A.

SakkuBai Naidu Neurogenetics Unit, Kennedy Krieger Institute, Johns Hopkins Medical Institutions, Baltimore, Maryland, U.S.A.

Kathryn N. North Institute for Neuromuscular Research, Children's Hospital at Westmead, Sydney, Australia

Lori L. Olson Medical University of South Carolina, Charleston, South Carolina, U.S.A.

Robert Ouvrier TY Nelson Department of Neurology and Neurosurgery, Children's Hospital at Westmead, Sydney, Australia

Roger J. Packer Neuroscience and Behavioral Medicine, Division of Child Neurology, Children's National Medical Center, The George Washington University, Washington, D.C., U.S.A.

Eric M. Pearlman Mercer University School of Medicine, Savannah, Georgia, U.S.A.

Frank S. Pidcock Department of Pediatric Physical Medicine and Rehabilitation, Johns Hopkins University School of Medicine, Kennedy Krieger Institute, Baltimore, Maryland, U.S.A.

Annapurna Poduri Division of Pediatric Neurology, Children's Hospital of Philadelphia, University of Pennsylvania, Philadelphia, Pennsylvania, U.S.A.

Michael R. Pranzatelli National Pediatric Myoclonus Center, Department of Neurology and Pediatrics, Southern Illinois University School of Medicine, Springfield, Illinois, U.S.A.

April Puscavage Johns Hopkins University School of Medicine, Kennedy Krieger Institute, Baltimore, Maryland, U.S.A.

Gerald V. Raymond Kennedy Krieger Institute, Johns Hopkins University School of Medicine, Baltimore, Maryland, U.S.A.

Anthony Redmond Academic Unit of Musculoskeletal Disease, University of Leeds, Leeds, U.K.

Tyler Reimschisel McKusick-Nathans Institute of Genetic Medicine, Johns Hopkins Hospital, Baltimore, Maryland, U.S.A.

Michael X. Repka Johns Hopkins Hospital, Baltimore, Maryland, U.S.A.

Mark Riddle Department of Psychiatry, The Johns Hopkins Hospital, Baltimore, Maryland, U.S.A.

James E. Rubenstein Johns Hopkins Medical Institutions, Baltimore, Maryland, U.S.A.

Monique M. Ryan Institute for Neuromuscular Research and Discipline of Paediatrics and Child Health, Children's Hospital at Westmead, Sydney, Australia

Shlomo Shinnar Departments of Neurology, Pediatrics, and Comprehensive Epilepsy Management Center, Montefiore Medical Center, Albert Einstein College of Medicine, Bronx, New York, U.S.A.

George K. Siberry The Johns Hopkins Hospital, Department of Pediatrics, Baltimore, Maryland, U.S.A.

Harvey S. Singer Departments of Neurology and Pediatrics, Johns Hopkins University School of Medicine, Baltimore, Maryland, U.S.A.

Constance Smith-Hicks The Johns Hopkins Hospital, Baltimore, Maryland, U.S.A.

Donna J. Stephenson Wilmington, Delaware, U.S.A.

Charlotte J. Sumner National Institute of Neurological Disorders and Stroke, National Institutes of Health, Bethesda, Maryland, U.S.A.

Traci D. Swink Marshfield Clinic, Marshfield, Wisconsin, U.S.A.

Rafael J. Tamargo Department of Neurosurgery, Johns Hopkins University School of Medicine, Baltimore, Maryland, U.S.A.

Gihan Tennekoon Division of Pediatric Neurology, Children's Hospital of Philadelphia, University of Pennsylvania, Philadelphia, Pennsylvania, U.S.A.

Elizabeth A. Thiele Harvard Medical School, Massachusetts General Hospital, Boston, Massachusetts, U.S.A.

William H. Trescher Kennedy Krieger Institute, Baltimore, Maryland, U.S.A.

Adeline Vanderver Department of Neurology, Children's National Medical Center, Washington, D.C., U.S.A.

Eileen P.G. Vining The John M. Freeman Pediatric Epilepsy Center, Johns Hopkins Hospital, Baltimore, Maryland, U.S.A.

John T. Walkup Division of Child and Adolescent Psychiatry, Johns Hopkins University School of Medicine, Baltimore, Maryland, U.S.A.

Jon Weingart Johns Hopkins School of Medicine, Johns Hopkins Hospital, Baltimore, Maryland, U.S.A.

Myson Yaster Departments of Anesthesiology, Critical Care Medicine, and Pediatrics, The Johns Hopkins Hospital, Baltimore, Maryland, U.S.A.

Kaleb Yohay Departments of Neurology and Pediatrics, Johns Hopkins Hospital, Baltimore, Maryland, U.S.A.

Michael E. Yurcheshen Department of Neurology, University of Rochester Medical Center, Rochester, New York, U.S.A.

Sina Zaim UMDNJ-New Jersey Medical School, Newark, New Jersey, U.S.A.

Andrew W. Zimmerman Kennedy Krieger Institute, Baltimore, Maryland, U.S.A.

1

Craniosynostosis

Benjamin S. Carson, Sr.
Department of Neurological Surgery, Johns Hopkins Medical Institutions, Baltimore, Maryland, U.S.A.

INTRODUCTION

Craniosynostosis, premature fusion of the coronal, sagittal, metopic, and/or lambdoidal sutures, may be primary or secondary to a wide range of poorly characterized genetic, nutritional, toxicological, and mechanical influences. Craniosynostosis also can be found when intracranial contents are markedly reduced, such as when patients are overshunted and sutures subsequently override and fuse or in cases of severe cerebral atrophy. The condition may be "isolated," involving a single suture, or "complex," involving multiple sutures. Approximately 100 different forms have been described. The manifestations have been classified as "nonsyndromic" and "syndromic." The latter have been linked to several chromosomes. Defects in fibroblast growth factor receptor (FGFR) genes have been identified by several groups. Apert, Pfeiffer, Jackson-Weiss, and Crouzon syndrome associate with mutations in FGFR genes. However, pathophysiology may be heterogenous because clinical features are not always associated with specific mutations (1).

Statistics regarding the incidence of craniosynostoses are difficult to assemble because cranial deformities often are not lethal, and are not always recognized at birth or recorded in adults. Studies have suggested a baseline of 0.2–0.5 cases per 1000 births. With lambdoidal craniosynostosis, anomalies in skull morphology usually precede complications such as visual impairment and increased intracranial pressure (ICP). Hydrocephalus frequently occurs with syndromic synostosis, and is rarely found in simple, nonsyndromic craniosynostosis, but increased ICP is not unusual. Elevated ICP appears to be the driving force behind the neurological deficits. The pressure may not be readily apparent on imaging studies or from clinical signs or symptoms.

A subset of the craniosynostoses, unilambdoidal synostosis, attracted particular interest in the early 1990s because several reports indicated a significant increase in the incidence, which was generally considered to be about 0.05 per 1000 births, or about 1% of the craniosynostosis cases. Pediatric neurosurgeons noted that lambdoidal craniosynostosis and positional plagiocephaly (sometimes referred to as "occipital plagiocephaly" and "functional plagiocephaly") had similar morphological characteristics. The suspected increase in lambdoidal synostosis was, in fact, an increase in positional plagiocephaly, an increase related to the American Academy of Pediatrics recommendations (in 1992) that healthy infants avoid the prone sleeping position. Asymmetric skull flattening tends to be perpetuated or accentuated by supine positioning of the infant; the head will turn to the flatter side by forces of gravity, or because of varying degrees of torticollis (2).

DIFFERENTIAL DIAGNOSIS

Pediatricians and family practitioners often request neurosurgical consultation for infants with abnormal head circumference in relation to standard growth curves, yet who are otherwise normal in growth and development, typically at about 6 months of age. An assessment model is shown in Fig. 1. Anomalies frequently are noted at birth; parents report a progressive worsening of the deformity and routinely express a concern about potential developmental problems. Differential diagnoses include torticollis, positional molding, and craniosynostosis. Other intracranial causes including tumors are less common. Positional molding may have clinical manifestations similar to that of an actual craniosynostosis, but the sutures appear open on plain x-rays and CT scans in such cases. Torticollis involves a shortened sternocleidomastoid muscle, which can result in flattening of the temporal and occipital region. The anterior deformity can be greater than the posterior deformity, and is on the side of the abnormality. The usually mild deformity improves with neck exercises and physical therapy. The muscle rarely needs to be divided or lengthened. Torticollis can cause or potentiate positional plagiocephaly.

The large majority of misshapen heads seen in primary care relate to positional plagiocephaly. These anomalies usually are mild and noticed at birth or soon thereafter. Anatomically, the occipital region in positional plagiocephaly is flattened with anterior compensatory changes and asymmetry in the ear position. Contralateral anterior flattening and unilateral anterior bossing generally are mild. Unilateral cases have compensatory growth in the contralateral parieto-occipital region, manifested by bossing and vertex elongation. This elongation is more prominent in bilateral deformities, which also have lateral parietal widening, and occipital flattening with anterior narrowing and increased frontal projection. Infants may sleep on their back and have slight flattening of the occipital region. These problems generally correct themselves as the infant grows and begins to roll over, although assistive devices are sometimes useful. Similar shaping can be seen in newborns with substantial developmental delays or torticollis, and in hypotonic infants who do not move their heads. Table 1 outlines the differential diagnosis between patients with lambdoidal synostosis and those with posterior plagiocephaly (3).

Figure 2 illustrates the effects of synostoses on the shape of the skull. A long, narrow, "keel"-shaped head, scaphocephaly, indicates sagittal synostosis. Unilateral and bilateral coronal synostoses are recognized by their anterior craniofacial deformities. A trigonocephaly-shaped forehead characterizes metopic synostosis.

Standard skull radiography historically has been used for preoperative information. More recently, advances in computer tomography (CT) imaging and three-dimensional (3D) reconstruction have been adopted as standard diagnostic tools. Reconstruction provides detailed information about the cranial anatomy and sutures that are not possible with routine radiographs.

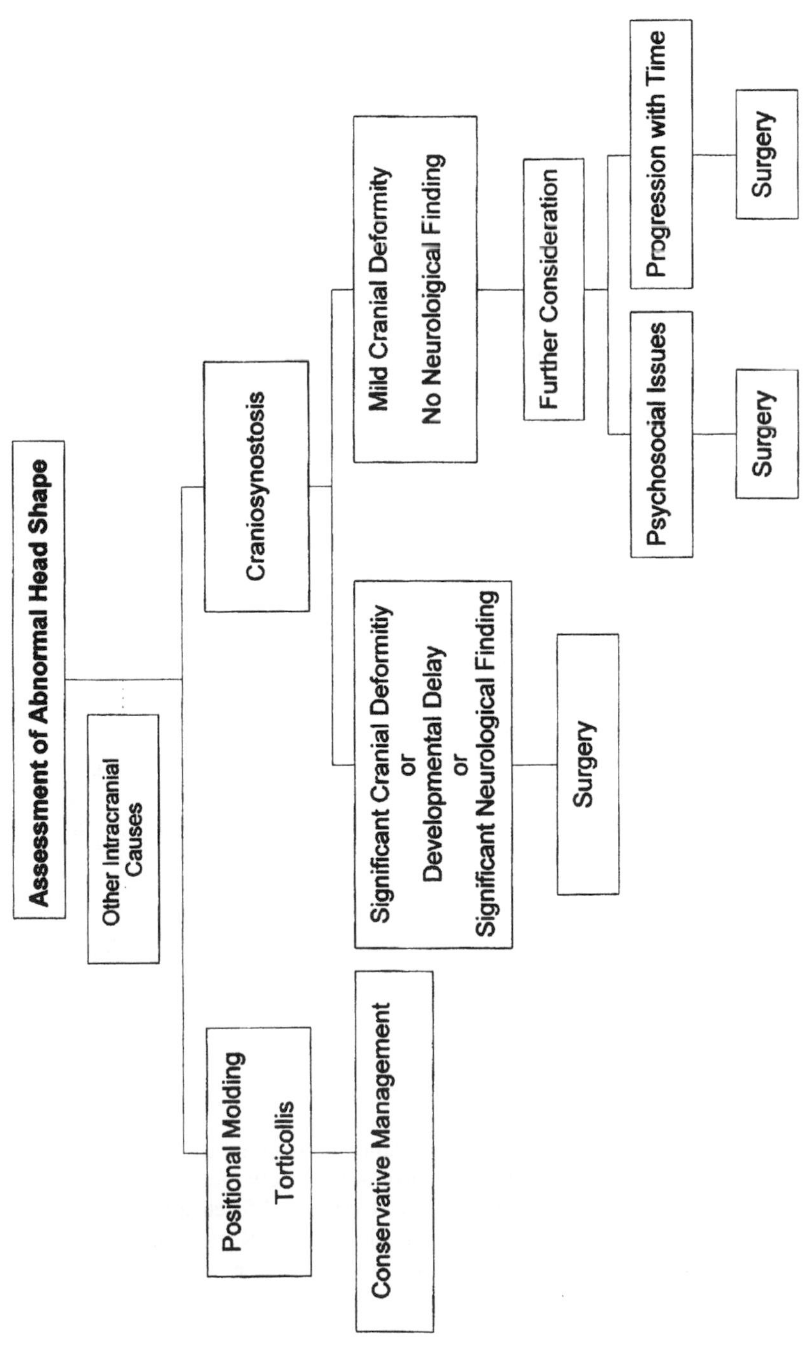

Figure 1 Assessment of abnormal head shape.

Table 1 Clinical Differences Between (Common) Positional Plagiocephaly and (Rare) Lambdoidal Craniosynostosis

Finding	Positional plagiocephaly	Lambdoidal craniosynostosis
Occipital bone	Flattening with little or no ridging	Flattening with ridge along suture. Frequently there is an ipsilateral inferior bulge
Ipsilateral ear position	Displaced anteriorly	Displaced posteriorly
Forehead	Ipsilateral bossing	Little or no bossing, but if present, it is usually contralateral
Head circumference	Usually increased	Normal or decreased
Anterior subarachnoid spaces	Usually increased	Normal

TREATMENT

Indications for procedures need to be considered by the craniomaxillofacial team for each case based on clinical signs, syndromic and genetic information, radiographic indicators, and whether the child is stable or developing symptoms. Positional plagiocephaly can be corrected by changing the child's position slightly during naps and sleeping. Frequently, neck exercises prescribed by an occupational therapist

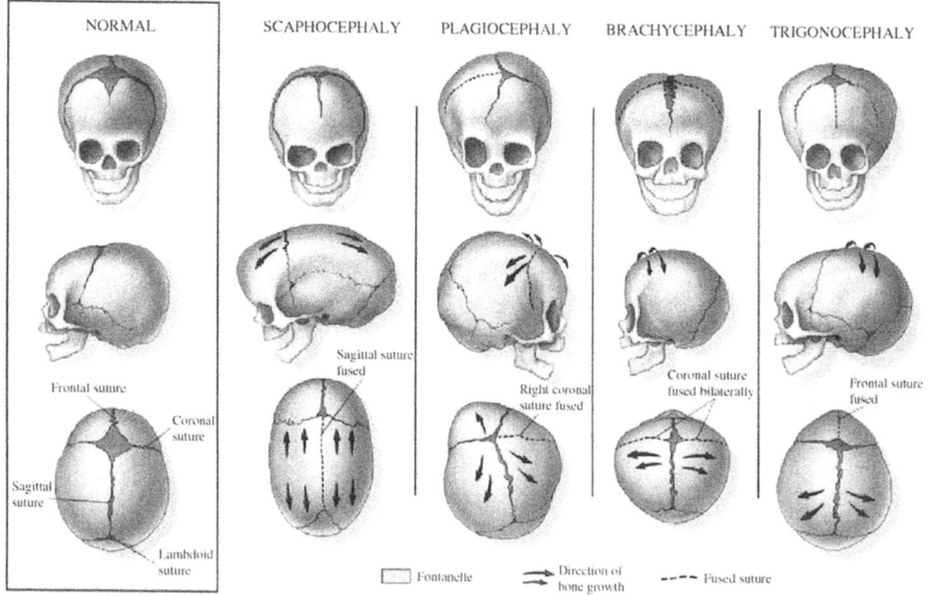

Figure 2 Illustrations of skull shapes and synostoses. Panel 2 (left to right): Typical elongated picture seen in sagittal synostosis. Panel 3: Anterior plagiocephaly characteristic of unilateral right coronal synostosis. Panel 4: Towering, bilateral widening, and forehead flattening with foreshortening characteristic of bilateral coronal synostosis. Panel 5: Keeled shape and biparietal widening characteristically seen with metopic synostosis. (Adapted from Vannier MW. Radiographic Evaluation of Craniosynostosis. In: Cohen, MacLean, eds. Craniosynostosis, Diagnosis, Evaluation, and Management. New York: Oxford University Press; 2000.)

are helpful. Many therapists know how to carve a pillow out of foam rubber that redistributes the weight of the head and is comfortable for the child. The costs are minor and the results appear to be excellent. Craniosynostosis is thought by some to be an aesthetic problem with infrequent consequences for brain function and development. Although clinical impressions have associated appearance with the adolescent's ability to socialize, school performance, and adult behavioral problems, studies have suggested that abnormal skull shapes do not directly affect intelligence test scores. Mental development, measured by intelligence quotient tests, in infants with nonsyndromic, single-suture craniosynostosis appears to be normal in the absence of increased ICP and other pathologies. In this regard, it is of interest to note the anthropological studies of the many civilizations that practised cranial deformation for cosmetic and political gains. Such practices imply that an abnormal skull shape does not interfere with normal intelligence, although one cannot conclude that the physiological results of congenital and cosmetic deformations are the same (4).

Apparently well-tolerated craniosynostosis, however, can abruptly worsen either spontaneously or following head injury. Skull base deformities can worsen to the point of affecting vision, hearing, and breathing, and oral occlusion. Anomalies in skull morphology usually precede complications such as visual impairment and increased ICP. Multiple-suture synostoses and syndromic synostoses frequently associate with increased ICP, hydrocephalus, and progressive mental impairment.

SURGICAL INTERVENTION

The cranium, cranial base, and facial region must be evaluated as growing structures. Brain development, vision, sinuses, and airway must also be considered. The craniomaxillofacial team also must evaluate midfacial growth in childhood and adolescence, as well as occlusion and mastication in the primary mixed and permanent dentition phase. A typical evaluation includes pediatric neurology, radiology, neurosurgery, anesthesiology, ophthalmology, and orthodontics. Major issues to be considered are: 1) frontal–orbital retrusion, usually manifest secondary to coronal synostosis affecting the frontal–orbital region; 2) posterior constraint occurring with growth anomalies in the parietal, occipital, and squamosal sutures; 3) posterior and anterior growth anomalies; and 4) midfacial anomalies. In addition, the evaluation frequently encounters Chiari malformations, hydrocephalus, hypertelorism, cleft palate, extraocular muscle movement, and ocular anomalies. Shunts further complicate reconstruction and increase opportunities for infection. Because abnormality at a single suture strongly influences the development of other areas in the craniofacial complex, there is a clinical impression that surgical correction during the neonatal period yields superior results, although in the absence of clinical or radiological signs of raised ICP, surgery may be delayed to 12–15 months (5).

Numerous approaches have been described, and many are being refined with advances in adsorbable plating materials, hardware, and microsurgical technology. Craniofacial surgeons have become more aggressive in trying to correct the suture and the associated deformities. Cranial vault remodeling involves excision of the frontal, parietal, and occipital bones, which are trimmed, shaped, relocated, and affixed with biomaterials. Specialized texts should be cited for details. Two new strategies, which currently are being evaluated, are outlined here.

In single-suture cases, the traditional aim has been to excise, or "strip," the fused suture in the hope that mechanical forces would automatically correct the deformities. Modifications include the use of biomaterials to prevent return of the sutures to their preoperative state, and to guide the desired remodeling. Recently, neurosurgeons have used an endoscope to perform extended strip craniectomies for single-suture craniosynostosis. In these cases, surgery is followed by 6–8 months of molding helmet therapy. The procedure involves less blood loss, operating time, and length of hospital stay, but it does not allow the surgeon to alter the calvarial shape or cephalic index. Outcome studies have been too short to evaluate the endoscopic procedures compared to cranial vault remodeling. Molding helmet therapy itself has been difficult to evaluate in prospective controlled trials.

Distraction osteogenesis of the mid-face alleviates many of the requirements of autogenous bone grafts and restriction of the soft-tissue envelope in remolding the mid-face. Potential advantages of distraction versus conventional LeFort III methods are claims of less dead space with a reduced infection potential, decreased blood loss, shorter operating times, and the allowance for gradual expansion of facial soft tissue. Modifications to the distraction procedure and hardware are the subject of several current studies.

REFERENCES

1. Cohen MM Jr, MacLean RE, ed. Craniosynostosis, Diagnosis, Evaluation, and Management. 2nd ed. New York: Oxford University Press, 2000.
2. Carson BC Sr, Munoz D, Gross G, Vander Kolk CA, James CS, Gates J, et al. An assistive device for the treatment of positional plagiocephaly. J Craniofacial Surg 2000;11:177–183.
3. Panchal J, Uttchin V. Management of craniosynostosis. Plast Reconstruct Surg 2003; 111:2032–2048.
4. Arnaud E, Meneses P, Lajeunie E, Thorne JA, Marchac D, Renier D. Postoperative mental and morphological outcome for nonsyndromic brachycephaly. Plast Reconstruct Surg 2002; 110:6–13.
5. Sun PP, Persing JA. Craniosynostosis. In: Albright AL, Pollack IF, Adelson PD, eds. Principles and Practices of Pediatric Neurosurgery. New York: Thieme, 1999:219–242.

2
Neurological Management of Myelomeningocele and Holoprosencephaly

Stephen L. Kinsman
Departement of Pediatrics, University of Maryland School of Medicine, Baltimore, Maryland, U.S.A.

INTRODUCTION

The management of nervous system malformations requires making the proper diagnosis followed by the recognition and treatment of potential complications. The intial step, essential to providing prognostic and anticipatory family guidence, is the accurate assessment of the severity of associated problems. This should be followed by the ongoing identification of complications, their proper treatment, and/or referral. This chapter reviews two common malformations, myelomeningocele (MMC) and holoprosencephaly. Principles learned and experience gained in the management of these two complex conditions can be readily applied to other malformations of the nervous system.

MYELOMENINGOCELE

Myelomeningocele (MMC), its treatment and management, can be viewed as a paradigm for the treatment of multiple complex health-challenging conditions, particularly those which exhibit problems throughout the lifespan. Management of MMC, with its gamut of nervous system dysfunction, requires neurological involvement from fetal life to adulthood (Table 1). It presents clinical situations involving fetal counseling, acute and sometimes life-threatening emergencies, issues of declining neuromotor function, and chronic problems such as headaches and back pain (see chapters on cerebral palsy, chiari malformations, hydrocehalus, learning disabilities, and headaches). Another distinguishing feature is the requirement for multidimensional and interdisciplinary treatment programs. No single medical, surgical, or rehabilitative specialty is truly equipped to handle all the problems encountered in the care of individuals with MMC. The standard of care remains multidisciplinary, or even better, interdisciplinary.

Table 1 Neurological Assessment of an Individual with MMC

1. Determination of the functional lesion level (sensory motor)
2. Assessment of hydrocephalus (shunted or unshunted, compensated or uncompensated)
3. Evaluation of brainstem and cerebellar function
4. Assessment of upper extremity function
5. Recognition of scoliosis and joint contractures
6. Participation in decision covering the use of adaptive equipment, such as ankle-foot orthoses and/or crutches (based on manual muscle testing, sensory considerations, and assessment of gait)
7. Assessment of the child's developmental gains, mental status, and cognitive function
8. Monitoring of family function and adaptation

The MMC is a complex embryonic malformation of the nervous system, which leads to structural and physiological abnormalities with a variety of disabilities. The functional neurological level, as established in the new born period, is a critical determinant in the management of MMC; provides the basis for prognosis (including functional outcome) and management decisions. Radiological levels of posterior vertebral spina bifida are less useful, since the direct correspondence of boney lesions with motor and/or sensory impairment is far from exact.

Mobility

In general, children with at least antigravity muscle strength or better in lumbar nerve root L3 will ambulate. Most will be able to walk indoors and outdoors, although a wheelchair may be required for longer trips. Others may have a greater requirement for the wheelchair in community and outdoor use. Children with higher levels of motor and/or sensory impairment (L1–L3) will ambulate with difficulty using high braces, such as reciprocating gait othoses (RGOs). Whether or not to pursue this degree of assistance to achieve some mobility must be weighed against time, energy, and financial considerations. Nonambulators (usually above L1) are wheelchair dependent.

Deterioration of functional motor level, upper extremity function, or appearance of scoliosis should prompt immediate assessment of the neuroaxis for progressive hydrocephalus, worsening of the Chiari II malfunction, increase in the size of a spinal cord syrinx, or tethered cord. A MRI of the entire neuroaxis is recommended. Consultation with neurosurgery is essential, since intervention for these complications may be necessary to prevent further deterioration. The appearance of abnormal neuromotor or other signs should always be present in the patients considered for neurosurgical intervention. When in doubt, serial examinations should be obtained over several months.

Hydrocephalus

Hydrocephalus is a dynamic condition that begins in utero in MMC, but becomes more manifest postnatally. The need for CSF shunting in the newborn period is reported to be as high as 80% in MMC. A clinical trial is currently underway to determine if fetal surgery designed to close the myelomeningocele defect results in a diminished need for CSF shunting. Nevertheless, the need for shunt revision remains high in this population and shunt function requires lifelong assessment. Shunt failure may be subtle and not associated with obvious symptoms/signs of increased intracranial pressure such as severe headache, vomiting, lethargy, and papilledema. Subtle symptoms of elevated pressure can include behavior change, decreased school performance, and chronic headache. The appearance of these findings should prompt further evaluation, no matter how long the individual has had a shunt in place. It is this author's opinion that individuals with MMC should never be considered shunt independent. In addition, individuals with MMC without CSF diversion (including adults) may manifest signs of symptomatic (acute or subtle) hydrocephalus at any time. Shunt failure with symptoms and signs of acute increased intracranial pressure is a medical emergency and can be a life-threatening problem.

Brainstem and Cerebellar Dysfunction

Dysfunction involving these regions is typically due to a Chiari II malformation; a combination of posterior fossa tightness and brainstem herniation. Up to 15% of newborns exhibit brainstem dysfunction including dysphagia, respiratory problems, and sleep apnea. Symptoms can present in either a gradually progressive or more acute stepwise fashion. Whether or nor posterior fossa decompression is beneficial over the long term is unresolved, but acutely this procedure often results in some improvement in symptoms/signs. Brainstem and/or cerebellar dysfunction can appear or worsen in adulthood. The possibility of increased intracranial pressure contributing to worsening of symptoms must always be considered. If there is any question about the presence of increased intracranial pressure exacerbating or causing brainstem/CB symptoms/signs, a shunt revision should be undertaken. Occasionally, tethered cord syndrome may be a contributing factor. When present, spinal cord untethering will be helpful.

Bladder/Bowel Impairment

Complications of neurogenic bladder lead to a major source of morbidity and mortality in MM, e.g., hydronephrosis and recurrent urinary tract infections (UTIs) causing renal damage and failure. Individuals born with a solitary kidney are at a particularly high risk. Renal sonogram is used to assess hydronephrosis and a voiding cystometrogram to identify vesiculoureteral reflux. Urological consultation is imperative in those patients with unexplained UTIs, hydronephrosis, and unstable bladders. Bladder outlet dys-synergy, hyper-reflexia, and high bladder filling pressures should prompt the initiation of clean intermittent catheterization (CIC) and anticholinergic medication (oxybutinin and newer agents). Sometimes temporary vesicostomy is required, especially when compliance with medical measures is not possible. Urinary tract infections should be treated promptly. It remains controversial whether asymptomatic bacturia in those on CIC should be treated. In our center, bacturia with a single organism of $> 100{,}000$ colonies/mL in association with a urine WBC count of >25 cells per HPF is treated with antibiotics. Unstable bladders with outlet dys-synergy and/or high pressures usually respond well to treatment with CIC and oxybutinin. In contrast, patients with atonic bladders (or very low outlet pressures) may benefit from sympathomimetic agents, although many do not achieve continence. Urological interventions with bladder neck injections or sling procedures have been used with mixed success. Many individuals with MM achieve continence with bladder augmentation surgery. Lastly, in individuals with significant issues of mobility, the placement of a continent stoma will allow bladder catheterization through an abdominal conduit.

Neurogenic bowel causes little morbidity but great morbidity in MM. Poor anorectal function leads to unsuccessful toilet training, fecal incontinence, and the potential for significant social disability. Neurogenic constipation further compounds the problem of bowel movement management in MM. The goal is regular, predictable, fecal evacuation in a manner that is acceptable and efficient for the patient and family. In the first few years of life, the focus is on stool consistency/bulk. First step interventions include the use of suppositories and enemas, along with stool softening and bulking agents. Evacuations should be done on the toilet to enhance later toilet training. Periodic bowel cleanouts may be required using either high volume enemas or osmotic solutions (Go-Lytely or others) delivered via nasogastric tube. As the child becomes more independent, these procedures become less acceptable. The MACE procedure, which creates an abdominal conduit into the cecum for the delivery of high volume fluids to the colon, has been very beneficial in producing fecal continence.

Cognition/Behavior/Family

A detailed discussion of development, cognition, behavior, and mental health of children with MMC is beyond the scope of this chapter. Mental retardation is present in about one-third of children with MMC; generally in the mild range (IQ 55–70). Individuals with normal intelligence and shunted hydrocephalus often have visual-motor and perceptional defects that lead to poor school performance. Behavioral and emotional issues are critical to the optimum functional outcome of an individual and need to be a component of all treatment plans. The impact of this condition on family functioning over the lifespan of the affected individual is profound and requires careful monitoring with interventions as needed; ideally from multiple perspectives in a longitudinal and coordinated manner.

HOLOPROSENCEPHALY

Holoprosencephaly (HPE) is another complex developmental malformation of the central nervous system that can lead to severe–profound impairment of global neurological function. The HPE is associated with two fundamental abnormalities; underhemispherization of the brain and cerebral underdevelopment with resultant microcephaly. The problems of HPE are typically more severe than those in MMC and include severe to profound cognitive impairment, oromotor dysfunction severe enough to inhibit growth and development, endocrine dysfunction, seizures, autonomic dysregulation (especially temperature instability), and disorders of motor tone. A motor dysfunction syndrome, classifiable as a mixed cerebral palsy, is usually present. Higher levels of neurological function can be seen, particularly in milder forms of HPE. Occasionally hydrocephalus is observed, even in the setting of severe microcephaly, and the presence of deteriorating function should prompt obtaining a head CT.

Step 1. Confirming the Diagnosis

The HPE is classified into three major types, although some investigators include a fourth type or middle interhemispheric fusion variant (MIHF). The most severe form, alobar HPE is characterized by a complete lack of cerebral hemispherization, resulting in a mono "hemisphere" with a single ventricle, and no evidence of an interhemispheric fissure. Deep cerebral structures, such as the caudate, putamen, and lentiform nuclei, are also fused due to a lack of midline brain structures. The severity and extent of this anatomic underdevelopment correlate roughly with the severity of functional impairment. The milder semilobar and milder still lobar HPE are characterized by lesser degrees of midline underdevelopment in a caudal to rostral gradient. Mild forms of lobar HPE are limited to the orbito-frontal lobes. The MIHF variant involves nonhemispherization of just the region of brain adjacent to the Rolandic fissure. Its characteristic MRI finding is underdevelopment or absence of the body of the corpus callosum with a seam of gray matter across the midline. The cerebral cortex rostral and caudal to the seam are either normal or exhibit neuronal migration defects.

Misdiagnosis is common, since interpretation of neuroimaging (from fetal ultrasound to postnatal MRI) has tended to focus on ventricular architecture rather than on the presence of midline noncleavage of gray matter structures. For confirmation of HPE, there must be some degree of cerebral hemispheric nonseparation (noncleavage). Many cases of alobar and semilobar HPE are accompanied by the presence of a dorsal cyst in the caudal most part of the supratentorial compartment. Additionally, most cases of HPE are associated with significant reductions in brain mass and microcephaly, unless hydrocephalus is present. Cases with normo- or macrocephaly must be diagnosed with caution; the destructive effects of hydrocephalus in malformations, such as agenesis of the corpus callosum with interhemispheric cyst, can lead to an anatomy that mimics HPE. Cases with HPE having a significant cortical mantle will demonstrate some degree of posterior callosal development.

Step 2. Search for an Etiology

All cases of HPE should have chromosomal analysis with G banding, as many chromosomal abnormalities can lead to HPE. To date, 11 chromosomal regions are known to be associated with HPE. It is this author's opinion that a geneticist should evaluate all children with HPE, as there are over a dozen syndromes associated with HPE. Syndrome delineation can lead to better genetic counseling, an important part of HPE management given the heterogeneous causes of the condition and their attendant differences in recurrence risk. Assessment for Smith–Lemli–Opitz syndrome is now available through metabolic testing for plasma sterols, including at least cholesterol and 7-dehydrocholesterol. Testing for other single gene mutations associated with HPE (at least six identified) is only available on a research basis.

Step 3. Outcome

An essential goal in dealing with families who have a child with HPE is to provide the latest information on etiology and prognosis. Most current textbooks in Neurology and Pediatrics focus their description on mortality and fail to describe the variation in neurological and medical morbidity. In my experience, families want a sense of how their child might function, regardless of how severe the impairment. Additionally, since mortality data are not population based, the validity of generalization is suspected. The HPE is a condition that, in its more severe forms, is associated with a high mortality rate. Nevertheless, our ability to predict the risk of mortality on an individual basis remains difficult and rarely is helpful for families regarding management and future planning. My approach is to first ask the family to tell me what they have been told about HPE and their child. Almost uniformally, they have received very grim information for obstetricians sonographers, and neonatologists. This "telling their story" sets the stage for our relationship and allows the family to discuss their values and priorities for their child and family. After this, I readdress the risk of mortality in a more general way and stress our inability to predict for specific individuals. We then discuss this uncertainty and how to manage it. Most deaths are from medical illnesses with a clear trend towards multisystem failure as a prelude to a terminal phase of illness. These latter problems are usually recognizable and permit further discussion on management and palliative. This frank approach and offer of assistance, if and when the time of a life-threatening illness occurs, puts most families at ease and allows them to focus on helping their child to stay healthy and function to the best of their potential.

Step 4. Complications

In general, there should be no progressive neurological deterioration in HPE and in most cases some developmental milestones are attained. Early medical issues relate to: (1) craniofacial aspects airway management due to cranofacial malfunctions, (2) issues of feeding and swallowing, (3) management of endocrine issues, (4) control of seizures, (5) maintenance of normal temperature, and (6) management of tone. If neurological and/or developmental regression occurs, one should search for structural or metabolic abnormalities. Occasionally, hydrocephalus has developed even in the setting of severe microcephaly. In this instance, CSF shunting has stabilized the condition. Episodes of hypoglycemia can lead to seizures and/or alterations of baseline function. A gastrostomy tube is beneficial when poor oromotor function with or without gastroesophageal reflux is present. Abnormalities of sodium balance can present as a diabetes insipidus-like disorder, particularly during intercurrent illness. Mild hypernatremia should be treated with liberalization of free water. Care must be utilized when treating with DDAVP to avoid over treatment with resultant hyponatremia and seizures. Disorders of temperature control are usually easily managed with environmental control and a warming blanket. Children with MIHF have greater cognitive and motor capabilities than those with "classical" HPE. Many are ambulatory, but often show signs of spastic diplegia. Endocrine and autonomic dysfunction is less common, but can be present.

Proper diagnosis of HPE is essential for an etiological search, attempt at prognosis, and in the follow up for potential complications. The neurologist is in a unique position to assist both the patient, and family. To do this properly, however, requires an ongoing long-term commitment. It is this author's opinion that complex conditions such as HPE are best managed in a longitudinal relationship in which education, support, and problem solving are essential components of the patient–physician relationship.

SUGGESTED READINGS

1. Botto LD, Moore CA, Khoury MJ, Erickson JD. Neural-tube defects. N Engl J Med 1999 Nov 11; 341(20):1509–1519.
2. Oakeshott P, Hunt GM. Long-term outcome in open spina bifida. Br J Gen Pract 2003 Aug; 53(493):632–636.

3. Plawner LL, Delgado MR, Miller VS, Levey EB, Kinsman SL, Barkovich AJ, Simon EM, Clegg NJ, Sweet VT, Stashinko EE, Hahn JS. Neuroanatomy of holoprosencephaly as predictor of function: beyond the face predicting the brain. Neurology 2002 Oct 8; 59(7):1058–1066.
4. Traggiai C, Stanhope R. Endocrinopathies associated with midline cerebral and cranial malformations. J Pediatr 2002 Feb; 140(2):252–255.

3
Spasticity/Cerebral Palsy

April Puscavage and Alec Hoon
Johns Hopkins University School of Medicine, Kennedy Krieger Institute, Baltimore, Maryland, U.S.A.

INTRODUCTION

Cerebral palsy describes a group of upper motor neuron syndromes secondary to a wide range of genetic and acquired disorders of early brain development. In addition to primary impairments in gross and fine motor function, there may be associated problems with cognition, seizures, vision, swallowing, speech, bowel/bladder, and orthopedic deformities. It is the most prevalent chronic childhood motor disability, affecting 2–3/1000 school aged children. Cerebral palsy is considered nonprogressive, but neurological findings may change or progress over time. Although comprehensive longitudinal studies are limited, the majority of children with cerebral palsy develop into adulthood, actively participating in societal life.

DIAGNOSIS/CLINICAL FEATURES

Cerebral palsy is a clinical diagnosis, made on the basis of significant delay in gross and/or fine motor function, with abnormalities in tone, posture, and movement on neurological examination. While the neurological abnormalities in cerebral palsy include loss of selective motor control, agonist/antagonist muscle imbalance, impaired balance/coordination, and sensory deficits, *diagnosis, classification, and treatment are often based on abnormalities in tone*. Children may have relatively pure spastic, rigid, or dystonic hypertonicity or mixed degrees of these three types. Position, posture, movement, anxiety, or illness may influence the determination of tone.

Spasticity, a velocity dependent increase in tonic stretch reflexes, is part of the upper motor neuron syndrome, including clonus, reflex overflow, hyperreflexia, positive Babinski, loss of manual dexterity, and spastic weakness. Spastic hypertonicity is commonly seen in association with white matter injury (e.g., periventricular leukomalacia) or widespread brain injury. While the neurophysiological mechanism(s) has not been conclusively determined, disturbed supraspinal control of spinal circuitry plays a major role in producing spasticity. Detrimental effects of spasticity include impaired movement, muscle tightness, contractures, impaired hygiene, disordered sleep and pain, and are the basis for many therapeutic interventions. *Spastic cerebral palsy* syndromes include diplegia, quadriplegia, and hemiplegia.

By contrast, rigid hypertonicity is bidirectional, elicited independent of velocity of stretch and without clonus. Dystonic hypertonicity, characterized by cocontraction of agonist–antagonist muscles and associated with twisting and repetitive movements, usually occurs during voluntary movement or with voluntary maintenance of a body posture. Dystonic hypertonicity is often associated with disorders of the basal ganglia and thalamus. *Extrapyramidal cerebral palsy* syndromes, with rigid or dystonic hypertonicity, are often categorized into dystonic, athetoid, choreic, and hemiballismic subtypes based on observation of movement as well as neurological examination.

In many children with cerebral palsy, there is mixed hypertonicity (*mixed cerebral palsy*). Treatment is often directed to the primary tone abnormality(ies). *Ataxic/hypotonic cerebral palsy* syndromes, a heterogeneous group of individually rare disorders often genetically mediated, have marked variability in motor outcome, and are not further discussed in this chapter.

THERAPY OVERVIEW

Children with cerebral palsy develop to their full potential when treatment programs optimize motor capabilities, minimize orthopedic deformities and address associated impairments. Neurologic interventions may be divided into medical, surgical, and rehabilitative components (Fig. 1). Specialists in orthopedics, neurosurgery, ophthalmology, gastroenterology, pediatric neurology, physical medicine and rehabilitation, child psychiatry, and pediatrics manage associated problems.

At the time of diagnosis, a thorough investigation of etiology should be completed (Tables 1 and 2), which may have important treatment, as well as prognostic and recurrence risk implications (4,6). For example, children with dystonic (or even "spastic diplegic") cerebral palsy may have dopa-responsive dystonia, with improved motor function using levodopa. Children with basal ganglia/thalamic injury from perinatal asphyxia may develop improved expressive speech and hand use with trihexyphenidyl (5), while those with spastic diplegia associated with prematurity may benefit from selective dorsal rhizotomy.

Medical therapies include oral medications such as baclofen, diazepam, and trihexyphenidyl as well as therapeutic botulinum toxin (Botox®) (3,7). Surgical interventions include orthopedic procedures such as tenotomies, tendon transfers and osteotomies, and neurosurgical procedures such as intrathecal baclofen, selective dorsal rhizotomy (SDR) and deep brain stimulation (DBS) (1). Rehabilitative specialists actively involved in treatment include physical and occupational therapists, speech-language pathologists, audiologists, psychologists, and special education consultants. Interventions used by therapists include NDT (neurodevelopmental treatment), serial casting, orthotic bracing, strength training, aquatherapy, hippotherapy, and technology systems such as augmentative communication and power mobility. Professionals cognizant of the effects of motor disability on other aspects of childhood development may be of great benefit in fostering social–emotional growth.

TREATMENT OF SPASTICITY

In infants with spasticity, intervention should begin as early as possible, with the primary focus to facilitate function. The initial approach is often rehabilitative, with an

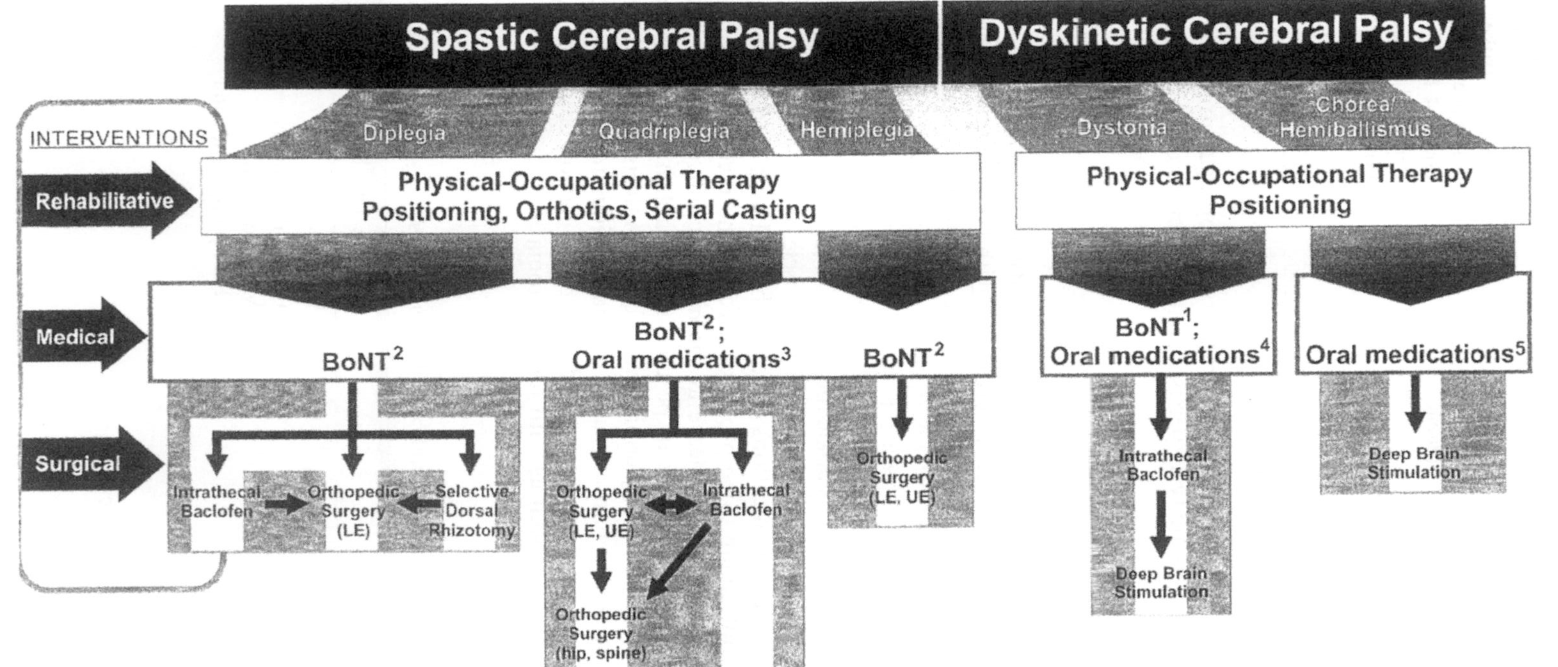

Figure 1 This algorithm is intended to provide an overview of the treatment options in children with cerebral palsy. While the general flow is from rehabilitative to medical and surgical interventions, over time most children receive an individualized combination of interventions, which may include treatment for both spasticity and dyskinetic findings. Physical and occupational therapy may consist of various treatments including strengthening programs appropriate positioning and orthotic use. [1]For focal dystonia; [2]for focal spasticity; [3]for generalized spasticity: diazepam (Valium®), baclofen (Lioresal®), tiazadine (Zanaflex®), dantrolene (Dantrium®), clonazepam (Klonopin®); [4]for generalized dystonia/athetosis: trihexyphendyl (Artane®), levodopa (Sinemet®), baclofen (Lioresal®), tetrabenazine; [5]for generalized chorea/hemiballismus: clonazepam (Klonopin®), reserpine, valproate (Depakene®), carbamazepine (Tegretol®), tetrabenazine, neuroleptics. BoNT = Botulinum neurotoxin; LE = lower extremities; UE = upper extremities.

Table 1 Etiology of Spastic Cerebral Palsy Syndromes

Spastic diplegia	Spastic quadriplegia	Spastic hemiplegia
PVL	PVL (severe)	Prenatal stroke
DRD	Brain malformations	Schizencephaly
HIV	Encephalomalacia	Grade 4 IVH
Hydrocephalus	TORCH	Perinatal stroke
Genetic (rare)	Hydrocephalus	Postnatal stroke
(Spinal cord)	Meningitis	
	Encephalitis	

experienced physical therapist showing parents/caregivers an approach to handling, stretching, and positioning. If spasticity is persistent, then a more comprehensive approach is required.

Spastic Diplegia

Spastic diplegia is characterized primarily by lower extremity hypertonia and limitations in ambulation, and etiologically most closely linked with prematurity. Diagnosis is usually established between 9 and 24 months of age. The focus of treatment is to diminish the effects of spasticity and weakness during the period of growth while motor circuits are actively developing. Medical management consists of a stretching program using daily exercises and splinting to prevent progressive loss of joint range of motion. Orthotic interventions such as ankle foot orthoses (AFOs) and hip abduction braces are used to provide a static stretch in tight muscles.

Therapeutic botulinum toxin injections followed by splinting and/or serial casting may be of benefit. Botulinum toxin produces selective and reversible chemodenervation by inhibiting acetylcholine release at the neuromuscular junction. By selectively weakening specific muscles, it can be used to reestablish balance from abnormal muscle forces across joints. Injections are safe, with effects lasting up to three to four months. It is most commonly used to treat equinus foot deformity, but may also be used in management of crouched gait, pelvic flexion contracture, and upper extremity deformities as well as with focal dystonia.

Table 2 Etiology of Extrapyramidal Cerebral Palsy Syndromes

Dystonia/athetosis	Chorea/hemiballismus
Dopa responsive dystonia	Kenicterus
Perinatal asphyxia	Perinatal asphyxia
Mitochondrial cytopathies	Mitochondrial
Glutaric aciduria, type 1	"Post-pump syndrome"
Methylmalonic acidemia	
Creatine deficiency	
Juvenile Huntington disease	
Pantothenate kinase associated degeneration	
Juvenile Parkinson disease	
Encephalitis	

Antispasticity medications may be used as adjunctive treatment to reduce hypertonicity in selected children. Commonly used medications include baclofen, benzodiazepines such as diazepam and clonazepam, tizanidine, dantrolene, and recently tiagabine. Beneficial effects on tone reduction must be weighed against non-selective action on all muscle groups and unwanted cognitive and other side effects. While these medications appear to enhance function in individual children, currently there are no double-masked studies showing that these medications improve motor capabilities.

A baseline evaluation from an orthopedic surgeon experienced with the management of children with cerebral palsy is useful for recommendations on nonsurgical interventions as well as for planning potential later surgery. Despite an early, well-coordinated treatment program, some children with spastic diplegia will require surgical intervention, commonly orthopedic and at times neurosurgical. The orthopedic management of spasticity is directed toward reducing deformity and facilitating function, utilizing tendon lengthenings/transfers, bony osteotomies, and joint fusion procedures. The initial procedures are frequently multilevel soft tissue, with later bony procedures as required. Computerized gait analysis for preoperative planning may be beneficial.

Intrathecal baclofen (ITB) and selective dorsal rhizotomy (SDR) are now used in many centers for children with spastic diplegia. Both are invasive procedures, but offer significant benefit in carefully selected patients. One significant difference is that ITB is reversible, while SDR is permanent.

Intrathecal baclofen therapy is the delivery of microgram amounts of baclofen, a GABA agonist, into the intrathecal space via an implanted, programmable pump. Intrathecal baclofen provides titratable reductions in spasticity using doses 100 times less than oral doses, and with a lack of adverse effects often associated with higher doses of oral baclofen. Prior to pump placement, a 50 μg bolus of baclofen is frequently given by lumbar puncture, with a 6–8 hr period of close observation for reductions in spasticity. At the time of pump insertion, catheter placement is important, with higher placement associated with greater benefit to the upper extremities. While there are reports of functional improvements in children with spastic diplegia using ITB, replication of findings in large prospective, randomized trials has not been done to date.

Effective management requires a team approach before, during, and after pump placement. Risks, treatment goals, and parental expectations of benefit should be completely outlined prior to surgery. After pump placement, ongoing surveillance for potentially serious side effects includes severe acute withdrawal secondary to, increased hypertonicity associated with catheter kinking or dislodgement; and CNS depression or loss of function from excessive dosing is required.

Selective dorsal rhizotomy is a surgical procedure in which 30–50% of sensory nerve fibers entering the lumbosacral cord are selectively cut, to reduce lower extremity spasticity and improve function. Some surgeons utilize intraoperative nerve stimulation to determine which rootlets to cut, while others feel this is not required. Selective dorsal rhizotomy has been recommended where there is significant spasticity, but motor strength is well preserved. The ideal patient is between 4 and 10 years of age, with relatively pure spastic diplegia, preservation of antigravity strength and selective motor control. While there are reported functional benefits with SDR, noted especially in former premature infants, long-term concerns including hip subluxation, spinal stenosis, and pain must be considered. As with ITB, families need to be well informed about risks and benefits.

Spastic (and Mixed) Quadriplegia

Children with spastic and mixed quadriplegia have four-limb hypertonicity and are frequently unable to sit independently. Treatment goals include improving comfort/positioning, reducing pain, slowing the progression of musculoskeletal deformities and at times improving function. Affected children may not be able to express sources of pain including muscle spasms as well as gastrointestinal reflux, which may contribute to abnormal posturing.

In children with quadriplegic syndromes, all efforts should be made to minimize hip and spine deformities, beginning with proper positioning and oral medications.

Although adductor tenotomy procedures are performed to prevent hip dislocation, many of these children will progress from subluxation to dislocation and require further surgery. While early scoliosis is treated with spinal orthoses, again a percentage of affected children will subsequently require spinal fusion. With this in mind, the active involvement of a tone management team and an experienced orthopedic surgeon would become integral to rehabilitative care.

For those children with intractable spasticity or severe mixed cerebral palsy, ITB has been of great benefit, significantly reducing hypertonicity and improving ease of care for families. Whether ITB reduces the need for subsequent orthopedic surgery has not been conclusively established.

Spastic Hemiplegia

Children with hemiplegic cerebral palsy represent a distinct group, frequently with characteristic findings in the contralateral hemisphere on MRI. Findings on clinical examination may be either arm or leg dominant. The majority of affected children walk independently, but may require interventions for lower and/or upper extremity impairments including splinting/orthotic intervention, therapeutic botulinum toxin, tendo-achilles lengthening for equines, and upper extremity surgical releases or transfers for contractures. Associated problems requiring treatment may include epilepsy, cortiosensory impairment and growth retardation on the affected side, and learning disabilities/mental retardation.

TREATMENT OF EXTRAPYRAMIDAL DISORDERS

Treatment for extrapyramidal syndromes often requires the combination of pharmacotherapy and rehabilitation including power mobility and communication systems.

Pharmacotherapy is determined on the basis of the observed movement disorder. In essence, in syndromes with athetosis or dystonia, upregulating dopamine by providing a dopamine precursor (levodopa, with carbidopa) or downregulating acetylcholine (trihexyphenidyl) may improve movement. In children with hyperkinetic components including chorea or hemiballismus, downregulating dopamine (reserpine, tetrabenazine, or potentially neuroleptics if very severe) or increasing GABA (benzodiazepines, anticonvulsants) may be beneficial. In our experience, drug therapy has been of greater benefit in dystonia and athetosis, with chorea and hemiballismus often difficult to control.

In children with dystonic cerebral palsy, ITB may reduce the dystonia and improve function. This requires high catheter placement, and considerable higher doses of baclofen than for spasticity. A promising direction for treatment is DBS, where electrodes are placed in specific nuclei in the extrapyramidal motor circuit including the globus pallidus and subthalamic nucleus. While some initial reports of improvement in dystonia are favorable, there are concerns about mechanical problems including electrode movement and breaks. To date, DBS has been infrequently employed in children with hyperkinetic movement disorders.

Children with extrapyramidal cerebral palsy are more likely than those with severe spasticity to have normal intelligence. However, this group may have difficulties with dysarthria or inability to speak. In this situation, assistive technology is an important component of therapy. Sophisticated devices can be designed to give children control of their environment from communication to mobility. Referral to specialized centers or teams is recommended to provide the optimum equipment, given the rapid advances in this area.

MEDICATION MANAGEMENT

While the possible range of side effects to oral medications is beyond the scope of this chapter, several generalizations can be made. Some medications have recognizable side effects, such as sedation from diazepam and seizures from acute baclofen withdrawal. Others become evident with repeated use, such as personality changes with trihexyphenidyl. As many of the medications used have not been thoroughly studied in childhood, clinicians should listen carefully to parental/caregiver concerns about any changes in their children after medication initiation.

Parents/caregivers will continue to administer medications if they see positive benefits, which should be an important determinant in clinician decision making with regard to use and dosing. A helpful additional aid is to keep community therapists masked as to onset and dosing of medications, utilizing their opinions as to changes in motor function with medication use/adjustments.

ASSOCIATED PROBLEMS

While this chapter is primarily directed toward medical management, it is important to recognize that affected children and their families may have a wide range of medical, financial, psychosocial, educational, and vocational needs, which may change over time. The identification of a person who can coordinate various aspects of care is of great benefit in overall management.

Furthermore, housing accessibility is critical for those children with more severe forms of cerebral palsy, both to optimize independence of the affected child, as well as to limit other impairments such as herniated disks from repeated lifting by caregivers. A practical recommendation is to find a dwelling on one floor, such as a ranch-style home.

COMPLEMENTARY ALTERNATIVE MEDICINE (CAM)

Families may use complementary alternative medicine, including acupuncture, craniosacral therapy, myofascial release, therapeutic taping, diet and herbal remedies, electrical stimulation, constraint-induced training, chiropractic treatments, massage and hyperbaric oxygen. While there are individual reports of improvements with various alternative therapies, some carry substantial risks. Furthermore, rigorous studies have not been conducted to assess efficacy. Prior to utilizing these therapies, cost, efficacy, and potential side effects should be carefully considered.

CONCLUSIONS

Despite the wide range of available interventions with demonstrated benefits in individual children, there is currently no clear consensus regarding the nature of optimal therapy(ies), as well as timing and duration of specific interventions (8–11). Further advances in treatment will require controlled trials, matched on etiological antecedents and using reliable, valid quantitative measurement systems to assess effectiveness.

ACKNOWLEDGMENTS

In addition to Drs. Singer and Kossoff, the authors acknowledge the thoughtful comments of numerous Kennedy Krieger Institute physicians, clinicians, and therapists, including Drs. Michael Johnston, Charles Silberstein, Frank Pidcock, Bruce Shapiro, Eric Levey, and Elaine Stashinko; Ms. Elsie Reinhardt, LaVerne Madden, Teresa Pesci.

WEB SITES OF INTEREST

1. http://www.wemove.org/kidsmove/. This WE MOVE web site offers information and support for healthcare professionals and others whose lives are affected by pediatric movement disorders.
2. http://www.ucp.org/main.cfm/81. United cerebral palsy (UCP) is the leading source of information on cerebral palsy and is a pivotal advocate for the rights of persons with any disability. As one of the largest health charities in America, UCP's mission is to advance the independence, productivity, and full citizenship of people with cerebral palsy and other disabilities.
3. http://www.hemikids.org/. The Children's Hemiplegia and Stroke Association, a non profit organization, offering support and information to families of infants, children, and young adults who have hemiplegia, hemiparesis, hemiplegic cerebral palsy, childhood stroke, infant stroke, or in utero stroke.
4. http://www.lissencephaly.org/. This web site is provided for the parents, siblings, physicians, and therapists of children born with lissencephaly (smooth brain), and other neuronal migration disorders.
5. http://www.eparent.com/. Exception Parent magazine's on-line resource, providing information, support, ideas, encouragement, and outreach for parents and families of children with disabilities, and the professionals who work with them.

REFERENCES

1. Albright AL. Neurosurgical treatment of spasticity and other pediatric movement disorders. J Child Neurol 2003; 18(suppl 1):S67–S78.
2. Butler C, Campbell S. Evidence of the effects of intrathecal baclofen for spastic and dystonic cerebral palsy. AACPDM Treatment Outcomes Committee Review Panel. Dev Med Child Neurol 2000; 42:634–645.
3. Edgar TS. Oral pharmacotherapy of childhood movement disorders. J Child Neurol 2003; 181:S40–S49.
4. Hoon AH, Johnston MV. Cerebral palsy. In: Asbury AK, McKhann G, McDonald WI, Goadsby PJ, McArthur JC, eds. Diseases of the Nervous System: Clinical Neuroscience and Therapeutic Principles. 3rd ed. New York: Cambridge University Press, 2002.
5. Hoon AH, Freese PO, Reinhardt EM, Wilson MA, Lawrie WT, Harryman SE, Pidcock FS, Johnston MV. Age dependent beneficial effects of trihexyphenidyl in children with extrapyramidal cerebral palsy. Ped Neurol 2001; 25:55–58.
6. Hoon AH, Belsito KM, Nagae-Poetscher LM. Neuroimaging in spasticity and movement disorders. J Child Neurol 2003; 18:S25–S39.
7. Koman LA, Paterson Smith B, Balkrishnan R. Spasticity associated with cerebral palsy in children: guidelines for the use of botulinum A toxin. Paediatr Drugs 2003; 5(1):11–23.
8. Patrick JH, Roberts AP, Cole GF. Therapeutic choices in the locomotor management of the child with cerebral palsy—more luck than judgement? Arch Dis Child 2001; 85: 275–279.
9. Siebes RC, Wijnroks L, Vermeer A. Qualitative analysis of therapeutic motor intervention programmes for children with cerebral palsy: an update. Dev Med Child Neurol 2002; 44:593–603.
10. Stanger M, Oresic S. Rehabilitation approaches for children with cerebral palsy: overview. J Child Neurol 2003; 18(Suppl 1):S79–S88.
11. Steinbok P. Outcomes after selective dorsal rhizotomy for spastic cerebral palsy. Childs Nerv Syst 2001; 17:1–18.

4
Hydrocephalus

Anthony M. Avellino
Division of Pediatric Neurosurgery, Children's Hospital and Regional Medical Center, University of Washington School of Medicine, Seattle, Washington, U.S.A.

INTRODUCTION

Hydrocephalus is the abnormal accumulation of cerebrospinal fluid (CSF) within the ventricles and subarachnoid spaces. It is often associated with dilatation of the ventricular system and increased intracranial pressure (ICP). The incidence of pediatric hydrocephalus as an isolated congenital disorder is approximately 1/1000 live births. Pediatric hydrocephalus is often associated with numerous other conditions, such as spina bifida, tumors, and infections. Hydrocephalus is almost always a result of an interruption of CSF flow and is rarely because of increased CSF production.

CLINICAL PATHOLOGY—SITE OF OBSTRUCTION

Historically, hydrocephalus has been classified as *obstructive* or *nonobstructive*, a somewhat misleading classification because all forms of hydrocephalus, except hydrocephalus ex vacuo (resulting from brain atrophy), involve some form of CSF obstruction. A more commonly used classification differentiates hydrocephalus between *communicating* or *noncommunicating* (Table 1). Traditionally, this classification was based on whether dye injected into the lateral ventricles could be detected in CSF extracted from a subsequent lumbar puncture. Currently, the term "noncommunicating hydrocephalus" refers to lesions that obstruct the ventricular system, either at the cerebral aqueduct of sylvius or basal foramina (i.e., basal foramina of Luschka and Magendie). The term "communicating hydrocephalus" refers to lesions that obstruct at the level of the subarachnoid space and arachnoid villi.

Lateral Ventricle

Choroid plexus tumors are rare in the pediatric population, with an incidence ranging from 1.5% to 3.9% of all pediatric CNS tumors. Most choroid plexus tumors are choroid plexus papillomas, which usually present within the first 3 years of life. The CSF production rates three to four times the normal rate have been documented in children with choroid plexus papillomas. Removal of the papilloma resolves the

Table 1 Causes of Hydrocephalus Based on Site of Obstruction

Lateral ventricle
Choroid plexus tumor
Intraventricular region glioma
Foramen of Monro
Congenital atresia
Iatrogenic functional stenosis
Stenotic gliosis secondary to intraventricular hemorrhage or ventriculitis
Third ventricle
Colloid cyst
Ependymal cyst
Arachnoid cyst
Neoplasms such as craniopharngioma, chiasmal-hypothalamic astrocytoma, or glioma
Cerebral aqueduct
Congenital aqueduct malformation
Arteriovenous malformation
Congenital aqueduct stenosis
Neoplasms such as pineal region germinoma or periaqueductal glioma
Fourth ventricle
Dandy–Walker cyst
Neoplasms such as medulloblastoma, ependymoma, astrocytoma, or brainstem glioma
Basal foramina occlusion secondary to subarachnoid hemorrhage or meningitis
Chiari malformations

hydrocephalus in approximately two-thirds of cases. The remaining third probably suffer from obstruction of the aqueduct and/or basal meninges and require a ventricular shunt presumably secondary to preoperative microhemorrhages or postoperative scarring of the arachnoid villae.

Foramen of Monro

Occlusion of one foramen of Monro can occur secondary to a congenital membrane, atresia, or gliosis after intraventricular hemorrhage (IVH) or ventriculitis. The resulting unilateral ventriculomegaly is often occult until early childhood, and may enlarge the ipsilateral hemicalvarium.

An iatrogenic functional stenosis of the foramen of Monro can develop in children with spina bifida whose hydrocephalus has been treated with a ventricular shunt. The contralateral nonshunted ventricle occasionally expands secondary to deformity of the foramen of Monro. If symptomatic, the patient can be treated with a shunt system having two ventricular catheters, each draining a separate lateral ventricle or an endoscopic fenestration of the septum pellucidum with one ventricular catheter draining both ventricles.

Third Ventricle

Cysts and neoplasms within the third ventricle commonly cause hydrocephalus. Colloid cysts are uncommon neoplasms that present superiorly and anteriorly within the third ventricle, and usually obstruct both foramina of Monro. Considered to be congenital lesions, they can become symptomatic at any age. However, they rarely present within the pediatric population, and are commonly symptomatic between the ages of 20 and 50 years. They can cause either intermittent, acute, life-threatening hydrocephalus or chronic hydrocephalus. They are customarily treated with resection via craniotomy, endoscopic resection, or stereotactic aspiration of the cyst.

Ependymal and arachnoid cysts within the third ventricle usually present with hydrocephalus in late childhood. Patients may present with bobble-head doll syndrome, a rhythmic head and trunk bobbing tremor at a frequency of two to three times per second. While endoscopic fenestration is a treatment option, they are often treated with a ventricular catheter fenestrated to drain both ventricles and the cyst.

The most common pediatric neoplasms that obstruct the third ventricle are craniopharyngiomas and chiasmal-hypothalamic astrocytomas. Hydrocephalus secondary to craniopharyngiomas usually resolves after surgical resection of the tumor. Hydrocephalus secondary to third ventricular region gliomas usually does not resolve after surgical resection, and ventricular shunt placement is often necessary.

Cerebral Aqueduct

The normal aqueduct of a neonate is 12–13 mm in length and only 0.2–0.5 mm in diameter. Thus, it is prone to obstruction from a variety of lesions, including congenital aqueductal malformations, pineal region neoplasms, arteriovenous malformations, and periaqueductal neoplasms.

Hydrocephalus secondary to aqueductal occlusion is generally severe and causes distension of the third ventricle and separation of the thalami, thinning of the septum pellucidum and corpus callosum, and compression of the cerebral hemispheres. Less than 2% of cases of congenital aqueductal stenosis are the result of the recessively inherited X-linked Bickers–Adams–Edwards syndrome, which is associated with flexion–adduction of the thumbs ("cortical thumbs").

Any pineal mass can obstruct the aqueduct and produce hydrocephalus. Many pineal region tumors, especially germinomas, are highly radiosensitive; and successful tumor irradiation as well as surgical resection may adequately treat the obstructive hydrocephalus.

Low-grade astrocytomas are the most common periaqueductal pediatric neoplasms that cause hydrocephalus. Historically, children with neurofibromatosis have often been diagnosed with "late-onset aqueductal stenosis." However, with the advent of magnetic resonance (MR) imaging, many of these children present with periaqueductal hyperintense T2 signals, indicating low-grade astrocytomas.

Fourth Ventricle

In infants, the fourth ventricle is the location for obstruction secondary to Dandy–Walker cysts or obliteration of the basal foramina. In older children, neoplasms are a common cause. Such occlusions result in the dilation of the lateral, third, and fourth ventricles above the obstruction. Dandy–Walker cysts are developmental abnormalities characterized by a large cyst in the fourth ventricle lined with pia-arachnoid and ependyma, hypoplasia of the cerebellar vermis, and atrophy of the cerebellar hemispheres. Over 85% of children with Dandy–Walker cysts have hydrocephalus.

Pediatric tumors associated with the fourth ventricle (e.g., medulloblastomas, ependymomas, astrocytomas, and brainstem gliomas) commonly present with hydrocephalus. Arachnoiditis secondary to either meningitis or subarachnoid hemorrhage can also occlude the basal foramina and cause obstructive hydrocephalus. In addition, infants with Chiari II malformations and myelomeningoceles have hydrocephalus secondary to blockage of CSF flow from basilar obstruction.

Arachnoid Granulations

Sclerosis or scarring of the arachnoid granulations can occur after meningitis, subarachnoid hemorrhage, or trauma. The subarachnoid spaces over the convexities enlarge, thus forming a condition often referred to as "external hydrocephalus." The radiographic imaging from this disorder is often confused with subdural effusions, which are typically bifrontal, or cerebral atrophy, which is rare in children with macrocephaly. Symptomatic external hydrocephalus is treated with a subdural/subarachnoid to peritoneal shunt.

CLINICAL FEATURES

Premature Infants

Hydrocephalus in premature infants is predominantly caused by posthemorrhagic hydrocephalus (PHH). Because the poorly myelinated premature brain is so easily compressed and the skull is so distensible, premature infants can develop considerable ventriculomegaly before their head circumference increases. Infants with PHH may have no symptoms or may exhibit increasing spells of apnea and bradycardia. Poor feeding and vomiting are uncommon signs of hydrocephalus in premature infants. If ventriculomegaly progresses and ICP increases, the anterior fontanelle becomes convex, tense, and nonpulsatile; and the cranial sutures splay and the scalp veins distend. As ventriculomegaly persists, the head develops a globoid shape, and the head circumference increases at a rapid rate. Head circumference increases 0.5 cm/week in sick premature infants, 1 cm/week in healthy premature infants, and up to 2 cm/week in premature infants with PHH (Table 2).

Table 2 Signs and Symptoms of Hydrocephalus in Children

Premature infants	Infants	Toddlers and older
Apnea	Irritability	Headache
Bradycardia	Vomiting	Vomiting
Tense fontanelle	Drowsiness	Lethargy
Distended scalp veins	Macrocephaly	Diplopia
Globoid head shape	Distended scalp veins	Papilledema
Rapid head growth	Frontal bossing	Lateral rectus palsy
	Macewen's sign	Hyper-reflexia-clonus
	Poor head control	
	Lateral rectus palsy	
	"Setting-sun" sign	

(From Elsevier from: P.P. Wang and A.M. Avellino. Hydrocephalus in children. In: Principles of Neurosurgery, 2nd edition, S.S. Rengachary and R.G. Ellenbogen (eds.). Elsevier Science, 2003.)

Full-Term Infants

The common causes of hydrocephalus in full-term infants include aqueductal stenosis, Chiari II malformation, Dandy–Walker syndrome, arachnoid cysts, neoplasms, vein of Galen malformations, and cerebral malformations (e.g., encephaloceles, holoprosencephaly, and hydranencephaly). Symptoms include irritability, vomiting, and drowsiness. Signs include macrocephaly, a convex and full anterior fontanelle, distended scalp veins, cranial suture splaying, frontal bossing, "cracked pot" sound on skull percussion over dilated ventricles (Macewen's sign), poor head control, lateral rectus palsies, and the "setting-sun" sign, in which the eyes are inferiorly deviated. Paralysis of upgaze and Parinaud's sign herald dilation of the suprapineal recess (Table 2).

Normal head circumference for full-term infants is 33–36 cm at birth. Head circumference increases by 2 cm/month during the first 3 months, by 1 cm/month from 4 to 6 months, and by 0.5 cm/month from 7 to 12 months. Head circumference increases that are progressive and rapid, crossing percentile curves on the head growth chart are a stronger diagnostic indicator of hydrocephalus than increases that are consistently above, but parallel to the 95% percentile curve.

Older Children

Hydrocephalus after infancy is usually secondary to trauma or neoplasms. The predominant symptom is usually a dull and steady headache, which typically occurs upon awakening. It may be associated with lethargy, and often improves after vomiting. The headaches slowly increase in frequency and severity over days or weeks. Other common complaints include blurred or double vision.

Children presenting with headaches, vomiting, and drowsiness are unfortunately often misdiagnosed as having early meningitis; thus, a head computerized tomography (CT) or MR imaging should be performed to rule out hydrocephalus, hematoma, or tumor before a lumbar puncture is attempted. Older children often present with decreased school performance and behavioral disturbances, as well as endocrinopathies (e.g., precocious puberty, short stature, and hypothyroidism).

Common signs include papilledema and lateral rectus palsies (unilateral or bilateral). Hyper-reflexia and clonus are also seen. Rarely, children with hydrocephalus may experience transient or permanent blindness if the posterior cerebral arteries are compressed against the tentorium. Treatment is urgent if the child becomes lethargic. If the hydrocephalus is severe, Cushing's triad of bradycardia, systemic hypertension, and irregular breathing patterns, as well as autonomic dysfunction, may occur. Cushing's triad is rare and often denotes very high ICP requiring emergency treatment (Table 2).

DIAGNOSIS

Historically, several imaging studies were commonly used before the advent of CT scans in 1976. Skull radiographs demonstrate several diagnostic signs, including cranial suture separation in infants, as well as a "beaten copper" appearance and enlarged sella in older children. Skull radiographs have since been supplanted by more modern imaging studies such as cranial ultrasonography, CT scanning, and

MR imaging that demonstrate increased ventricular size, the site of pathological obstruction, and may show transependymal resorption.

TREATMENT

The treatment of hydrocephalus can be divided into nonsurgical approaches and surgical approaches, which in turn can be divided into nonshunting or shunting procedures. The goals of any successful management of hydrocephalus are: (1) optimal neurological outcome and (2) preservation of cosmesis. The radiographic finding of normal-sized ventricles should not be considered the goal of any therapeutic modality.

Nonsurgical Options

There is no nonsurgical medical treatment that definitively treats hydrocephalus effectively. Even if CSF production were to be reduced by 33%, ICP would only modestly decrease by 1.5 cm H_2O pressure. Historically, acetazolamide and furosemide have been used to treat hydrocephalus. Although both agents can decrease CSF production for a few days, they do not significantly reduce ventriculomegaly. Acetazolamide, a carbonic anhydrase inhibitor, is needed in large doses (25 mg/kg/day divided into three daily oral doses), and potential side effects include lethargy, poor feeding, tachypnea, diarrhea, nephrocalcinosis, and electrolyte imbalances (e.g., hyperchloremic metabolic acidosis, which may require treatment with a systemic alkalizer). While acetazolamide has been used historically to treat premature infants with PHH, recent studies have shown it to be ineffective in avoidance of ventricular shunt placement and to be associated with increased neurological morbidity.

Surgical—Nonshunting Options

Whenever possible, the obstructing lesion that causes the hydrocephalus should be surgically removed. For example, the resection of tumors in the vicinity of the third and fourth ventricle often treats the secondary hydrocephalus. Unfortunately, in most cases of congenital hydrocephalus, the obstructive lesion is not amenable to surgical resection.

For CSF obstruction at or distal to the aqueduct (e.g., tectal plate tumors, acquired aqueductal stenosis, or posterior fossa tumors), a potential surgical treatment is the endoscopic third ventriculostomy. By surgically creating an opening at the floor of the third ventricle, CSF can be diverted without placing a ventricular shunt. Recent studies report a high success rate for endoscopic third ventriculostomies among pediatric patients with hydrocephalus secondary to aqueductal stenosis. While earlier studies demonstrated that third ventriculostomies are of intermediate value in patients with congenital aqueductal stenosis (i.e., < 1 year of age) and myelomeningoceles, recent studies suggest that these patients also have high success rates with this procedure. Communicating hydrocephalus is not an indication for a third ventriculostomy.

Surgical—CSF Shunts

Table 3 lists common indications for ventricular shunt placement.

Table 3 Indications for Ventricular Shunt Placement

Congenital hydrocephalus
Persistent posthemorrhagic hydrocephalus
Hydrocephalus associated with myelomeningocele
Hydrocephalus associated with Dandy–Walker cyst
Hydrocephalus associated with arachnoid cyst
Hydrocephalus associated with posterior fossa tumor
Treatment of trapped fourth ventricle secondary to intraventricular hemorrhage or meningitis

Components

The CSF shunts are usually silicone rubber tubes that divert CSF from the ventricles to other body cavities where normal physiologic processes can absorb the CSF. Shunts typically have three components: a proximal (ventricular) catheter, a one-way valve that permits flow out of the ventricular system, and a distal catheter that diverts the fluid to its eventual destination (i.e., peritoneal, atrium, or pleural space). Most shunts have built-in reservoirs that can be percutaneously aspirated for CSF.

Most shunt valves are pressure-differentiated valves, i.e., they are designed to open at designated pressures and remain open as long as the pressure differential across the valve is greater than the opening pressure. However, some shunts are flow -controlled, where the valve mechanism attempts to keep flow constant in the face of changing pressure differentials and patient position. Valves come in a variety of different pressure and flow settings depending on the manufacturer. A recent advance in shunt valve technology has been the introduction of programmable valves. These permit the neurosurgeon to adjust the opening pressure settings of the implanted shunt valve without the need to subject the child to an additional surgical procedure to change valves.

Shunt Complications

Shunt complications and failure remain a significant problem in treating hydrocephalus. The goal in treatment of hydrocephalus with a shunt is to decrease intracranial pressure and associated cerebral damage and simultaneously prevent complications associated with the ventricular shunting procedure. Shunt complications fall into three major categories: (1) mechanical failure of the device, (2) functional failure because of too much or too little flow of CSF, and (3) infection of the CSF or the shunt device. A list of shunt complications is outlined in Table 4. The two most common complications are infection and obstruction.

Shunt Infection

Despite the numerous measures used to decrease the risk of infection, in general, approximately 1–15% of all shunting procedures are complicated by infection. This rate seems to remain constant despite a host of precautions employed, which include the use of systemic and intrashunt antibiotics, iodine-impregnated transparent surgical drapes, covering incisions with Betadine-soaked sponges, glove changes, and using only instruments to handle shunt hardware. Premature infants have an increased risk. Approximately three-quarters of all shunt infections become evident within one month of placement. Nearly 90% of all shunt infections are recognized

Table 4 Shunt Complications

Common complications	Uncommon complications			
	Cranial	Subcutaneous	Peritoneal	Atrial
Infection	Subdural hygroma	Shunt migration	Peritonitis	Endocarditis
Obstruction	Subdural hematoma	Shunt disconnection	Pseudocysts	Nephritis
Inadequate flow or	Hemiparesis	Shunt fracture	Perforation	
overdrainage	Hematoma		Hernias	

(From: P.P. Wang and A.M. Avellino. Hydrocephalus in children. In: Principles of Neurosurgery, 2nd edition, S.S. Rengachary and R.G. Ellenbogen (eds.). Elsevier Science, 2003.)

within one year of the last shunt manipulation, as it is believed that most bacteria are introduced at the time of surgery.

The offending organism is most often a member of the skin flora. *Staphylococcus epidermidis* causes approximately 60% of shunt infections, *Staphylococcus aureus* is responsible for 30%, and coliform bacteria, Propionibacteria, Streptococci, or *Haemophilus influenzae* cause the remainder. In general, Gram-positive organisms correlate with a better prognosis than Gram-negative organisms.

Common symptoms include irritability and anorexia. Common signs include low-grade fever and elevated C-reactive protein. *S. aureus* infections often present with erythema along the shunt track. Infected ventriculoatrial shunts may present with subacute bacterial endocarditis and shunt nephritis, an immune-complex disorder that resembles acute glomerulonephritis.

The literature regarding the usefulness of prophylactic antibiotics is conflicting. Several prospective, randomized, trials demonstrated statistically significant improvement in shunt infection rates when children were treated with systemic oxacillin, systemic trimethoprim–sulfamethoxazole, or intraventricular vancomycin. However, similar studies using systemic methicillin or cephalothin demonstrated no significant advantage. Regardless of this, prophylactic antibiotics, such as cefazolin, vancomycin, or oxacillin, are routinely used in clinical practice.

The most effective and widely used treatment of a shunt infection is to remove the infected shunt hardware and either place no hardware (if tolerated) or place an external ventriculostomy drain. The patient is then treated with the appropriate intravenous antibiotics based on culture and sensitivity results. When the infection is cleared [i.e., (1) 5–7 consecutive daily CSF cultures that are negative, (2) CSF white blood cell count $< 50\,\text{mm}^3$, and (3) CSF protein $< 500\,\text{mg/dL}$], a new ventricular shunt system is implanted and the external ventriculostomy is removed. In the case of some bacterial infections, it is possible to eradicate the infection without removing the shunt. However, in situ treatment of shunt infections is fraught with hazards and does not uniformly lead to success.

Shunt Obstruction

Shunt obstruction is another common complication. The clinical presentation can vary greatly. Shunt devices are to be viewed as mechanical devices that can become obstructed or malfunction anywhere in their course and anytime during their lifetime. The most common scenarios occur weeks, months, or years after insertion, when choroid plexus or debris has occluded the proximal ventricular catheter tip. Another common shunt malfunction scenario is the child who has obstructed his distal catheter or has outgrown his peritoneal catheter, and presents with an obstruction after the distal catheter tip has slipped out of the peritoneal cavity. In addition, shunt valves can malfunction, and shunt tubing can break, disconnect or dislodge from its previous location.

Common symptoms of shunt obstruction depend on the age of the child. A child with a shunt malfunction often presents with signs and symptoms of increased ICP. Infants with a shunt malfunction usually present with irritability, poor feeding, increased head circumference, and/or inappropriate sleepiness. Children with a shunt malfunction usually present with headache, irritability, lethargy, nausea, and/or vomiting. However, it is important to inquire if the signs and symptoms that the child is presenting with are the same as those during a shunt malfunction in the past. The child can present with waxing and waning symptoms, or can alternatively present with a progressively worsening picture that does not improve until the shunt is revised. A child complaining of pain with a clinical picture consistent with shunt obstruction should not be given narcotics because of possible respiratory depression or arrest.

When a shunt malfunction is suspected, neuroimaging studies should be obtained after a careful history and physical examination. A head CT, as well as anteroposterior and lateral skull, chest, and abdominal radiographs are obtained to evaluate for increased ventricular size and shunt hardware continuity. Even though a majority of children with a shunt malfunction present with increased ventricular size on neuroimaging studies, there are those whose ventricular size does not change because of decreased brain compliance (i.e., "stiff ventricles"). In these children, a shunt tap through the reservoir or valve is indicated to test the adequacy of CSF flow and the intracranial pressure. Children who are diagnosed with a shunt malfunction are taken promptly to the operating room for shunt revision.

The shunt itself can be examined for evidence of obstruction. The presence of a fluid collection in the subcutaneous tissue in proximity to the shunt track is suggestive. The shunt valve can be "pumped" (i.e., compressed several times against the skull), which may provide useful information. A collapse of the valve without quick refilling of CSF may indicate a shunt obstruction. Finally, the shunt reservoir can be accessed by a 23- or 25-gauge butterfly needle. The presence of spontaneous flow with good respiratory variations up the tubing or in a manometer connected to the butterfly indicates patency of the ventricular catheter. The ICP can be measured simultaneously. If there is no CSF flow up the manometer and the ventricles are large, a presumed shunt obstruction is confirmed. In some institutions, a nuclear medicine patency study may be performed to evaluate a presumed shunt malfunction, by occluding the valve and injecting through the butterfly needle a radioactive isotope, such as indium [111In] into the reservoir. The radioactive isotope can then be traced from the ventricular system, through the shunt device, and into the distal collection site.

Uncommon Shunt Complications

Table 4 lists several uncommon shunt complications. Subdural hygromas and hematomas may develop after the insertion of a ventricular shunt into a child with very large ventricles and a thin cerebral cortical mantle. Treatment of symptomatic subdural hygromas and hematomas consists of changing the shunt valve to a higher pressure setting and/or by introducing a catheter into the subdural effusion and connecting it to the distal shunt system. Ventricular catheter migration out of the ventricular system occurs if the shunt has not been properly fixed at the burr hole site where it exits the skull.

Abdominal pseudocysts can develop around the distal end of the peritoneal catheter. They often develop in young children secondary to indolent bacterial infections. In addition to presenting with a clinical picture of a shunt infection, the patient may also complain of abdominal pain and distension. They can be diagnosed by an abdominal ultrasound or CT scan. The cysts may be percutaneously aspirated, and the fluid can be cultured. Given the indolent nature of the likely infections, treatment is no different from any other shunt infection. Ascites, similarly, may be indicative of an indolent infection, or it may be secondary to CSF overproduction and/or inadequate peritoneal absorption.

Hernias can also develop within 3 months of shunt insertion, and are treated like any other hernia. Perforation of intraperitoneal organs is a rare but well-recognized complication.

Treatment of Posthemorrhagic Hydrocephalus (PHH)

Premature infants weighing 0.5–1.5 kg often develop IVH that obstructs the CSF pathways. First, serial lumbar punctures and/or ventricular taps are performed to normalize ICP; approximately 5–15 mL of CSF must be removed daily to adequately temporize the PHH. The infant's ICP can be assessed by palpation of the anterior fontanelle and detection of the cranial suture splaying; and ventriculomegaly can be followed by serial cranial ultrasounds. If the infant's weight is 1–1.5 kg, a ventriculosubgaleal shunt or a ventricular catheter and subcutaneous reservoir can be placed. Ventriculosubgaleal shunts can safely temporize PHH while avoiding external drainage or frequent CSF aspirations. A ventricular catheter connected to a subcutaneous reservoir can be accessed for daily CSF aspirations with a risk of infection of less than 5%. A ventriculoperitoneal shunt should be considered when the CSF is cleared of posthemorrhagic debris, CSF protein is <1000 mg/dL, the infant weighs >1.5 kg, and the infant has persistent PHH.

Treatment of Hydrocephalus Associated with Myelomeningocele

Approximately 85% of infants with myelomeningoceles develop symptomatic hydrocephalus, and approximately 50% have obvious hydrocephalus at birth. Treatment is usually with a ventriculoperitoneal shunt, although recent evidence suggests that endoscopic third ventriculostomies may have a useful role. Historically, shunt placement is deferred until after the myelomeningocele is repaired; however, contemporary evidence suggests that the risks of shunt complications are not significantly increased if the shunt is placed at the same time as the myelomeningocele closure. In many centers, the shunt is placed in neonates with ventriculomegaly at the time of the myelomeningocele closure with the hope that a shunt will prevent a CSF leak from the repaired myelomeningocele site.

Treatment of Hydrocephalus Associated with a Dandy–Walker Cyst

To treat hydrocephalus secondary to a Dandy–Walker cyst, a contrast study can be performed to determine if the lateral ventricles communicate with the cyst. With no communication, at least two shunts are necessary, one to decompress the cyst and one to drain the ventricular system. With communication, a single shunt in either the lateral ventricle or the cyst could adequately treat the hydrocephalus, although some centers recommend simply shunting both the cyst and ventricle as the initial treatment. A decompressed Dandy–Walker cyst can yield dramatic radiographic results (i.e., cerebellar hemispheres that seem to be severely atrophic are often in reality only severely compressed).

PROGNOSIS

The prognosis of pediatric hydrocephalus is dependent more on the underlying brain morphology as well as other factors such as IVH, ventriculitis, and perinatal ischemia, than on the severity of the hydrocephalus and ventriculomegaly. The 5-year survival rate of children with congenital hydrocephalus is approximately 90%. Normal intellect has been reported to range from 40% to 65%, but obviously varies widely with each specific etiology.

Before the advent of the CT scan, several studies attempted to investigate the prognosis of shunted vs. nonshunted hydrocephalic children. In 1963, Foltz and Shurtleff performed a 5-year study of 113 hydrocephalic children of whom 65 were shunted early, and 48 were not operated on. They found that shunted children had a significantly better survival and a higher percentage had an IQ of at least 75. In 1973, Young and colleagues performed an outcome analysis on a series of 147 shunted hydrocephalic children. They found a correlation between the width of the child's cerebral mantle and IQ in that the IQ distribution approached a normal pattern when a cerebral mantle width of 2.8 cm was achieved.

Since the introduction of CT and MR imaging, there have been several studies investigating the outcomes of hydrocephalus secondary to specific etiologies. In 1985, Op Heij and colleagues followed children with congenital nonobstructive hydrocephalus and found that IQ was normal (> 80) in 50% of cases and abnormal (< 55) in 28%. There was no correlation with head circumference or degree of ventriculomegaly. They concluded that the degree of intellectual impairment had less to do with the severity of the hydrocephalus and more to do with the severity of underlying anomalies in the central nervous system and defects in the cytoarchitecture of the neocortex.

Infants with PHH have a significantly higher mortality rate when compared with low-birth-weight infants without PHH. The correlation between severity of PHH and neurological disabilities is less clear.

Historically, the mortality for infants with Dandy–Walker malformation approached 20–30%. However, in 1990, Bindal and colleagues demonstrated a mortality rate of 14% in their series. Lower IQ and neurological developmental delay are seen in children with Dandy–Walker malformations, but they are thought to be related to the associated anomalies in the central nervous system.

SUMMARY

Signs and symptoms of progressive hydrocephalus depend on age. Symptomatic ventricular shunt malfunction should be evaluated, recognized, and treated promptly to avoid undue morbidity. Ventricular shunt infection currently occurs in 1–15% of children who have shunts placed or revised, and the majority of infections are detected within the first 1–6 months after a shunt procedure. The prognosis of pediatric hydrocephalus is dependent primarily on the underlying brain morphology.

REFERENCE

1. Wang PP, Avellino AM. Hydrocephalus in children. In: Rengachary SS, Ellenbogen RG, eds. Principles of Neurosurgery. 2d ed. United Kingdom: Elsevier Science, Chapter 8, 2003. (Portions of this chapter were reprinted with permission from Elsevier.) In press.

SUGGESTED READINGS

1. Albright AL. Hydrocephalus in children. In: Rengachary SS, Wilkens RH, eds. Principles of Neurosurgery. London: Wolfe Publishing, Chapter 6, 1994:6.1–6.23.
2. Dandy WE, Blackfan KD. An experimental and clinical study of internal hydrocephalus. JAMA 1913; 61:2216–2217.

5
Scoliosis

Leslie A. Morrison
Department of Neurology, University of New Mexico, Albuquerque, New Mexico, U.S.A.

INTRODUCTION

Scoliosis is a lateral and rotational curvature of the thoracic and lumbar spine measuring greater than 10°. Three major categories exist. The first, idiopathic scoliosis, accounts for 80% of cases with a predilection for adolescent females. The second category, neuromuscular scoliosis, describes an acquired deformity that results from neurologic impairment of either a peripheral or central nature. The third category involves those forms with congenital onset or that are attributable to other connective tissue and musculoskeletal disorders. Children with severe neurological impairment are at high risk for the development of scoliosis, especially within certain diagnostic groups. For example, 90% of boys with Duchenne muscular dystrophy (DMD) will develop scoliosis. In cerebral palsy, the incidence is highest in those most severely affected, usually with quadraplegic, hemiplegic, and dystonic forms of CP.

DIAGNOSIS AND EVALUATION

The neurologist's role in the evaluation of the child with scoliosis is to uncover disorders of the central or peripheral nervous system that might have additional implications for prognosis or management. Most patients with scoliosis, however, have the idiopathic form of scoliosis or scoliosis due to obvious neurologic (Table 1) or musculoskeletal (Table 2) causes that do not require further diagnostic investigation. The most common problem, therefore, is to separate those with idiopathic scoliosis from those with scoliosis due to occult neurologic impairment. In most cases of idiopathic scoliosis, curvature appears in preadolescence. For those with scoliosis due to underlying neurologic causes, the appearance of curvature can occur early. It is therefore incumbent upon pediatricians, neurologists, and other pediatric subspecialists to have a high index of suspicion in patients with both new or long standing scoliosis.

Neurologic evaluation entails a careful history with attention to back or leg pain, changes in bowel or bladder function, and weakness or sensory changes. The clinical examination should focus on the any focal features of the neurologic

Table 1 Neurological Conditions with an Enhanced Risk for Scoliosis

Central nervous system: brain	*Peripheral nervous system*
Cerebral palsy	Poliomyelitis
Congenital brain malformation	Spinal muscular atrophy
Degenerative diseases of brain	Brachial plexopathies
Tumors	Genetic or acquired neuropathies
Vascular malformations	Disorders of neuromuscular junction
Stroke	Myopathies (congenital and inflammatory)
Genetic disorders	Muscular dystrophies
Traumatic brain injury	*Central nervous system: spinal cord*
Central nervous system: spinal cord	Friedreich's ataxia
Tumors, vascular malformations	Congenital muscular dystrophies
Myelodysplasias, acquired myelopathies	Mitochondrial encephalomyopathies
Traumatic spinal cord injury	Myotonic dystrophy type I

evaluation, particularly a difference between upper and lower extremities, manifesting with signs of weakness, spasticity, incoordination, disproportionate tendon reflexes, or extensor toe responses. Concave curves to the left, multiple, or complex curves predict higher risk of underlying neurological disorders. Sensory examination should focus on uncovering features of a sensory level, suspended sensory deficit of spinothalamic modalities suggestive of a syrinx, or local sensory deficits characteristic of radiculopathy. Scoliosis is a common early feature of Friedreich's ataxia, where diffuse areflexia, extensor toe responses, and abnormal Romberg testing are prominent. Abnormalities of bowel or bladder function should be evaluated with examination of sacral reflexes. Ancillary tests that might be of value include EMG and somatosensory evoked potentials; the latter may be useful as preoperative baseline studies for interoperative monitoring. Spinal cord MRI studies are invaluable in investigating a possible mass or syrinx; in occasional circumstances as, for example when metal rods preclude MR imaging, CT or standard myelography may also have a role.

Orthopedic evaluation entails inspection for symmetry in standing and forward bending, and determination of whether the curvature is fixed or flexible. Spine radiographs are obtained with standing posterior–anterior and lateral films; if the child is unable to stand, they are obtained in anterior–posterior seated or supine positions. Curvatures are named for the side and region of the convexity, measured

Table 2 Musculoskeletal and Genetic Causes of Scoliosis

Musculoskeletal disorders	*Genetic syndromes*
Rheumatoid arthritis	Rett
Leg length discrepancy	Neurofibromatosis
Injury to vertebrae	22q11.2 deletion syndrome
Infection of vertebrae	Marfan syndrome
Tumors of vertebrae	Osteogenesis imperfecta
Postthoracotomy	Achondroplasia
Hemivertebrae and other vertebral malformations	Aicardi syndrome
Klippel–Feil syndrome	Ehlers–Danlos
Postrhizotomy	

by the method of Cobb, and assigned a severity ranking by Risser or other scales. Curves of 10–30° are considered mild, and over 60° severe. Curves may be multiple. Periodic re-evaluation determines the rate of progression, and whether intervention is required.

Frequent use of radiographs in neonatal units will detect most cases of congenital scoliosis. Operative treatment is recommended prior to progressive development of deformity and secondary changes. Vertebral anomalies are the most common cause. Whether or not a localized vertebral anomaly is identified, 20–50% of cases of congenital scoliosis are associated with spinal cord abnormalities. In view of the high association of renal malformations with vertebral anomalies, renal ultrasonography is recommended whenever vertebral abnormalities are identified.

TREATMENT

Non-surgical

With progressive scoliosis, initiation of treatment typically begins at 20–25° of curvature. The type of treatment depends on age and skeletal maturity, degree and location of curve(s), underlying diagnosis and prognosis, general health, and parents' and child's wishes.

Exercise

Although stretching, other exercises and wheelchair positioning may alleviate some of the discomfort or pain caused by scoliosis, these measures do not halt the progression of the curvature. Exercise and sports are not contraindicated, and in most cases can be encouraged unless painful. Orthotics may need to be removed for sports.

Orthotics

In idiopathic scoliosis, bracing is sufficient to control moderate curves in skeletally immature patients. Several types of brace are available, many of which can be concealed under clothing. Braces worn 18–23 hr per day stabilize or improve curves in patients with curvatures of 25–45° in 70% or more of appropriate cases of idiopathic scoliosis. Braces must be worn until skeletal maturity or surgery. In neuromuscular scoliosis, the function and deformities of children may limit the use of commercially available devices; instead custom-molded polypropylene body jackets (Thoraco-Lumbo-Sacral Orthosis, TLSO) are used. In patients with impaired balance or strength, the use of a TLSO may improve sitting, balance, and upper extremity function.

Bracing has several disadvantages, however. Chief among these is discomfort : in many cases, the brace is restrictive and hot, even in the best of circumstances. Obesity may preclude use of a brace, reducing mobility and restricting pulmonary capacity. Skin breakdown, dermatitis, and infection can also occur. The brace may interfere with immediate access to vagus nerve stimulators, baclofen pumps, and venous catheters. The need for prolonged wearing times and concern over cosmetic appearance limit compliance. Social isolation and stigmatization may warrant counseling.

Surgical

The timing and type of surgery depend on the patient's age, rate of progression, skeletal maturity, symptoms, underlying diagnosis, degree and location of curvature, and cardiopulmonary function. In idiopathic scoliosis, curves that exceed 40–50° prior to the onset of skeletal maturity usually require surgery to prevent progression and to diminish spinal deformity. In neuromuscular scoliosis, surgery is highly dependent upon etiology and rate of progression. For example, because scoliosis is relentlessly progressive in most cases of Duchenne muscular dystrophy, surgery is recommended as soon as a progression of curvature can be established, generally at 20–30°. This generally occurs within 2–5 years of wheelchair dependence, so the recognition of the earliest stages of curvature warrants special prospective monitoring. An indication for surgical intervention for children with idiopathic scoliosis requires assessment of rate of progression and stage of skeletal maturation, since progression tends to cease at the time of epiphyseal closure. The intent is to correct operatively those with the worst curves while the degree of angulation is less severe. In contrast to idiopathic scoliosis, progression of curvature in children with scoliosis due to neuromuscular causes may continue beyond the time of skeletal maturity. Earlier operative intervention may be required if there is congenital onset, rapid progression of scoliosis or pelvic obliquity, or when progressive pulmonary dysfunction could increase surgical risk if delayed as in Duchenne muscular dystrophy.

Preoperative evaluation may include spinal imaging with MRI or CT myelography, and somatosensory evoked potentials. Screening for potential anesthetic risks with this long and difficult surgery with pulmonary, cardiologic, hematologic, and nutritional assessment may also be warranted. Preoperative MRI is especially important to assess whether non-orthopedic approaches, such as decompression of Chiari I malformation, might result in slowing of the rate of progression. The reduction of a tethered cord in myelomeningocele patients is unlikely to improve scoliosis, but documentation of this finding is helpful in postoperative care and prognosis. Identification of spinal cord anomalies including tumors, syringomyelia, diastematomyelia, or impingement upon the spinal canal will affect surgical approaches.

Patient and family education includes a discussion of risks and benefits of the surgery. Patients may have increased sitting or standing height, and improved self-esteem due to diminished deformity. Potential risks include anesthetic complications, bleeding, postoperative pain, pulmonary complications, infection, and even death. Morbidity and mortality are highest in neuromuscular cases. Because children in wheelchairs may have an increased sitting height, transportation needs may be altered by the procedure. Changes in body mechanics can impair the independent ability to perform many simple tasks such as arising from the floor, or important self-care activities such as feeding and personal hygiene.

If a neuromuscular diagnosis is suspected, it may be an opportune time to obtain a muscle biopsy. Preoperative consultation with a pediatric anesthesiologist is required for many muscle disorders, such as central core myopathy, where there is enhanced risk for malignant hyperthermia.

Operative Approaches

The choice of posterior fixation only, or posterior and anterior fixation combined, is a complex matter that includes assessment of the severity of curvature, number of segments over which the angulation occurs, level of skeletal maturity, and the degree of planned correction. Addition of an anterior approach with discectomy and bone grafts between vertebral bodies increases the potential correction, and removal of the growth plate can alter later growth as necessary. Anterior spinal fusion is, however, associated with greatly increased operative morbidity. Sometimes the surgery can be done in two stages to minimize complications associated with a long procedure with large fluid shifts. In some cases of a short segment severe curvature, anterior access can be accomplished with an endoscopic approach using minimally invasive instruments. An anterior approach to shorten the vertebral column by removal of the discs and portions of one or more vertebral bodies may be necessary in cases where significant lordosis is to be corrected. Without this intervention, there is a risk that excessive traction on the posterior elements can lead to ischemic changes in the spinal cord. In the earliest version of posterior spinal fusion, a "Harrington rod" was placed and secured at both ends; this procedure has been replaced by a variety of segmental procedures where wires or hooks are affixed to posterior elements of the spine at multiple locations. The advantage is substantial; with modern techniques the patients can be mobilized much sooner and usually do not require postoperative external fixation to achieve a good fusion.

In many centers, continuous intraoperative monitoring of the posterior columns with somatosensory evoked potentials, or the corticospinal tract with cortical evoked motor potentials, provides the surgeon with an ongoing assessment of spinal cord function.

A 50-year natural history study of untreated idiopathic scoliosis by Weinstein et al. concluded that the chief long-term problem is back pain and cosmetic. With more severe curves, however, and in patients with other neurologic impairments, the consequences of unrepaired scoliosis can be more significant, and include confinement to bed with persistent pain and potential for visceral complications. Whenever possible, careful positioning in wheelchairs equipped with three-point lateral trunk supports, molded backs, special seats and seat covers to minimize pressure points, and tilt-in-space options to relieve pressure are all of value. Pain management is fundamental.

SUMMARY

Idiopathic scoliosis can usually be successfully treated with bracing or surgical methods. Children with congenital or neuromuscular scoliosis are more challenging to treat because of associated medical, orthopedic, and neurological disorders. Surgeons and families may opt for conservative management with bracing, but ultimately surgical arthrodesis with instrumentation is often necessary. The ideal outcome requires both careful patient selection and preoperative evaluation.

SUGGESTED READINGS

1. Campbell's Operative Orthopaedics. 10th ed. Copyright © 2003 Mosby, Inc.
2. DeLee and Drez's Orthopaedic Sports Medicine, 2nd ed. Copyright 2003 Elsevier.
3. Weinstein SL, Dolan LA, Spratt KF, Peterson KK, Spoonamore MJ, Ponseti IV. Health and function of patients with untreated idiopathic scoliosis: a 50-year natural history study. JAMA 2003; 289:559–567.

6
Chiari Malformations

Jon Weingart
Johns Hopkins School of Medicine, Johns Hopkins Hospital, Baltimore, Maryland, U.S.A.

INTRODUCTION

Chiari malformations are hindbrain herniation syndromes that occur in children and adults. The classification scheme (i.e., Chiari I, II, III, and IV) describes the relationship of the posterior fossa contents to the foramen magnum (Table 1). This classification scheme does not imply a spectrum of increasing severity of the anatomical abnormality or the clinical significance (i.e., a Chiari I does not progress to a Chiari II). Chiari I and II are the only clinically relevant types.

Anatomically, Chiari I and II differ in the degree of herniation of the posterior fossa contents through the foramen magnum. In Chiari I, only the cerebellar tonsils are descended or herniated through the foramen magnum. The extent of tonsillar hernitaion can vary from a few millimeters to greater than a centimeter. The radiographic diagnosis uses tonsillar ectopia of greater than 3–5 mm below the foramen magnum as a diagnostic criterion. Recently, Milhorat has focused on the importance of a decrease in the CSF spaces surrounding the cerebellum and brainstem at the foramen magnum, suggesting that tonsillar descent of less than 3 mm may be clinically relevant in some patients.

In Chiari II malformations, the lower brainstem, inferior cerebellar hemispheres, cerebellar vermis, and cerebellar tonsils descend through the foramen magnum. Chiari II malformations are associated with myelomeningocele and spina bifida. For this reason, these patients often have associated hydrocephalus and/or tethered spinal cords that can exacerbate the symptoms related to the Chiari II

Table 1 Classification of Chiari Malformations

Type I	Displacement of cerebellar tonsils below foramen magnum
Type II	Displacement of the cerebellar vermis, fourth ventricle, and lower brainstem below foramen magnum
Type III	Displacement of cerebellum and brainstem into a high cervical meningocele
Type IV	Cerebellar hypoplasia

malformation and thus must be evaluated when considering the best treatment for a patient.

The clinical presentation of children with Chiari I or II malformations varies depending on the age of the child and the presence of other associated findings such as syringomyelia, hydrocephalus, or tethered cord. The treatment is symptom-driven; that is, asymptomatic patients, in general, do not need treatment.

CLINICAL PRESENTATION

The symptoms and signs are varied and age-dependent (Table 2) and secondary to cranial nerve dysfunction, cerebellar dysfunction, and/or spinal cord dysfunction usually secondary to a syrinx. A syrinx is a fluid filled cavity within the spinal cord that develops in the setting of a Chiari malformation secondary to the obstruction of CSF flow at the foramen magnum. Symptom complexes in individual patients may vary despite similar anatomy on the MRI.

The majority of children born with a myelomeningocele will also have a Chiari II malformation and hydrocephalus. In infants, the Chiari II malformation can be life threatening. Brainstem and cranial nerve dysfunction can produce apneic episodes and respiratory compromise, the former occurring in association with agitation. Children with Chiari II tend to be poor feeders and have weak cries. Examination reveals nystagmus, spasticity in the upper extremities, and fixed neck

Table 2 Clinical Signs and Symptoms in Children with Chiari Malformations

	Chiari I	Chiari II
Infant		Stridor Apnea-episodic Decreased gag reflex Aspiration Fixed neck extension (retrocollis) Weak cry Nystagmus Increased tone Upper extremity weakness
Childhood	Headache Neck pain Ataxia or balance problems Scoliosis	Headache Neck pain Nystagmus Increased tone Upper extremity weakness Aspiration GE reflux Decreased cough reflux
Adolescence		Headache Neck pain Ataxia or balance problems Scoliosis Suspended sensory loss (due to syrinx) Hand or arm atrophy

extension or retrocollis. These children often have other health problems and are failing to thrive, which can make evaluation difficult and the clinical picture confusing. Despite surgery in this patient group, many of these children continue with symptom progression and die due to progressive disease. It is essential to rule out hydrocephalus or shunt malfunction in a symptomatic infant as treatment of the hydrocephalus can reverse the clinical course.

After 1 year of age, the apnea spells are much less frequent. Although sequelae of cranial nerve dysfunction, such as aspiration or recurrent pneumonia, can be seen, motor symptoms become more common. These include an impact on motor development of the upper extremities and the appearance of spasticity. As the child gains language function, headache or neck pain become more common. The character of the headache is fairly consistent between Type I and II malformations and across ages. The location is occipital, suboccipital, and posterior neck. The pain can radiate to behind the eyes and is often described as a feeling of pressure. Exercise, straining, coughing, or any valsalva maneuver will bring on the pain, which tends to pass over a short period of time. Not uncommonly, parents note complaints of headache or pain during upper respiratory infection or asthma attacks. Since headaches in patients with Chiari malformations can occur in other locations on the head, one should not dismiss the diagnosis of this disorder just because the headache is atypical.

In middle and late childhood, the clinical presentation is very similar to adolescence. Pain, headache, and motor symptoms predominate. Motor symptoms include spasticity, weakness, and balance problems. Symptoms secondary to a syrinx begin to appear in this age group. These symptoms include sensory loss, hand and arm weakness, change in leg function, and extremity or torso pain that is often burning in character. The development of scoliosis can be due to formation of a syrinx.

The diagnostic test of choice is the MRI scan. The radiological evaluation should include at least the brain and cervical spine. In the Chiari II malformation, the whole spine should be imaged. Similarly, in a patient with scoliosis and a Chiari malformation, the entire spine should be imaged. The purpose of this extensive imaging evaluation is to evaluate for hydrocephalus, syrinx, tethered spinal cord, or other skull base anomalies associated with Chiari malformations. An additional helpful study is a cine-MRI that evaluates CSF flow across the foramen magnum. In patients with Chiari malformations, the reduced flow is found posterior to the cerebellum. The radiological evaluation is important because it helps guide the proposed treatment that may address associated findings rather than the Chiari malformation itself.

TREATMENT

The decision to treat, when to treat, and what to treat is very dependent on the severity of the symptoms and the clinical presentation. For patients in whom pain or headache is the only symptom, medical management is the first line of therapy (see Chapter 20 on headaches). In patients who fail medical management or who have loss of neurologic function, surgical management is indicated. Currently, there is no standard operative procedure. Accepted procedures range from a bony decompression only to a bony decompression with dural patch grafting, intradural dissection, and tonsillar manipulation.

The Asymptomatic Patient with Chiari I Malformation

With the wide use of MRI scanners, children will occasionally be diagnosed with Chiari malformation and syringomyelia before they have symptoms. In a 1998 survey of pediatric neurosurgeons, 81% of respondents favored observation with yearly neurological exams and MRI scans. It is not clear whether these children should restrict their activity. In the survey, a third of respondents would place activity restrictions, primarily avoidance of contact sports. If a follow-up MRI demonstrates progression of a syrinx, 61% of responding pediatric neurosurgeons would recommend surgical intervention.

Chiari II Malformation and Myelomeningocele

This group can be very challenging to manage due to the complexity of the myelomeningocele patient. As an infant, the symptoms of apnea and swallowing problems can be life threatening. Prior to decompressing the Chiari malformation, the child must be evaluated for hydrocephalus. If a shunt is already in place, the function of the shunt should be evaluated. The hydrocephalus should be treated first, as often this will result in symptom resolution and improvement in neurological function. In the absence of hydrocephalus, an infant with progressive symptoms and abnormal neurological function should undergo a posterior fossa decompression.

In childhood and adolescence, in addition to assessing for hydrocephalus, the lower spine should be imaged to rule out a tethered spinal cord. If a tethered cord is found, consideration of first untethering the spinal cord should be given. Patients can have improvement of their Chiari symptoms with cord untethering.

Chiari Malformation with Syrinx

Obstruction to CSF flow at the foramen magnum is the cause of syrinx development in the setting of a Chiari malformation. For symptomatic patients, posterior fossa decompression is the optimal surgical treatment. In the majority of patients, reestablishing CSF flow at the foramen magnum results in spontaneous collapse of the syrinx. The majority of syrinxes will collapse within a few weeks of posterior fossa decompression, though it can take longer. If the syrinx does not collapse, then surgical drainage of the syrinx is indicated.

Syrinx Without Chiari Malformation

This group of patients is included here because if a syrinx is diagnosed then a Chiari malformation should be looked for with a brain MRI. If tonsillar ectopia is not identified then surgical treatment should be aimed at the syrinx itself. Primary surgical treatment involves shunting the syrinx either into the subarachnoid or pleural space. One study described a group of patients with syringomyelia and no tonsillar ectopia who were treated successfully with posterior fossa decompression. He identified abnormalities in the posterior fossa anatomy on MRI scans and found intradural abnormalities at the foramen magnum at the time of surgery. Cine-flow MRI scanning might be helpful in this group of patients to try and identify an alteration in CSF flow at the foramen magnum. A measurable obstruction to CSF flow would support a posterior fossa decompression as the first surgical treatment.

OUTCOMES

The goal of surgical treatment is symptomatic improvement and stabilization or improvement in neurologic function. Unfortunately, prospective studies looking at outcomes after surgery do not exist. The majority of patients improve but the durability of that improvement is not well delineated in the literature. Symptom recurrence several years after surgery is reported as high as 40–45%. Nevertheless, the progressive nature of the symptoms in patients with Chiari malformations can significantly affect the patient's quality of life and surgical treatment should be offered to these patients.

SUGGESTED READINGS

1. Haroun RI, Guarnieri M, Meadows JJ, Kraut M, Carson BS. Current opinions for the treatment of syringomyelia and Chiari malformations: survey of the Pediatric Section of the American Association of Neurological Surgeons. Pediatr Neurosurg 2000; 33:311–317.
2. Iskander BJ, Hedlund GL, Grabb PA, Oakes WJ. The resolution of syringohydromyelia without hindbrain herniation after posterior fossa decompression. J Neurosurg 1998; 89:212–216.
3. Krieger MD, McComb JG, Levy ML. Toward a simpler surgical management of Chiari I malformation in a pediatric population. Pediatr Neurosurg 1999; 30:113–121.
4. Milhorat TH, Chow MW, Trinidad EM, Kula RW, Mandell M, Wolpert C, Speer MC. Chiari I malformation redefined: clinical and radiographic findings for 364 symptomatic patients. Neurosurgery 1999; 44:1005–1017.
5. Oldfield EH, Muraszko K, Shawker TH, Patronas NJ. Pathophysiology of syringomyelia associated with Chiari I malformation of the cerebellar tonsils. J Neurosurg 1994; 80:3–15.
6. Tubbs RS, Elton S, Grabb P, Dockery SE, Bartolucci AA, Oakes WJ. Analysis of the posterior fossa in children with the Chiari I malformation. Neurosurgery 2001; 48:1050–1055.
7. Weinberg JS, Freed DL, Sadock J, Handler M, Wisoff JH, Epstein FJ. Headache and Chiari I malformation in the pediatric population. Pediatr Neurosurg 1998; 29:14–181.

7
Status Epilepticus

Elizabeth A. Thiele
Harvard Medical School, Massachusetts General Hospital, Boston, Massachusetts, U.S.A.

INTRODUCTION

Status epilepticus (SE) is considered a medical emergency, and is defined by the International League Against Epilepsy (ILAE) as "an epileptic condition that occurs whenever a seizure persists for a sufficient length of time or is repeated frequently enough that recovery between attacks does not occur." The concept of how long a seizure lasts prior to being considered SE has changed over time, and continues to be controversial. Initial definitions, such as by Aicardi and Chevrie, suggested a duration of 1 hr; however, with increased understanding of the pathophysiology of seizures from animal models this time period has shortened. Many pediatric epileptologists now propose that 5–10 min of continued seizure activity be considered SE.

Status epilepticus can be associated with significant morbidity both in children and adults, and in children the mortality from SE has been reported to be as high as 10%. The prognosis of SE depends on etiology, age of the child, and duration of SE. Status epilepticus occurs commonly in all age groups, including children. In population-based studies, the incidence of SE in children has ranged from 10 to 41 per 100,000. Several studies have shown that SE is more common in younger children, with other risk factors including symptomatic etiology and partial seizures. In the United States, 70% of children under one year of age who are diagnosed with epilepsy initially present with status epilepticus. In children with epilepsy, approximately 20% have an episode of SE within 5 years of diagnosis. Five percent of children with febrile seizures present with SE.

ETIOLOGY

The classification of SE using the International Classification of Epileptic Seizures is based on seizure onset as either partial (focal) or generalized, and can occur with any seizure type (Table 1). The SE can be further classified by phenotype of the seizure (absence, myoclonic, tonic, clonic) and whether consciousness is preserved or impaired (simple vs. complex). The SE can also be classified by etiology including symptomatic (acute and remote), remote symptomatic with acute precipitant,

Table 1 Classification of Status Epilepticus

Generalized status epilepticus
Convulsive (tonic clonic)
Nonconvulsive (NCSE, absence, petit mal)
Partial status epilepticus
May be NCSE
Simple (no alteration of awareness)
Somatomotor—epilepsia partialis continuum
Complex (altered awareness)
Pseudo-status epilepticus
Pseudoseizures, psychogenic SE

progressive encephalopathy, cryptogenic, idiopathic, and febrile SE. Childhood SE is associated with a variety of etiologies (Table 2). The etiology of SE is an important determinant of outcome. In children, the most common etiology is infection with fever, which accounts for approximately 50% of pediatric SE.

Table 2 Etiologies of Status Epilepticus in Childhood

Neonates (first month of life)
Birth injury (anoxia, hemorrhage)
Infection
Congenital abnormalities
Inborn errors of metabolism
Amino acidurias
Lipidoses
Metabolic disorders
Hypoglycemia
Hypocalcemia
Hyponatremia
Early childhood ($<$ 6 years)
Birth injury
Febrile convulsions
Infection
Metabolic disorders
Trauma
Neurocutaneous syndromes
Neurodegenerative disorders
Tumors
Idiopathic
Children and adolescents
Birth injury
Trauma
Infection
Neurodegenerative disorders
Tumor
Toxins
Idiopathic
Epilepsy with inadequate drug levels

An episode of SE can be divided into four stages: (1) incipient (premonitory, prodromal), 0–5 min after seizure onset; (2) early stage, 5–30 min after seizure onset; (3) late (or established) stage, 30–60 min after seizure onset; (4) refractory stage, greater than 60 min. The concept of premonitory, prodromal, or incipient SE has been introduced to identify a situation that may lead to SE. Prehospital treatment with agents such as rectally administered diazepam can then be given to hopefully prevent progression into SE. The stages are used to help determine course of treatment, and are based in part by understanding the neurometabolic changes which occur during seizures leading to potential neuronal injury.

THERAPY

Initial Evaluation and Management

The initial evaluation of a child having ongoing seizure activity includes the assessment of the child's airway and ventilation; the initial management involves steps necessary to maintain these functions. The child's circulation should be assessed and intravenous access should be obtained. Vital signs and pulse oximetry should be closely followed. Available directed history of the seizure episode and the child's previous medical history should be obtained and the child examined. Blood glucose concentration should be checked with a dextrostick to allow rapid detection of hypoglycemia. Further diagnostic studies are selected as indicated based on the above information as well as child's age. Blood laboratory evaluation including electrolytes, calcium, magnesium, and phosphorous level may be helpful in determining cause, particularly in the setting of intercurrent illness or other cause of metabolic abnormality; complete blood count may reveal an elevated white blood cell count resulting from infection or the seizure activity itself. If the child is on anticonvulsant medications for an already recognized seizure disorder, drug levels should be determined, as low levels could be associated with increased seizure activity and SE.

Following stabilization of the child, additional history should be obtained, including course of current seizure activity (time and nature of onset, phenotypic characteristics including any focality), duration of seizure activity prior to medical attention, mental status after cessation of seizure activity; fever or intercurrent illness, prior history of seizures, head injury, intoxication or toxic exposure, CNS abnormality or illness, birth history and developmental delay, and other medical history. A rapid directed examination should be performed looking for signs of sepsis or meningitis, evidence of head or other CNS injury, and evidence of neurocutaneous syndromes. Further investigations should be considered if clinically indicated. Spinal fluid analysis should be performed if meningitis is suspected based on clinical presentation, history, and age. If there is a concern of increased intracranial pressure or a structural lesion that would contraindicate lumbar puncture, antibiotics should be administered and neuroimaging obtained prior to lumbar puncture.

Neuroimaging is generally indicated for SE after assuring the child is stable clinically, particularly if the child does not have a history of previous seizures or if the cause of SE is unknown. If readily available, MRI is a preferred imaging modality, but CT scan would allow detection of conditions needing urgent intervention such as hemorrhage, edema, or mass lesion. An EEG should be considered if there is any concern that the child may have ongoing seizure activity, either related to continued altered awareness or focality on examination, or if there is a concern of pseudoseizure. An EEG may also be necessary if neuromuscular paralysis is used in treatment of SE, or if suppressive therapy is required for refractory SE.

Pharmacologic Management of SE

Several medications have been shown to be effective in treating SE (Table 3). The ideal medication would be a drug that is safe and easily administered, acts rapidly, is effective for many hours, and produces minimal sedation. Unfortunately, many of the anticonvulsant medications currently used to treat SE can cause significant respiratory and cardiac suppression when given in doses recommended for SE; therefore, the child should continue to be closely monitored for airway patency, ventilation, and circulatory stability. Treatment should be initiated as soon as the patient is stabilized. Several protocols have been developed for the treatment of SE, and a practice parameter for pediatric SE is currently under development in the United States (Table 4).

Benzodiazepines

Diazepam. Due to high lipid solubility, diazepam rapidly enters the brain and has a prompt anticonvulsant effect. However, due to rapid tissue redistribution, it loses this effect in 20–30 min, and therefore another agent to maintain seizure control must follow it. Availability in a rectal formulation allows administration without IV access, which allows earlier treatment, even before medical assistance is available.

Lorazepam. Lorazepam is currently the medication of choice in the initial management of SE in both children and adults. Although lorazepam enters the brain slightly less rapidly than diazepam, due to a smaller volume of distribution it has longer-lasting anticonvulsant activity than diazepam. Lorazepam is less sedative than diazepam, and associated with less respiratory suppression.

Midazolam. Although it has a shorter half-life than other benzodiazepines, midazolam has an important role in the management of SE. If IV access is not available, midazolam can be given IM, where it is fairly well absorbed due to its water solubility in acidic solutions. At physiologic pH it then becomes lipid soluble, allowing fairly rapid penetration into the CNS. Due to a shorter half-life, midazolam

Table 3 Medications Used in Treating SE

	Loading dose		$T_{1/2}$ elimination
Lorazepam	0.1 mg/kg/dose	Repeat prn at 10–15 min intervals Maximum 4 mg/dose	16 hr
Diazepam	0.2–0.5 mg/kg/dose	Repeat q 15–30 min to maximum 10 mg	36 hr
Midazolam	0.05–0.2 mg/kg IV, 0.2 mg/kg IM or 0.15–0.2 mg/kg IV followed by continuous infusion of 1 mcg/kg/min	Repeat q 10–15 min to10 mg;	1.5–3.5 hr
Fosphenytoin	20 phenytoin equivalents/kg		20–50 hr
Valproate	15–20 mg/kg		6–16 hr
Phenobarbital	20 mg/kg		60–180 hr

Table 4 Pediatric Status Epilepticus Treatment Algorithm

Early stage (5–30 min after seizure onset)		
1. Assess airway, breathing, circulation (ABCs)		
2. Lorazepam	0.1 mg/kg IV	Maximum dose: 4 mg
OR (if no IV access)		
Midazolam	0.2 mg/kg IM	Maximum dose: 10 mg
Diazepam	0.5 mg/kg PR	Maximum dose: 20 mg
(if seizure does not stop in 5–10 min, repeat dose and begin Fosphenytoin)		
3. Fosphenytoin	20 mg PE (phenytoin equivalents)/kg IV or IM	
4. Phenobarbital	20 mg/kg IV	
Late, established SE (30–60 min after seizure onset)		
5. Maximize fosphenytoin	Give additional 10 mg PE/kg IV or IM	
6. Valproic acid	20–25 mg/kg IV	
7. Pyridoxine (B6)	200 mg IV	
Refractory stage (>60 min after seizure onset)		
Use one of the following:		
8. Midazolam	0.2 mg/kg IV followed by 0.02–0.4 mg/kg/hr	
9. Pentobarbital	2–10 mg/kg IV followed by 0.5–1 mg/kg/hr	
10. Propofol	1–2 mg/kg IV over 5 min followed by 2–3 mg/kg/hr	
11. Isoflurane	0.5–1.0% MAC	

(Adapted from JJ Riviello, with permission.)

is either given as repeated doses (or continuous infusion), or followed by another longer acting agent.

Fosphenytoin and Phenytoin

Fosphenytoin is a prodrug of phenytoin that is rapidly converted to phenytoin by blood and organ phosphatases. Its chemical properties allow it to be administered without the propylene glycol carrier required for phenytoin, which is responsible for many of the potentially severe side effects of IV phenytoin administration. Fosphenytoin (or phenytoin) begins to act 10–30 min after IV administration. Given in a loading dose, these drugs reach a therapeutic level fairly rapidly, without significant respiratory depression or sedation. Following resolution of SE, fosphenytoin treatment can be converted to oral phenytoin maintenance therapy.

Phenobarbital

Phenobarbital can be used for SE in all age groups, and continues to be the medication of choice for neonatal seizures. Since respiratory and CNS depression are common side effects, phenobarbital is typically used to treat SE only after benzodiazepines and phenytoin have failed.

Sodium Valproate

An intravenous formulation of sodium valproate (Depacon™) is now available and may be effective in the treatment of SE in children and adults. It can be given as a loading dose, with subsequent maintenance dosing, and is not significantly sedating.

Refractory Status Epilepticus

If SE continues for 30–60 min despite nominal treatment with anticonvulsants, it is then considered refractory SE. The child should receive further treatment in an intensive care unit setting, and airway should be protected and ventilation controlled via intubation. Aggressive pharmacologic therapy should be applied with the goal of immediately stopping SE. Options include high dose barbiturates (pentobarbital and phenobarbital), benzodiazepines (midazolam, lorazepam, and diazepam), as well as other IV anesthetic agents including thiopental, lidocaine, and inhalational anesthetics including isoflurane and propofol.

Pentobarbital has been the most widely used agent in refractory SE, usually titrated to suppression of EEG background. Midazolam is better tolerated and less sedating, although the frequency of breakthrough seizures may be higher. Careful EEG monitoring should be used, and drugs titrated until clinical and electrographic seizures are controlled. Maintenance drug therapy should be instituted prior to weaning aggressive therapy, in order to prevent seizure recurrence.

Prognosis

Status epilepticus can be associated with significant morbidity both in children and adults, and in children the mortality from SE has been reported as high as 10%. The prognosis of SE depends on etiology, type of SE, age of the child, and duration of SE. Generalized tonic clonic SE can be associated with morbidity including subsequent seizures as well as developmental deterioration; absence SE typically has few if any lasting sequelae. Outcomes of SE in childhood are better with either febrile or idiopathic SE than symptomatic SE.

SUGGESTED READINGS

1. Gaitanis J, Drislane FW. Status epilepticus: a review of different syndromes, their current evaluation, and treatment. Neurologist 2003; 9:61–76.
2. Riviello JJ. Pediatric status epilepticus. Seizure supplement. Ann Emer Med 2003; In press.
3. Shorvon S. Status Epilepticus: Its Clinical Features and Treatment in Children and Adults. Cambridge: Cambridge University Press, 1994.
4. Working Group on Status Epilepticus, Epilepsy Foundation of America. Treatment of convulsive status epilepticus. JAMA 1993; 270:854–859.

8

The Evaluation of a Child with a First Seizure

John M. Freeman
Pediatrics and Neurology, Johns Hopkins Hospital, Baltimore, Maryland, U.S.A.

INTRODUCTION

A seizure is a transient alteration in motor function, sensation, or consciousness due to an electrical discharge in the brain. "Seizure-like episodes" are terrifying to the families, frightening to medical personnel, and usually benign to the affected child. The most important aspect of management of a child with a first seizure-like episode is reassurance: *do not just do something, stand there and be reassuring*!

IMPORTANCE OF HISTORY IN DIAGNOSIS OF AN EPISODE

A child does not present with a first seizure, but rather with a first recognized "episode." It is the physician's duty to determine whether this first episode was an epileptic seizure or whether it was something else (Fig. 1). Since neither an EEG or a scan can diagnosis a seizure, the only way of making this differentiation is by a careful history. A careful history includes a description of:

1. *What happened during the event? Did she stiffen? Did she turn her head or eyes in one direction? To which side? Did she shake? On one side or both? Did the shaking start in the face? In the hand? In the leg? Somewhere else? Did it seem to start all over at the same time? How did it progress? How long did it last?*

Timing the observer's memory of the event from start to finish may provide a better estimate of the spell's duration than asking the observer to estimate the duration. Make the observer aware that the seizure ended at the termination of the shaking, not after the sleep-like postictal state that often follows a major seizure. Having the observer imitate the event often comes closer to what happened than asking for a verbal description. The onset of the spell is very important, but unfortunately the onset may not have been observed, or the observer may not be available or may be unreliable.

2. *Did he stare into space or jerk? If during the spell the child stared into space and looked blank rather than stiffening or shaking, how did he look? Did the staring*

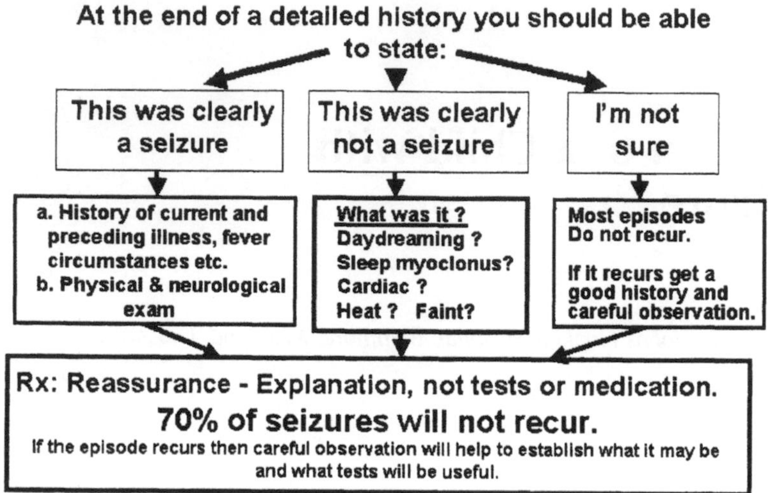

Figure 1 Evaluation of a first seizure.

start suddenly? In mid sentence? Was there a warning? Could you call her during the spell and would he respond? Could your touch elicit a response? Did this happen in school where he may have been daydreaming, or was he watching TV? Did he do anything else—did he smack his lips? Pick at his clothes? Wander about the room? Did he act confused? Has it happened before? Does it happen frequently, or only on rare occasions?

Absence seizures occur frequently (many a day) and the first one is rarely recognized, whereas partial complex seizures (temporal lobe seizures) occur less frequently, often last longer, and are often associated with automatisms such as lip smacking, picking at clothes, or aimless wandering.

3. *What was happening before the event? Was she sick? Did she have a fever? Was the episode part of an acute illness? Had this illness and fever been going on for several days or weeks? Does she have an underlying chronic illness or a progressive illness?*

What was occurring at the time of the event or before the event may be as important as what happened during the event. For example, the child who was having blood drawn, felt dizzy, was sweaty, lost consciousness, and then had a generalized seizure had what is termed "convulsive syncope." She had a seizure, but it was related to fainting and has very different implications, evaluation and management than the child who just had shaking out of the blue. These questions will help to resolve the time-line of the illness, and perhaps help to determine an etiology of the seizure, if there was an etiology. Most seizures are idiopathic (of unknown etiology). Fever itself may cause "febrile seizures," but fever and illness may also trigger the seizures of epilepsy.

4. *What happened after the event? Was the child arousable? Did the child sleep? Was he able to talk? Was his speaking clear or was it thick—like a drunken person? Did she have trouble finding the correct words? Did he have weakness on one side or in one part of the body (Todd's paralysis)? Postictal speech difficulties may help with lateralization of the seizure.*

5. *What was happening in the child's life around the time of the episode? Psychological factors in the child's school, family, or social life may lead to episodes that may appear to be seizures. Were there possible psychological factors that could have led to the event? Were there unusual family stress, divorce, or school problems? Are there other things, medical or psychological, which could precipitate an alteration in awareness or a change in motor function?*

At the end of this very detailed and careful history, the event should be classified as a definite seizure, a paroxysmal event that was not a seizure, or an event whose nature is uncertain.

A careful history can usually and reliably differentiate an "epileptic" seizure (i.e., a seizure due to an electric discharge from the brain) from other paroxysmal events even after only a single episode. Seizures themselves come in two forms: febrile and nonfebrile, in various forms.

Evaluation of First Seizures

Febrile Seizures

When a seizure has been diagnosed, the determination that it was a febrile seizure depends on the age of the child and the height and rapidity of rise of the fever. Febrile seizures occur in 2–5% of all children aged 6 months to 5 years of age. They can be very frightening, but are benign. They are rarely followed by nonfebrile seizures (epilepsy) and virtually never require extensive evaluation or therapy. After the seizure, the child will return to normal. The seizure may be a subtle, brief stiffening, or may be focal or generalized tonic–clonic jerking. They are rarely prolonged, but status epilepticus can occur. Several febrile seizures occurring on the same day, with fever, are considered a single febrile seizure and require the same evaluation and have the same prognosis.

The recommendations of the American Academy of Pediatrics (AAP) are summarized in Table 1. Again, the diagnosis of a febrile seizure always needs a good history. Assessment of its significance requires a good physical and neurological examination. Most children with a first febrile episode (or seizure) do not need to have blood work a CT scan, an MRI scan, or an EEG. Meningitis may present with a seizure. In children under 18 months of age, the signs of meningitis may be subtle and when the child has had prior antibiotics, the physician should consider the possibility of meningitis; otherwise, a lumbar puncture is unnecessary. Neither the AAP nor the author recommends continuous or intermittent anticonvulsant therapy after a febrile seizure.

Table 1 Evaluation of a First Febrile Seizure

	Sometimes	Usually	Always
History			X
Physical and neurological examination			X
Lumbar puncture	>18 months	12–18 months	<12 months
EEG	No		
Blood studies	No		
Imaging	No		
Counseling of parents			X

The most important therapy for a child after a first febrile seizure is counseling the distraught parents. The author tells parents that the outcome for the child is good, although febrile seizures may recur. The child will not die, swallow the tongue, or injure himself, nor will he suffer brain damage as a result of the seizure. Parents typically have many questions about this diagnosis, and time is needed to answer them. However, this discussion is difficult in the busy emergency room at a time when the parents are very upset. The private physician should repeat the counseling a few days later. Referring them to the author's book about seizures (written for parents) is often very helpful. The AAP's guidelines for the evaluation of febrile seizures are for neurologically healthy children between 6 months and 5 years of age who have had a single febrile seizure. The author recommends an identical evaluation for those children who have prior neurological impairment.

Nonfebrile Seizures

Nonfebrile seizures are also common in children and may be partial (simple or complex) or generalized—tonic, clonic, or both. The hallmark of nonfebrile seizures is an alteration of motor or sensory function or of awareness in a child who does not have a fever. However, fevers may trigger nonfebrile seizures by lowering the child's seizure threshold. Since the physician is unlikely to treat a child after either a first febrile seizure or a nonfebrile seizure triggered by fever, the distinction between the two after a first episode is neither possible nor important. Practice parameters have also been issued for the evaluation of nonfebrile seizures in children.

Evaluation after a First Nonfebrile Seizure

Recommendations for the evaluation of a child after a first nonfebrile seizure have recently been published by the Quality Standards Subcommittee of the American Academy of Neurology, the Child Neurology Society, and the American Epilepsy Society. These recommendations are summarized in Table 2. A careful history, physical and neurological examination should always be performed. As discussed above, a careful history can, with great reliability, differentiate a seizure from other paroxysmal events. Routine laboratory screening with blood counts, glucose, electrolytes, calcium, etc. are rarely useful and should be done only when the child's history or

Table 2 Evaluation of a First Nonfebrile Seizure

	Sometimes	Usually	Always
History			X
Physical and neurological examination			X
Lumbar puncture	Rarely		
EEG			Recommended by guidelines. But not by author
Blood studies	Based on history		
Imaging	Sometimes based on history	Unless emergency preferable	
Counseling of parents			X

clinical findings make the physician suspicious of an ongoing or underlying process. Toxicology should be done when there is suspicion of drug ingestion. A lumbar puncture is rarely useful. Magnetic resonance imaging (MRI) is always preferable to computerized axial tomography (CT scan). Although MRIs are more sensitive, they are rarely rapidly available or necessary after a first episode. If the child has a "high risk" condition such as recent trauma with other neurological findings, sickle cell disease, or a bleeding disorder or if a focal seizure occurred in a child less than 33 months of age, an emergent CT scan may be indicated.

The Subcommittee also recommends an EEG as part of the initial evaluation of a nonfebrile seizure "to determine the epilepsy syndrome, determine the need for imaging, and for predicting the prognosis." The author disagrees with this recommendation. He believes that these factors are unimportant after a first seizure since they do not reliably diagnose a syndrome nor predict prognosis. An EEG might be more useful if and when a seizure recurs.

Thus, the emergency room evaluation for both febrile seizures and nonfebrile seizures need only be minimal. There is little need for blood work, CT, or MRI scanning. The EEGs are not needed after a febrile seizure, and probably will not be helpful after a nonfebrile seizure. In every child a good history and physical as well as neurological examination are mandatory. The use of testing should be reserved for the unusual child with a suspicious history or physical examination. No anticonvulsant therapy is indicated after a febrile seizure. Usually none is indicated after a first nonfebrile seizure, either.

Management after a First Episode

Although the guidelines for the evaluation of febrile and nonfebrile seizure differ, there is general agreement that no medication is needed after the first seizure of either type. However, a discussion and explanation of what happened and its meaning are always needed to calm the parent's fears and misconceptions.

If it was a nonfebrile seizure, the parents should be reassured. Most first seizures will not recur with or without medication and this should be emphasized. The episode was likely to have been very frightening to the parents. Generalized tonic–clonic seizures are often associated with some tonic contractions of the chest and some cyanosis. Observers often believe that the child will swallow her tongue, die, or suffer brain damage because of the lack of oxygen. None of these statements are true, but the medical system must explain that truth to the panic-stricken parents at the time the child is first seen. All of this should be repeated when calmness prevails.

If the event clearly was not a seizure, reassure the parents. Explain to the parents what caused the episode. The parents were just as frightened as if it had been a seizure since they believed that it was a seizure and need just as much reassurance. Fainting has many causes, most benign. Daydreaming is readily recognized when appropriately considered. Sleep myoclonus is common but only occurs in sleep. The appropriate work-up should be done if necessary but the parents can be reassured, regardless of the nature of the event.

If the nature of the episode was unclear, reassure the parents. They will be relieved that the episode was a seizure or anything else serious. Tell them that if it occurs again it will be critical for them to carefully observe the circumstances and the order in which things happen. Assure them that if a similar episode recurs their child will recover just as he has after this episode and with a better history you can rethink the diagnosis. Most such episodes will not recur. The most important role of the physician managing a child and the family after a first seizure is to provide appropriate information about what seizures are and what they are not.

In particular, the following should be emphasized:

- Reassurance about swallowing the tongue, suffering hypoxic damage to the brain and dying should be given.
- Limitations on the activities of daily living, riding bikes, swimming are unreasonable even after a first seizure. In the majority of children, a second seizure will not occur.
- Testing is necessary only if there is something alarming about the child's history or the examination. If the child has a new neurological deficit, recent substantial head trauma with loss of consciousness or if there is evidence of progressive loss of motor or cognitive function, then the physician should consider if further testing would be helpful.

What if the initial impression is incorrect and the event really was a seizure? Diagnosing epilepsy at the time of the first seizure is not necessarily a benefit to the parent or the child, since early treatment does not prevent further seizures or alter the long-term course. Most progressive diseases will progress and result in further seizures. Neither diagnosing them early nor missing them until they are more clearly present will have much impact on the child's outcome or life. There will be ample time to use medication. Reassurance is the best treatment for initial seizures.

SUGGESTED READINGS

1. Freeman JM. Letter to editor. Neurology 2001; 56:574.
2. Freeman JM. Less testing is needed in the emergency room after a first afebrile seizure. Pediatrics 2003; 111:194–196.
3. Freeman JM, Vining EPG, Pillas DJ. Seizures and Epilepsy in Childhood: A Guide. 3rd ed. Baltimore: Johns Hopkins Press, 2002.
4. Hirtz D, Ashwal S, Berg A, Bettis D, Camfield C, Camfield P, Crumrine P, Elterman R, Schneider S, and Shinnar S. Practice parameter: evaluating a first non-febrile seizure in children. Report of the Quality Standards Subcommittee of the American Academy of Neurology, The Child Neurology Society, and the American Epilepsy Society. Neurology 2000; 55:616–623.
5. Sharma S, Riviello JJ, Harper MB, Baskin MN. The role of emergent neuroimaging in children with new-onset afebrile seizures. Pediatrics 2003; 111:1–5.
6. Stroink H, van Donselaar CA, Geerts, AT, Peters AC, Brouwer OF, Arts WF. The accuracy of the diagnoses of paroxysmal events in children. Neurology. 2003; Mar 25;60(6):979–982.
7. Provisional Committee on Quality Improvement, Subcommittee on Febrile Seizures. Practice guideline: the neurodiagnostic evaluation of the child with a first simple febrile seizure. Pediatrics 1996; 97(5):769–775.
8. Provisional Committee on Quality Improvement, Subcommittee on Febrile Seizures. Practice parameter: long-term treatment of the child with simple febrile seizures. Pediatrics 1999; 103(6):1307–1309.

9
Neonatal Seizures

Ann M. Bergin
Childrens Hospital, Department of Neurology, Boston, Massachusetts, U.S.A.

INTRODUCTION

Neonatal seizures may be the first sign of cerebral dysfunction in the newborn, and may alert the clinician to the presence of an underlying neurological injury, and/or possibly reversible systemic disorder. These symptomatic seizures represent the majority of seizures in the neonate, although epileptic syndromes, both benign and "malignant" may also present at this age. The precise incidence of neonatal seizures is unknown and estimates vary depending on a number of factors, including the retrospective or prospective nature of the data reported, the definition used to define a neonatal seizure, and the source of diagnostic information. Estimates range from 1.8/1000 live births up to 5.1/1000 live births.

Developmental immaturity influences many aspects of diagnosis, management, and prognosis of seizures in the newborn. For instance, clinical seizure patterns in the neonate reflect the "reduced connectivity" in the neonatal brain—with prominence of focal ictal characteristics, and rarity of generalized patterns of clinical seizures. Many physiological processes are immature, leading to altered drug handling compared to older children, and the immature brain may be more susceptible to developmental effects of anticonvulsant medications.

CLINICAL FEATURES

Careful observation of the clinical characteristics of paroxysmal movements in the newborn allows differentiation of more or less concerning patterns. Among the many repetitive, rhythmic, and jerky movements made by normal newborns, those movements and behaviors provoked by stimulation, and/or eliminated by passive flexion or soothing touch are unlikely to represent seizures. Generalized tonic–clonic seizures are rare in infants. Certain patterns of movement are more likely to be accompanied by electrographic seizure. These include: (1) focal clonic movements, which may occur unilaterally, sequentially in different limbs, or simultaneously but asynchronously; (2) focal tonic movements, such as a sustained limb posture, or tonic horizontal eye deviation (generalized tonic movements are generally not accompanied by seizure on EEG); (3) generalized, but not focal or multifocal myoclonic events; (4) autonomic events such as apnea, often with associated tachycardia rather than bradycardia (particularly in term newborns), and/or pupillary dilatation. Many newborns may have more than one seizure type. Other movements commonly seen in the encephalopathic newborn, such as "bicycling" or "boxing" movements and oromotor movements are not consistently accompanied by electrographic seizure. Whether these movement patterns are associated with electrographic discharges in deep structures remains controversial. They are generally not treated with anticonvulsant medications.

The diagnosis of seizure in the newborn depends on informed observation for suggestive events and the identification of accompanying electrographic seizure. Once the presence of electrographic seizure has been identified, underlying etiologies, particularly reversible causes must be sought. The details of the clinical history are most important in directing the initial evaluation. For instance, a history of traumatic delivery, with good Apgar scores in a term infant raises the possibility of intracranial hemorrhage. The age at onset of seizure may suggest likely etiologies. Hypoxic–ischemic encephalopathy (HIE), which is the single most common cause of neonatal seizures, usually causes seizures within the first 24 hr of life. When seizures present after the first 48 hr of life, and particularly after a period of initial well being, infection and biochemical disorders should be considered. Seizures occurring later (e.g., >10 days of life) are more likely to be related to disorders of calcium metabolism (rare now in the United States), malformation, or neonatal epilepsy syndromes, which may be benign (e.g., benign familial neonatal seizures) or severe [e.g., early infantile epileptic encephalopathy (EIEE)]. Multiple possible etiologies may be identified in a neonate with seizures (Table 1), such as HIE with hypoglycemia, hypocalcemia, or intracranial hemorrhage, and each must be treated appropriately.

Evaluation should include EEG and neuroimaging. The EEG can provide direct confirmation that suspicious clinical events represent electroclinical seizures if the event is captured during EEG recording. In the event that the suspicious event does not occur during a brief recording, the presence of epileptiform features and/or focal abnormalities supports the diagnosis of neonatal seizure. The goal of neuroimaging is the identification of intracranial hemorrhage, focal or distributed parenchymal injury, or structural developmental abnormalities. Cranial ultrasound can be performed at the bedside and is effective in identifying intraventricular and many parenchymal hemorrhages, but has limitations in its ability to detect focal infarcts, developmental abnormalities, and convexity hemorrhages. CT or MRI yields more information but usually require skilled transportation from the neonatal intensive care unit to the radiology suite, and may need to be deferred, at least initially, until the infant is stabilized.

THERAPY

Treatment of the newborn with seizures involves general supportive measures, management of any underlying disorder, and often requires treatment with anticonvulsant medication. Seizures themselves and treatment with anticonvulsant medication may impair respiratory drive and the ability to maintain adequate circulation. Therefore, supportive management to ensure maintenance of adequate ventilation and perfusion is imperative. Further discussion of this important area is beyond the scope of this chapter, and the reader is referred to other sources on general neonatal medical management. Apart from recommendations for acute

Table 1 Neonatal Seizures: Etiologies to Consider

Vascular and perfusion abnormalities
Hypoxic–ischemic injury
Stroke
Sinovenous thrombosis
Intracranial hemorrhage
Intraventricular
Parenchymal
Subdural
Subarachnoid
CNS infection
Malformations and other structural lesions
Neuronal migration disorders
Cerebral dysgenesis
Neurocutaneous disorders, e.g., Sturge–Weber syndrome, tuberous sclerosis
Acute metabolic disorders
Hypoglycemia
Hypocalcemia
Hypomagnesemia
Inborn errors of metabolism
Aminoacidopathies
Organic acidurias
Peroxisomal diseases
Mitochondrial disorders
Epilepsy syndromes
Benign familial syndromes
Severe neonatal epileptic encephalopathies
Pyridoxine (B6)-dependent seizures

treatment of the most common acute reversible metabolic abnormalities such as hypoglycemia and hypocalcemia (Table 2), the management of specific underlying disorders will not be addressed.

The decision to treat neonatal seizures with anticonvulsant drugs depends on the risk of acute seizure-related respiratory or cardiac decompensation in a critically ill newborn, as well as the potential for long-term seizure-related neurological injury balanced against the potential adverse effects of anticonvulsant medications. Some newborns may not need treatment with anticonvulsant medication, for instance, those with seizures due to reversible and appropriately treated metabolic derangements, or those with rare, short-lived events. However, in considering a decision not to treat, it is important to recognize that a significant proportion of newborns with electroclinical seizures have additional clinically silent electrographic seizures.

Table 2 Initial Management of Acute Metabolic Disorders

Hypoglycemia	10–15% dextrose, 2–3 mL/kg IV
Hypocalcemia	5% calcium gluconate, 2 mL/kg IV
Hypomagnesemia	2–3% magnesium sulfate, 2 mg/kg IV

This is particularly likely in premature infants and those with severe encephalopathy. Prolonged EEG monitoring is helpful in identifying the presence of unsuspected electrographic seizures. The importance of these subclinical events in the genesis of seizure-related neuronal injury is unknown at present. In the setting of severe neonatal encephalopathy, these events may be prolonged and refractory to treatment, and efforts to eliminate them may be limited by systemic vulnerability to the circulatory effects of anticonvulsant medications.

A number of factors alter the pharmacokinetics of the anticonvulsant drugs in neonates. Physiological immaturity delays drug elimination, and asphyxial injury to the liver and kidney may further delay metabolism. Maturation of the various pathways involved in drug metabolism occurs at variable rates over the first weeks of life, and recovery from perinatal injury improves hepatic and renal function. Overall, there is a dramatic increase in the ability to eliminate the commonly used anticonvulsant drugs, so that changes in dosing are required to maintain therapeutic drug levels over the first weeks of life.

When anticonvulsant treatment is indicated, phenobarbital is the drug most commonly used as first-line therapy. Other first-line options include benzodiazepines (diazepam, lorazepam), and phenytoin or, if available, its prodrug fosphenytoin. There have been few studies comparing the efficacy of these drugs in the treatment of neonatal seizures. Painter et al. compared treatment with phenobarbital and phenytoin and found no difference in efficacy between the two drugs, with fewer than 50% of infants achieving control with either drug. Typical initial doses of the first-line drugs are provided in Table 3, and additional discussion of the individual drugs is given below.

Phenobarbital: Phenobarbital affects $GABA_A$ receptors to enhance GABA-related inhibition. It may also inhibit excitatory amino acid transmission and block voltage-activated calcium currents. It is a weak acid, with low lipid solubility. Phenobarbital is subject to protein binding, and it is the unbound (free), unionized fraction that is active. Alterations in acid–base balance in the newborn may impact efficacy of the drug for this reason. Phenobarbital is metabolized in the liver and excreted by the kidney. Its half-life is long, from 100 to 300 hr, or longer in premature infants, but declines to 100 hr or less over the first weeks of life. An initial intravenous (IV) loading dose of 20 mg/kg may be followed by increments of 5–10 g/kg IV to a total of 40 g/kg, with higher doses associated with improved efficacy. Careful monitoring of cardiac and respiratory function may be required in vulnerable infants.

Table 3 Anticonvulsant Drug Doses for Initial Management of Neonatal Seizures

Drug	Initial dose	Maintenance
Phenobarbital	20 mg/kg IV. Consider further 5–10 mg/kg increments to a total of 40 mg/kg	Check drug levels—may not need further doses for many days. 3–4 mg/kg/day
Phenytoin	20 mg/kg IV. Fosphenytoin: 20 mg PE/kg IV (see text)	3–4 mg/kg/day divided bid to qid
Benzodiazepines	Lorazepam: 0.05–0.1 mg/kg IV. Diazepam: 0.3 mg/kg IV	

Phenytoin/Fosphenytoin: Phenytoin acts by blockade of voltage-dependent sodium channels, probably by binding to inactivated channels and stabilizing the inactive state. This decreases the tendency of neurons to high frequency, repetitive firing and therefore their excitability. Phenytoin is a weak acid and is poorly soluble in water. High lipid solubility results in rapid entry to the brain, but it is quickly redistributed and levels decline, requiring continued administration to restore brain levels. It is protein bound, though to a lesser degree in newborns than in older children and adults. Phenytoin is metabolized in the liver and eliminated in the kidney. Its half-life varies with concentration, increasing with higher concentrations due to decreased clearance as levels increase. An intravenous loading dose of 20 mg/kg of phenytoin administered at no greater than 1 mg/kg/min (to avoid cardiac arrhythmia and hypotension) is followed by a maintenance dose of 2–3 mg/kg/day IV divided between 2 and 4 doses. Fosphenytoin is a prodrug of phenytoin. Its advantages are its higher water solubility and lower pH, which, in addition to the lack of toxic vehicles required for its formulation, reduce local irritation of skin and blood vessels at the site of infusion. Fosphenytoin is converted to phenytoin by plasma phosphatase enzymes in neonates as in adults. Dosing is in "phenytoin equivalents" (PE), i.e., a loading dose of fosphenytoin is 20 mg PE/kg IV.

Benzodiazepines: Diazepam and lorazepam, like other benzodiazepines, bind to the postsynaptic $GABA_A$ receptor to enhance GABA-activated inhibitory chloride currents. At high levels, benzodiazepines may also influence voltage-gated sodium channels and calcium channels. Benzodiazepines are lipid soluble. Differential lipid solubility confers some advantage on lorazepam, which is less lipid-soluble and therefore is not redistributed away from the brain as rapidly as is diazepam. Benzodiazepines are metabolized in the liver, and the majority of the drug is excreted in the urine. The plasma half-life of both lorazepam and diazepam is approximately 30 hr, and may be longer in premature and/or asphyxiated newborns. Onset of action is within minutes for both drugs, however, duration of action is longer for lorazepam (up to 24 hr). Diazepam may be more effective as a continuous infusion. Lorazepam is given IV at a dose of 0.05–0.1 mg/kg. Diazepam dose is 0.3 mg/kg IV. An infusion rate of 0.3 mg/kg/hr IV has been described. Benzodiazepines are usually used as second- or third-line agents in neonatal seizures, but may also be used as an initial treatment for their earlier onset of action, in anticipation of the effect of a concurrent dose of phenobarbital.

Other Anticonvulsants: Upward of 90% of neonatal seizures will be controlled by the combined use of the above anticonvulsant medications. Many other drugs have been used in an attempt to control refractory cases. Support for their use is based on reports of efficacy in small, uncontrolled series.

Midazolam is a short-acting benzodiazepine that has been used as a continuous IV infusion (0.1–0.4 mg/kg/hr) after an initial loading dose (0.15 mg/kg).

Lidocaine has been used, mostly in Europe, as an IV infusion of 4 mg/kg/hr with decreasing doses over 4–5 days. This drug has a narrow therapeutic range, and may induce seizures at higher levels.

Paraldehyde (no longer available in the United States) has been used as an IV bolus of 400 mg, followed by a further bolus of 200 mg. This drug is excreted by the lung and is used with caution in pulmonary disease. Paraldehyde can dissolve plastic tubing, which should therefore be avoided when administering this agent.

Orally administered anticonvulsants that have been used adjunctively include *carbamazepine* (10 mg/kg initially, followed by 15–20 mg/kg/day), *primidone* (loading dose 15–25 mg/kg followed by 12–20 mg/kg/day), and *valproic acid* (3 of 6 neonates developed hyperammonemia). Of the new anticonvulsants, there is a case report of a single newborn with refractory seizures of unknown etiology that responded to the introduction of *lamotrigine* (4.4 mg/kg/day).

Medications Other than Anticonvulsants

Pyridoxine: A trial of pyridoxine (100 mg IV) should be considered in refractory neonatal seizures without a history of perinatal complications, particularly if there is excessive discontinuity for age in the background EEG activity. A history of rhythmic intrauterine movements, or a family history of another child with refractory epilepsy should also raise the possibility of pyridoxine-dependent seizures.

Folinic Acid: Rare cases of refractory neonatal seizures have been associated with an unknown biochemical marker in the CSF on high-pressure liquid chromatography assays. These cases have responded to oral supplementation of folinic acid. A dose of 2.5 mg bid has been effective in newborns.

Treatment with anticonvulsant medication is often associated with resolution of clinical seizures. However, it is increasingly clear that electrographic seizures may continue, without clinical correlate, after anticonvulsant medication is initiated in a substantial subgroup of newborns (estimates vary from 30% to 80%). Continuous or serial EEG recordings to detect ongoing electrographic seizures should be strongly considered.

No guidelines exist as to appropriate duration of anticonvulsant treatment for newborns with seizures. There is a trend toward shorter therapy, taking into account the short-lived nature of precipitating causes, the recovery from acute hypoxic–ischemic encephalopathy in many instances, and the possible detrimental effect of anticonvulsants on the immature brain. A single dose of phenobarbital may result in therapeutic levels persisting over a number of days. Additional doses may not be needed in the above instances, if seizures do not recur. Newborns with persistent, difficult to control seizures, persistently abnormal EEG, and/or persistently abnormal neurological examination should be considered for longer-term treatment following discharge from hospital.

PROGNOSIS

The underlying etiology and severity of brain injury at the time of seizures is the best predictor of long-term prognosis, emphasizing the importance of full and accurate diagnosis. Mortality associated with neonatal seizures has declined with improvements in perinatal and neonatal care, and is 20% or less. Morbidity rates have changed less, partly due to increased numbers of survivors among ill premature newborns, who have a greater risk of neurological sequelae. Overall, the risk of abnormal neurological outcome (motor and/or cognitive abnormality) is approximately 25–35%. The likelihood of postneonatal epilepsy is 15–20%. Besides etiology, the presence, severity and persistence of abnormality of the EEG background activity may be helpful in predicting abnormal outcome.

The role of neonatal seizures themselves in generating brain injury and long-term sequelae remains controversial, as is the role of clinically silent electrographic seizures. The immature brain appears to be more resistant to seizure-related excitotoxicity than the mature brain. However, subtle alterations in connectivity and cell number in the immature brain exposed to neonatal seizures may predispose to later seizure-related injury.

SUMMARY

Neonatal seizures are an important marker of neonatal brain injury, and may themselves contribute to long-term neurological sequelae. The goals of clinical management include, correct identification of suspicious clinical events, EEG confirmation, immediate supportive therapy and correction of reversible precipitating conditions, and accurate diagnosis of the underlying etiology. Anticonvulsant therapy is appropriate in many, but not necessarily all cases, and decisions regarding initiation and duration of such therapy should be individualized. Results of ongoing in vivo, in vitro and clinical research will hopefully clarify the differential roles of various etiologies and seizures themselves, as well as offering new opportunities and approaches for neuroprotection in these vulnerable infants. Early in vivo studies suggest that topiramate, one of the new anticonvulsant agents, may hold promise of neuroprotection and/or antiepileptogenic effect in immature rats.

SUGGESTED READINGS

1. Holmes GL, Lombroso CT. Prognostic value of background patterns in the neonatal EEG. J. Clin. Neurophysiol. 1993; 10:323–352.
2. Koh S, Jensen FE. Topiramate blocks perinatal hypoxia-induced seizures in rat pups. Ann Neurol 2001; 50:366–372.
3. Lombroso CT. Neonatal seizures: a clinician's overview. Brain Develop. 1996; 18:1–28.
4. Mizrahi EM, Kellaway P. Characterization and classification of neonatal seizures. Neurology 1987; 37:1837–1844.
5. Mizrahi EM, Kellaway P. Diagnosis and Management of Neonatal Seizures. Lippincott Raven, 1998.
6. Mizrahi EM, Watanabe K. Symptomatic neonatal seizures. In: Roger J, Bureau M, Dravet Ch, Genton P, Tassinari CA, Wolf P, eds. Epileptic Syndromes in Infancy, Childhood and Adolescence. 3rd ed. John Libbey, 2002:15–31.
7. Scher MS. Neonatal seizures and brain damage. Pediatr Neurol 2003; 29:381–390.
8. Volpe JJ. Neonatal seizures. Neurology of the Newborn. 4th ed. Philadelphia: WB Saunders, 2001:178–214.

10
Absence Seizures

Edwin C. Myer
VCU Health System, Department of Neurology, Richmond, Virginia, U.S.A.

INTRODUCTION

Absence seizures usually occur in children and on occasion may not be recognized because of their association with a typically normal neurological and cognitive examination. Various types of absence seizures occur including typical childhood absence seizures, juvenile absences, and atypical absence seizures. In most cases, the seizures are of abrupt onset and patients are neurologically and intellectually normal. In atypical absences, however, neurological impairment may occur. In the past, these seizure types were diagnosed under the heading of "petit mal" which is still unfortunately used at times and usually describes all seizures without a clear convulsion. The etiology of absence epilepsy is unclear, but may involve abnormal oscillatory rhythms in the $GABA_B$ and T-type calcium channels of the thalamus.

DIAGNOSIS

Childhood absence seizure onset is generally between 5 and 10 years and can frequently occur as a staring spell, loss of awareness, or unconsciousness interpreted by observers as daydreaming (Table 1). The most typical presentation is a blank expression or stare for up to several seconds. Absence seizures can be sometimes misdiagnosed as attention deficit disorder syndrome since these events are frequent and usually noticed by the teacher. Seizures can occur multiple times during the day. Some mild tonic movements such as eye blinking and automatisms (semipurposeful behaviors) with involuntary movements can be seen. Autonomic symptoms such as pupil dilatation, flushing, incontinence, and diaphoresis can occur. Ninety percent of children outgrow their absences within 2–5 years, often at puberty.

Juvenile absence epilepsy presents typically at an older age (age 7–16) and generalized tonic–clonic seizures are frequently the presenting symptom, as opposed to childhood absence in which the larger convulsions are rare. The absence seizures usually are not daily but can occur in clusters. Automatism components with involuntary movements and visual hallucinations occur similarly to childhood absence. Prognosis is usually favorable, although seizures may be lifelong.

Table 1 Comparison of Childhood Absence, Juvenile Absence, and Juvenile Myoclonic Epilepsy

	Childhood	Juvenile
Age of onset	5–10 Years	Puberty
Frequency	Multiple daily	Rarely daily
EEG epileptiform activity	3 Hz spike-wave	3.5–4 Hz spike-wave
Medications	Ethosuximide, valproate, lamotrigine	Valproate, ethosuximide, lamotrigine, topiramate
Therapy length	Short[a]	Short or prolonged
Genetic	8	3.5
Prognosis	Favorable	Favorable

[a] Generally short duration of treatment would be 2 years seizure free. Specific duration of treatment is variable; average age of cessation is 10.6 years.

A typical absences can occur associated with Lennox Gastaut Syndrome. Other seizure types such as myoclonic, tonic, and generalized tonic–clonic are frequent. Myoclonic astatic epilepsy may also be a feature. Seizures are typically much more difficult to control, and may be resistant to anticonvulsants.

EVALUATION

In suspected typical childhood absences, hyperventilation will help and provoke the absences in the office setting. The classic EEG pattern is generalized 3 Hz spike and slow-wave complexes (Fig. 1) with an otherwise normal background, slowing to

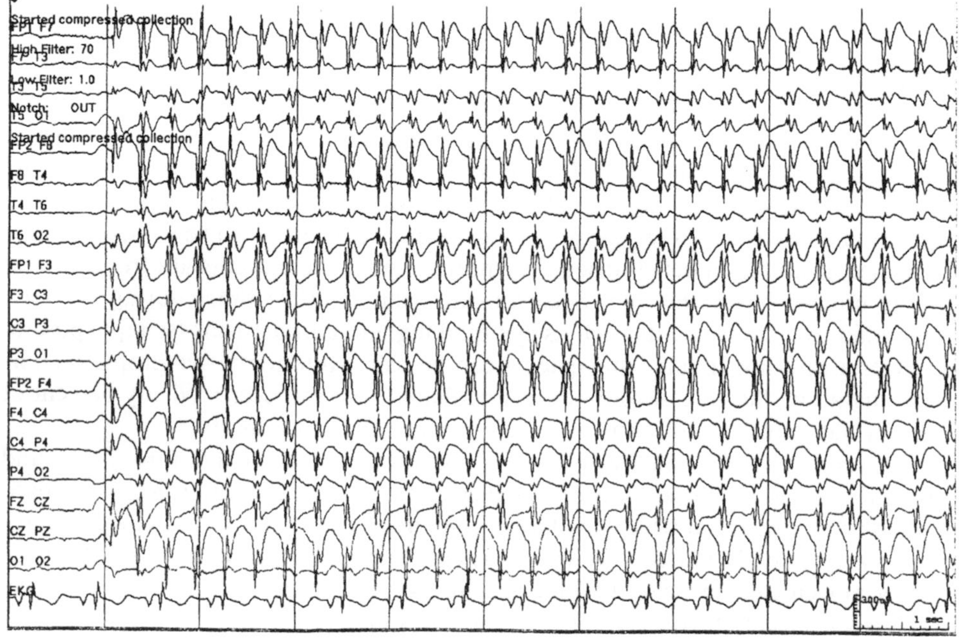

Figure 1 EEG in typical absence epilepsy.

2–2.5 Hz at the end of the abrupt-onset burst. On occasions some slowing can occur, but intermittent delta with sharp activity is rare. Clinically, during a several second burst of 3 Hz spike-wave discharges, the child will typically have a brief alteration in consciousness.

In juvenile absence epilepsy, the EEG will show mild background slowing with occipital intermittent rhythmic delta activity. Spike-wave activity is usually somewhat faster at 3.5–4.0 Hz. In atypical absences, the delta activity is slower at 1.5–2.5 Hz with background slowing and interictal multifocal spikes and sharp waves.

TREATMENT

Because of the recurrent seizures (of which many are not noticed by family or teachers), in the majority of children of school age, treatment is usually beneficial and outweighs risks of anticonvulsants. In juvenile absence epilepsy, the risk of generalized tonic–clonic seizures often influences strongly the decision to treat. Making the correct diagnosis early can be invaluable as several medications such as carbamazepine, gabapentin, vigabatrin, and tiagabine can make absence epilepsy significantly worse if attempted.

First-line medications for absence seizures are either ethosuximide (Zarontin™) or valproic acid (Depakote™), with an approximately 70% chance of either seizure freedom or a dramatic reduction. Ethosuximide is initiated in doses of 10–20 mg/kg/day but may be increased to 30 mg/kg/day as needed. Ethosuximide is a T-type calcium channel blocker available since 1960. This agent is available in 250 mg pills and 250 mg/5 cm^3 suspension. Although the half-life of ethosuximide is prolonged, due to possible nausea and gastrointestinal upset, a divided dose twice per day is suggested. Other rare side effects include lupus erythematous, rash and Steven Johnson Syndrome, thyroiditis, and aplastic anemia (recurrent blood work is indicated).

Valproic acid (Depakote™ or Depakene™) may be a better choice for juvenile absence epilepsy due to its protective effects against generalized tonic–clonic seizures (not typically seen with childhood absence). Valproic acid is started at 5–10 mg/kg/day, divided twice to three times per day, increasing weekly to 20–30 mg/kg/day. It is available as 125, 250, and 500 mg tablets (including 250 and 500 mg extended release formulations), 125 mg sprinkle capsules, and 250 mg/5 cm^3 syrup. Blood levels as high as 130 mg/dL are well tolerated and may be necessary for seizure control. Dose-related side effects include rare hepatic dysfunction, thrombocytopenia pancreatic involvement, and bone marrow suppression. These rare side effects can be life threatening and repeated blood work is necessary. Common side effects include weight gain, hair thinning, and tremor. The combination of ethosuximide and valproic acid may be beneficial.

Other medication options do exist should ethosuximide and valproic acid prove unsuccessful. Clonazepam (Klonopin™) can be helpful, started at 0.03 mg/kg increasing to 0.1–0.3 mg/kg/day, given twice a day. It is available only as tablets (0.5, 1, and 2 mg). Side effects are mostly sedation, mood changes, and dependence.

Newer medications have also been successfully used including lamotrigine, topiramate, and zonisamide. Lamotrigine (Lamictal™) is started at a low dose 1–2 mg/kg/day (or lower when used in combination with valproic acid) and increased very slowly every 1–2 weeks to as high as 15–20 mg/kg/day. Lamotrigine is available as 25, 100, 150, and 200 mg tablets, and 5 and 25 mg chewable–dispersible tablets. Side effects include a rash and Steven Johnson Syndrome, but seem to be lower with slow titration. When weight gain is a concern, lamotrigine may be a reasonable alternative to valproic acid.

Topiramate (Topamax^{TM}) has also been reported successful. Normal initial starting doses (1 mg/kg/day divided twice a day) and increasing slowly to a maximum of 10 mg/kg/day are the format we prefer. It is available as 25, 50, and 100 mg tablets, and 15 and 25 mg sprinkle capsules. Side effects of topiramate include kidney stones (1.5%), ataxia, cognitive slowing at high doses and particularly in polypharmacy, oligohydrosis, and hyperthermia.

Zonisamide (Zonegran^{TM}) was approved in the United States in 2000 and also has some beneficial effects on absence epilepsy. Zonisamide also works on t-type calcium channels, similarly to ethosuximide. Doses typically begin at 2 mg/kg/day, /day, increasing to 5–10 mg/kg/day, dosed once a day (due to a long half-life). At this time, zonisamide is only available as a 100 mg capsule, which limits its use in children. The capsule can be opened into 30 cm^3 of water or juice and mixed together. Side effects include kidney stones (3–4%), rash, oligohydrosis, and rarely behavioral changes.

Patients with typical childhood absence epilepsy can be treated for until approximately 2 years seizure-free with a normal EEG. At that point, discontinuation of medicines can be attempted. Most patients will have a remission rate of 8%. Juvenile epilepsy has a remission rate that is lower and deciding on withdrawing anticonvulsants may be a more difficult decision. In atypical absences, treatment will probably require lifelong therapy not just for control of these particular seizures but the other seizure types.

SUGGESTED READINGS

1. Engel J. Seizures and Epilepsy. F. A. Davis Company, 1989.
2. Levy R, Mattson RH, Meldrum BS, eds. Antiepileptic Drugs 4th ed. Raven Press, 1995.
3. Mattson RH. Idiopathic Generalized Epilepsies. Epilepsia Vol. 44, Supplement 2, 2003.
4. Rojer J, Bureau M, Dravel C, Dreifuss FE, Perret A, Wolf P, eds. Epileptic Syndromes in Infancy, Childhood, and Adolescence. 2nd ed. John Libbey, 1992.
5. Wyllie E, ed. The Treatment of Epilepsy: Principles and Practice. 3rd ed. Lea & Febiger.

11
Febrile Seizures

Shlomo Shinnar
Departments of Neurology, Pediatrics, and Comprehensive Epilepsy Management Center, Montefiore Medical Center, Albert Einstein College of Medicine, Bronx, New York, U.S.A.

INTRODUCTION

Febrile seizures are the most common form of childhood seizures. Febrile seizures are defined as by the International League Against Epilepsy as a "seizure occurring in childhood after the age of one month, associated with a febrile illness not caused by an infection of the central nervous system, without previous neonatal seizures or a previous unprovoked seizure, and not meeting the criteria for other symptomatic seizures." This is similar to the definition adopted by the National Institutes of Health Consensus Conference in 1980, except that the lower age limit has been moved from 3 to 1 month of age. While they are most common between 6 months and 5 years of age, they can occur in younger and somewhat older children. Note that the definition does not require the child to be febrile at the time of the seizure, although the event must be in the context of a febrile illness.

Febrile seizures are further divided into simple and complex. Simple febrile seizures are relatively brief (< 10–15 min), generalized seizures without recurrence within the same febrile illness. A febrile seizure is considered complex if it is prolonged (≥ 10 or ≥ 15 min in different studies), focal, or multiple within the same illness. The issue of whether a child is neurologically normal or not does not enter into the definition. Complex features are relatively common and occur in a quarter to a third of febrile seizures.

In North America and Western Europe, approximately 2–5% of all children will experience a febrile seizure by age 7. In Japan, however, 9–10% of all children experience at least one febrile seizure. Interestingly, there is no increased risk of epilepsy in Japan compared with North America and Western Europe attesting to the generally benign nature of febrile seizures. In all these countries, despite differences in the risk of having a febrile seizure, the peak incidence of febrile seizure onset is between 18 and 22 months, and the majority of cases occur between 6 months and 3 years of age.

Factors that predispose a child to have a febrile seizure during the first few years of life include a family history of febrile seizures in a first or second degree relative, attendance at day care, developmental delay, and a neonatal nursery stay of

> 30 days. While children with one or more of these factors are at increased risk of having febrile seizures, more than half the cases occur in children with no known risk factors.

Clearly, not every 18 month old with a febrile illness experiences a seizure. The most important factors associated with an increased risk of having a seizure during a febrile illness are the peak temperature (as distinct from the temperature at the time of the seizure), and a family history of febrile seizures in a first or second degree relative. The nature of the illness was also relevant. Children with gastroenteritis are less likely to experience a febrile seizure than are children with otitis media or an upper respiratory tract infection.

DIAGNOSTIC EVALUATION

The diagnostic evaluation of a child who presents with a seizure in the context of a febrile illness is primarily aimed at excluding other types of acute symptomatic seizures. The major concern is to exclude infection as the cause. Between 2% and 5% of children who present with seizures and fever will turn out to have meningitis rather than a febrile seizure. Risk factors for meningitis include focal or prolonged seizures, suspicious findings on neurological or physical examination, and a visit for medical care within the previous few days. Lumbar puncture is therefore recommended in all children with a complex febrile seizure, particularly a prolonged or focal one.

In 1996, the American Academy of Pediatrics issued guidelines for the evaluation of a child with simple febrile seizures between age 6 months and 5 years. It recommended that a lumbar puncture should be strongly considered in an infant less than 12 months of age. Since the signs of meningitis may be subtle in the 12–18 month age group, a careful assessment is mandatory. A lumbar puncture is not necessary in a child above 18 months of age if the history and physical examination are not suspicious for meningitis. In children older than age 5, one must also consider a lumbar puncture to exclude encephalitis, as febrile seizures in this age group are relatively uncommon. It is important to realize that "having a source" for the fever is not a useful criterion in the decision about whether to do a lumbar puncture. The most common source of an otitis media would be *Streptococcus pneumo* or *Hemophilus flu*, which are also the most common organisms involved in meningitis. The clinical appearance of the child is most important.

While commonly done, in the absence of suspicious history (e.g., vomiting or diarrhea) or abnormal physical examination findings, routine serum electrolytes, glucose, calcium, phosphorus, magnesium, and a complete blood count are of limited value in the evaluation of a child with febrile seizures above 6 months of age. In younger children, more detailed laboratory investigations may be helpful in selected cases.

More sophisticated neurodiagnostic studies such as the electroencephalogram (EEG) and neuroimaging studies, while very useful in the diagnostic evaluation of children with afebrile seizures, are of very limited value in the evaluation of febrile seizures. EEG abnormalities are relatively common, particularly in older children with febrile seizures, and are not useful in guiding therapy, as they do not predict either febrile seizure recurrence or development of epilepsy. This is true for both simple and complex febrile seizures with the exception of status epilepticus.

Neuroimaging studies are also of limited usefulness in evaluation of the child with a seizure and fever. They are not needed prior to performing a lumbar puncture in children. Neuroimaging studies are primarily used when it is unclear if the child had a febrile seizure, especially when the neurological examination is worrisome. In cases of febrile status epilepticus (seizures lasting longer than 30 min) neuroimaging is usually indicated as part of the evaluation of status epilepticus. An MRI within a few days of the episode of febrile status epilepticus is being used to identify whether or not hippocampal damage has occurred in the research setting, but at the moment there is insufficient data to use the results to guide clinical care.

While genetic factors are important, there are no specific tests beyond taking a good family history. The known genetic mutations are mostly in sodium channels and account for less than one percent of cases. While this is a rapidly evolving field, formal genetic testing is not part of the routine clinical evaluation of children who exclusively have febrile seizures at this time.

THERAPY

The approach to the treatment of febrile seizures has changed over the last few decades. These changes have been driven by three factors. First, the recognition that the vast majority of febrile seizures are benign has occurred. Second, there has been an increasing recognition that chronic therapy with antiepileptic drug (AED) therapy is associated with a variety of cognitive and behavioral side effects. Lastly, we have realized that chronic and intermittent AED therapy, while effective to some degree in preventing recurrent febrile seizures, do not alter the risk of subsequent epilepsy. For this reason, especially in children with simple febrile seizures, reassurance and counseling rather than drugs are the preferred treatment options. In this section, we will first review the available treatment options and then present an approach to the management of the child with both simple and complex febrile seizures (Table 1).

Chronic prophylaxis with phenobarbital or valproate will reduce the risk of recurrent febrile seizures. However, it does not reduce the risk of subsequent epilepsy and is associated with significant morbidity and is therefore no longer recommended. Carbamazepine and phenytoin are ineffective in preventing further febrile seizures. There are insufficient data on any of the newer antiepileptic drugs to justify their use in this setting at the present time.

Intermittent treatment with benzodiazepines given orally or rectally at time of fever reduces the risk of recurrent febrile seizures. It must be given every time the

Table 1 Treatment of the Child with Simple and Complex Febrile Seizures

Chronic AEDs (phenobarbital and valproate)
Not indicated
Diazepam (oral or rectal) at the time of fever
Not routine for simple febrile seizures
Consider for complex or multiple simple febrile seizures
Rectal diazepam at the time of seizure
First-line therapy for prolonged febrile seizures
Rapid, simple, safe, and effective

child has an intercurrent illness, which can become an issue given the frequency of febrile illnesses in early childhood. There is also the theoretical concern about sedation masking signs of more serious illness such as meningitis. Even when effective, it does not reduce the risk of subsequent epilepsy. Furthermore, children who have a seizure as the first manifestation of their febrile illness are both at higher risk to have another one and least likely to benefit. This treatment does have a limited role in selected cases with frequent recurrences.

Antipyretics at time of illness are commonly prescribed. Data from controlled clinical trials suggest that this treatment is no more effective than placebo in preventing recurrence. While antipyretics are generally benign and may make the child more comfortable, recommendations for their use should recognize their relative lack of efficacy and avoid creating undue anxiety and guilt feelings in the parents.

Abortive therapy with rectal diazepam (dose based on weight) at the time of seizure does not alter the risk of recurrence but is effective in preventing prolonged febrile seizures, which are often the main concern. It is provided as 2.5, 5, 10, and 20 mg rectal gel formulations and in packages of two. Children with prolonged febrile seizures are good candidates for this form of therapy. Rectal diazepam can also be used in cases with a high risk of recurrence, for families who live far away from medical care and for families where the parents are very anxious. In these cases it avoids the need for chronic or intermittent therapy unless a seizure actually occurs and lasts more than 5 min.

No treatment. In many cases, particularly those with simple febrile seizures, reassurance and education about the benign nature of the condition are all that is needed. The American Academy of Pediatrics 1999 practice parameter recommends no treatment for children with simple febrile seizures.

The specific treatment option chosen depends on the goals of therapy and specific features individual to each case. For simple febrile seizures, the American Academy of Pediatrics recommends no treatment except reassurance; a recommendation the author fully agrees with. In parents who live far away from medical care or who are particularly anxious, a prescription for rectal diazepam may be appropriate and further minimize anxiety and risk. There is less consensus on the treatment of complex febrile seizures. However, even in this setting, chronic AED therapy is very, very rarely appropriate. For children with complex febrile seizures, current therapeutic options include no treatment, which is appropriate in many cases, intermittent diazepam at the time of fever, and rectal diazepam should a seizure occur and last longer than 5 min.

As treatment does not alter long-term outcome and only very prolonged febrile seizures have been causally associated with subsequent epilepsy, a rational goal of treatment would be to prevent prolonged febrile seizures. Therefore, when treatment is indicated, particularly in those at risk for prolonged or multiple febrile seizures or those who live far away from medical care, rectal diazepam used as an abortive agent at the time of seizure would seem the most logical therapeutic option.

The above discussion assumes the child is not actively convulsing at the time of decision making which will be true in the vast majority of cases. If a child arrives in the emergency department in the midst of a seizure, they should be treated using the current pediatric status epilepticus protocol, which is covered in Chapter ___. A child who is in the emergency department for the evaluation of an illness and starts seizing should be managed more conservatively and only needs emergency treatment if the seizure persists beyond 5 min.

PROGNOSIS

Morbidity and Mortality. The morbidity and mortality associated with febrile seizures is extremely low, even in the case of febrile status epilepticus. Several large series of febrile status epilepticus reported no deaths and no new neurological deficits following febrile status. Three different studies have found no differences in IQ scores, academic achievement, and behavioral measures between children with febrile seizures and either sibling or population-based controls. These favorable cognitive and behavioral outcomes included children with both simple and complex febrile seizures as well as children with febrile status epilepticus.

Recurrent Febrile Seizures. Approximately one-third of children who have a febrile seizure will have at least one recurrence. Risk factors for recurrent febrile seizures are summarized in Table 2. Children with two or more risk factors have a 30% recurrence risk at 2 years; those with three or more risk factors have a 60% recurrence rate. Half of all recurrences are within the first 6 months and 90% occur within 2 years. A complex febrile seizure is not associated with an increased risk of recurrence in most studies. However, complex features tend to persist if recurrences occur. In particular, children who have a prolonged initial febrile seizure and have a recurrence are likely to have a prolonged recurrent seizure as well. Conversely, the child whose initial febrile seizure is simple in nature and has a second febrile seizure, the chances it will be prolonged are small. Thus, we can reliably identify at the time of the first febrile seizure those children at risk for prolonged recurrences who would be candidates for abortive therapy.

Epilepsy and Febrile Seizures. If followed for many years, eventually between 2% and 10% of children with febrile seizures of all types will develop epilepsy. The risk of developing epilepsy after a single febrile seizure is not substantially different than that in the general population. With the possible exception of very prolonged febrile seizures, the relationship between febrile seizures and subsequent epilepsy does not appear to be causal. Rather, children with an underlying predisposition to seizures are more likely to also experience a febrile seizure when in the appropriate age window.

Risk factors for epilepsy following febrile seizures are summarized in Table 2. Of these, neurodevelopmental abnormality and a family history of epilepsy are risk factors for epilepsy whether or not there is a history of febrile seizures. It is important to note that, a short duration of recognized fever prior to seizure onset is associated with not just a higher risk of subsequent febrile seizures but of epilepsy. This is the only risk factor that is the same when comparing risk factors for recurrent febrile seizures and for subsequent epilepsy.

Table 2 Risk Factors for Febrile Seizures and Epilepsy

Febrile seizures	Epilepsy
Young age of onset	Neurodevelopmental abnormality
Family history of febrile seizures	Family history of epilepsy
Low temperature at occurrence	Complex febrile seizures
Short duration of fever	Short duration of fever
	Number of febrile seizures

Febrile Seizures and Mesial Temporal Sclerosis. This a very controversial topic. Retrospective studies from adult epilepsy surgery programs report that many patients with mesial temporal sclerosis (MTS) and intractable temporal lobe epilepsy have a history of febrile seizures in childhood. Prospective studies have failed to find this association. Recent studies utilizing imaging within 72 hr of the event may provide the answer to this seeming contradiction. These studies suggest that very prolonged febrile seizures lasting more than 60 min may cause acute hippocampal damage that in some cases will evolve to MTS. Febrile status epilepticus lasting 30 min accounts for approximately 5% of febrile seizures, and seizures lasting 60 min or more are 2%. Thus, even large prospective studies are unlikely to have the power to detect this phenomenon. Conversely, it is unlikely to account for the majority of cases of MTS. A multicenter prospective imaging study of children with very prolonged febrile seizures is currently underway to attempt and answer this vexing question. In the meantime, the available data support prevention of prolonged febrile seizures as a rational treatment approach.

CONCLUSIONS

In summary, febrile seizures are the most common seizure type and have a mostly benign prognosis. Both human and animal data demonstrate that brief febrile seizures are benign and not associated with long-term sequelae. Treatment is usually not needed for either simple or complex febrile seizures. Given our current state of knowledge, a rational plan of treatment focuses on counseling and on preventing prolonged febrile convulsions. Prolonged febrile convulsions are the only ones that have been causally implicated with adverse outcomes.

While the data are reassuring, the clinician needs to recognize that febrile seizures are a very frightening event. Parents need to be reassured that the child will not die during a seizure, a fear that seems to be widespread. They also need to be provided information about the prognosis and management of febrile seizures.

SUGGESTED READINGS

1. American Academy of Pediatrics. Provisional Committee on Quality Improvement. Practice parameter: the neurodiagnostic evaluation of the child with a simple febrile seizure. Pediatrics 1996; 97:769–775.
2. American Academy of Pediatrics, Committee on Quality Improvement, Subcommittee on Febrile Seizures. Practice parameter: long-term treatment of the child with simple febrile seizures. Pediatrics 1999; 103:1307–1309.
3. Baram TZ, Shinnar S, eds. Febrile Seizures, San Diego CA: Academic Press, 2002.
4. Berg AT, Shinnar S, Darefsky AS, Holford TR, Shapin ED, Salomon ME, Gain EF, House WA. Predictors of recurrent febrile seizures. Arch Ped Adolesc Med 1997; 151:371–378.
5. Knudsen FU. Febrile seizures: treatment and prognosis. Epilepsia 2000; 41:2–9.
6. Verity CM, Greenwood R, Golding J. Long-term intellectual and behavioral outcomes of children with febrile convulsions. N Engl J Med 1998; 338:1723–1728.
7. Shinnar S, Glauser TA. Febrile seizures. J Child Neurol 2002; 17:S44–S52.
8. Shinnar S. Febrile seizures and mesial temporal sclerosis. Epilepsy Curr 2003; 3:115–118.

12
Lennox–Gastaut Syndrome

Adeline Vanderver and William Davis Gaillard
Department of Neurology, Children's National Medical Center, Washington, D.C., U.S.A.

INTRODUCTION

Defined by Gastaut in 1966, but first recognized in 1939 by Lennox, Lennox–Gastaut syndrome (LGS) has attracted considerable interest in the last half century. Responsible for less than 5% of childhood epilepsies, this catastrophic epilepsy consists of a typical triad of intractable seizures (tonic axial, atonic, myoclonic, and atypical absence), characteristic EEG abnormalities (bursts of slow spike and wave during the awake state and 10 Hz—fast rhythms with bursts of slow polyspikes during sleep state), and cognitive delay. Its disabling course and refractory nature give it an importance out of proportion to its incidence. Its often-cryptogenic nature is a continuing enigma.

DIAGNOSIS

The diagnosis of LGS is clinical and rests on a constellation of clinical characteristics and electrographic findings.

Characteristic Seizures

Children with LGS have multiple seizure types, and their epilepsy is medically intractable with high frequency of seizures. The onset is in childhood, typically between 1 and 8 years with greatest frequency between 3 and 5 years. Seizures most commonly include tonic axial seizures, often nocturnal during non-REM sleep and associated with autonomic phenomena. Frequently described seizures include atonic and tonic seizures resulting in drop attacks, and prolonged atypical absence with automatisms sometimes accompanied by generalized seizures. Complex partial seizures may occur. Other seizure types may occur and predominate, such as in the myoclonic variant, or evolve, such as the increased frequency of generalized tonic–clonic convulsions in adolescence.

Seizures are exacerbated by inactivity and drowsiness. Seizures usually occur multiple times a day, are usually brief but may be repetitive or prolonged. Tonic or atypical absence status may occur frequently in some patients. Frequent falls because of repeated seizures are disabling in many children with LGS and may result in injury.

Characteristic EEG Findings

Electroencephalographic tracings are not diagnostic, as in some epilepsy syndromes, but are characteristic of the diagnosis. The background is abnormal, with lower than age appropriate frequency of the posterior basic rhythm and intrusion of slow activity generally. During wakefulness, generalized, bisynchronous slow spike-and-wave and polyspike-and-wave discharges (1–2.5 Hz) are seen, maximal over anterior head regions. These may occur in bursts or as near continuous activity, and are most often irregular in frequency, distribution, and amplitude. This pattern may be asymmetric and intermixed with bursts of faster activity. Hyperventilation may increase the frequency of slow spike-and-wave discharges, but photic stimulation produces no paroxysmal activation. During sleep, bursts of generalized fast spikes are seen at 10 Hz or more, maximal in non-REM sleep, and are the electrographic correlate of nocturnal tonic seizures. They may obscure normal sleep architecture and, while not the pattern of electrographic status epilepticus of sleep (ESES), may occupy up to 50% of the recording. Generalized spikes, and in some patients multifocal spikes, can be seen throughout the recording. Early on, these EEG abnormalities are often not seen but may evolve. This may make the diagnosis initially unclear.

Neuropsychologic Disturbances

Mental retardation is almost universal in LGS, with fewer than 10% of patients preserving near-normal intellectual functioning. Children may appear normal or near normal at onset with an abrupt deterioration following the onset of uncontrolled seizures, or may have a preceding encephalopathy, including infantile spasms. Overall, cognition progressively deteriorates, compounded by repeated trauma from falls and the effects of multiple anticonvulsants. Behavior problems abound and include autistic spectrum disorders, aggressiveness, and hyperactivity.

EVALUATION—ETIOLOGY

The differentiation of LGS from other catastrophic onset childhood epilepsies is important for prognosis and management. The seizure pattern may not appear characteristic initially and suggestive EEG patterns may not appear for several months. Therefore, it is not unreasonable to pursue diagnostic testing that may be suggested by the individual's presentation—for example, that of progressive myoclonic epilepsy in a patient in whom the initial presentation includes myoclonic seizures. Very few patients with LGS, however, have documented abnormalities of metabolism. There are rare cases ascribed to Leigh encephalomyelopathy. Other metabolic diseases are exceptional. Concerns that LGS may be related to a developmental channelopathy or be an immune-mediated process have yet to be substantiated.

In some series, 17–30% of patients with LGS have a history of infantile spasms. Therefore, central nervous system insults known to predispose to infantile spasms have been implicated in the pathogenesis of LGS. These include congenital infections, sequela of neonatal hypoglycemia, hypoxic–ischemic encephalopathy, and traumatic brain injury.

Structural abnormalities are the most common underlying etiology of symptomatic LGS. Rarely, brain tumors have been known to cause LGS, although this raises the difficulty of differentiating true LGS from secondary bilateral synchrony. Tuberous sclerosis or other neurocutaneous syndromes are found in children with LGS, but not as frequently as in association with infantile spasms. Developmental brain malformations are the most common structural lesion to be reported in LGS, especially subcortical band heterotopia, bilateral perisylvian syndrome, and focal cortical malformations. It is therefore important to perform magnetic resonance imaging when considering the diagnosis of LGS, as there are reported cases of seizure reduction with focal surgical resection of lesions. Other types of neuroimaging, including PET and SPECT scans, have not been uniformly helpful and are currently better research than diagnostic tools. The majority of cases of LGS remain cryptogenic despite extensive metabolic evaluation and neuroimaging. Evaluation aimed at maximizing supportive care, such as neuropsychological assessment to identify baseline neurodevelopmental state and aid in appropriate educational placement are also important.

It is helpful to differentiate LGS from other seizure syndromes, especially from myoclonic astatic epilepsy (Doose syndrome), that may have a more favorable prognosis. Children with myoclonic astatic epilepsy have the occurrence of multiple types of generalized seizures suggestive of LGS (i.e., atonic–astatic seizures, myoclonic seizures, atypical absences, generalized tonic clonic) and an EEG pattern sometimes reminiscent of LGS with interictal slow spike-and-wave discharges. However, it is always idiopathic, axial tonic seizures are rare or absent, onset is younger than in LGS (typically between 18 months and 4 years), EEG demonstrates photosensitivity, and there is a strong genetic predisposition. Prognosis for seizure control and developmental outcome is more benign than in LGS. Similarly, an entity named atypical benign partial epilepsy of childhood occurs in children between 2 and 6 years, with prominent nocturnal partial seizures, myoclonic, and atonic seizures without tonic seizures. Electroencephalogram is remarkable for diffuse slow spike and wave in sleep and 3-Hz spike wave in the waking record. Seizures remit in late childhood in most patients and developmental regression is limited. Other seizure types that may be mistaken for LGS include frontal lobe epilepsy and multifocal epilepsy with rapid propagation.

TREATMENT

The therapy of LGS is disappointing, complicated by the variety of seizure types and the occasional worsening of seizure control and cognitive functioning with polypharmacotherapy. Carbamazepine and phenytoin may exacerbate atypical absence and atonic seizures. Phenobarbital, in causing drowsiness, may worsen seizure frequency.

Until the introduction of the more recent antiepileptic drugs (AEDs), valproic acid was regarded as the mainstay of treatment of LGS. Valproic acid is still often regarded as a drug of choice because of its broad spectrum of activity; however, seizure control is achieved in only 10–30% of patients.

Lamotrigine is used in this patient population. In a double-blind placebo-controlled study, lamotrigine resulted in a decrease in seizure frequency of $> 50\%$ in 33% of patients vs. 16% of patients on placebo. Multiple other studies suggest similar efficacy in children with refractory epilepsy, especially for drop seizures. The risk of rash, especially in interaction with valproic acid, a frequently used anticonvulsant in this population, warrants careful titration as doses are increased.

Felbamate is used successfully in this patient population. Early reports on the use of felbamate in LGS suggested a response with seizure reduction of >50% in 50% of children with LGS. Also, more recent studies in which a subgroup of patients had the diagnosis of LGS, suggest that felbamate continues to be efficacious in 41% of children with refractory epilepsy after 3 years of follow-up. There is also some suggestion that add-on felbamate therapy may decrease the seizure frequency by increasing levels of valproic acid. Although felbamate and lamotrigine are both efficacious, especially for injury causing drop attacks, both are associated with serious idiosyncratic or hypersensitivity reactions leading to interest in newer anticonvulsants.

Topiramate has a broad spectrum of action and few therapy-limiting adverse events. An initial double-blind randomized study revealed a decrease in seizure frequency of >50% in 33% of children with target doses of approximately 6 mg/kg/day vs. 8% in controls. A follow-up open label study after adjustment of mean anticonvulsant doses to 10 mg/kg/day demonstrated a reduction in seizures of ≥50% in 43–45% of patients and drop attacks were decreased by ≥50% in 55–57% of patients. Another multicenter study found seizure reduction of >50% in 40% of patients with a mean dose of 4.1 mg/kg/day. A more recent open, multicenter study, however, recorded a response rate as defined above of only 25%, although this is discrepant with other reports of topiramate efficacy as add-on therapy in LGS.

These three anticonvulsant agents have been shown to decrease seizure frequency including drop attacks by about half in as much as one-half of children when used as adjunctive agents. Because seizures remain intractable, other options are often considered. Less well-documented therapies include zonisamide. A small subgroup of patients with LGS in a study of zonisamide as an adjunctive agent in pediatric epilepsy had a "response" of 25–50%, although effectiveness is not clearly defined. Levetiracetam is also used, although there is limited data regarding efficacy.

Benzodiazepines, especially clobazam and nitrazepam, are used with some success. A small study recently suggested that nitrazepam may be at least as efficacious as other anticonvulsant drugs, decreasing seizure frequency by ~50% in more than 60% of patients. Use of these drugs is limited by the development of tolerance and physiologic dependence. The ketogenic diet has also been used with some success in many centers although there are no well-documented studies of this therapy specifically for LGS.

Surgical options have been explored. Prospective studies show a modest reduction in seizure frequency after vagal nerve stimulator implantation. This therapy may be helpful in limiting drop attacks and therefore may lead to improvement in quality of life. Corpus callosotomy has also been used to reduce tonic seizures that result in injury secondary to falling, with some moderate success. Both these measures are palliative. The recognition of episodes of nonconvulsive status, which may occur frequently in these patients, is important. The use of steroids in this situation has been occasionally used when more conventional therapies have failed.

Very few patients have complete seizure control and none of these therapies appears to have altered the progress of intellectual decline. Anticonvulsant management should aim to minimize polypharmacotherapy and accumulated toxicity. When possible, AEDs should be limited to one or two agents (unless switching medications where the child would be on three AEDs during transition). Treatment of LGS has therefore remained inherently frustrating for both physicians and families.

PROGNOSIS

Prognosis in children with LGS is defined mainly by neurodevelopmental outcome and refractory seizures. An underlying etiology, when discovered, also determines prognosis. Other important considerations, such as the mortality due to status epilepticus, are not particular to this seizure syndrome. Seizure types evolve as the child matures, most typically into more complex partial, and generalized tonic–clonic seizures, although the nocturnal seizures persist into adolescence. Mental retardation and behavior disorders persist in a static fashion, although greater demands on an older child or changes in polypharmacotherapy may occasionally make the encephalopathy appear progressive.

In a retrospective analysis of prognosis in children meeting criteria for LGS, the long-term intellectual and neurological outcome was poor. Over the course of an average follow-up period of 16 years, 38% of the patients lost the ability to speak, 21% were nonambulatory and 96% had ongoing seizures. Four independent risk factors for severe mental retardation were identified by multivariate analysis: nonconvulsive status epilepticus; a previous diagnosis of West syndrome; a symptomatic etiology of epilepsy; and an early age at onset of epilepsy. Patients with LGS and their families continue to bear the burden of a debilitating epileptic encephalopathy.

SUMMARY

Lennox–Gastaut syndrome is a clinically defined epileptic encephalopathy of childhood characterized by multiple seizure types, which remain refractory to medical and surgical intervention, suggestive electroencephalogram patterns, and significant mental retardation.

SUGGESTED READINGS

1. Beaumoir A, Blume W. The Lennox Gastaut Syndrome. In: Roger J, Genton P, Bureau M, Tassinari CA, Dravet Ch, Wolf P. eds Epileptic Syndromes in Infancy, Childhood and Adolescence. 3d ed. UK: John Libbey Ltd., 2002:113–135.
2. Cilio MR, Kartashov AI, Vigevano F. The long term use of felbamate in children with severe refractory epilepsy. Epilepsy Res 2001; 47(1–2):1–7.
3. Frost M, Gates J, Helmers SL, et al. Vagus nerve stimulation in children with refractory seizures associated with Lennox–Gastaut Syndrome. Epilepsia 2001; 42(9):1148–1152.
4. Glauser TA, Levisohn PM, Ritter F, et al. Topiramate in Lennox–Gastaut syndrome: open label treatment of patients completing a randomized controlled trial. Epilepsia 2000; 41(S1):S86–S90.
5. Hoffman-Riem M, Diener W, Benninger C, et al. Non convulsive status epilepticus—a possible cause of mental retardation in patients with Lennox Gastaut syndrome. Neuropediatrics 2000; 31(4):169–174.
6. Jensen PK. Felbamate in the treatment of Lennox–Gastaut syndrome. *Epilepsia* 1994; 35(suppl 5):S54–S57.
7. Mikaeloff Y, de Saint-Martin A, Mancini J, et al. Topiramate: efficacy and tolerability in children according to epilepsy syndromes. Epilepsy Res 2003; 53:225–232.
8. Motte J, Trevathan E, Arvidsson JF, et al. Lamotrigine for generalized seizures associated with the Lennox Gastaut syndrome. New Eng. J Med 1997; 337(25):1807–1812.

9. Sachdeo RC, Glauser TA, Ritter F, et al. A double-blind, randomized trial of topiramate in Lennox–Gastaut Syndrome. Neurology 1999; 52(9):1882–1887.
10. Siegel H, Kelley K, Stertz B, et al. The efficacy of felbamate as add-on therapy to valproic acid in the Lennox Gastaut syndrome. Epilepsy Res. 1999; 34(2–3):91–97.

13

Landau–Kleffner Syndrome (LKS) and Epilepsy with Continuous Spike-Waves During Slow-Wave Sleep (CSWS)

William H. Trescher
Kennedy Krieger Institute, Baltimore, Maryland, U.S.A.

INTRODUCTION

In 1957, Landau and Kleffner reported a group of children with a syndrome of acquired epileptic aphasia (Landau–Kleffner syndrome, LKS) and in 1971, Patry et al. described the syndrome of epilepsy with continuous spike-waves during slow-wave sleep (CSWS). These syndromes can be relatively distinct and the International League Against Epilepsy has recognized them as separate syndromes. An overlap of symptoms of these conditions has led to a developing view that these disorders may be related to each other with the common feature of electrical status epilepticus in sleep (ESES). Furthermore, they may be related to the less severe condition of benign childhood epilepsy with central–temporal spikes.

CLINICAL FEATURES

In the relatively pure form of LKS, children usually do not have antecedent developmental or neurological abnormalities. Loss of language usually occurs in a subacute or stuttering pattern. Onset is usually between 3 years and 8 years of age. Seizures, typically partial or generalized tonic–clonic, occur in 70–80% of individuals and may precede or develop around the same time as the language deterioration. The language impairment usually appears as a receptive aphasia or verbal auditory agnosia (VAA) with intact hearing. Reading, writing, and use of visual cues often are preserved initially, but may deteriorate over time. Associated features include hyperactivity, inattention, irritability, and mild motor apraxia. Routine imaging studies are generally normal, although tumors, neurocysticercosis, congenital hemiparesis, a history of encephalitis and other conditions have been reported in association with LKS. A hereditary predisposition is uncommon. The seizures are usually easily controlled, but the language impairment is often more refractory to treatment. Aphasia persists in more than half of cases. Adverse factors for language recovery include: younger age on onset, longer duration of ESES, and spread of the spikes bilaterally.

In the syndrome of CSWS, onset is between 4 years and 14 years of age. Most children have seizures, which may be partial, generalized tonic–clonic, as well as myoclonic, atonic, or atypical absence. Seizures, when they occur, develop as early as the first year of life, often preceding the onset of ESES by 1–2 years. Language impairment is typically an expressive aphasia rather than VAA. Global cognitive deterioration, behavioral dysfunction, and motor impairments are more severe than with LKS. Approximately one-third of children have a history of antecedent neurological problems or abnormalities on imaging studies.

Precise diagnosis of these conditions may be difficult because many cases described in the literature and possibly a greater number of children presenting to clinicians do not manifest classic symptoms, but rather have intermediate forms of these disorders. Further complicating diagnosis, approximately one-third of children with autistic spectrum disorder (ASD) experience language regression, albeit at a much earlier age than the loss of language associated with LKS. While the incidence of epilepsy among children with autistic ASD is no different between those with and without regression, there is some evidence to suggest that the incidence of epileptiform discharges on EEG is greater among those with language regression compared to those without regression. The term Landau–Kleffner variant often is used to characterize those children with infantile autism with language regression and coincident epileptiform discharges, but this designation is not universally accepted.

DIAGNOSIS

The key to diagnosis is recognition of the clinical syndrome of a loss of language function with or without a deterioration of cognitive abilities and behavior. The diagnosis may be overlooked when seizures do no occur. Routine daytime EEGs that include at least 20–30 min of sleep may capture ESES, but caution is advised in the event of a negative daytime study in the setting of cognitive, behavioral, or language deterioration. A full overnight EEG may be necessary to make the diagnosis. Once the diagnosis is established, further evaluation may be necessary to determine if predisposing conditions that may be contributing to the disorder. History and physicial examination should be comprehensive to evaluate for evidence of antecedent brain injury, infection, immunological dysfunction, and prior developmental abnormalities. High-resolution magnetic resonance imaging (MRI) is important to evaluate for structural abnormalities with particular emphasis on adequate coronal views through the hippocampus. Audiological evalution is necessary to rule out hearing loss. Early involvement of a neuropsychologist and a speech language pathologist is absolutely critical to fully evalutate of baseline cognitive and language function and to monitor the course of treatment. These specialists are necessary to work with the schools to create an appropriate educational program for the child.

The defining feature of LKS or CSWS is paroxysmal spike-wave activity, which is often continuous and generalized, or at least bilateral on EEG. This EEG activity is induced during sleep and called ESES. A fair degree of variability exists, however, and the EEG discharges may be discontinuous, unilateral or focal, and sometimes associated with sharp-wave, polyspikes or polyspike-and-slow-wave activity. Typically, this activity is more prominent during non-REM (rapid-eye-movement) sleep and markedly attenuated during REM sleep and when the individual is awake. The paroxysmal EEG activity may last for months to years. Careful analysis of the electrographic spike-wave activity often reveals that LKS is associated with a temporal spike focus and CSWS a frontal focus. Greater dysfunction seems to be associated with bilateral spread of the epileptiform discharges. Additionally, the extent of epileptiform activity has been defined by the spike-wave index, which is the percentage of the time of slow-wave sleep time occupied by continuous spike-wave activity. In most cases of CSWS, the spike-wave index is greater than 85%, but some individuals may otherwise meet criteria for the disorder with a slightly lower spike-wave index. In LKS, the spike-wave index may be lower, but still above 50%.

TREATMENT

The major goal of therapy is to reverse the deterioration of cognitive and language function and to suppress ESES. The seizures associated with LKS usually are not severe and generally respond well to a variety of antiepileptic medications. The seizures that accompany CSWS may be more difficult to control, but seizures are not the major problem for either of these disorders. In contrast, cognitive and language dysfunction, as well as the associated ESES, do not respond well to standard antiepileptic medications, but no controlled treatment studies of LKS or CSWS are available. Furthermore, the variable natural history of the disorders complicates assessment of the small case series and case treatment reports.

Of the conventional antiepileptic medications, sodium valproate, ethosuximde, and various benzodiazepines, particularly clobazam, have shown benefit in some cases, but the responses have been inconsistent. Newer agents such as lamotrigine, levetiracetam, and vigabatrin have also shown benefit, but it should be emphasized that these are usually in isolated case reports. Conversely, isolated reports document that carbamazepine, phenytoin, and phenobarbital may exacerbate these conditions, but the data to support this conclusion are limited.

Corticosteroids or ACTH (adrenocorticotropic hormone) administered in high doses generally is considered the most effective treatment for the language and cognitive dysfunction. In absent evidence of superiority of one form of treatment, corticosteroids are preferred. Relapse rates are high with attempts to taper the steroids and multiple treatment courses may be necessary. The side effects of steroids, including weight gain, hypertension, immunosuppression and infection, glucose and electrolyte abnormalities, cataracts, and avascular necrosis of the hip, often limit continued treatment. Additionally, steroids may significantly worsen behavior, which can be difficult to distinguish from the effects of the underlying disorder. Conversion to an every other day treatment regimen or once per week pulse steroids administered over two days helps to minimize side effects. In isolated reports, intravenous immunoglobulin and the ketogenic diet have proved beneficial.

Benzodiazepines may have a specific role in the treatment of these disorders. Intravenous administration of diazepam can suppress the electrical status epilepticus, but the effect is relatively short in duration, usually hours to days. Long-term suppression of the ESES can sometimes be achieved with a relatively high-dose bolus of diazepam followed by prolonged administration of oral diazepam. A suggested protocol that we have used with success is diazepam (1 mg/kg) administered per rectum, followed by oral administration of 0.5 mg/kg per day for 3 weeks. Benzodiazepines seem to be most effective when administered in conjunction with another antiepileptic medication, such as sodium valproate.

When medical therapy fails, surgical treatment may be an option but stringent criteria should be applied to the selection of candidates. Recovery of language function may occur after temporal lobectomy, but due to the risk of removing eloquent cortex, the procedure of multiple subpial transactions (MST) should be considered. The best outcome from surgery for LKS occurs when the child has: (1) normal cognitive and language development prior to the onset of symptoms; (2) relative preservation of nonverbal cognitive function prior to surgery; (3) evidence of a unilateral focus of the diffuse or bilateral discharges; and (4) duration of CSWS of less than 3 years.

PROGNOSIS

The long-term prognosis for both LKS and CSWS in guarded, but definitive predictions are difficult to make as most of the information comes from case reports and small case series with various treatment regimens. Overall, less than half of all children regain language function sufficiently to allow return to a regular school environment. Somewhat better outcomes may be associated with surgical treatment, but selection criteria have limited this option to an extremely small subset of children.

SUMMARY

The LKS and CSWS are rare disorders of young children, characterized by a subacute deterioration of language, which tends to be a receptive aphasia in LKS and an expressive aphasia in CSWS. Varying degrees of cognitive, behavioral, and motor dysfunction are associated with the aphasia. Seizures occur in most children with these disorders, but are not the major challenge for treatment. The impaired language and cognitive dysfunction are correlated with the extent of electrical status epilepticus during sleep, which can be difficult to treat. Benzodiazepines given in conjunction with sodium valproate and corticosteroids are currently considered the most effective treatments. Surgery, in the form in multiple subpial transactions, may benefit a highly selected subset of patients.

DIAGNOSIS AND TREATMENT OF SUBACUTE LANGUAGE REGRESSION, WITH OR WITHOUT SEIZURES

Evaluation:

1. History and physical examination with screening CBC, metabolic studies to evaluate for hepatic, renal, or immunological dysfunction.
2. An EEG, to include a minimum of 30 min of slow-wave sleep, and consider an overnight study to evaluate all stages of sleep.
3. The MRI of the brain with adequate visualization of the hippocampus.
4. Consider SPECT, PET, MRS, magnetoencephalography for localization of regions of cerebral dysfunction.

Suggested treatment course after diagnosis:

1. Administer diazepam 1 mg/kg per rectum, followed by 0.5 mg/kg/day for 3 weeks.

2. Coincident with diazepam administration, begin sodium valproate at 5–10 mg/kg/day in 2–3 divided doses, gradually increasing dose over 1–2 weeks to 20 mg/kg/day. Higher doses (at least 60 mg/kg/day) may be necessary.
3. If above regimen does not suppress ESES after 1 month, begin prednisone 2–3 mg/kg/day for 1 month with gradual taper over 3 months. Longer treatment or repeat courses of treatment may be necessary. Consider every other day regimen or weekly pulse steroids.
4. If above does not prove beneficial, consider: addition of ethosuximide to sodium valproate; or substitution of lamotrigine or levetiracetam for sodium valproate.
5. Consider ketogenic diet.
6. Consider IVIG 400 IU/kg.
7. If ESES and language dysfunction and ESES persist for greater than 6–12 months, consider referral for surgical evaluation.

SUGGESTED READINGS

1. Ballaban-Gil K, Tuchman R. Epilepsy and epileptiform EEG: association with autism and language disorders. Ment Retard Dev Disabil Res Rev 2000; 6:300–308.
2. De Negri M. Electrical status epilepticus during sleep (ESES). Different clinical syndromes: towards a unifying view? Brain Dev 1997; 19:447–451.
3. Deonna TW. Acquired epileptiform aphasia in children (Landau–Kleffner syndrome). J Clin Neurophysiol 1991; 8:288–298.
4. Galanopoulou AS, Bojko A, Lado F, Moshe SL. The spectrum of neuropsychiatric abnormalities associated with electrical status epilepticus in sleep. Brain Dev 2000; 22: 279–295.
5. Jayakar PB, Seshia SS. Electrical status epilepticus during slow-wave sleep: a review. J Clin Neurophysiol 1991; 8:299–311.
6. Morrell F, Whisler WW, Smith MC, Hoeppner TJ, de Toledo-Morrell L, Pierre-Pouis SJC, Kanner AM, Buelow JM, Ristanovic R, Bergen D, Chez M, Hasegawa H. Landau–Kleffner syndrome—treatment with subpial intracortical transection. Brain 1995; 118:1529–1546.
7. Smith MC, Spitz MC. Treatment strategies in Landau–Kleffner syndrome and paraictal psychiatric and cognitive disturbances. Epilepsy Behav 2002; 3:24–29.
8. Tassinari CA, Rubboli G, Volpi L, Meletti S, d'Orsi G, Franca M, Sabetta AR, Riguzzi P, Gardella E, Zaniboni A, Michelucci R. Encephalopathy with electrical status epilepticus during slow sleep or ESES syndrome including the acquired aphasia. Clin Neurophysiol 2000; 111(Suppl 2):S94–S102.

14
Juvenile Myoclonic Epilepsy

Traci D. Swink
Marshfield Clinic, Marshfield, Wisconsin, U.S.A.

INTRODUCTION

Juvenile myoclonic epilepsy (JME) is an idiopathic generalized epilepsy (IGE) syndrome that typically appears in the second decade of life. Herpin wrote the first detailed description of a patient with JME in 1867. In 1957, Janz and Christian published their article on 47 patients with "impulsive petit mal." The term JME was introduced by Lund in 1975 and is the term currently recognized by the International League Against Epilepsy. The JME is estimated to account for 5–10% of all epilepsies.

CLINICAL FEATURES

There are a number of different epilepsy syndromes within the IGEs (Table 1). JME, childhood absence epilepsy (CAE), epilepsy with generalized tonic–clonic seizures on awakening (GTCA), and juvenile absence epilepsy (JAE) can present in late childhood and adolescence. The JME is characterized by myoclonic, generalized tonic–clonic, and/or absence seizures. The typical age of onset is between 12 and 18 years of age (range 8–24).

Myoclonic seizures are the hallmark of JME and occur in all patients. Myoclonic seizures occur as the only seizure type in only a small percentage of patients (3–12%). Myoclonic jerks are characterized by sudden, brief, bilateral symmetric, and synchronous muscle contractions that affect predominantly the shoulders and upper extremities. The jerks can be single or repetitive and consciousness is preserved. Many patients do not recognize these jerks as seizures until they manifest with a generalized tonic–clonic (GTC) seizure. Prior to diagnosis, the jerks may be interpreted as nervousness, clumsiness, or tics/twitches. A careful history with specific questioning for the presence of myoclonic jerks is critical to making a correct diagnosis of JME, as many patients may not volunteer these symptoms. Even with careful questioning, some patients are diagnosed only after documentation of myoclonic seizures by video EEG monitoring. In many cases, myoclonic seizures precede the onset of generalized tonic–clonic seizures, sometimes by several years.

Absence seizures are reported to occur in as many as 40% of patients with JME but are typically infrequent, of short duration, and not associated with automatism,

Table 1 Idiopathic Generalized Epilepsy Syndromes (Listed in Order of Age of Onset)

Benign neonatal familial convulsions
Benign neonatal convulsions
Benign myoclonic epilepsy of infancy
Childhood absence epilepsy
Juvenile absence epilepsy
Juvenile myoclonic epilepsy
Epilepsy with grand mal seizures on awakening
Other generalized idiopathic epilepsies not defined above

particularly when onset is after 10 years of age. It is important to distinguish the myoclonic jerks and absence seizures of JME from myoclonic absence epilepsy, a much rarer form of generalized epilepsy that develops in early or middle childhood and has a much poorer prognosis both in terms of response to treatment and overall cognitive impairment. The JME may evolve out of CAE when the patient reaches adolescence.

Generalized tonic–clonic seizures are very common in JME, occurring in 87–95% of patients. The GTC seizures occur most frequently on awakening and are often preceded by a series of myoclonic jerks.

DIFFERENTIAL DIAGNOSIS

The JME is a distinct epilepsy syndrome with a well-defined age on onset, characteristic electroencephalographic pattern, and response to therapy. The JME should be distinguished from the progressive myoclonic epilepsies and other IGEs with onset in adolescence, as treatment strategies differ depending on the epilepsy syndrome (Table 2).

The electroencephalogram (EEG) is the most valuable tool for diagnosing JME. A sleep deprived EEG yields a higher rate of abnormal results and should be performed whenever possible when evaluating adolescents with new onset seizures. Video EEG with recording on awakening can be extremely helpful when JME is suspected, particularly in patients who do not provide a typical history of myoclonus. The characteristic interictal EEG pattern consists of generalized 4–6 Hz polyspike and wave complexes, often with frontocentral predominance; however, many patients have slower 3–4 Hz spike and wave complexes. The resting background is typically normal in patients with JME. Photosensitivity is common with precipitation of electrographic polyspike and wave complexes as well as myoclonic seizures. As many as 30–50% of patients may have subtle asymmetric EEG abnormalities in addition to typical generalized fast polyspike and wave complexes, these findings should not deter from or delay the diagnosis of JME.

The characteristics of the EEG of myoclonus are repetitive, medium to high amplitude, fast 10–16 Hz polyspikes, followed by 1–3 Hz slow waves. The electrographic seizure can last longer than the clinical seizure and the number of spikes is more closely related to the intensity of the myoclonic jerks rather than the duration of the myoclonus.

Treatment with appropriate anticonvulsant drugs may normalize the EEG; however, even on medication, recording on awakening and with sleep deprivation

Table 2 Idiopathic Generalized Epilepsy Syndromes of Childhood and Adolescence

Feature (Age of onset)	JME (Second decade)	CAE (First decade)	JAE (Second decade)	GTCA (Second decade)
Myoclonus	Required for diagnosis, 5% myoclonus only	Rare	15% of patients	Rare, often hypnagogic when present
Absence	Occur in 10–33% of patients but infrequent	Required for diagnosis but fewer/day than CAE	Required for diagnosis	Less common than JAE and JME
Tonic–clonic	95% of patients	40% of patients but infrequent	80% of patients	Required for diagnosis
EEG	Polyspike and wave, 4–6 or 8–12 Hz	3 Hz spike and wave	Generalized spike and polyspike and wave	Generalized spike and polyspike and wave
Hyperventilation-induced discharges	Rare	Common	Common	Rare
Photosensitivity	Common	15% of patients	Rare	Common
Prognosis	Favorable but life long	40% remission by adolescence	Favorable but remission less frequent than CAE	Favorable but often life long

often reveals the characteristic EEG features. Extra effort should be taken to document EEG abnormalities when counseling adolescents with a history of generalized seizures about discontinuing medication given the high incidence (90%) of seizure recurrence after withdrawal of medications in patients with JME.

The neurological examination reveals no abnormalities in patients with JME. Routine MRI studies are normal as well. Quantitative MRI and 18F-2-deoxyglucose PET studies in patients with JME have found regional differences supporting the idea that individuals with JME may have abnormalities of cortical organization and abnormal patterns of cortical architecture that may also be associated with subtle cognitive dysfunction.

TREATMENT

The goal of treatment for patients with JME differs somewhat from other forms of childhood idiopathic epilepsy in that patients with JME typically do not "outgrow" their seizures. Lifelong anticonvulsant therapy and monitoring for complications related to seizures and medications are usually necessary. In addition to appropriate anticonvulsant drug therapy, considerable time and effort should be spent counseling patients on appropriate lifestyle choices that minimize the risks of seizure recurrence such as sleep deprivation, alcohol consumption, noncompliance with medications, and stress. Issues involving pregnancy, the potential for teratogenic effects from seizures and anticonvulsant medications, and hereditary issues should be discussed early in the diagnostic process and reviewed frequently with patients and their families. Women in particular should be counseled on birth control, folic acid supplementation, and the hormonal influences of epilepsy.

Valproic acid (VPA) remains the drug of choice for most patients with JME with the majority of patients experiencing good control of all three seizure types at relatively low doses. While no randomized clinical trials have been conducted using any medications for JME, open case studies with VPA have shown a 41–88% seizure-free rate for patients receiving VPA, either as an add-on medication or as monotherapy. Therapeutic doses typically range from 20 to 30 mg/kg (range 10–70 mg/kg) and most patients are well controlled with blood levels of 40–100 μg/mL. When seizures recur on VPA it is usually due to noncompliance, sleep deprivation, other drugs or alcohol consumption, or stress. Several formulations of VPA exist. Most patients prefer long-acting preparations and new extended release formulations offer most patients the convenience of once a day dosing with effective seizure control.

Supplementation with a minimum of 1 mg of folic acid (range 1–4 mg) is strongly recommended for women taking VPA to reduce the risks of neural tube defects in offspring. We typically recommend 4 mg/day of folic acid for women of childbearing age. Neural tube defects are associated with up to 4% of pregnancies in patients receiving VPA monotherapy and up to 9% of pregnancies result in major birth defect. There appears to be a pharmacogenetic susceptibility to the teratogenic effects of VPA and folic acid supplementation does not prevent NTDs in susceptible women. The VPA has a relatively low incidence of neurocognitive side effects. The most common side effects are weight gain, anorexia, nausea, alopecia, tremor, and rash. Rare but serious complications include hepatic failure, pancreatitis, thrombocytopenia, hyperammonemia, polycystic ovarian disease, stupor, and encephalopathy. Liver function testing is recommended before beginning therapy with VPA and periodically during treatment. Unfortunately, periodic screening of liver functions may not detect an adverse effect and discontinuation of VPA may not prevent fulminant hepatic failure in susceptible patients.

Increasing awareness of and concern for the reproductive health of women with epilepsy have generated much interest in evaluating newer AEDs for the treatment of JME. Lamotrigine (LMT) is an excellent alternative to VPA, but possibly less effective. Studies of LMT have shown it to be effective for most of the seizures types in JME but may exacerbate some seizures, particularly the myoclonic jerks. When LMT is added to other anticonvulsant medications, particularly VPA, better control may be achieved. Most adolescent patients respond to doses ranging from 200 to 400 mg/day for monotherapy. When used in combination with VPA, doses of 100–200 mg are often sufficient. Caution should be used when adding LMT to VPA due to the increased risk of life-threatening rash and clinicians are advised to not to exceed the recommended initial doses and dose escalation schedule.

Ethosuximide when used in combination with VPA or LMT can be effective in patients whose absence seizures are not adequately controlled with VPA or LMT monotherapy. Alone it provides no coverage for generalized tonic–clonic or myoclonic seizures. Ethosuximide can be initiated at doses of 250 mg/day in older children and adolescents and increased weekly to desired effect. Most patients require dosages ranging from 500 to 1000 mg/day.

Topiramate (TPM) and zonisamide (ZNS) both have been shown to have broad-spectrum properties and could be considered in patients with JME who have failed or cannot tolerate first- or second-line therapy. A recent pilot study comparing TPM to VPA monotherapy in patients with JME found TPM to be equally as efficacious as VPA at relatively modest dosages. The TPM can be initiated at dosages of 25–50 mg/week and titrated every one to two weeks to desired effect. Most patients respond to dosages in the range of 200–600 mg/day. The ZNS is initiated at dosages of 50–100 mg/day and increased every one to two weeks to desired effect. Total dosages range between 100 and 600 mg/day. Levetiracetam (LEV) has also shown some promising results in IGEs and seems to control the generalized tonic–clonic seizures and myoclonic seizure for some patients. The LEV can be initiated at 250–500 mg/day and increased weekly to desired effect with most patients responding at dosages of 1000–4000 mg/day. While there is no class I evidence regarding TPM, ZNS, or LEV in JME, these medications should be considered if first- or second-line therapies fail. Less is known regarding the hormonal and reproductive effects of these newer AEDs. A serious discussion of issues related to reproductive health and pregnancy must take place between health-care providers and female patients with JME.

Clonazepam (CZP) can also be effective in the treatment of JME. It is most commonly utilized as a low dose add-on therapy when GTC seizures are well controlled with other AEDs but myoclonic seizures persist. It is much less effective when used as monotherapy and in some cases may eliminate the warning myoclonus before a GTC seizure, resulting in increased risk of injury.

Clinicians need to be aware of the potential for some AEDs to aggravate seizures in JME resulting in increased seizure frequency, increased seizure severity, or the appearance of a new seizure type. Carbamazepine (CBZ) and phenytoin (PHT) both appear to have this potential with CBZ having the strongest aggravating potential, whereas the aggravating effect of PHT appears less prominent. Newer AEDs such as vigabatrin (VGB) and LMT also have the potential to aggravate myoclonic seizures and it is important that this potential is discussed with patients when prescribing newer medications. Finally, the ketogenic diet has been shown to be effective in treating all three seizure types common to JME and may be useful in refractory patients but rarely is indicated given the high response rate of JME to AED therapy.

In general, I use either VPA or LMT in monotherapy as first-line therapy, followed by the combination in polytherapy. Should these choices fail, I would then consider TPM, ZNS, or LEV as monotherapy as equivalent second-line choices. If unsuccessful, VPA in combination with TPM, ZNS, or LEV may have a role before trying CZP or the ketogenic diet.

SUMMARY

The JME carries an excellent prognosis for the majority of patients who understand that their disorder is lifelong, requires treatment with antiepileptic medications to control the seizures, and who understand the importance of healthy lifestyle choices to minimize seizure recurrence. With appropriate education, counseling and medical treatment, 86–90% of patients will be seizure free or well controlled on medication.

SUGGESTED READINGS

1. Bourgeois B. Chronic management of seizures in the syndromes of idiopathic generalized epilepsy. Epilepsia 2003; 44(suppl 2):27–32.
2. Delagado-Escueta AV, Enrile-Bascal F. Juvenile myoclonic epilepsy of Janz. Neurology 1984; 34:285–29.
3. Janz D. Junvenile myoclonic epilepsy: epilepsy with impulsive petit mal. Cleve Clin J Med 1989; 56(suppl 1):23–33.
4. Wheless J, Sankar R. Treatment strategies for myoclonic seizures and epilepsy syndromes with myoclonic seizures. Epilepsia 2003; 44(suppl 11):27–37.
5. Wyllie E, ed. The Treatment of Epilepsy: Principles and Practice. Lippincott Williams &Wilkins, 2001.

15
Progressive Myoclonic Epilepsy

Joan A. Conry
George Washington University School of Medicine, Children's National Medical Center, Washington, D.C., U.S.A.

INTRODUCTION

Progressive myoclonic epilepsy (PME) is a syndrome (not a specific disease) with myoclonic seizures and progressive neurological decline. The diagnosis of PME is based on the presence of a degenerative process which includes myoclonic seizures and progressive neurological dysfunction and which does not fit into any of the other myoclonic epilepsy syndromes. (Table 1). Myoclonic seizures are seen in a variety of epileptic syndromes, some benign and some malignant.

All patients with PME at some point in the illness must have myoclonic seizures, which characteristically are brief shock like "jerks" involving the extremities and/or the head/neck and trunk. Myoclonic seizures can also consist of "negative myoclonus" which consist of a brief loss of tone and may be described as a "drop." In addition to myoclonic seizures, patients with PME usually also have tonic or tonic–clonic seizures.

All patients also must have "progressive neurological decline." The progressive neurological deterioration most often involves cerebellar degeneration and/or progressive dementia. In children, a typical cerebellar syndrome of trunkal ataxia, appendicular tremor, and hypotonia may be difficult to recognize until late in the disease. Subtle presentations in young children include developmental delay and failure to acquire motor milestones, in addition to a flat affect and nystagmus. An actual loss of milestones and deterioration in neurological function may occur months or even years after "developmentally delay" is diagnosed.

In this treatment focused text, much of the intervention and therapy in PME is centered on making a diagnosis and treating seizures symptomatically. Since PME is a collection of diseases, the most common causes and diagnostic criteria will be discussed so the rationale for diagnostic studies is clarified. The most common identified causes of PME will be discussed in the next section.

UNVERRICHT–LUNDORG DISEASE

Unverricht–Lundborg disease, also known as Baltic myoclonus or Mediterranean myoclonus, is an autosomal recessive disorder which is prevalent in Finland (1 in

Table 1 Classification of Myoclonic Epilepsies

Early myoclonic epilepsy
Benign myoclonic epilepsy in infants
Severe myoclonic epilepsy in infants
Myoclonic astatic epilepsy
Epilepsy with myoclonic absences
Eyelid myoclonia with absence
Juvenile myoclonic epilepsy
Progressive myoclonic epilepsy
Myoclonic seizures not otherwise classified

20,000). The onset of symptoms is in late childhood (8–13 years), with myoclonic jerks, which are often stimulus sensitive, as the presenting symptom. The seizures evolve to severe myoclonic seizures and tonic–clonic seizures. The degenerative cerebellar symptoms (ataxia, dysarthria, and tremor) and cognitive decline are mild and present much later than the seizures. Affected patients may survive into adulthood. Histological markers, when present, are membrane-bound vacuoles with clear contents in eccrine glands. The defect is a mutation in the cystatin B gene, which is found on chromosome 21. Treatment is symptomatic.

MITOCHONDRIAL EPILEPSY WITH RAGGED RED FIBERS (MERRF)

Mitochondrial epilepsy with ragged red fibers (MERRF) is a mitochondrial disease which may present either in childhood or adulthood. MERRF either is sporadic or is transmitted via mitochondrial (maternal) inheritance. The initial symptoms are medically refractory myoclonic seizures and tonic–clonic seizures. Progressive ataxia and dementia are variable but may occur relatively early in the disease. The presence of myopathy, sensorineural hearing loss or optic atrophy should raise the index of suspicion. The defect is a defect in mitochondrial DNA resulting in an abnormal transfer RNA *Lys* gene. If the mother is affected, there is a 100% recurrence rate. However, the clinical course may vary from mild to severe. Diagnosis is made by demonstration of ragged red fibers on muscle biopsy. Unfortunately, the muscle histology may be normal especially early in the disease. Repeat biopsy later in the illness may reveal ragged red fibers as more mitochondria become severely involved. Treatment is supportive.

LAFORA BODY DISEASE

Lafora body disease is an autosomal recessive disorder which usually presents between 10 and 18 years of age. Tonic–clonic seizures in a neurologically normal child are the initial symptoms, with myoclonic seizures which initially may respond to medications. The clinical course is rapidly progressive, with the development of severe seizures, stimulus sensitive myoclonus, disabling ataxia, and severe dementia. Death usually occurs within 10 years of clinical onset. Polyglucosan bodies (Lafora bodies) can be seen in many tissues, especially the excretory ducts of eccrine sweat glands. The genetic defect is the EPM2A gene on chromosome 6q23-25 which codes for a protein tyrosine phosphatase (laforin).

Lafora body disease is clinically different from Unverricht–Lundborg disease because of the rapidly progressive neurological decline in Lafora body disease. Histologically, they have different inclusions. The genetic defect has been identified in both and they are clearly different diseases.

NEURONAL CEROID LIPOFUSCINOSIS (NCL)

Neuronal ceroid lipofuscinosis (NCL) is an autosomal recessive disorder with onset at multiple ages and with varied initial symptoms. Depending on the age of onset, NCL is known as Santavuori–Haltia disease (infantile onset, 0–2 years), Jansky–Bielschowsky disease (late infantile onset, 2–4 years), Batten's disease or Spielmeyer–Vogt–Sjogren disease (juvenile onset, 4–10 years) or Kuf's disease (adulthood). Severe tonic–clonic or myoclonic seizures, developmental delay, and visual impairment are the presenting symptoms in the infantile and late infantile variants. A movement disorder, psychiatric or behavioral symptoms or visual loss may be the initial symptoms in older patients (juvenile onset and adults). The rate of progression of disease is more fulminant with younger presentations. Nonetheless the disease is relentlessly progressive and ultimately fatal. Diagnostic studies supportive of the diagnosis are the electroretinogram, which may be abnormal early, and visual evoked potentials, which initially may be "giant" then disappear. Typical intracellular fingerprint, curvilinear, or granular inclusions may be seen in multiple tissues, including skin, conjunctiva, muscle, leukocytes, or rectal mucosa. Although the underlying genetic defect has not been identified, genetic markers have been identified for at least 10 subtypes with defects on chromosome 16 (juvenile) or chromosome 13 (late infantile). No definitive therapy is available.

SIALIDOSIS (CHERRY-RED SPOT MYOCLONUS SYNDROME)

Two variants of Sialidosis are known. Sialidosis type I is caused by a deficiency of *N*-acetylneuraminidase and causes PME. Sialidosis type II is due to a deficiency of both *N*-acetylneuraminidase and beta galactosidase, and is also known as Mucolipidosis Type I.

Sialidosis Type I is a rare cause of PME. Transmission is autosomal recessive inheritance. A macular cherry-red spot may be seen although not all patients have cherry-red spots. The symptoms typically appear in adolescence, with tonic–clonic seizures and myoclonic seizures. Facial myoclonus and intention myoclonus may be present. Progressive visual loss ensues. The development of cerebellar symptoms is late and slow. Dementia may be mild or absent. The patient may live 10–40 years after onset of symptoms. The diagnosis is made by demonstrating a deficiency in *N*-aeetylneuraminidase and normal beta-galactosidase in leukocyte lysosomal enzymes. No definitive therapy is available.

UNCOMMON CAUSES OF PME

Several other diseases may present as PME (with myoclonic seizures, cerebellar degeneration, and dementia). These include mitochondrial disorders other than MERRF, biotin responsive encephalopathy, childhood onset Huntington's disease, infantile neuroaxonal dystrophy, Hallervorden–Spatz disease, and Alper's disease. Atypical presentations of several lysosomal enzyme defects may also present as PME.

DIAGNOSIS

The diagnosis of PME is usually suspected after the patient has demonstrated refractory seizures, including myoclonic seizures, as well as a degenerative CNS process or severe infantile encephalopathy. As discussed in the first section, recognition of cerebellar dysfunction is difficult in infancy. Relatively common disorders with myoclonic seizures which may be confused with PME include Lennox Gastaut syndrome, juvenile myoclonic epilepsy, or slow virus infections such as SSPE or Jacob–Creutzfleld. Progressive myoclonic epilepsy may initially be diagnosed as a behavioral disorder, learning problem, or psychiatric disease. The appearance of myoclonic seizures or cognitive deterioration should signal the possibility of misdiagnosis.

Several red flags should raise the possibility of a diagnosis of PME. In the history, the presence of developmental delay is significant. The child may not ever have acquired motor or mental milestones, so regression may not have occurred. A plateau in acquisition of milestones is significant, as the child may not have actually lost milestones yet. A description of all seizure types is essential. A family history of any neurological impairment may be significant.

On examination, findings which may point to a diagnosis of PME are abnormal tone, impaired visual skills, nystagmus, and tremor in addition to ataxia and tremor. A comprehensive exam for any major organ abnormality is required.

Diagnostic studies may be extensive, but should start with BEG, MRI, and MR spectroscopy. The MRI may demonstrate cerebellar or generalized atrophy, and serial MRIs may reveal progressive atrophy. The MR spectroscopy may demonstrate a lactate peak. Ophthalmologic consultation may reveal visual impairment as well as a cherry-red spot, optic atrophy, or abnormal retinal pigment.

Metabolic and electrophysiological studies which may point to a specific diagnosis are listed in Table 2. If the child's clinical course continues to support a diagnosis of PME, the definitive diagnosis may require biopsy. Muscle biopsy should be obtained for light microscopy, electron microscopy, and respiratory chain enzymes. A skin biopsy can often be performed in conjunction with the muscle biopsy. Other tissues to be considered (based on the clinical course) are conjunctiva, rectal mucosa, liver, and bone marrow. A nondiagnostic biopsy does not exclude a diagnosis of many of the disorders discussed above.

Table 2 Diagnostic Screening Laboratory and Electrophysiologic Studies for PME

Metabolic studies
Lactate, pyruvate, urine organic acids, plasma amino acids, plasma acylcarnitine, NH_3, uric acid, renal function studies, liver function studies, CBC and differential
Electrophysiological studies
Electroencephalography (EEG), electroretinogram (ERG), visual evoked response (VER), brainstem audio evoked response (BAER). Electrocardiogram (ECG)

More specific metabolic or genetic tests may be obtained, depending on the clinical course and results of the studies above. Unfortunately, in many cases, a diagnosis of a specific disease may be made only at autopsy, if then.

TREATMENT

Treatment is supportive, directed at specific symptoms. The seizures in these patients are extremely difficult to treat, often requiring combinations of medications. For myoclonic seizures, the drug of choice remains valproic acid. The target dosage of valproic acid is 20–60 mg/kg/day, starting with 10–20 mg/kg/day and increasing as tolerated. Many clinicians start carnitine when valproic acid is used in a patient with suspected metabolic disease. The target dosage is 50–100 mg/kg/day. Most (if not all) patients, especially those less than 2 years of age, should be given a trial dose of intravenous pyridoxine (100 mg) early in the course of the illness. Nitrazepam and clonazepam have been used with limited success, due to side effects (sedation, drooling) and the development of tolerance.

Several of the newer antiepileptic medications have shown some efficacy, including zonisamide and topiramate. In an uncontrolled clinical trial, zonisamide (mean dose 5.7 mg/kg/day, range 2–10) produced a dramatic reduction of myoclonic seizures in 50% of patients, and a significant reduction of total seizures in 75%. In most "responders," a reduction in myoclonic seizures was paralleled with a reduction in ataxia. The efficacy of topiramate in PME is not reported, even in small clinical trials. However, efficacy of topiramate in Lennox Gastaut syndrome has been well documented, and the use of topiramate in Infantile Spasms has also been reported. The maximum dosage used in infantile spasms has been reported as high as 24 mg/kg/day, with a rapid rate of titration (dosage increases every 2–3 days). Levetiracetam may be effective in PME since it is structurally similar to piracetam (which is effective in myoclonic seizures). Case reports indicate that it is effective in Unverricht–Lundborg disease. The dose range for myoclonic seizures is not known, but for partial seizures is 20–60 mg/kg/day. Corticotrophins (ACTH, prednisone) may induce a remission but have limited long-term utility. Alternative treatments including the ketogenic diet and/or the vagus nerve stimulator are effective in some patients.

Several antiepileptic medications may exacerbate myoclonic seizures, including carbamazepine, phenytoin, and tiagabine. Lamotrigine and vigabatrin are effective in some patients and exacerbate seizures in others.

Cofactors and vitamins are used in many of these patients. The efficacy of complementary medications is reported using a change in global neurological function (not seizure frequency) for outcome. Conclusions about efficacy are limited by the paucity of interpretable results.

SUMMARY

The most common disorders which belong to the progressive myoclonic epilepsies are Unverricht–Lundborg disease, mitochondrial epilepsy with ragged red fibers (MERRF), Lafora body disease, neuronal ceroid lipofuscinosis (NCL), and Sialidosis (cherry-red spot myoclonus syndrome). A definitive diagnosis can be made in Unverricht–Lundborg disease, Lafora body disease, and Sialidosis, and a presumptive diagnosis (by electron microscopy, respiratory chain enzyme analysis, or chromosomal linkage) can be made in some cases of MERRF and NCL. Unfortunately, a definitive diagnosis cannot be made in many patients who fall into the PME spectrum. The prognosis is poor and depends on the underlying disease. These are all degenerative diseases with medically refractory seizures. In view of the fact that most cases of clearly diagnosed PME are either autosomal recessive or mitochondrially (maternally) transmitted genetic disorders, a definitive diagnosis for genetic counseling is essential even in those patients who are declining rapidly.

SUGGESTED READINGS

1. Berkovic SF, Engle J, Pedley TA, eds. Progressive myoclonic epilepsies. In: Progressive Myoclonic Epilepsies in Epilepsy: A Comprehensive Textbook. Philadelphia: Lippincott-Raven, 1997:2455–2467.
2. Conry J. Progessive myoclonic epilepsies. J Child Neurol 2002; 17:S80–S84.
3. Leppick IE. Classification of the myoclonic epilepsies. Epilepsia 2003; 44(suppl 11):2–6.
4. Wheless JW, Sankar R. Treatment strategies for myoclonic seizures and epilepsy syndromes with myoclonic seizures. Epilepsia 2003; 44(suppl 11):27–37.

16
Intractable Epilepsy

Eric H. Kossoff
The Johns Hopkins Hospital, Baltimore, Maryland, U.S.A.

INTRODUCTION

In both community practices and academic centers caring for children with epilepsy, it is not uncommon for 10–30% of patients to have seizures that defy control with standard anticonvulsant drugs. Who are these children? In a study by Berg, intractable seizures occurred more commonly in patients with cryptogenic or symptomatic generalized syndromes (e.g., Lennox–Gastaut). In addition, the presence of focal slowing on electroencephalogram (EEG), high initial seizure frequency, and either acute symptomatic or neonatal status epilepticus were positively correlated with an increased likelihood of having intractable epilepsy.

How is intractability defined? The definition varies, but most definitions in the literature describe those patients who fail to respond to two or more antiepileptic drugs at maximally tolerated doses. In one large study of adults by Kwon, approximately 50% of patients became seizure-free with the first anticonvulsant chosen; but if it failed, only 11% became seizure-free (without intolerable side effects) with a second agent. Beyond that, only 3% responded to the third anticonvulsant. In our experience, the percentages are probably similar for children, although there is always the possibility of epilepsy being outgrown. Because results after a patient fails a second agent are discouraging, further options need to be strongly considered and this may require referral to a pediatric epilepsy center.

DIAGNOSTIC OPTIONS

All children presenting to our epilepsy center for evaluation of intractable epilepsy are asked several questions in order to provide appropriate advice and management. A careful history can occasionally reveal clues to finding the most effective therapy. All materials including prior EEGs, magnetic resonance imaging (MRI), and medication and seizure records are reviewed in depth. An algorithm for approaching these children is presented in Fig. 1.

The first, most important question is "Does the child actually have epilepsy?" Many children referred for a second opinion may have a nonepileptic cause for their spells, including sleep myoclonus, movement disorders, vasovagal syncope, or

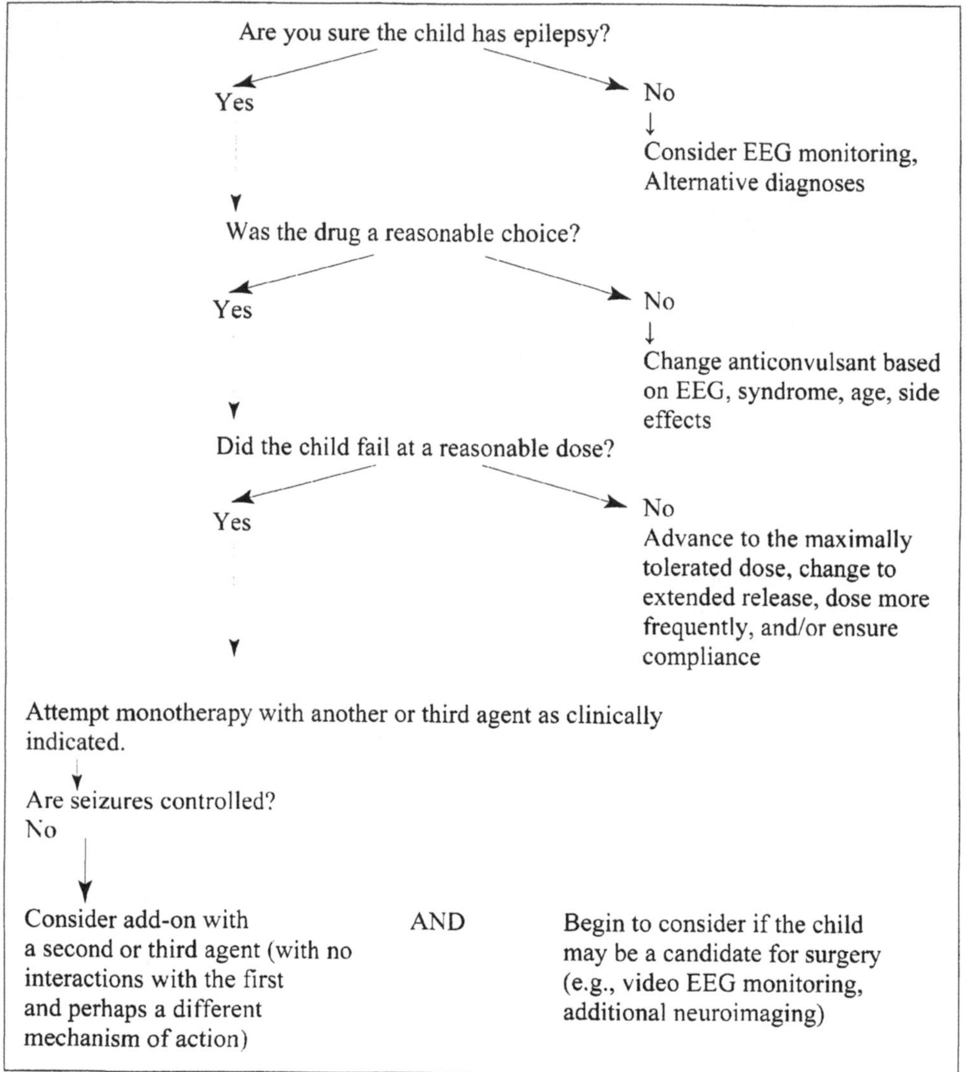
Are you sure the child has epilepsy?
Yes
No
Consider EEG monitoring, Alternative diagnoses
Was the drug a reasonable choice?
Yes
No
Change anticonvulsant based on EEG, syndrome, age, side effects
Did the child fail at a reasonable dose?
Yes
No
Advance to the maximally tolerated dose, change to extended release, dose more frequently, and/or ensure compliance
Attempt monotherapy with another or third agent as clinically indicated.
Are seizures controlled?
No
Consider add-on with a second or third agent (with no interactions with the first and perhaps a different mechanism of action)
AND
Begin to consider if the child may be a candidate for surgery (e.g., video EEG monitoring, additional neuroimaging)

Figure 1 Algorithm for intractable epilepsy-1.

pseudoseizures (Table 1). Failure to respond to medications in combination with multiple normal EEGs should arouse concern for a possible nonepileptic cause for recurrent events. In many cases, home videos obtained by the family can help with the diagnosis. Ambulatory EEG can be helpful at times. Nevertheless, it is frequently necessary to admit the child for a prolonged video-EEG monitoring period to capture an event and make a definitive diagnosis.

For the majority of cases in which epilepsy is assumed to be the diagnosis, the next question is: "What specific type of epilepsy does the child have?" Although at the time of writing of this chapter, the International League Against Epilepsy classification of seizure types is being changed, several basic principles apply. Knowing if the child has partial or generalized epilepsy can sometimes change an "intractable"

Table 1 Major Nonepileptic Causes for Unusual Events

Neonates
Jitteriness
Clonus
Apnea
Sleep myoclonus
Benign shuddering attacks
Infants
Sleep myoclonus
Sandifer syndrome (gastroesophageal reflux)
Breath-holding spells
Stereotypies
Children/adolescents
Syncope
Tics (vocal and motor)
Migraines
Sleep disturbances (including narcolepsy)
Attention deficit disorder
Vertigo
Pseudoseizures

patient into one who is easily controlled. Often an inappropriate choice of an anticonvulsant has been made (e.g., carbamazepine for a generalized epilepsy syndrome or phenobarbital for infantile spasms) because the data or history are misleading or incomplete. A history of paradoxical worsening to a standard anticonvulsant can give clues to this situation. Again, video-EEG monitoring may be necessary if the seizure type is unclear despite parental history and routine EEG.

If reasonable anticonvulsants were chosen for the seizure type, we next ask: "Were drugs pushed to toxicity?" Many children are tried for only brief periods on low doses of an anticonvulsant and then are switched to a different agent. Anticonvulsants require a minimum of 6–8 weeks to determine efficacy. In many children, anticonvulsants are added in polytherapy in rapid succession over weeks as the child continues to have daily seizures, and the parents and physician become impatient. Trying to determine which particular agents were helpful is nearly impossible in this situation.

We advocate choosing a low dose of a single anticonvulsant first, then increasing the dose as tolerated for seizure control. Anticonvulsant levels are statistical concepts, can be misleading, and only estimate the therapeutic range, typically for adults. Levels can be helpful to monitor compliance, but are rarely useful otherwise. Once a child has reached a dose in which side effects occur (e.g., sedation, dizziness, mood changes), we may lower the dose and add a second drug, and discontinue the first when the new anticonvulsant is at a reasonable dose. A second trial of monotherapy is usually beneficial. Other options include polytherapy, with use of anticonvulsants with different mechanisms of action, side effect profiles, and limited drug–drug interactions. If polytherapy is attempted, treating with low (rather than maximal) doses of multiple agents simultaneously has no clear role.

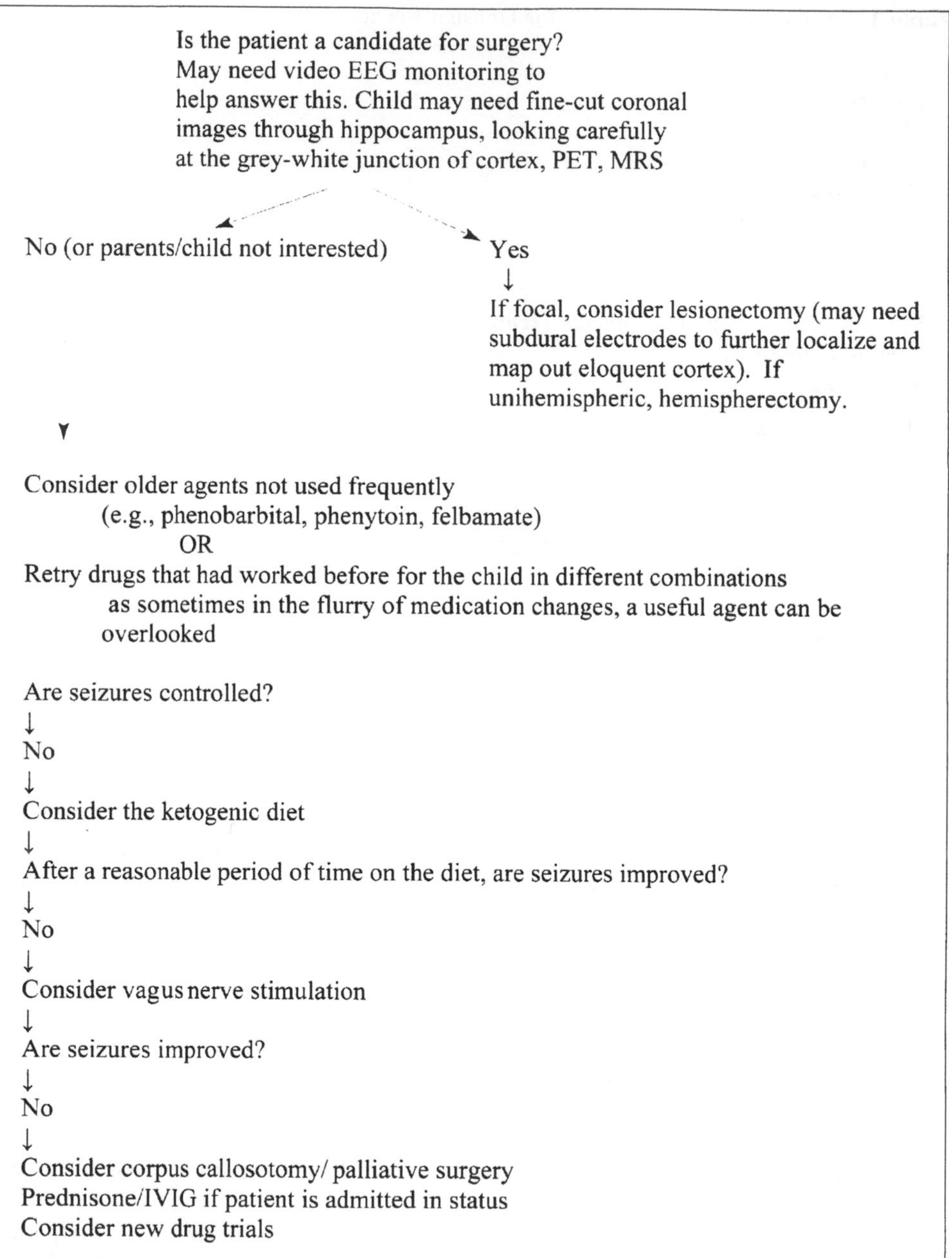

Is the patient a candidate for surgery?
May need video EEG monitoring to
help answer this. Child may need fine-cut coronal
images through hippocampus, looking carefully
at the grey-white junction of cortex, PET, MRS
No (or parents/child not interested)
Yes
↓
If focal, consider lesionectomy (may need
subdural electrodes to further localize and
map out eloquent cortex). If
unihemispheric, hemispherectomy.
Consider older agents not used frequently
(e.g., phenobarbital, phenytoin, felbamate)
OR
Retry drugs that had worked before for the child in different combinations
as sometimes in the flurry of medication changes, a useful agent can be
overlooked
Are seizures controlled?
↓
No
↓
Consider the ketogenic diet
↓
After a reasonable period of time on the diet, are seizures improved?
↓
No
↓
Consider vagus nerve stimulation
↓
Are seizures improved?
↓
No
↓
Consider corpus callosotomy/ palliative surgery
Prednisone/IVIG if patient is admitted in status
Consider new drug trials

Figure 2 Algorithm for intractable epilepsy-2.

TREATMENT

For the truly intractable patient, who has failed several anticonvulsants either due to poor efficacy or intolerable side effects, further medication options have limited efficacy (Fig. 2). There have been just as many anticonvulsants introduced in the past decade as in all years prior (Table 2). Although monotherapy is always the goal,

Table 2 Anticonvulsants Introduced Since 1993

Anticonvulsant	Trade name	Formulations	Special circumstances (not all currently FDA approved)	FDA approved in children?	Side effects
Felbamate	Felbatol™	Tablets (400, 600 mg), liquid (600/5 cc^3)	Juvenile myoclonic epilepsy, Lennox Gastaut syndrome	Yes (>2 yo)	Weight loss, hepatotoxicity, sleep disturbances, aplastic anemia (1:7900)
Gabapentin	Neurontin™	Tablets (600, 800 mg), capsules (100, 300, 400 mg), liquid (250/5 cc^3)	Pain, postherpetic neuralgia, few side effects and interactions, renally excreted	Yes (>3 yo)	Weight gain, leg edema
Lamotrigine	Lamictal™	Tablets (25, 50, 150, 200 mg), chewable–dispersible tablets (2, 5, 25 mg)	Lennox Gastaut, absence, juveniles myoclonic epilepsy, approved for monotherapy	Yes (>2 yo)	Rash (increased risk with combination valproate), requires slow titration
Topiramate	Topamax™	Tablets (25, 100, 200 mg), sprinkle caps (15, 25 mg)	Lennox Gastaut, infantile spasms	Yes (>2 yo)	Cognitive side effects, weight loss, renal stones, glaucoma (28:800,000), oligohydrosis
Tiagabine	Gabitril™	Tablets (2, 4, 12, 16 mg)	Spasticity	Yes (>12 yo)	Can worsen generalized seizures
Levetiracetam	Keppra™	Tablets (250, 500, 750 mg), liquid (500 mg/5 cc^3)	Myoclonic epilepsy, myoclonus	No	Behavioral changes, irritability, rare psychosis
Oxcarbazepine	Trileptal™	Tablets (150, 300, 600 mg), liquid (300 mg/5 cc^3)	Less side effects and interactions than carbamazepine	Yes (>4 yo)	Hyponatremia
Zonisamide	Zonegran™	Capsules (25, 50, 100 mg)	Refractory partial epilepsy, Lennox Gastaut, progressive myoclonic	No	Renal stones, oligohidrosis, weight loss

rational polytherapy may be necessary in these patients, as discussed above. There is little scientific evidence for any particularly beneficial combinations; however, ethosuximide and valproate, lamotrigine and valproate, and lamotrigine and topiramate have anecdotally been reported as effective.

A trial with older agents that are not typically considered nowadays because of the advent of many newer anticonvulsants can also be considered. Phenobarbital, phenytoin, primidone, ethosuximide, and long-acting benzodiazepines (e.g., clonazepam, clorazepate) are well-studied agents that certainly have their share of adverse reactions, but also have proven efficacy. We will often retry agents previously believed to be failures that were used in polytherapy years ago. Occasionally, these drugs will work well either in monotherapy, different combinations, or as the child has grown older.

Some newer agents with more significant side effect profiles may be worth the risk as well. For example, felbamate has a risk of aplastic anemia with dose initiation, which has limited its use. This has not been seen in children, however, and felbamate can be very efficacious, particularly for Lennox Gastaut syndrome. Vigabatrin, not available in the United States, is certainly worth attempting for intractable infantile spasms, especially if comorbid tuberous sclerosis exists. Irreversible visual field defects have limited its use long-term, but in some children the risk–benefit ratio makes vigabatrin worthwhile, and for infantile spasms the duration of therapy may be short enough to avoid visual defects. Lastly, although the pipeline of new anticonvulsants has slowed somewhat recently, many pediatric epilepsy centers are still investigating agents in development for use on a research basis.

Once a reasonable trial of anticonvulsants has been attempted, it is imperative to determine if the child is a candidate for epilepsy surgery. Surgery can be curative rather than just reduce seizures; nevertheless, the risks are significant. Recent evidence in adults suggests that if an epileptic focus is located in the temporal lobes, surgery is superior to medical management after 1 year, with 58% seizure-free at this time compared to 8% in the medical group. Evidence from children and even infants is equally strong, with approximately 60% seizure freedom with surgery. Parents must be willing to accept the potential for motor, language, cognitive, or visual deficits as well as possible mortality. In order to proceed with surgery, we seek a "convergence of evidence." Routine and video-EEG, clinical history, MRI, neurologic exam (occasionally showing focal deficits), and sometimes PET or MR spectroscopy data should all converge towards a uniform epileptogenic focus to be targeted. If not, bilateral subdural electrodes may need to be placed on the surface of the brain for better localization of the region or laterality of epileptogenicity.

Once the area is identified, baseline neuropsychologic testing and occasionally a Wada procedure to lateralize memory and language will be performed. Subdural grid electrodes placed over the region of interest are often required for a 1-week monitoring period before resection to delineate both epileptogenic and functional cortex. The smallest resection possible is always strived for, but in cases of intractable unihemispheric epilepsy (e.g., Rasmussen's syndrome, hemimegalenephaly, large congenital infarctions), a total hemispherectomy may be advised.

If the child is not a candidate for surgery, or the family and child do not wish to take the risk of loss of function, alternatives to further medication trials do exist and can be very beneficial. Whereas some would argue that these alternatives should be tried earlier than traditionally considered because of their relatively low side effect profile, they typically remain treatments of last resort. The ketogenic diet has been available as a dietary option since the 1920s, but starvation as a treatment for epilepsy was even described in the Bible. This high-fat, adequate-protein, low-carbohydrate therapy requires careful calorie and fluid management. The entire family must be invested in the process and we require the family to take classes in its management. Traditionally, children are admitted for a 48-hr fast, followed by gradual introduction of the ketogenic diet as an eggnog preparation. Even children with intractable epilepsy may show significant seizure reduction. In a large retrospective study at our institution, we found greater than 50% seizure reduction in 50% of patients and greater than 90% in 27%. Well-established side effects include constipation, slowed weight gain and growth, hyperlipidemia (reversible), and kidney stones (6%). A current trial of the Atkins diet, a therapy with less protein and calorie restriction that also induces ketosis, is underway as well.

Vagus nerve stimulation has emerged over the past decade as another tool for intractable epilepsy. This therapy has been approved by the FDA since 1997, but is not officially approved for use in children under age 12. More than 25,000 patients have been implanted and more than 7000 of these patients were under age 18 at surgery. The device is implanted in the operating room. It is then programmed over the ensuing months. Standard stimulation settings of 30 sec on and 5 min off are initially programmed, but can be adjusted as needed. The vagus nerve stimulator is theorized to stimulate the nucleus solitarius and locus ceruleus, but its effects on the brain and EEG patterns are less clear. Efficacy is typically a 25–40% seizure reduction, similar to most new anticonvulsants. However, side effects are few and limited generally to voice change and hoarseness. In addition, a small magnet that causes an immediate stimulation to occur can be used to try and abort seizures, allowing the child and family a unique form of acute therapy. Reports of behavioral improvement have also been described in the recent literature.

Corpus callosotomy can also be performed for intractable nonfocal epilepsy, commonly atonic seizures. Callosotomies have been used since 1940 and are either partial (anterior two-thirds) or complete in two stages. This therapy specifically benefits atonic seizures, but is more palliative than curative according to reports, with an approximate 8% seizure-free rate described. Side effects include transient left-sided neglect, mutism, and apraxia. In catastrophic cases where a child is in persistent status epilepticus, the use of intravenous solumedrol or immunoglobulin has been described as a potential immunomodulating therapy. There is little scientific evidence for steroids other than in infantile spasms outside of anecdotal reports.

SUGGESTED READINGS

1. Berg AT, Shinnar S, Levy SR, Testa FM, Smith-Rapaport S, Beckerman B. Early development of intractable epilepsy in children: a prospective study. Neurology 2001; 56: 1445–1452.
2. Freeman JM, Vining EP, Pillas DJ, Pyzik PL, Casey JC, Kelly LM. The efficacy of the ketogenic diet-1998: a prospective evaluation of intervention in 150 children. Pediatrics 1998; 102:1358–1363.
3. Karceski S, Morrell M, Carpenter D. The expert consensus guideline series: treatment of epilepsy. Epilepsy Behav 2001; 2:A1–A50.
4. Kwan P, Brodie MJ. Effectiveness of first antiepileptic drug. Epilepsia 2001; 42:1255–1260.
5. Vining EPG, Freeman JM, Pillas DJ, Uematsu S, Carson BS, Brandt J, Boatman D, Pulsifer MB, Zuckerberg A. Why would you remove half a brain? The outcome of 58 children after hemispherectomy—The Johns Hopkins Experience 1968–1996. Pediatrics 1997; 100:163–171.

6. Wheless JW, Maggio V. Vagus nerve stimulation therapy in patients younger than 18 years. Neurology 2002; 59(suppl 4):S21–S25.
7. Wiebe S, Blume WT, Girvin JP, Eliasziw M. A randomized, controlled trial of surgery for temporal-lobe epilepsy. N Engl J Med 2001; 345:311–318.

17
Infantile Spasms

Eric H. Kossoff
The Johns Hopkins Hospital, Baltimore, Maryland, U.S.A.

INTRODUCTION

Infantile spasms is an epilepsy syndrome associated with acquired mental retardation that affects infants usually between the third and eighth month of life. It was recognized as far back as 1841 when Dr. West described a condition afflicting his infant son. It is a generalized seizure disorder characterized by clusters of sudden flexor or extensor jerks. Spasms are often initially misdiagnosed as colic or gastroesophageal reflux before they increase in frequency and severity. In many children, loss of developmental milestones can occur. West syndrome specifically is the triad of infantile spasms, psychomotor regression, and the electroencephalogram (EEG) pattern of hypsarrhythmia. The incidence of infantile spasms is low, but the disorder is not uncommon, with approximately 1 per 3000 births.

DIAGNOSIS AND EVALUATION

The etiology of infantile spasms warrants careful investigation, with from 50% to 70% of patients having a defined cause (symptomatic), including metabolic conditions, perinatal asphyxia, Down syndrome, cerebral infarction, structural malformations, and tuberous sclerosis. Relatively fewer cases are defined as having a cryptogenic (unclear) etiology. The diagnosis is confirmed by EEG, showing a chaotic pattern of multifocal spikes without normal background rhythms, otherwise known as hypsarrhythmia.

TREATMENT

Many treatments have been proposed for ameliorating infantile spasms, but very few have been demonstrated to be consistently effective (Table 1). Only 11 randomized, controlled trials have been reported in the literature, comprising a total of 477 patients. A recent Cochrane review of the literature from 1960 to 2000 stated "there is still little evidence available on the optimum treatment for infantile spasms." However, a practice parameter from the American Academy of Neurology and the Child

Table 1 Efficacies of Anticonvulsants in Reports for New-Onset Infantile Spasms

Medication	Seizure free by 3–6 months (%)	Side effects
ACTH	50–86	Hypertension, GI upset, irritability, glaucoma, death, use only short-term
Vigabatrin	36–76	Visual field constriction
Valproate	40–63	Hepatic toxicity
Lamotrigine	33	Rash, slow titration
Topiramate	45	Cognitive effects, renal stones
Zonisamide	33	Renal stones, anhydrosis
Clonazepam/nitrazepam	33–50	Increased salivation, dependence, sedation

Neurology Society was recently be published giving general recommendations. On the basis of existing medical literature, a suggested algorithm for an approach to new-onset infantile spasms is presented (Table 2).

ACTH

ACTH (adrenocorticotropic hormone) has been used for infantile spasms since the 1950s. The proposed benefit may lie from reduction of neuronal excitability, and the influence of endogenous steroids on decreasing the level of insulin, and thus both

Table 2 Algorithm for Infantile Spasms

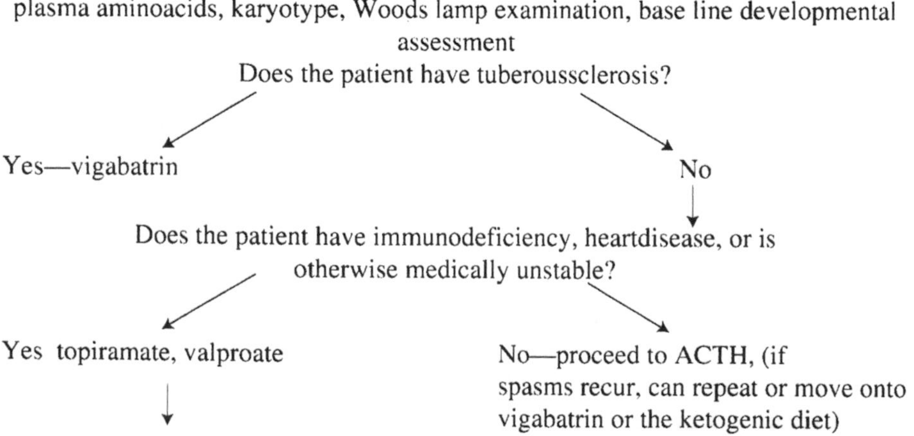
New-onset-infantile spasms?
Obtain MRI, EEG with 100 mg IVB6 injection, lumbar puncture, urine organic acids, plasma aminoacids, karyotype, Woods lamp examination, base line developmental assessment
Does the patient have tuberoussclerosis?
Yes—vigabatrin
No
Does the patient have immunodeficiency, heartdisease, or is otherwise medically unstable?
Yes topiramate, valproate
No—proceed to ACTH, (if spasms recur, can repeat or move onto vigabatrin or the ketogenic diet)
Consider use of the ketogenic diet, vigabatrin, topiramate, valproate or prednisone based on individual preferences.

reducing norepinephrine and increasing dopamine neurotransmission. The combination of these effects seems to reduce seizure sensitivity. Studies have revealed a 50–86% effectiveness of ACTH in eradicating spasms in infants. We use the Snead protocol; ACTH 150 units/m^2/day divided twice a day for 1 week, then 75 units/m^2/day divided once a day for 1 week, occasinally 75 units/m^2/day divided every other day for 2 weeks, occasionally tapering over the next several weeks. Other approaches include higher doses for longer periods of time, but the superiority of one approach over another is unclear. At this time, ACTH remains the agent of first choice for new-onset infantile spasms.

However, ACTH is not without its problems. In particular, it is a temporary therapy. Unlike more traditional anticonvulsants, ACTH cannot be continued long term. Spasms can occasionally recur after ACTH is discontinued, but after perhaps one or two repeated treatment courses (each usually lasting 4 weeks), it must be abandoned to avoid the side effects of chronic steroids. These side effects can include hypertension, susceptibility to infection, cerebral atrophy, obesity, edema, gastric ulceration and hemorrhage, hyperphagia, glaucoma, and irritability. Mortality can be as high as 5%. All these difficulties can be seen even with the first course of ACTH. Also, ACTH is quite expensive, costing approximately $745 for a 3-week course.

Vigabatrin

Vigabatrin is another recent medication that has become available. Vigabatrin was introduced in 1994 for the treatment of partial epilepsy. It works by irreversibly inactivating GABA-transaminase allowing higher levels of the inhibitory neurotransmitter. The dose recommended is 100 mg/kg/day divided twice daily, titrated up from 25 to 50 mg/kg/day over a 7–day period. Vigabatrin has been shown to have promise in infantile spasms, with 48–76% efficacy by 2 weeks. Some experts recommend the specific usage of vigabatrin first line for infantile spasms secondary to tuberous sclerosis.

Vigabatrin is also not without side effects. The potential side effects of visual field constriction, loss of acuity, and color vision may be irreversible according to some studies. In infants, it may be years before adequate ophthalmologic testing could reveal the retinal damage. It is unclear whether this response is total dose related or not, and an electroretinogram (ERG) is recommended if therapy continues beyond 6 weeks. Because of this side effect, the U.S. FDA withdrew the drug from the market. It is currently available in Canada, Mexico, and abroad, but may return to the United States hopefuly soon.

Ketogenic Diet

The ketogenic diet has been proposed for predominantly recalcitrant infantile spasms. Livingston originally described the use of the diet in this population with success. Indeed, before the use of ACTH, the ketogenic diet was thought to be the most useful therapy. The potential benefit of the ketogenic diet for infantile spasms makes sense given on the current basic science literature. As discussed earlier, elevated cortisol with decreased insulin, resulting from ACTH administration, may be neuroprotective. The ketogenic diet has been shown to have similar effects on these hormones. However, the indirect effect of the ketogenic diet on corticotropin releasing hormone specifically, although logical, remains to be proven.

From 1996 to 2000, 23 children with infantile spasms, aged 5 months to 2 years were started on the ketogenic diet at our institution. These children had mostly intractable seizures, with an average of 541 spasm clusters per month (range 60–3000) and had been previously exposed to an average of 3.3 antiepileptic medications (range 0–7). At 3–12 months, 38–53% of all patients currently on the diet were >90% improved (3 were seizure free at 12 months); 67–100% were >50% improved. The ketogenic diet has been used at our institution as first-line therapy in five patients, with >90% seizure freedom in three. A multicenter pilot study of the ketogenic diet for new-onset infantile spasms is being planned. Please refer to the chapter on the ketogenic diet for further information.

Other Approaches

Other than these agents, the practicing child neurologist has very few proven options. Sodium valproate and clonazepam have had only limited success in abolition of spasms, and are not thought to be particularly efficacious in comparison to ACTH. There is some evidence for the use of pyridoxine (vitamin B6) for infantile spasms, but the data are sparse. We advise an EEG with 100 mg intravenous B6 provided concurrently; should the EEG improve dramatically then pyridoxine would be continued. Newer drugs, such as topiramate, lamotrigine, zonisamide, and ganaxolone have all been tested for infantile spasms in case series but have only limited efficacy (similar to the natural history of resolution of infantile spasms) with their particular set of side effects. There is no evidence for the adjunctive use of any of these anticonvulsants for infantile spasms.

PROGNOSIS

Although some studies show that early therapy is associated with a better long-term seizure and developmental outcome, the data are quite limited. The majority of the prospective evidence would suggest that there is no specific therapy that is more likely to improve either long-term seizure or cognitive outcome. Half of children go on to have Lennox Gastaut syndrome; 80–90% of children will have mental retardation regardless of how prompt the therapy is, with better cognitive outcome for those without a specific etiology (cryptogenic patients). Mortality can be as high as 20%.

SUMMARY

Infantile spasms is a relatively common epilepsy syndrome affecting young infants and often with devastating results. The current gold standard therapy remains ACTH at this time. However, vigabatrin and the ketogenic diet may become more useful agents in the future. Other therapies are of little proven value. With significant morbidity, the need for additional therapies for infantile spasms is clearly imperative.

SUGGESTED READINGS

1. Elterman RD, Shields WD, Mansfield KA, Nakagawa JA. Randomized trial of vigabatrin in patients with infantile spasms. Neurology 2001; 57:1416–1421.

2. Hancock E, Osborne JP, Milner P. The treatment of West syndrome: a Cochrane review of the literature to December 2000. Brain Dev 2001; 23:624–634.
3. Hrachovy RA, Frost JD Jr, Kellaway P, Zion T. A controlled study of ACTH therapy in infantile spasms. Epilepsia 1980; 21:631–636.
4. Kossoff EH, Pyzik PL, McGrogan JR, Vining EPG, Freeman JM. Efficacy of the ketogenic diet for infantile spasms. Pediatrics 2002; 109:780–783.
5. Mackay M, Weiss S, Snead OC. Treatment of infantile spasms: an evidence-based approach. Int Rev Neurobiol 2002; 49:157–184.
6. Snead III OC, Benton JW, Myers GJ. ACTH and prednisone in childhood seizure disorders. Neurology 1983; 33:966–970.
7. Vigevano F, Cilio MR. Vigabatrin versus ACTH as first-line treatment for infantile spasms: a randomized, prospective study. Epilepsia 1997; 38:1270–1274.
8. Mackay MT, Meiss SK, Adama-Webber T, et.al. Practice parameter: medical treatment of infantile spasms: report of the American Academy of Neurology and the Child Neurology Society. Neurolory, 2004; 62:1668–1681.

18

Benign Epilepsy with Centrotemporal Spikes

James E. Rubenstein
Johns Hopkins Medical Institutions, Baltimore, Maryland, U.S.A.

INTRODUCTION

Benign epilepsy with centrotemporal spikes (BECTS) is also still frequently referred to as benign rolandic epilepsy. It is the most common of the idiopathic partial epilepsies of childhood (IPEC) and ranks second in incidence behind only childhood absence epilepsy (CAE) in children under 15 years of age. It is classified as "benign" by the International League Against Epilepsy (ILAE) because it has a generally favorable prognosis and is almost always outgrown by age 18 regardless of anticonvulsant intervention.

DIAGNOSIS AND EVALUATION

Age of onset is from 2 to 13 years, with 80% beginning between 5 and 10 years, and peak onset at 9 years. Consistent with the observation that BECTS has a strong genetic basis, studies show a positive family history in 20–30%. The electroencephalographic (EEG) findings in families appear to have an autosomal dominant pattern. The gene for BECTS is located on chromosome 15q14 and there is incomplete penetrance. There is an association with perinatal difficulties, central nervous system infection, head trauma, or other possible causes in only 10% of cases. The affected children are by definition neurologically intact, with normal clinical examination and normal neuroimaging. There is an association between mild behavioral and learning difficulties and the presence of centrotemporal spikes with and without seizures.

Nocturnal seizures are the norm, occurring in 75% of patients as the only seizure timing. There can be variability in frequency and severity from a single, brief event or rare episodes in 67% up to frequent events or rarely status epilepticus. Children report hemisensory and motor phenomena of the facial and oral structures, and motor findings in the limbs (which may be unilateral or generalized). With the nocturnal-only presentation of BECTS frequently seizures, may be unwitnessed or only suspected based on atypical enuresis or fatigue in the morning.

Interictal characteristics of the EEG in BECTS include high amplitude, centrotemporal sharp waves that may be bilateral or unilateral, semirhythmic at times, and are superimposed on a normal background. These sharp waves are more likely to spread from the perirolandic region when they are higher in voltage. They are not altered or modified by eyelid movement, hyperventilation, or photic stimulation. As awake readings will miss up to 80% of findings, the EEG must encompass some periods of sleep.

Differential diagnosis includes focal cortical lesions that may mimic the BECTS phenotype, such as migrational disorders, symptomatic arachnoid cysts, glial scarring, and cavernous hemangiomas. However, in a child with a classic history, EEG, and normal neurologic examination, an MRI is not necessary.

TREATMENT

The diagnosis of BECTS results in one of the most interesting management decisions in pediatric epilepsy practice because there is clear evidence that remission occurs regardless of the decision to treat with anticonvulsants and a large proportion of affected individuals have seizures only at night. This complicates the usual conundrum for the clinician, who is challenged by the patient and/or the parent(s) to answer the three key questions: who, how, and for how long?

Early onset, focal seizures, and shorter initial interepisode interval are thought to be predictors of seizure recurrence, and hence may lead to a decision to intervene in approximately half the cases. However, if seizures are infrequent and brief, families may choose to avoid treatment. The recommendation to avoid sleep deprivation is always warranted for patients with BECTS.

Fortunately, the seizures themselves are almost always responsive to low-dose monotherapy with carbamazepine. With nocturnal-only seizures, the use of an extended-release preparation at night (e.g., Carbatrol™ or Tegretol XR™) is an option. Valproate, phenytoin, gabapentin, and lamotrigine have also been reported as helpful. The choice of medication should be individualized based on potential side effects.

There is general agreement based on the natural history of BECTS that anticonvulsant therapy after age 16 is unwarranted. It may be somewhat problematic, however, to discontinue anticonvulsant treatment at age 16 because teenagers approaching driving age may be reluctant to risk seizure recurrence by terminating treatment. This requires the patient, parents, and the clinician to carefully review the clinical course in order to make an informed choice.

SUMMARY

Benign epilepsy with centrotemporal spikes (BECTS) is the most common idiopathic partial epilepsy syndrome in childhood, ranking second only to childhood absence epilepsy in incidence under the age of 15 years. It has a classical EEG pattern of high amplitude centrotemporal sharp waves that may be bilateral or unilateral, accentuated by sleep. There is a likely autosomal dominant pattern of inheritance with incomplete penetrance. Affected individuals are neurologically normal. The syndrome is generally outgrown with or without anticonvulsants by age 18 years, but treatment with low-dose carbamazepine can be beneficial if desired.

SUGGESTED READINGS

1. Bouma PA, Bovenkerk AC, Westendorp RG, Brouwer OF. The course of benign partial epilepsy of childhood with centrotemporal spikes: a meta-analysis. Neurology 1997; 48:430–437.
2. Croona C, Kihlgren M, Lundberg S, Eeg-Olofsson O, Eeg-Olofsson KE. Neuropsychological findings in children with benign childhood epilepsy with centrotemporal spikes. Dev Med Child Neurol 1999; 41:813–818.
3. Loiseau P, Duche B, Cordova S, et al. Prognosis of benign childhood epilepsy with centrotemporal spikes : a followup study of 168 patients. Epilepsia 1988; 29:229–235.
4. Neubauer BA, Fiedler B, Himmelein B, et al. Centrotemporal spikes in families with rolandic epilepsy: linkage to chromosome 15q14. Neurology 1998; 51:1608–1612.
5. Saint-Martin AD, Carcangiu R, Arzimanoglou A, Massa R, Thomas P, Motte J, Marescaux C, Metz-Lutz MN, Hirsch E. Semiology of typical and atypical Rolandic epilepsy: a video-EEG analysis. Epileptic Disord 2001; 3:173–182.
6. Weglage J, Demsky A, Pietsch M, Kurlemann G. Neuropsychological, intellectual, and behavioral findings in patients with centrotemporal spikes with and without seizures. Dev Med Child Neurol 1997; 39:646–651.

19
Rasmussen's Syndrome

Eileen P.G. Vining
The John M. Freeman Pediatric Epilepsy Center, Johns Hopkins Hospital, Baltimore, Maryland, U.S.A.

INTRODUCTION

Rasmussen's syndrome (RS) is a chronic encephalitis that leads to a progressive unilateral seizure disorder, functional decline, and hemiplegia. Although Rasmussen and colleagues originally described this syndrome in 1958 in the context of possible viral encephalitis, similar to Kozhevnikov's epilepsy (tick-borne encephalitis with a similar scenario of epilepsia partialis continua), no consistent viral etiology has ever been identified. It is currently believed to be an autoimmune disease, based both on the pathology that has been elucidated and response to therapy.

ETIOLOGY

The original pathological description of perivascular round cell infiltration, microglial nodules, astrocytosis, and spongy degeneration suggested a viral "footprint," and although recent infectious illness was seen in about half of the original patients, determined efforts to isolate viruses or their DNA/RNA have been unsuccessful. The tissue from affected patients has not been able to infect other animals or cell cultures and electron microscopy has not identified viruses. More recent attempts using polymerase chain reaction (PCR) have demonstrated a wide array of findings, but no consistent picture, with CMV, HSV1, and EBV variably implicated.

Interest in the immunologic basis of RS emerged in the 1990s. Rogers and colleagues reported elevated levels of antibodies to a glutamate receptor (GluR3). They, and others, hypothesized that these antibodies could be highly neurotoxic. This led to a very complex hypothesis concerning the unihemispheric nature of RS. They proposed that there was a focal disruption of the blood–brain barrier that permitted GluR3 antibodies to interact with the glutamate receptors. Theorizing that if these antibodies could be eliminated, patients would improve, they treated a number of patients with plasmapheresis. The initial patient, and many others, responded initially to this therapy with a decrease in seizures and improved function. However, over time repeated pheresis did not maintain this improvement and children deteriorated.

More recently, interest has turned to a cellular mechanism leading to the inflammatory response. This theory evokes an extensive lymphocytic infiltration by CD8 killer T cells. There is an extensive astroglial reaction, microglial activation, and cytolysis. There is also a marked increase in cytokines.

CLINICAL ASPECTS

Although RS is considered a disorder of childhood and one that affects only a single hemisphere, there have been reported instances of Rasmussen-like conditions that have begun in adulthood or that have involved both hemispheres. Classically, seizures begin in the early school years, with a range of onset from the second year of life to mid-teens. The initial seizure can be partial, generalized, or even an episode of status epilepticus. Seizures then typically evolve over time to produce a multifocal or unilateral condition of epilepsia partialis continua that is seen in slightly more than half of individuals with RS.

The progression of a seizure is quite different from the well-understood Jacksonian march. Instead, one sees the clinical manifestations of separated areas of cortex firing independently. One can see the foot jerk, then the shoulder, then the thigh, then the hand, and then the face, with no contiguous march along the homunculus. It can almost be visualized as a popcorn effect: suddenly a seizure pops from one area, then another. This is also not like polymyoclonus, because the clonic activity can remain active in one area, but be rhythmically clonic at a different frequency in another area of the body. Another, somewhat less common presentation involves the basal ganglia and one can see expressions of dystonia and choreoathetosis in the setting of RS as well. Invariably, the process continues, resulting in hemiplegia or hemiparesis, homonymous hemianopia and functional deterioration.

There is no diagnostic test that is invariably conclusive. Neuroimaging has shown considerable utility because over time some degree of atrophy becomes apparent. Recent work has suggested that one can assess a hemispheric ratio from MRI studies to determine the degree and rate of atrophy of the hemisphere, with some evidence that most of the atrophy occurs in the first year of the disease. However, there is huge variability in RS and some individuals present with extensive atrophy at the time of their first seizure while others display a much slower course of progression. This can often lead to delays in diagnosis. Other newer modalities may be useful, including magnetic resonance spectroscopy (MRS) in which *N*-acetyl-aspartic acid (NAA), a marker of neuronal death or injury, has been shown to be decreased beyond what would be expected based simply on atrophy. Other modalities such as diffusion-weighted imaging may also be helpful in the future.

Electroencephalography is also not specific. At best, it would show slowing over the affected hemisphere with multifocal spikes. At worst, because it can create doubt of the diagnosis, seemingly independent discharges can be seen bilaterally. With careful analysis, large asymmetries are usually apparent, and the spike from the truly abnormal hemisphere can often be seen to be leading the contralateral spike by milliseconds.

Some debate continues about the utility of brain biopsy. We do not believe it is useful because we are aware of the pathology that can show normal tissue intimately adjacent to inflamed tissue. Even with use of MRI-guided biopsy we know that the biopsy can still be negative, sometimes interfering with the appropriate management of the condition. Several years ago, serum for GluR3 antibodies was routinely sent.

Unfortunately, this was never available on a standardized basis and the literature is clear that the test can be positive in some control individuals and negative in some with proved RS. At this time, the diagnosis remains clinical: unilateral progressive epilepsy in the setting of atrophying brain.

TREATMENT

The progress of RS is inexorable, but variable. Aggressive medical management with anticonvulsant medication is uniformly unsuccessful. Seizures can be contained to some degree, but they cannot be stopped; it is imperative that the physician pays careful attention to the amount of side effects produced by the medications, often for very little additional benefit. Certainly, with the concern that RS may be viral-related, numerous attempts to treat with antiviral agents have been made with little success. The use of immunomodulatory therapy has increased over the last decade, influenced by the further understanding of the pathogenesis of the condition. Plasmapheresis may produce a rapid, but unsustainable, improvement in the child's condition and this may be important to the immediate management of devastating seizures. Various steroid protocols have been suggested, but again, none appear to offer sustained relief and there are the obvious problems inherent in the prolonged use of such treatment. Intravenous immunoglobulin (IVIg) is also a reasonable, albeit again short-term approach, for most individuals. There are various protocols suggested, including: monthly cycles of high-dose IVIg (0.4 g/kg/day for 5 days) followed by maintenance therapy (0.4 g/kg/day each month) after the patients' conditions began to improve.

Unfortunately, the only therapy that has shown consistently favorable results is surgery. There are a variety of approaches that appear to be useful, ranging from the hemidecorticectomy procedure used at Hopkins to functional hemispherectomy and the recently described hemispherotomy technique. Results appear quite similar with 80–90% of children experiencing either complete relief from seizures or negligible auras. There is morbidity and mortality associated with this surgery and it should not be minimized. Problems include infection in about 5–10% and a need for shunt placement in about 20% of patients. On the other hand, improvement in function is often dramatic. This is clearly related to the elimination of seizures, but in addition, motor function also may actually improve in spite of the dense hemiplegia. This perhaps relates to the stability and predictability of the deficit, rather than the unpredictability of motor function in the setting of recurring seizures. Postoperatively, the decline in intelligence appears to stabilize and some children actually improve. This may depend considerably on whether the right or left hemisphere is involved and the ultimate impact on language. It is perhaps also related to the extent of rehabilitation services available to the child. We believe it is important for children and parents to participate in a network of other families in order to better understand the problems and solutions that may arise.

THE FUTURE

Improvement in care for patients with RS lies along many avenues. Certainly, a better understanding of the pathogenesis will lead to better therapies. This may include novel strategies such as immunoablation with high-dose cyclophosphamide, in which one attempts to eliminate the entire host population of "sensitized" T cells, or the use of other immunosuppressive agents such as tacrolimus. Improved neuroimaging may provide us with additional strategies to assess the impact of therapy. Surgical strategies need constant refining, in order to eliminate the 10–20% of children who appear to be left with residual tissue or "nondisconnected" tissue. Finally, rehabilitation must improve with better strategies to improve gait; programs that might involve computer-assisted devices to improve hand and finger function; and finally improved understanding of the cognitive, language, and behavioral problems these children face so that they can function as productive, capable, and happy adults.

SUGGESTED READINGS

1. Bien CG, Bauer J, Deckwerth TL, Wiendl H, Deckert M, Wiestler OD, et al. Destruction of neurons by cytotoxic T cells: a new pathogenic mechanism in Rasmussen's encephalitis. Ann Neurol 2002; 51:311–318.
2. Gordon N. Rasmussen's encephalitis. Dev Med Child Neurol 1997; 39(2):133–136.
3. Leach JP, Chadwick DW, Miles JB, Hart IK. Improvement in adult-onset Rasmussen's encephalitis with long-term immunomodulatory therapy. Neurology 1999; 52:738–742.
4. Villemure J-G, Andermann F, Rasmussen TB. Hemispherectomy for the treatment of epilepsy due to chronic encephalitis. In: Andermann F, ed. Chronic Encephalitis and Epilepsy. Boston: Butterworth-Heineman, 1991:235–244.
5. Vining EPG, Freeman JM, Pillas DJ, Uematsu S, Carson BS, Brandt J, et al. Why would you remove half a brain? The outcome of 58 children after hemispherectomy—The Johns Hopkins Experience 1968–1996. Pediatrics 1997; 100:163–171.
6. Vining EPG. Rasmussen's syndrome. In: Kotagal P, Luders HO, eds. The Epilepsies: Etiologies and Prevention. San Diego: Academic Press, 1999:283–288.

20
Treatment of Tourette Syndrome

Harvey S. Singer
Departments of Neurology and Pediatrics, Johns Hopkins University School of Medicine, Baltimore, Maryland, U.S.A.

OVERVIEW

The Gilles de la Tourette syndrome (TS) is a chronic, inherited neuropsychiatric disorder characterized by the presence of involuntary motor and phonic tics that wax and wane. Although once considered a rare disorder, the prevalence of TS may be as high as 3.5% of school-aged children. In addition to tics, individuals with TS often have a variety of concomitant psychopathologies including obsessive compulsive disorder (OCD), attention deficit hyperactivity disorder (ADHD), learning difficulties, and sleep abnormalities. Although the presence of neurobehavioral problems is not required for the diagnosis of TS, their clinical impact on the patient may be more significant than the tics themselves. Tourette syndrome is an inherited disorder (specific gene and mode of inheritance remain unclear), but nongenetic environmental factors can influence tic frequency and severity. Pathophysiologically, tics arise within cortico-striatal-thalamo-cortical pathways and likely represent a dysfunction of synaptic neurotransmission.

Diagnosis

Formal diagnostic criteria include: (a) onset of symptoms before age 21; (b) the presence of multiple motor and at least one vocal tic (not necessarily concurrently); (c) a waxing and waning course, with tics evolving in a progressive manner; (d) the presence of tic symptoms for at least 1 year; (e) the absence of a precipitating illnesses (e.g., encephalitis, stroke, or degenerative disease) or association with potential tic-inducing medication; and (e) the observation of tics by a knowledgeable individual. Tics, the essential component of the syndrome, are manifest in a variety of forms, with different durations and degrees of complexity. Common characteristics of tics include: brief voluntary suppression; exacerbation by anxiety, excitement, anger, or fatigue; reduction during absorbing activities or sleep; and fluctuation over time. Premonitory urges or sensations, such as a tickle, itch, discomfort, or "feeling," are reported in some TS patients before they make a tic movement or vocalization.

Outcome

Although TS was originally proposed to be a lifelong disorder, its course may be quite variable, and some patients may have a spontaneous remission or marked improvement independent of the use of tic-suppressing medications. Investigators used a mathematical model to assess the time course of tic severity over the first two decades, which suggested that maximum tic severity occurs between the ages of 8 and 12 years and is then followed by a steady decline in symptoms. In a study of 58 teenager/young adults, tics virtually disappeared in 26%, diminished considerably in 46%, remained stable in 14%, and increased in 14%. Early tic severity is not a good predictor of later tic severity, but some authors have suggested that the presence of only mild tics through adolescence was a good indicator of mild tics in adulthood. Nevertheless, even cases with severe tics in childhood had the potential for a good outcome.

EVALUATION AND EDUCATION

Although approaches to the assessment and treatment of individuals with TS may vary, there are several important steps (Table 1). All patients with tics should be evaluated to assure the proper diagnosis and to eliminate the possibility that tics are secondary to another medical condition. Personal interview of the patient and parent and the use of standardized parent/teacher questionnaires are helpful in identifying the presence of comorbid psychopathology and academic problems. Further, it is essential to identify the level of adaptive functioning, degree of impairment, and extent of distress associated with tics and with each comorbid condition. The physician should educate the patient and family about the characteristics of the disorder, that tics wax and wane, have periodic fluctuations, and are variable. It should be emphasized that tics are involuntary and not secondary to stress or an underlying psychological problem. The effect of environmental factors should be clarified and the controversial role of infection noted. The purpose of symptomatic therapy must be carefully reviewed, and its goals of targeting specific symptoms defined. Finally, physicians must emphasize that they are there to provide long-term treatment.

TREATMENT

Treatment is individualized on the basis of the functional impairment resulting from tics and/or comorbid problems, sources of support, capacities for coping, and challenges associated with various stages of development. Medications should

Table 1 General Principles for Evaluation of Patient with Tics

(1) Document tics
(2) Take history and perform physical examination
(3) Assess for comorbid psychopathology and academic problems
(4) Identify degree of impairment and extent of distress for tics and each comorbid condition
(5) Educate the patient and family
(6) Establish consensus about need for treatment
(7) Discuss available therapy
(8) Emphasize your availability to provide long-term treatment

Table 2 Treatment Decisions

General
1. Clarify patient's difficulties (tics or comorbid problems)
2. Define what symptoms require pharmacotherapy
If tics are causing significant psychosocial or physical problems, consider Rx
3. Remember, tic-suppressing medications do not generally treat comorbid issues
4. A conservative approach is recommended
Observation or nonpharmacologic

be targeted and reserved for only those problems that are functionally disabling and not remediable by nondrug interventions. For many families, education about the diagnosis, outcome, genetic predisposition, underlying pathophysiologic mechanism, and availability of tic-suppressing pharmacotherapy often obviate or delay the need for medication. Discussing and treating comorbid symptoms as separate entities from tics has enabled families and health-care specialists to focus on individual needs more effectively. Finally, reassuring the family, providing clear and accurate information, and allowing adequate time for questions and responses enhance the ability of patients and family members to cope with issues surrounding this disorder (Table 2).

Treatment of Tics

Initiation of tic-suppressing pharmacotherapy is restricted to those patients whose tics are causing psychosocial (i.e., loss of self-esteem, peer problems, difficulty in participating in academic, work, family, social, and after-school activities, and disruption of classroom settings) or musculoskeletal/physical problems. All other patients are counseled and observed for progression of symptoms. In general, a conservative approach is strongly recommended. Physicians considering behavioral or pharmacologic treatments should be aware of the natural variability and waxing and waning of tics, the large placebo response, and the strong influence of other comorbid psychopathologies on outcome.

Nonpharmacological Therapy

Classroom strategies of potential benefit include education of teachers and fellow students, providing optional study breaks, and eliminating unnecessary stressful situations. In addition, a variety of behavioral treatments (conditioning techniques, massed negative practice, awareness training, habit reversal, relaxation training, biofeedback, and hypnosis) have been proposed as alternative therapeutic approaches for tics, but few have been adequately evaluated. In my practice, behavioral approaches are considered in highly motivated individuals who wish to avoid medications, or as an adjunctive therapy in those with stressful life situations or in whom increasing the medication dose may result in excessive side effects. There is little or no supporting scientific evidence for the use of alternative dietary therapies (i.e., vitamins, herbs, protein supplementation, elimination diets, and others), or acupuncture.

Pharmacotherapy

If tic-suppressing medication is indicated, a two-tiered approach is generally recommended that is broadly divided into an initial "milder" (nonneuroleptic) medication

Table 3 Principles of Tic Pharmacotherapy

1. Start with low doses and increase gradually
2. Evaluate efficacy and monitor for side effects
3. Use monotherapy whenever possible
4. Use Tier 1 medications first, especially for milder tics
5. Obtain predrug EKG, when indicated, for Tier 2 medications
6. Taper medication after appropriate treatment periods

group and a second neuroleptic/atypical neuroleptic group. The goal of treatment is not to suppress movements entirely, but to reduce them to the point at which they no longer cause a significant psychosocial disturbance. Therapeutic agents should be prescribed at the lowest effective dosage and the patient should be carefully followed, with periodic evaluations to determine the need for continued therapy (Table 3). Generally, after several months of successful treatment, I consider a gradual taper of the medication during a nonstressful time. Typically, in school-aged children, the summer vacation is a good time to begin the taper. Although a variety of medications are prescribed for tic suppression (Table 4), only pimozide and haloperidol are approved by the FDA for TS.

First Tier Pharmacotherapy.

Clonidine. In individuals with milder tics, especially in those with behavioral problems (i.e., ADHD, poor frustration tolerance, and aggressive outbursts), I first

Table 4 Medications for Tic Suppression

Tier 1	
	Unproven
Clonidine (Catapres)	Gabapentin
Guanfacine (Tenex)	Topiramate
Baclofen (Lioresal)	Levetiracetam
Clonazepam (Klonopin)	
Tier 2	
	Unavailable in the U.S,
Pimozide (Orap)	Tetrabenazine (Nitoman)
Fluphenazine (Prolixin)	Sulpiride
Risperidone (Risperidol)	Tiapride
Olanzepine (Zyprexa)	
Quetiapine (Seraquel)	
Haloperidol (Haldol)	
Trifluoperazine (Stelazine)	
Ziprasidone (Geodon)	
In selected situations	
Botulinum toxin	
Pergolide (Permax)	
Nicotine patch	
Experimental	
Delta-9-tetrahydrocannabinol	
Transcranial magnetic stimulation	

prescribe the α-2-adrenergic receptor agonist clonidine (primarily activates presynaptic autoreceptors and reduces norepinephrine release and turnover). If there are no side effects to a morning test dose of 0.05 mg, the dose is increased to 0.05 mg BID. Doses are gradually increased about every 5–7 days up to a daily dose of 0.1–0.4 mg. Response to treatment may be delayed for 6–8 weeks. For the treatment of comorbid ADHD, clonidine should be used TID to QID (typical dose 0.05 mg QID). The most common side effect is drowsiness, which often resolves spontaneously. Dry mouth, itchy eyes, postural hypotension, bradycardia, headaches, nocturnal unrest, euphoria, and a mild withdrawal syndrome (increased tics, anxiety, and irritability) are occasionally reported. Clonidine is also available as a transdermal patch, but in active children, it may be difficult to keep the patch in place and there may be local skin hypersensitivity reactions. Clonidine should be gradually tapered to avoid rebound tic exacerbation and hypertension.

Guanfacine. Guanfacine is a longer acting α-2-adrenergic receptor agonist that is more selective for postsynaptic 2a receptors located in the prefrontal cortex. Several investigators have expressed a preference for the use of guanfacine over clonidine because it is less sedating. Preliminary studies have suggested a role as a tic-suppressing medication and in the treatment of ADHD. The initial dose is 0.5 mg at bedtime with gradual increases, as needed, to final doses up to 3 mg per day in two divided dosages. Guanfacine is generally well tolerated; the most common side effects are sedation, fatigue, and headaches.

Baclofen. Baclofen, which contains both GABA and phenylethylamine moieties, has been variably effective as a treatment for TS. In a double-blind, placebo-controlled crossover study, baclofen in doses of 20 mg TID statistically improved overall well-being, but did not reduce motor or vocal tic activity.

Clonazepam. Clonazepam, a benzodiazepine, is widely used for tics despite confirmation of a tic-suppressing effect in only limited studies. I personally use it only as an adjunctive medication in anxious patients. Side effects include drowsiness, dizziness, fatigue, and altered behavior. It may be habit-forming.

Second Tier Pharmacotherapy. If an individual fails initial therapy or presents with severe tics, medications in the Tier 2 (classical neuroleptic or atypical neuroleptics) category should be initiated. Neuroleptics, D2 dopamine receptor antagonists, are the most effective tic-suppressing agents (about 70–80% effective), but side effects may limit their usefulness. Complications that may occur even with low doses tend to be similar with most neuroleptic medications: sedation, drowsiness, dysphoria, movement abnormalities (acute dystonic reactions, bradykinesia, akathisia, tardive and withdrawal dyskinesias, tardive TS), depression, aggression, "fog states," weight gain, EKG abnormalities, endocrine dysfunction, and poor school performance with or without school phobia. A variety of neuroleptic and atypical neuroleptic agents have been suggested as tic-suppressing therapy, although few have been adequately evaluated. My personal preferences are to use monotherapy and start with pimozide and then use fluphenazine, risperidone, olanzepine, and haloperidol in that order. In individuals with significant behavioral issues, the use of atypical neuroleptics as the initial Tier 2 therapy should be considered.

Classical Neuroleptics.

Pimozide. Pimozide, a diphenylbutylpiperidine derivative, is a D2 receptor antagonist that also blocks calcium channels. Two double-blind studies have compared the efficacy and safety of pimozide and haloperidol. In both, pimozide was either equal to or more effective than haloperidol at suppressing tics and had fewer serious side effects. Before starting pimozide, an EKG should be obtained in order to detect a prolonged Q-T interval, a contraindicating factor. Electrocardiographic changes induced by pimozide include Q-T lengthening, U waves, and alteration of T-waves (flattening, notching, or inversion). This medication is started at 0.5–1 mg/day given at bedtime. The dose is gradually increased, if necessary, in 1-mg increments on a weekly basis and used in a BID dosing schedule. A general target range is 2–6 mg/day. day. The use of macrolide antibiotics (clarithromycin, erythromycin, troleandomycin, and ditromycin), azole antifungals (ketoconazole, itraconazole), and protease inhibitors should be avoided. Grapefruit juice may also inhibit the metabolism of pimozide, resulting in increased serum concentrations of this medication. Long-term treatment with pimozide is more effective in controlling the course of tics than its use solely to treat an exacerbation. If pimozide is ineffective, I switch to fluphenazine.

Fluphenazine. Fluphenazine is an antagonist at both D1 and D2 dopaminergic receptors. Several studies have shown that this medication is an effective tic-suppressing agent that may have fewer side effects than other neuroleptics. Treatment is started with a dose of 1 mg at bedtime and increased in a similar fashion to pimozide, by 1 mg every 5–7 days, while the patient is monitored for a therapeutic response or side effects. A typical daily dose is 2–4 mg/day.

Haloperidol. Haloperidol, a butyrophenone and D2 blocking agent, was first documented to be an effective tic suppressor more than 40 years ago. Although it is probably the most widely used agent, in my experience the observed frequency of side effects is greater than with other agents in this category. The therapeutic tic effect with haloperidol is seen at low doses. Medication is started at 0.5 mg/day and increased by small amounts every week, to a target range of about 1–5 mg/day.

Others. Another less commonly used neuroleptic, *trifluoperazine*, may also have beneficial effects. *Sulpiride* and *tiapride* are substituted benzamides that are free of anticholinergic and noradrenergic effects. Both of these selective D2 antagonists have been shown to be beneficial in studies performed in Europe, but neither is available in the United States.

Atypical Neuroleptics. These newer antipsychotic agents (risperidone, olanzapine, ziprasidone, quetiapine) are characterized by a relatively greater affinity for 5HT2 receptors than for D2 receptors and the potential for fewer extrapyramidal side effects than typical neuroleptics. Substantial variations in receptor affinity profiles for subtypes of dopamine, serotonin, and adrenergic receptors exist among these agents, suggesting that there may be important differences in clinical effects. Risperidone and olanzapine have been studied most extensively.

Risperidone. This benzisoxazol derivative acts at low doses on 5-HT2 receptors, while at higher doses, it is a potent D2 antagonist. It also has moderate to high affinity for α-1-adrenergic, D3, D4, and H1-histamine receptors. Several studies have suggested that risperidone may be effective for some patients and that it compares favorably with pimozide. It has also been suggested that risperidone may be most beneficial in patients with comorbid OCD. Risperidone is started at 0.5 mg/day, given at night, and increased as necessary at 5- to 7-day intervals to a maximum of about 3 mg/day in two divided doses. Side effects include weight gain, fatigue, photophobia, and, rarely, extrapyramidal problems.

Olanzepine. Olanzepine exhibits moderate to high affinity for D2, D4, 5-HT2A, 5-HT2C, and α-1-adrenergic receptors and also binds to D1 receptors. Several small studies with olanzepine have shown improvement of tics. The initial dose is 2.5 mg at bedtime and, if necessary, dose is gradually raised to 5–10 mg/day in divided doses. Side effects include weight gain and mild sedation.

Other Atypical Neuroleptics. In preliminary studies, *ziprasidone* was significantly more effective than placebo in suppressing tic symptoms in patients with TS. The starting dose is 5 mg in the evening with gradual increases to 40 mg in divided doses, if tolerated. An EKG should be performed before and after starting treatment to detect possible cardiac conduction abnormalities. Case reports have suggested that *quetiapine* may be an effective treatment for tics.

Other Dopaminergic Pharmacotherapies.

Dopamine Antagonists. Tetrabenazine is a benzoquinolizine derivative that depletes the presynaptic stores of catecholamines and blocks postsynaptic dopamine receptors. Several studies have confirmed a tic-suppressing effect at doses of 25–100 mg/day. The combined use of tetrabenazine and a classical neuroleptic may permit the use of lower doses of each medication with fewer side effects, which include sedation, depression, Parkinsonism, insomnia, anxiety, and akathisia. The medication is not routinely available in the United States.

Dopamine Agonists. Pergolide, a mixed D1/D2/D3 dopamine receptor agonist, has been shown to improve tics at a dose about one-tenth of that used in treating Parkinson's disease, i.e., 0.1–0.3 mg/day in divided doses. Side effects were mild and electrocardiograms showed no difference from control. The mechanism of action is speculated to involve presynaptic rather then postsynaptic striatal or cortical dopamine receptors. Major side effects include nausea, syncope, sedation, and dizziness.

Other Nondopaminergic Therapies. The distribution and interaction of classical neurotransmitters within frontal–subcortical structures make it possible for a variety of neurotransmitters, in addition to dopamine, to be involved in the pathobiology of TS. Hence, it is not surprising that multiple nondopaminergic therapies have been proposed for the treatment of tic disorders, but very few have been adequately evaluated, including nicotine; donepezil, a noncompetitive inhibitor of acetylcholinesterase; delta-9-tetrahydrocannabinol, the major psychoactive ingredient of marijuana; and a variety of antiepileptic agents.

Botulinum toxin (Botox). Botulinum toxin which reduces muscle activity by inhibiting acetylcholine release at neuromuscular junctions, has been used successfully in treating dystonic motor and vocal tics. Botox (mean dose of 500 units) has been injected into a variety of regions including face, back, shoulder, cervical, upper thoracic, and vocal cords. Benefits appeared in 3–4 days and lasted a mean of 14 weeks. Careful consideration must be given to the proper selection of the targeted tic.

Treatment of Comorbid Problems

ADHD

Similar to treatment in any child with this problem, a variety of behavioral and educational approaches should be implemented before pharmacotherapy is considered. Psychostimulant medications are generally regarded as the treatment of choice for

ADHD and their use in children with TS is not contraindicated. Alternative medications for the treatment of ADHD symptoms in children with TS include clonidine, guanfacine, atomoxetine, desipramine, and nortriptyline. In the occasional situation where a stimulant is required for attendance in school or performance at work and tics remain constant, stimulants and tic-suppressing medications are used simultaneously.

OCD

In TS patients with OCD, pharmacologic and cognitive-behavioral therapy should be considered. Several selective serotonin reuptake inhibitors may be beneficial (see chapter on OCD).

Other Behavioral Disorders

Episodic outbursts (rage), argumentativeness, disruptive behaviors, conduct problems, anxiety, and mood disorders are relatively common in patients with TS. In many, these difficulties are comingled with tics, ADHD, and OCD presenting a major challenge for the family and physician. In complex cases, it is essential that the affected patient receives the proper evaluation and care from a multidisciplinary team of specialists.

SUGGESTED READINGS

1. Müller-Vahl KR. The treatment of Tourette's syndrome: current opinions. Expert Opin Pharmacother 2002; 3:899–914.
2. Robertson MM. Tourette syndrome, associated conditions and the complexities of treatment. Brain 2000; 123:425–462.
3. Sandor P. Pharmacological management of tics in patients with TS. J Psychosomatic Res 2003; 55:41–48.
4. Singer HS. The treatment of tics. Current Neurol Neurosci Reports 2001; 1:195–202.

PATIENT RESOURCE

1. Tourette Syndrome Association. 42–40 Bell Boulevard, Bayside, NY, U.S.A.

21
Chorea in Children

Lori C. Jordan
Department of Neurology, Johns Hopkins University School of Medicine, Baltimore, Maryland, U.S.A.

Harvey S. Singer
Departments of Neurology and Pediatrics, Johns Hopkins University School of Medicine, Baltimore, Maryland, U.S.A.

INTRODUCTION

Chorea (Latin for "dance") is a hyperkinetic movement disorder usually due to basal ganglia injury or dysfunction. Movements are brief, irregular, unpredictable, and flow from one body part to another in a random fashion. Occasionally, they may be incorporated into a more purposeful movement to avoid social embarrassment. Chorea can occur in isolation, but usually appears in conjunction with slow, writhing, distal movements called athetosis (i.e., choreoathetosis). Initially, described in the Middle Ages and thought to be psychogenic, chorea was subsequently shown to have numerous etiologies. Sydenham's chorea (SC, or rheumatic chorea, chorea minor, St. Vitus' dance) remains one of the most common causes of acute chorea in children.

DIAGNOSIS/CLINICAL FEATURES

Chorea is associated with a variety of conditions that affect the nervous system (Table 1). In childhood, it may occur as part of paroxysmal dyskinesias, immune-mediated conditions (SC, systemic lupus erythematosus, antiphospholipid antibodies), hereditary disorders (ataxia telangiectasia, benign familial), metabolic abnormalities (hyperthyroidism, mitochondrial abnormalities, congenital disorders of glycosylation), postcardiopulmonary bypass, drug or toxin exposures, infections, neoplasm, vascular, and degenerative disorders. A suggested evaluation for a child presenting with acute chorea is presented in Table 2.

THERAPY

Treatment, if possible, should be directed to the underlying disease process, especially if the disorder is amenable to therapy. Medications for the clinical sign of

Table 1 Differential Diagnosis of Chorea

Inherited
Wilson's disease
Neuroacanthocytosis
Benign familial chorea
Huntington's disease
Ataxia telangectasia
Immunologic
Sydenham's chorea
Systemic lupus erythematosus
Antiphospholipid antibody
Chorea gravidarium
Infectious
Lyme disease
Syphilis
Encephalitis
Drug related
Tardive dyskinesia
Anticonvulsants (phenytoin, lamotrigine)
Tricyclic antidepressants
Neuroleptic withdrawal
Metoclopramide
Fluphenazine
Levadopa
Cocaine
Amphetamines
Petroleum intoxication
Oral contraceptives
Metabolic disturbance
Mitochondrial cytopathy
Amino acidopathy
Organic aciduria (glutaric, propionic)
Creatine deficiency
Hyperthyroidism
Hypoparathyroidism
Hypocalcemia
Pregnancy
Post-traumatic
Anoxic brain injury
Kernicterus
Vascular
Stroke
Moyamoya
Postpump chorea (after cardiac surgery)

chorea are symptomatic, not curative. Pharmacotherapy for the suppression of chorea is based, in part, on correcting neurotransmitter abnormalities proposed for the pathophysiology of chorea, i.e., reduced levels of gamma-aminobutyric acid (GABA) and acetylcholine (ACh), and/or hyperinnervation of dopamine receptors (see Table 3). Thus, rational therapy may include the use of different medications that act to enhance the effects of GABA and ACh or diminish dopaminergic stimulation.

Table 2 Basic Evaluation of Acute Chorea[a]

Serum electrolytes including calcium
Complete blood count and peripheral blood smear
Sedimentation rate
ASO and DNase B titers
Anticardiolipin antibodies
Antinuclear antibody
TSH
Ceruloplasmin and copper levels
Toxicology screen
MRI of brain

[a] Additional testing as indicated by history and physical examination.

In children, most of the scientific literature on the treatment of chorea is based on studies in Sydenham's chorea (SC). To date, there have been no randomized, controlled studies evaluating the treatment of chorea, except in Huntington's chorea.

The following sections on therapy are divided into (A) pharmacologic approaches based on the correction of neurotransmitter abnormalities, (B) possible surgical approaches, and (C) results of treatment in SC.

Pharmacologic Approaches Based on the Correction of Neurotransmitter Abnormalities

Drugs That Increase GABA

GABAergic neurons in the striatum, globus pallidus interna (GPi), and substantia nigra pars reticulata (SNpr) have been implicated in hyperkinetic movement disorders such as chorea and tardive dyskinesia. Medium-sized spiny neurons (MSSN) containing GABA are the major output pathways from the striatum, and neurons in the GPi and SNpr project to the thalamus, superior colliculus, and reticular formation, establishing important inhibitory efferent pathways from the basal ganglia.

Valproic Acid. Valproic acid is thought to act by enhancing GABA levels in the striatum and substantia nigra. In multiple small studies and case reports, valproic

Table 3 Treatment of Chorea Based on Neurochemistry

Pathologic mechanisms	Role of medication
Reduced Ach	*Increase Ach* Lecithin? Choline?
Reduced GABA	*Increase GABA* Valproic acid Clonazepam
Excess DA	*Diminish DA* Pimozide Haldol Tetrabenazine Reserpine Carbamazepine (mechanism?)

acid in doses of 10–20 mg/kg/day have been used successfully to treat chorea. In general, no serious side effects were noted, but hepatotoxicity and thrombocytopenia have been reported with valproic acid use in other disorders.

GABAmimetic Drugs. Clonazepam is a long-acting benzodiazepine that has been used to treat chorea with some success. Benzodiazepines act on the $GABA_A$ receptor–chloride ion channel complex and increase the frequency of ion channel opening, acting as indirect GABA agonists. Case reports document improved choreiform movements at relatively low clonazepam doses, 1–5 mg/day. Tolerance may develop after a period of months, necessitating dose escalation or a drug holiday. Side effects of clonazepam may include dry mouth and sedation.

Drugs That Increase ACh

Large aspiny cholinergic interneurons within the striatum innervate GABAergic MSSN and tend to counterbalance the influences of dopamine and glutamate. Trials of cholinergic precursors, such as choline and lecithin, for chorea have been limited and results modest. An unpleasant fishy odor is noted in patients ingesting lecithin.

Drugs That Diminish Dopaminergic Activity

Dopamine-Depleting Agents. Reports dating back to the 1970s suggest that tetrabenazine may be helpful in selected patients with chorea. Tetrabenazine acts by preventing the presynaptic release of dopamine, so-called monoamine depletion, as well as blocking dopamine receptors on postsynaptic terminals. Tetrabenazine treatment in 5 pediatric patients with chorea significantly improved movements in 80%, although high doses (up to 275 mg/day or 25 mg/kg/day) were often necessary (Chatterjee). Medication was continued for at least several months and side effects commonly reported in adults, such as depression, parkinsonism, hypotension, acute dystonic reaction, and neuroleptic malignant syndrome, were not present. Tetrabenazine is not approved for use in the United States, but can be obtained from Canada for selected cases. Reserpine, another dopamine-depleting agent, is effective for chorea in some patients. Reserpine is longer acting than tetrabenazine and side effects may include hypotension, depression, and parkinsonism.

Dopamine Antagonists. Dopamine antagonists including the typical neuroleptics haloperidol, pimozide, and chlorpromazine have been efficacious in treating chorea. Early case reports describe rapid improvement of abnormal movements within a few days, using low doses of haloperidol, from 0.5 to 2 mg twice daily. Other authors have suggested that pimozide may have a lower risk of inducing neuroleptics side effects, such as sedation, parkinsonism, weight gain, school phobia, hepatocellular dysfunction, leukopenia, and tardive dyskinesia.

Carbamazepine has also been used to treat chorea, but its mechanism of action is unknown. Some authors have postulated that it stimulates cholinergic pathways and others have implicated structural similarity to tricyclic antidepressants and phenothiazines.

Surgical Therapy

Surgical approaches for the treatment of chorea are unproven. Deep brain stimulation (DBS) of the thalamus and pallidotomy have been performed in a small number of cases with mixed results.

Therapy in Sydenham's Chorea

Since treatment is symptomatic and not curative, the decision to initiate therapy in patients with SC is based on the degree of patient disability, whether due to chorea, behavioral, or psychiatric symptoms. Numerous neuropsychiatric problems are seen in association with SC, including emotional lability, irritability, attention deficit hyperactivity disorder (ADHD), obsessive compulsive disorder (OCD), and psychosis, and specific therapy may be required to address these issues (see appropriate chapters).

Studies in patients with SC have shown improvement of chorea with the use of anticonvulsants. In limited trials, there were no significant differences between valproic acid and carbamazepine in the time to clinical improvement, time to complete remission, duration of therapy, or recurrence rates. Other therapies have included neuroleptics, such as haldol and pimozide. In most patients, chorea improved dramatically and the duration of therapy, although variable, ranged from 3 to 6 months.

Immunomodulatory therapies, such as corticosteroids, plasmapheresis, and intravenous immunoglobulin (IVIG), have been used to treat SC. Therapy is based on the premise that SC is an immune-mediated disorder. Case reports and retrospective reviews of corticosteroid therapy in SC suggest that they may shorten the time to recovery. These data, however, should be interpreted with caution, because there were few studies and these were retrospective or uncontrolled. A prospective, uncontrolled trial of intravenous methylprednisolone followed by oral prednisone for refractory SC was just published (Cardoso). Results in five patients appear promising. Several patients with recalcitrant SC have received IVIG or plasmapheresis therapy, the latter resulting in fewer recurrences of chorea. In summary, because patient numbers are so small, firm conclusions cannot be drawn regarding the efficacy of immunomodulatory therapies.

The only clear consensus in the treatment of SC is the recommendation for prophylactic penicillin to prevent re-infection with group A beta-hemolytic streptococcus (GABHS) and potential cardiac problems. Secondary prophylaxis with penicillin has been shown to prevent the recurrence of rheumatic fever and chorea. For dosing and additional information, consult the American Academy of Pediatrics guidelines.

PROGNOSIS

Prognosis for children with chorea clearly depends upon its etiology. Chorea secondary to a cerebral infarction is unlikely to remit, whereas chorea secondary to medication often subsides soon after the medication is withdrawn. The natural history of Sydenham's chorea presents symptoms for 3–6 months followed by spontaneous remission; the recurrence rate for SC is between 10% and 25%. Clinicians obviously must be mindful of an individual patient's prognosis when counseling families about the risks and benefits of treatment.

SUMMARY

Chorea, particularly Sydenham's chorea, remains an important public health problem in many parts of the world. Chorea is among the most challenging neurologic disorders to treat. There is still no consensus regarding appropriate treatment other than penicillin prophylaxis for SC. A decision to treat chorea should be based upon patient disability and an awareness of the risk-benefit and side effect profiles of the various treatment options. Studies to date are limited and comprise primarily case reports and retrospective reviews. The limited data, however, support pharmacologic therapy as the logical first step, with anticonvulsants such as valproic acid or carbamazepine as the initial drugs of choice in most circumstances. Polytherapy may be necessary, and rational drug combinations would include a dopamine receptor blocker (higher risk of tardive dyskinesia) or a GABAmimetic drug such as clonazepam. Immunomodulatory and surgical therapies remain investigational. Additional large, randomized, controlled studies are needed to further explore therapy for chorea.

SUGGESTED READINGS

1. American Academy of Pediatrics: 2003 Red Book. Report of the Committee on Infectious Diseases. 26th ed. Elk Grove Village: American Academy of Pediatrics, 2003:581–584.
2. Cardoso F, Maia D, Cunningham MC, Valenca G. Cesar M, et al. Treatment of Sydenham chorea with corticosteroids. Movement Disord 2003; 18(11):1374–1377.
3. Chatterjee A, Frucht SJ. Tetrabenazine in the treatment of severe pediatric chorea. Movement Disord 2003; 18(6):703–706.
4. Garvey MA, Swedo SE, Shapiro MB, Parker C, Allen AJ, Dows, Leonard HL. et al. Intravenous immunoglobulin and plasmapheresis as effective treatments of Sydenham's chorea. Neurology 1996; 46:A147.
5. Jordan LC, Singer HS. Sydenham chorea in children. Curr Treatment Opt Neurol 2003; 5:283–290.
6. Marques-Dias MJ, Mercadante, MT, Tucker, D, Lombroso, P. Sydenham's chorea. Psych Clin N Amer 1997; 20(4):809–820.
7. Moore, DP. Neuropsychiatric aspects of Sydenham's chorea: a comprehensive review. J Clin Psych 1996; 57(9):407–414.
8. Swedo, SE. Sydenham's chorea: a model for childhood autoimmune neuropsychiatric disorders. JAMA 1994; 272(22):1788–1791.
9. Special Writing Group of the Committee on Rheumatic Fever, Endocarditis, and Kawasaki Disease of the Council on Cardiovascular Disease in the Young of the American Heart Association. Guidelines for the diagnosis of rheumatic fever: Jones criteria, 1992 update. JAMA 1992; 268:2069–2073.
10. Thompson TP, Kondziolka D, Albright AL. Thalamic stimulation for choreiform movement disorders in children: report of two cases. J Neurosurg 2000; 92:718–721.

22
Dystonia (DRD, Primary, and Secondary)

Jonathan W. Mink
University of Rochester, Departments of Neurology, Neurobiology & Anatomy, and Pediatrics, Rochester, New York, U.S.A.

INTRODUCTION

Dystonia is a syndrome of sustained muscle contractions, frequently causing twisting and repetitive movements or abnormal postures. Historically, dystonia has been divided into primary (idiopathic) and secondary etiologies. Primary dystonias are disorders in which dystonia is the only feature, is the primary feature and accompanied only by other movement disorders (e.g., myoclonus or parkinsonism), or the cause is either a specific genetic mutation or is unknown. The two most important types of primary dystonia in children are dopa-responsive dystonia (DRD) and idiopathic torsion dystonia associated with the DYT1 mutation. Secondary dystonias are those disorders in which the dystonia is due to another identifiable cause. The most important etiologies of secondary dystonia in children are listed in Table 1.

DIAGNOSIS AND EVALUATION

The etiology of dystonia warrants careful investigation. It is critical for the neurologist to witness the abnormal postures and movements to be certain that the movement disorder is indeed dystonia. A home video demonstrating the presence and range of symptoms is critical. This is especially true when the dystonia is intermittent. Because of the large number of etiologies, comprehensive testing can be time consuming and expensive. A rational, tiered diagnostic approach, tailored to the individual patient and influenced by the presence of accompanying neurologic signs, temporal course, family history, and other factors is recommended. Most, but not all, secondary dystonias have additional neurologic signs or symptoms. Perhaps the most important entity to diagnose is DRD because it is readily treated. A therapeutic trial of levodopa can often make the diagnosis of DRD.

SPECIFIC DISORDERS AND TREATMENT

Treatment of dystonia varies depending on the etiology. In the following sections, treatment of DRD, primary dystonia, and secondary dystonia will be considered separately.

Table 1 Causes of Secondary Dystonia

Heredodegenerative and metabolic disorders
Dentatorubropallidoluysian atrophy (DRPLA)
Gangliosidoses
Glutaric aciduria
Huntington disease
Lesch-Nyhan
Metachromatic leukodystrophy
Methylmalonic acidemia
Mitochondrial disorders
Niemann-Pick Type C
Neuronal degeneration with brain iron accumulation (NBIA), including pantothenate kinase associated neurodegeneration (PKAN)*
Spinocerebellar ataxia (esp. SCA-3)
Wilson disease
Structural brain lesions
Acute disseminated encephalomyelitis
Infection
Perinatal hypoxia-ischemia
Stroke
Tumor
Drugs/toxins
Dopamine blockers
e.g., haloperidol, pimozide, chlorpromazine, metoclopramide, prochlorperazine, risperidone
Antiepileptics
e.g., carbamazepine, phenytoin
Psychogenic

Dopa-Responsive Dystonia

Dopa-responsive dystonia is a syndrome characterized by childhood onset of progressive dystonia with sustained dramatic response to low doses of levodopa. The DRD is also known as *hereditary progressive dystonia with diurnal fluctuations* or Segawa syndrome. The DRD typically presents between 1 and 12 years of age with a gait disturbance involving foot dystonia. In untreated older children, there is development of diurnal fluctuation with worsening of symptoms toward the end of the day and marked improvement in the morning. It is important to recognize the entity of DRD because it responds dramatically to low doses of levodopa. The DRD can be misdiagnosed as cerebral palsy. Thus, it is important to consider DRD in the child with abnormal movements that might otherwise appear to be cerebral palsy if there is prominent dystonia and a progressive rather than static course. With appropriate diagnosis and treatment, children with DRD can lead normal lives. The goal of drug therapy in DRD is complete remission of symptoms.

Pharmacologic Treatment

Carbidopa/Levodopa. Carbidopa/levodopa is the mainstay of treatment in DRD. A starting dose is 1 mg/kg/day of levodopa, which can be increased gradually until there is complete benefit or dose-limiting side effects. Most individuals respond to 4–5 mg/kg/day in divided doses, but some authors have suggested doses up to 10 mg/kg/day. If there is no response to a dose of 600 mg/day, it is highly unlikely that DRD is the correct diagnosis. Carbidopa/levodopa should be given as 25/100 mg tablets. They can be crushed and dissolved in an ascorbic acid solution or in orange juice and used within 24 hr. The 10/100 tablets contain insufficient carbidopa to prevent nausea in most patients. The most common side effects are somnolence, nausea and vomiting, decreased appetite, dyskinesia, and hallucinations. Nausea and vomiting can be reduced by given additional carbidopa, available in 25 mg tablets. Dyskinesia may occur upon initiation of treatment or in older individuals who are treated with relatively higher doses of levodopa. Dyskinesia can be reduced or eliminated by reducing the dose of levodopa. If dyskinesia is present with the initiation of treatment, reduce the dose. If inadequate benefit at the lower dose, it can usually be increased again slowly without recurrence of dyskinesia. Motor complications of levodopa therapy that are seen in Parkinson disease do not occur in DRD.

Trihexyphenidyl. The dosing of trihexyphenidyl for treatment of DRD is not well established. Starting dose should be 0.5 mg/day in children <4 years old and 1 mg/day in older children. The dose should be increased by 1 mg every 3–7 days in a t.i.d. schedule until benefit or side effects. In DRD, there is benefit from relatively low doses compared to those used to treat other forms of dystonia. Trihexyphenidyl should be considered as second-line treatment in DRD because it does not reverse the biochemical defect of decreased dopamine synthesis in DRD. Side effects are uncommon at low doses.

Other Approaches. Tetrahydrobiopterin may be a useful treatment in DRD due to GTP-cyclohydrolase I deficiency, but it is not readily available and has not been well studied. Dosing information is not available.

Primary Dystonia

The major form of primary dystonia in children is childhood onset, generalized, idiopathic torsion dystonia, formerly known as *dystonia musculorum deformans.* This disorder is inherited as an autosomal dominant condition with incomplete (30%) penetrance. A GAG deletion at the DYT1 locus on chromosome 9 causes most autosomal dominant, early-onset primary generalized dystonia in Ashkenazi Jewish families (90%) and also in non-Jewish populations (50–60%). In childhood-onset idiopathic torsion dystonia, symptoms usually begin in a limb with a mean onset age of 12.5 years. Onset is usually before 28 years of age, but seldom before age 6. The legs are commonly affected before the arms and symptoms typically become generalized within 5 years. Diagnosis is based on identifying a GAG deletion in the DYT-1 gene; genetic testing is available commercially.

Pharmacologic Treatment

Trihexyphenidyl. Anticholinergic medications are the most consistently effective in treatment of primary dystonia. Most available data and experiences are with trihexyphenidyl. Children typically tolerate higher doses than do adults and may find maximum benefit with doses of 60 mg per day or more. To avoid side effects, trihexyphenidyl should be started at 1 mg/day at bedtime and increased by 1 mg each week until the desired benefit is obtained or side effects develop. The usual maintenance dose varies from 6 to over 60 mg/day divided three times per day. The most common side effects of trihexyphenidyl are sedation, dry mouth, decreased concentration and memory, hallucinations, constipation, and blurred vision. Chorea can develop with high doses. Sudden cessation should be avoided because it can precipitate mental status changes.

Baclofen. Baclofen is somewhat less effective than trihexyphenidyl in most children, but can be helpful in diminishing pain due to dystonia. It can provide additional benefit when used in combination with trihexyphenidyl. A typical starting dose is 5 mg at bedtime. The dose should be increased slowly until desired benefit or side effects occur. The usual maintenance dose is 10–60 mg per day in three divided doses, but some older children obtain maximum benefit at doses as high as 180 mg per day. The most common side effect is sedation. Sudden cessation can precipitate seizures or psychosis and should be avoided.

In patients with good benefit from oral baclofen, but who cannot tolerate the effective dose due to side effects, intrathecal baclofen may be an option. There are few data available on the use of intrathecal baclofen in primary dystonia and the use of this therapy in primary dystonia is controversial.

Other Medications. Several other medications may be effective in a minority of children with primary dystonia. These include clonazepam (gradually increase to maximum of 0.2 mg/kg/day in three divided doses), carbamazepine (start at 10 mg/kg/day in two divided doses and increase as tolerated to maximum benefit), dopamine antagonists such as haloperidol (start at 0.05 mg/kg/day and increase to maximum of 0.1 mg kg day in two divided doses), carbidopa/levodopa, and botulinum toxin. Botulinum toxin injections are highly effective in focal and segmental dystonias due to the limited number of muscles involved. It plays a smaller role in treatment of generalized dystonia because of the large number of involved muscles. However, it can be quite helpful in reducing symptoms when isolated problematic muscle groups are targeted.

Nonpharmacologic Treatment

Promising neurosurgical treatments of dystonia include thalamotomy, pallidotomy, and deep brain stimulation (DBS) of the globus pallidus pars interna. Thalamotomy was the most frequently performed ablative procedure in the past. However, when performed bilaterally, there is a high incidence of dysarthria and dysphagia. The benefits of thalamotomy are highly variable. More recently, pallidotomy has been preferred to thalamotomy because of the lower morbidity. Direct comparison has not been performed, but data suggest that pallidotomy is more effective than thalomotomy in DYT-1 dystonia. However, the benefits may be temporary. Thalamotomy may be more effective for secondary dystonia. Most recently, pallidal DBS has been used to treat DYT1 dystonia with promising early results. The effects of DBS are similar to those of pallidotomy, but DBS is programmable and does not involve a destructive lesion. The long-term effects of pallidal DBS on dystonia are not yet known.

Physical and occupation therapy can be helpful in maximizing the function of individuals with primary generalized dystonia. Bracing may be helpful in some cases.

Secondary Dystonia

Some secondary dystonias may also respond to levodopa and therefore, a trial of levodopa is recommended for any child in whom dystonia is a prominent component of their neurologic syndrome. There are many causes of secondary dystonia (Table 1). In most cases, treatment depends on the etiology. When possible, the best approach is to treat the underlying cause. For example, if the cause is a medication or other toxin, the best course is to eliminate that agent. If available, specific treatment for the underlying metabolic disturbance should be employed. In cases where there is no known primary treatment or when symptoms persist despite treatment of the underlying cause, symptomatic treatment can be employed. There are relatively few data on the efficacy of various agents in the treatment of secondary dystonia. The medications described above for primary dystonia may be effective in secondary dystonias. Empirical treatment with carbidopa/levodopa, trihexyphenidyl, baclofen, carbamazepine, or a combination should be considered.

In the case of tardive dystonia, dopamine depletors such as reserpine or tetrabenazine can be effective. Reserpine should be started at a dose of 20 μg/kg daily and increased gradually until benefit is achieved or side effects occur. It can take a week or more to see the effect of a dose change. A typical maintenance dose is 0.25 mg per day divided twice daily, but higher doses may give additional benefit if tolerated. The most common side effects are sedation, depression, orthostatic hypotension, and parkinsonism. Tertrabenazine is also effect in tardive dystonia, but is not available in the United States. The starting dose of tetrabenazine is 12.5 mg at bedtime. The dose should be increased gradually until there is benefit or side effects occur. The effective maintenance dose varies widely from 25 to 200 mg per day divided three times daily. The most common side effects are sedation and depression.

Perhaps the most common secondary dystonia is the acute dystonia reaction that typically occurs in response to a dopamine antagonist. Anticholinergic medications are the most effective; benztropine and diphenhydramine are the most commonly used agents to treat acute dystonia reactions. Benztropine should be given in a dose of 0.02–0.05 mg/kg IM or IV (maximum dose 2 mg) acutely. It should be continued at 0.02–0.05 mg/kg PO (maximum dose 2 mg) twice daily for 1–3 days to prevent recurrence. Diphenhydramine should be given in a dose of 1.0–1.25 mg/kg IM or IV (maximum dose 50 mg) acutely. It should be continued at 1.0–1.25 mg/kg PO (maximum dose 50 mg) every 6–8 hr as needed for 1–3 days to prevent recurrence. After occurrence of an acute dystonia reaction, re-exposure to a dopamine antagonist should be avoided if possible.

PROGNOSIS

The prognosis of dystonia in children depends on the cause. The prognosis for DRD is excellent with life-long benefit from low doses of carbidopa/levodopa. Often, the symptoms diminish in the 3rd decade of life and it may be possible to decrease the levodopa dose. Primary dystonia is typically progressive to a point at which point there is usually a plateau. This typically occurs in the 3rd to 4th decade of life. Benefit from medication is symptomatic only. There is no known treatment for the underlying cause. DBS is promising and may confer long-lasting benefit, but there are insufficient data at this time. The prognosis for secondary dystonia depends entirely on the cause and availability of primary treatment for the underlying etiology. Some conditions are fatal (e.g., Huntington disease) and others are transient (e.g., acute dystonia reaction). Symptomatic treatment of secondary dystonia is not expected to alter the natural history of the underlying disease.

Table 2 Commonly Used Medications in Treatment of Dystonia

Medication	Dose	Most common side effects
Carbodopa/levodopa	Start: 1 mg/kg/day Maintenance: 4–5 mg/kg/day divided t.i.d	Somnolence, nausea and vomiting, decreased appetite, dyskinesia, hallucinations
Trihexyphenidyl	Start: 1 mg q.h.s Maintenance: 6–60 mg/day divided t.i.d.	Sedation, dry mouth, decreased concentration and memory, hallucinations, constipation, blurred vision
Baclofen	Start 5 mg q.h.s. Maintenance: 10–60 mg/day divided t.i.d.	Sedation, weakness

SUMMARY

Dystonia has many causes and many treatment options (Table 2). Some forms of dystonia, such as DRD, are readily treated with complete benefit expected. Because the symptoms of DRD respond entirely in most cases, it is important to always consider this diagnostic possibility. Other forms of dystonia are more difficult to treat and may require empirical trials of multiple medications to achieve maximum benefit. Many medications are tolerated at higher doses in children than in adults, so dosing is usually guided by degree of benefit and severity of side effects. Stereotaxic surgical treatments are promising, particularly for primary dystonia due to the DYT1 mutation.

SUGGESTED READINGS

1. Bandmann O, Wood NW. Dopa-responsive dystonia—the story so far. Neuropediatrics 2002; 33:1–5.
2. Burke RE, Fahn S, Marsden CD. Torsion dystonia: a double-blind, prospective trial of high-dosage trihexyphenidyl. Neurology 1986; 36:160–164.
3. Fahn S, Hallett M, DeLong MR, ed. Dystonia 4. Philadelphia: Lippincott Williams & Wilkins, 2004.

23
Tremor in Childhood

Leon S. Dure, IV
Division of Pediatric Neurology, Department of Pediatrics,
The University of Alabama at Birmingham, Birmingham, Alabama, U.S.A.

INTRODUCTION

Tremor in childhood, although considered rare, is frequently seen among patients referred to pediatric neurologists. In a series of 684 children with movement disorders, the incidence of tics was 39%, dystonia 24%, tremor 10%, chorea 5%, myoclonus 2%, akinetic-rigid syndromes 2%, and mixed disorders 8%. Although not generalizable data, it is of interest that there is very little published regarding this entity in childhood.

DIAGNOSIS/CLINICAL FEATURES

Tremor is defined as an involuntary rhythmical reciprocal oscillatory movement of a body part, typically around a joint. It may occur at rest (rest tremor) or with action. Action tremors are further divided into those occurring while maintaining a posture (postural tremor) and those that are kinetic. Kinetic tremors occur while reaching for a target or performing a movement, and include intention tremors.

Various tremors have been characterized syndromically according to their clinical phenotype and where possible, by neurophysiologic measures. Physiologic tremor is present in all individuals, with low amplitude and a frequency of 6–12 Hz. It is typically maximal while maintaining a posture. When such a tremor is visible at high frequency and of short duration in an otherwise normal individual, it is denoted an enhanced physiologic tremor. Essential tremor (ET) is likewise monosymptomatic, typically occurring as an isolated finding. However, ET is prominent with action and postural maneuvers. The frequency may be from 4 to 11 Hz, and usually involves the hands and head. Intention tremor, often considered synonymous with cerebellar dysfunction, is a kinetic tremor that interferes with directed movements, typically worsening as a reaching task is near completion. Parkinsonian tremor is rarely seen in childhood, and is seen only at rest, with a frequency of 4–6 Hz. Parkinsonian tremor may also appear if a posture is held for some seconds. A rubral, or Holmes' tremor manifests as a slow (<4.5 Hz) tremor at rest with a concomitant higher frequency intention tremor. Finally, psychogenic tremor is one that is characterized primarily by sudden onset, an unusual combination of kinetic, postural, and/or resting components, a variable distribution and frequency, and a decrease in tremor activity with distraction.

The clinical phenotype of tremor in childhood is similar to that in adults, although neurophysiologic comparisons are lacking (Table 1). Nonfamilial tremors are rare in childhood. Rest tremor is seldom seen in children, with the exception of parkinsonism that may be drug-induced, associated with dopamine pathway disorders, basal ganglia degenerative disorders, and structural or metabolic abnormalities. Kinetic or postural tremors due to cerebellar disease and rubral lesions parallel the incidence of the underlying diseases that occur in this age group. Despite a dearth of research in this area, ET is probably the most common type seen in childhood. Essential tremor is characterized by a hand tremor that is present during the maintenance of a posture and during active movements (handwriting, drinking liquids). Patients may also have involvement of the head, voice, and occasionally the legs. Familial forms are transmitted as an autosomal dominant trait, but some cases are sporadic. Essential tremor has also been reported in carriers of the fragile X mutation.

In newborn infants, jitteriness is a rhythmic tremor that may be seen in up to 40% of children during the first few hours of life. Etiologies for tremors involving the head include spasmus nutans, the bobble-head doll syndrome, and an isolated head tremor of childhood. Tremor is a known side effect of multiple pharmacological agents including anticonvulsant drugs, lithium, and adrenergic agents, among others (Table 2). A syndrome of transient tremor has been reported in infants who have received supplemental vitamin B12 for megaloblastic anemia. Tremor can also be a manifestation of a conversion reaction with the features previously described for psychogenic tremor.

EVALUATION

In the evaluation of tremor, a complete history, physical and neurologic examinations are indicated, as they can provide clues as to whether a tremor is essential or symptomatic. Family history of tremor can be helpful, but actual examination of the biological parents is often required. Assessment of exacerbating factors such as exercise or anxiety can help focus the diagnosis, as they may suggest an enhanced physiologic tremor. Chronicity and family history will help in the diagnosis of

Table 1 Classification of Tremors

Type	Frequency (Hz)	Features
Physiologic	6–12	Mainly postural
Essential	4–11	Postural and kinetic
Parkinsonian	4–6	Rest
Cerebellar	<5	Kinetic (intention)
Rubral/Holmes'	2–4.5	Rest and kinetic
Drug induced	2–11	Kinetic and postural
Psychogenic	4–10	Variable

Table 2 Drugs That May Cause Tremor

Anticonvulsants	Phenytoin Carbamazepine Valproic acid/divalproex
Antidepressants	Tricyclic antidepressants
Sympathomimetic agents	Epinephrine, other β2-agonists Theophylline
Neuroleptics (Parkinsonian tremor)	Haloperidol, other typical antipsychotics Atypical antipsychotics
Others	Chemotherapeutic agents—vincristine, Ara-C Immunosuppressants—cyclosporine

essential tremor, while the presence of other medical or neurologic conditions will generally indicate that tremor is sign of a comorbid process. The sudden onset of tremor with variation in distribution, frequency, or amplitude is more consistent with a conversion disorder.

Ancillary studies to perform in the evaluation of childhood tremor should be dictated by the degree of suspicion for a symptomatic process. Since patients with longstanding tremor and a family history of similar tremor in all likelihood would have an essential tremor, little further investigation is necessary. However, if there is historical or clinical evidence that tremor is coexistent with systemic or CNS pathology, then an evaluation should proceed to identify the underlying cause. In these instances, thyroid function testing, liver function studies, toxic exposures to drugs or heavy metals, ceruloplasmin levels, and brain imaging may be warranted.

TREATMENT

Before attempting a therapeutic intervention, it is of paramount importance to determine the etiology of a tremor. Although the cause of tremor ultimately may not be discernible, treatable causes such as Wilson's disease, thyrotoxicosis, or toxin exposures must be addressed. Additionally, there are no published studies of controlled treatment interventions in childhood tremor, nor are there FDA approved medications with indications for childhood tremor. Hence, since therapeutic interventions in childhood tremor have not been well studied, it is incumbent on the treating physician to assess whether the degree of disability or impairment related to the tremor warrants pharmacotherapy. Likewise, evaluation of the goals of therapy is a necessary component of a treatment plan.

Essential Tremor

There are no published series of treatment strategies in childhood ET. In general, younger children seldom require more than education and perhaps modifications in school regarding handwriting. Adolescents, however, will often request a treatment trial in order to avoid exhibiting tremor in public. In this author's experience, pharmacologic agents such as primidone, β-adrenergic blockers, and topiramate have proven useful, as they have in adults. Clonazepam and botulinum toxin have been successfully used in adults with ET, but their use in childhood has not been

Table 3 Drugs Used to Treat Essential Tremor

Drug	Dosage	Potential side effects
Propranolol, atenolol, other β-blockers	5–10 mg starting dose, increasing as tolerated BID	Hypotension, orthostasis, depression, may aggravate preexisting reactive airways disease
Primidone	125 mg/day increasing to 250 mg TID	Sedation, hypersensitivity, ataxia
Botulinum toxin	Variable	Weakness, pain upon administration
Clonazepam	0.25–0.5 mg BID, increasing as tolerated	Sedation, ataxia, paradoxical activation
Topiramate	1–3 mg/kg/day increasing slowly to 2.5–4.5 mg/kg BID	Sedation, anorexia, weight-loss, cognitive slowing

reported (Table 3). In terms of pharmacologic dosages, the treating physician is urged to start at a low dose and titrate upward depending on treatment effect. The appearance of side effects should be weighed against previously defined treatment goals.

Other Tremors

The use of agents to treat other tremors is based on anecdotal evidence of improvement. Other than attempts at using dopaminergic agonists such as carbidopa/levodopa for the management of Holmes' tremor, no specific recommendations can be made. Although carbidopa/levodopa may be helpful for rest tremor, its use is often limited by gastrointestinal side effects. Other agents to try for management of tremor would include primidone, propranolol, and clonazepam. However, the treatment of symptomatic tremor is often only marginally effective.

SUMMARY

For the clinician faced with a child manifesting tremor, every attempt should be made to consider a reasonable differential diagnosis. However, most cases of childhood tremor do not require specific therapy, but rather treatment of an underlying cause if it exists. In children with tremor of a severity to result in some degree of disability or impairment, therapeutic options exist, although they have yet to be studied carefully in children. The clinician is urged to carefully weigh the potential risks when considering a drug intervention, and to develop reasonable expectations with respect to possible outcomes.

SUGGESTED READINGS

1. Brown P, Thompson PD. Electrophysiological aids to the diagnosis of psychogenic jerks, spasms, and tremor. Move Disord 2001; 16:595–599.
2. Deuschl G. Differential diagnosis of tremor. J Neural Trans Suppl 1999; 56:211–220.

3. Deuschl G, Bergman H. Pathophysiology of nonparkinsonian tremors. Mov Disord 2002; 17(suppl 3):S41–S48.
4. Findley LJ, Koller WC. Essential tremor: a review. Neurology 1987; 37:1194–1197.
5. Louis ED, Dure LS, Pullman S. Essential tremor in childhood: a series of nineteen cases. Mov Disord 2001; 16:921–923.
6. Ondo W, Jankovic J. Essential tremor. CNS Drugs 1996; 6:178–191.
7. Zesiewicz TA, Hauser RA. Phenomenology and treatment of tremor disorders. Neurol Clin 2001; 19:651–680. vii.

24
Myoclonus

Michael R. Pranzatelli
National Pediatric Myoclonus Center, Department of Neurology and Pediatrics, Southern Illinois University School of Medicine, Springfield, Illinois, U.S.A.

INTRODUCTION

Myoclonus is one of the more challenging movement disorders to conceptualize and treat. Effective therapy is rooted in a thorough understanding of the pathophysiology, neurophysiology, and pharmacology of myoclonus. Many good review articles and chapters have been written, but the focus of this chapter is a practical synopsis for the busy clinician.

DIAGNOSIS/CLINICAL FEATURES

Myoclonus affects all age groups and may be disabling or mild and require no treatment. It is a brief involuntary muscle jerk originating in the central nervous system. Myoclonus may appear as an isolated finding or as a symptom of many diseases. Physiologic myoclonus occurs episodically throughout life as hypnic (sleep) jerks and hiccoughs (singultus).

Myoclonus may be epileptic or nonepileptic. Cortical reflex myoclonus, reticular reflex myoclonus, and the myoclonic jerks that presage a generalized seizure in patients with primary generalized epilepsy are examples of epileptic myoclonus. Nonepileptic myoclonus includes dystonic and segmental myoclonus, essential myoclonus, exaggerated startle, myoclonic tics, normal physiologic phenomena, and periodic movements of sleep.

Action or movement-induced myoclonus is the most common clinical type. Reflex myoclonus is activated by sound, light, touch, or passive movement of a limb. Movement-induced myoclonus may be activated by the intention of an action or the action itself. The same individual may manifest spontaneous, action-induced, and sensory-induced myoclonus.

Electromyography (poly-EMG) can be used to confirm the clinical distinction between "positive" and "negative myoclonus." Postural lapses correspond to a silent period on EMG. This brief lack of muscle activity that sometimes follows a muscle discharge has been called negative myoclonus, or asterixis, in contradistinction to the muscle discharges denoted as positive myoclonus. Many patients have both types.

EMG bursts are briefer in epileptic (< 50 msec) than in nonepileptic (50–200 msec) positive myoclonus.

Sophisticated back-averaging techniques are required to document cortical, subcortical, and segmental myoclonus, but certain distinctions can be made clinically. Cortical myoclonus is focal and distal and typically found in the distal extremities. Patients with subcortical myoclonus have both proximal and distal generalized myoclonus, involving both agonist and antagonist muscle groups. Segmental myoclonus may be limited to muscles innervated by a few or multiple spinal segments.

The possible etiologies of myoclonus could fill multiple pages and are beyond the scope of this article. The designation "essential" is used to indicate absence of other neurological abnormalities. Symptomatic myoclonus may be genetic (hereditary or sporadic) or acquired (e.g., from drugs or toxins). All of the major disease categories give rise to myoclonus. The presence of neuropathy, myopathy, ocular abnormalities, other movement disorders, and non-CNS organ involvement may help focus laboratory studies and narrow an otherwise extensive investigation. Most of the effort of diagnostic evaluation should be directed at uncovering potentially reversible disorders.

The context in which myoclonus occurs is often a powerful diagnostic clue. Co-occurrence of opsoclonus signals opsoclonus–myoclonus syndrome, which is paraneoplastic at least 50% of the time. The tumor, which is usually an occult neuroblastoma, is often found only as a result of the neurological presentation. Epilepsy and myoclonus may occur as progressive myoclonus epilepsy (PME), a progressive syndrome of various diverse etiologies, or juvenile myoclonus epilepsy (JME), a single, nonprogressive disorder. Mitochondrial disorders, Unverricht–Lündborg disease (EPM1), and Lafora disease (EPM2A) are the most common forms of PME in the United States. Progressive myoclonus ataxia (PMA) is only one form in which myoclonus and ataxia may be combined. The "serotonin syndrome" is the prototype of drug-induced myoclonus, which is usually caused by unfortuitous combination of serotonergic agents in individuals with neuropsychiatric disorders. Myoclonus in sleep is part of normal physiology in rapid eye movement (REM) sleep, but appears during NREM sleep in neonatal sleep myoclonus, a benign and usually transient condition. "Status myoclonus," an acute state of severe, uncontrolled myoclonus, requires prompt treatment to prevent renal failure from rhabdo-myolysis and death.

THERAPY

The foregoing information lays the foundation for devising a treatment strategy, but there are other considerations (Table 1). Does the myoclonus require any treatment? In patients with multiple neurologic problems or more than one dyskinesia, what is the most significant problem? Assessing the impact of myoclonus on the activities of daily living is second only to the underlying etiology in importance.

Pharmacologic Therapy

Although gamma-aminobutyric acid (GABA), glycine, and serotonin seem to be the primary neurotransmitters in the mechanism of human myoclonus, few direct manipulations of neurotransmitter pathways or receptors have been applied or are available in the treatment of myoclonus. Most of these are subsumed under the heading of antiepileptic drugs (AEDs).

Table 1 Considerations in Choosing a Treatment Strategy

Anticipated future needs
Cognitive abilities
Contributing factors
Current therapy
Etiologic diagnosis
Functional assessment
General health
Level of independence
Major limitations
Need for rehabilitation
Patient/parental attitudes
Physician attitudes
Prior interventions
Realistic goals
Risk for aspiration and choking
Risk for pregnancy

Antiepileptic Drugs (AEDs)

The AEDs have remained the principal pharmacologic treatment of myoclonus for decades (Table 2). Newer AEDs have not supplanted the "big three": clonazepam, primidone, and valproic acid. However, the new additions are most welcome. The AEDs may have synergistic effects in myoclonus, especially those with different mechanisms of action. Not all are antimyoclonic. In patients with epilepsy, especially intractable seizures, certain AEDs alone or in combination, may be promyoclonic. Others may contribute to the pathology, such as toxic effects of phenytoin on the cerebellum, a presumed site of pathology in PME.

For those who treat many patients with epilepsy, the greatest obstacle to treating myoclonus is applying the goal of monotherapy. In the more severe and chronic forms of myoclonus, monotherapy is seldom effective, and patients may require three or more medications. In progressive disorders, a mere 20% clinical improvement is considered a good response and may be functionally significant. Polytherapy still carries attendant risks for oversedation and drug–drug interactions, but it is a reality in myoclonus therapy.

Table 2 Antiepileptic Drugs for Myoclonic Disorders

Antimyoclonic	Unstudied	Sometimes promyoclonic[a]	Often promyoclonic[a]
Clonazepam	Clobazam[b]	Gabapentin	Carbamazepine
Ethosuximide	Eterobarb[b]	Lamotrigine	Oxcarbazepine
Felbamate	Remacemide[b]	Lorazepam	Phenytoin
Levetiracetam	Stiripentol[b]	Pregabalin[b]	
Phenobarbital	Tiagabine	Vigabatrin[b]	
Primidone	Topiramate		
Valproic acid			
Zonisamide			

[a] In epileptic patients.
[b] Not available in the United States.

When patients are referred to our center for myoclonus, we often find them on drugs that are not antimyoclonic. This is usually a result of treatment for concomitant epilepsy. However, it is important to choose antiepileptic medications for their antimyoclonic potential as well. This usually means removing phenytoin and carbamazepine-like drugs and replacing them with clonazepam, valproate, primidone, or other antimyoclonic drugs. Occasionally, a patient will have a history of status epilepticus when such changes are attempted and we leave their regimen alone.

Development of tolerance is a significant problem in the treatment of myoclonus regardless of the specific agent being used. The period of responsiveness may be months to years. Caution is indicated when the dose of clonazepam is increased due to tolerance, as choking on secretions may result at higher doses in individuals with PME.

Weight gain on valproate, an important drug for EPM1, can be massive in wheelchair-bound patients. Co-administration of a very small dose of topiramate may offset this effect.

Nonantiepileptic Drugs

Nonantiepileptic drugs as a group are the second line of symptomatic therapy for myoclonus, often reserved for special circumstances (Table 3). Usually they can be combined with antiepileptic drugs. None of these medications are FDA-approved for myoclonus. The pharmacologic treatment of autoimmune myoclonus serves as an example of therapy unrelated to AEDs or other neuropsychotropic drugs. Opsoclonus–myoclonus syndrome is best treated with immunotherapy, such as corticotropin (ACTH), intravenous-immunoglobulins (IVIG), or chemotherapy. Symptomatic treatments for the sleep disorder and rage attacks, such as trazodone, can be co-administered.

Intramuscular injection of botulinum toxin temporarily alleviates painful segmental myoclonus. In preventing the release of acetylcholine at the neuromuscular junction, botulinum toxin may block involuntary movement but will preserve strength. The effects last from weeks to months, but the injections can be repeated. Both botulinum toxins A (Botox) and B are used clinically. The current trend is toward lower doses than those recommended initially.

Table 3 Non-AEDs for Myoclonic Disorders

Drug	Indication
Acetazolamide	PMA
Baclofen	PME
Beta-adrenergic blockers	Essential myoclonus
Chloral hydrate	PME
Depo-estrogen	Perimenstrual exacerbation of myoclonus
5-Hydroxytryptophan[a]/carbidopa	Posthypoxic myoclonus
Piracetam[b]	Cortical myoclonus
Lisuride[b]	Photosensitive myoclonus
Midazolam	Opiate-induced myoclonus in cancer patients
Trihexyphenidyl	Myoclonus-dystonia

[a] A physician may prescribe under the manufacturer's IND in the United States for this specific indication only.

[b] Not available in the United States.

Nonpharmacologic Therapy

Vitamins, cofactors, dietary restriction, and chelation for metabolic disorders are examples of being able to treat myoclonus by reversing the underlying disorder. Together they constitute the most important category of nonpharmacologic therapy. Biotin can reverse the symptoms of biotinidase deficiency or other causes of biotin deficiency. Implementation of the ketogenic diet early in the course of EPM 2A may bypass a metabolic defect in carbohydrate metabolism.

Transcranial magnetic stimulation (TMS) is a noninvasive, safe, and painless way to stimulate the human motor cortex in humans. Repetitive TMS (rTMS) can be used to transiently inactivate different cortical areas to study their functions. Modulation of cortical excitability by rTMS has therapeutic potential in myoclonic disorders, because low-frequency stimulation (1 Hz) reduces cortical excitability. rTMS is currently investigational and not widely available, however, the equipment is not extremely costly or expansive and may well find its way into the clinical setting. The patient sits in a chair and a coil is lowered over the head. Although only cortical structures are currently accessible, rTMS seems capable of affecting activity in cortically linked deep brain structures.

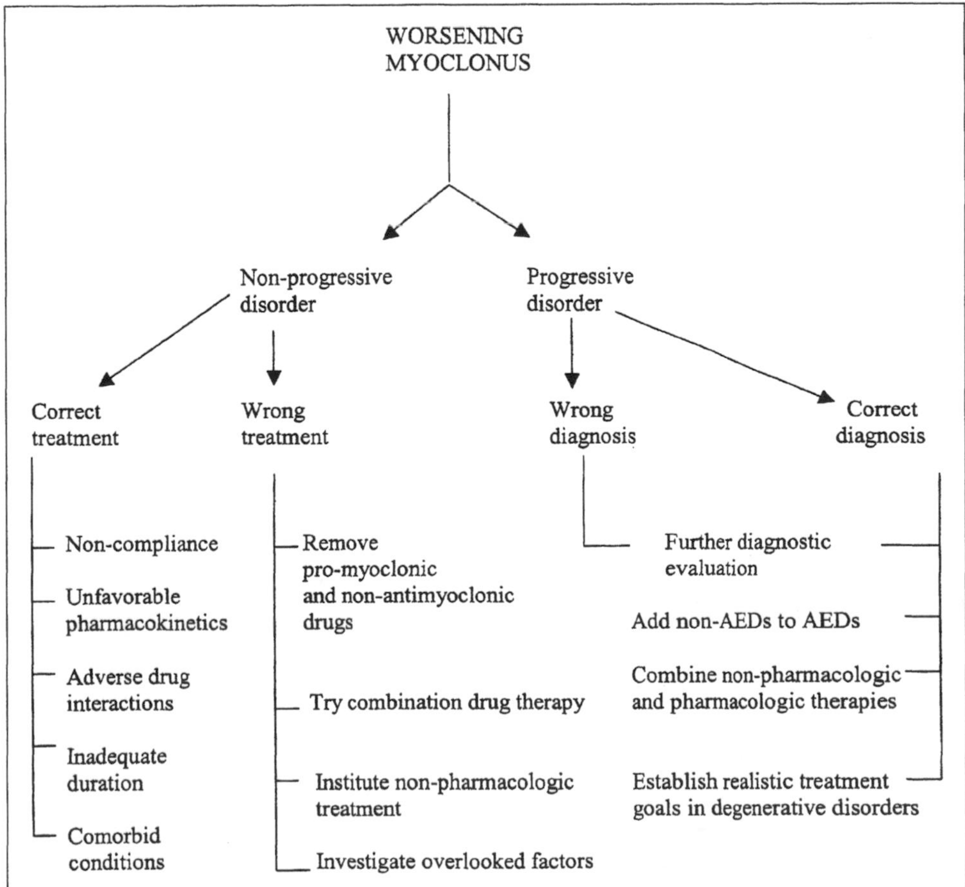

Figure 1 Troubleshooting flow chart. Lack of treatment response requires re-evaluation and should prompt re-thinking the diagnosis and a search for exacerbating factors. (*Continued*)

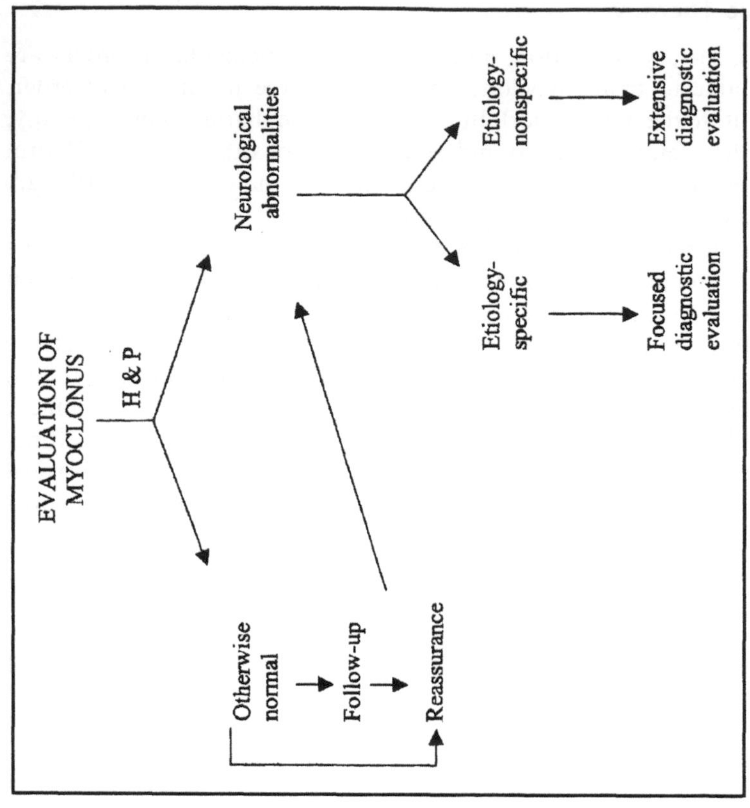

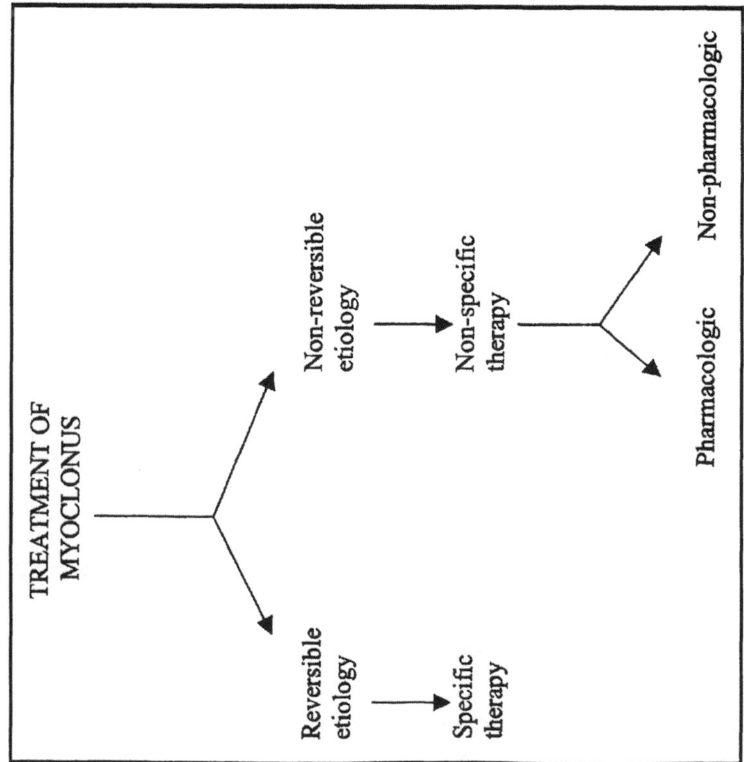

Figure 1 *(Continued)*

Possible Reasons for Treatment Failure

Myoclonus may fail to respond or increase as a result of misdiagnosis, mistreatment, or a refractory condition (Fig. 1). Persistence is the key to accurate diagnosis and treatment. It may be necessary to revisit the initial diagnosis, assess for overlooked factors, and verify that the drug regimen is being followed.

Exacerbating factors are frequently overlooked or not mentioned: dietary, hormonal, lifestyle, and psychosocial factors. Comorbid illnesses, such as anxiety, depression, or other affective disorders may compromise myoclonus treatment. An undiagnosed sleep disorder is common in some of the more severe myoclonic disorders, and poor sleep may increase myoclonus. Poor physical health caused by inactivity, obesity, or injuries from falls. A good general physical examination is a simple necessity.

Pharmacotherapy may be inadequate for many reasons. The drug may be ineffective or used at the wrong doses. Several weeks are required to properly evaluate treatment successes or failures; avoid too sudden changes. Further dose increases beyond the typical ceiling dose may be indicated in individuals with a partial drug response without side effects. Many different pharmacokinetic factors may be at play.

As a general rule, subcortical and segmental myoclonus are difficult to treat. It should also be remembered that in progressive disorders, the neural substrate for drug responsiveness may be lost, so that medications do not work as expected. In that situation, it is important to set realistic treatment endpoints.

Quality of Life Issues

It is easy to lose sight of quality of life issues in our focus on the medical aspects of myoclonus (Table 4). However, patients and their families carry a burden of living with a chronic disease, whether or not it is progressive, often without prospects for significant improvement. Severe myoclonus may rob adolescents of the necessary "breaking away" from parents, which leads to maladaptive behaviors and habitual family conflicts. Isolation, inactivity, and a decline in physical strength result in marginalization and reduced quality of life. Perhaps confidence is the most essential element to reinforce because it carries over so prominently into activities of daily living. When we cannot cure myoclonus, we must at least improve the way individuals with myoclonus feel about themselves. With gene therapy on the forefront, we must keep them in the best possible mental and physical shape. Different approaches should be taken at the same time.

PROGNOSIS

The prognosis of myoclonus depends on its etiology. It may resolve, remain static, or worsen. On the one end of the spectrum, benign neonatal sleep myoclonus usually resolves during infancy. While essential myoclonus does not resolve, it typically does not increase much over time, in contrast to PME, which by definition, worsens steadily. Even with PME, the prognosis varies considerably, ranging from lethality within 7–10 years in Lafora disease to a reasonably normal lifespan in EPM1. The myoclonus of biotin deficiency remits so long as the patient remains on biotin replacement therapy. In opsoclonus–myoclonus syndrome, myoclonus may remit, reappear during relapses, or progress depending on inflammatory activity of the

Table 4 Improving Quality of Life in Patients with Severe Myoclonus

Goal	Means
Continue education	Tutors
Counter depression	Pharmacologic and nonpharmacologic
Decrease strife	Counsellor/psychiatrist, individual, and family
Encourage independent living	Assisted living; visiting health aide
Establish medical contingencies for travel	Take emergency drugs on vacations
Increase safety in wheelchair	Wheelchair seat belt
Improve quality of sleep	Sleep study; treat depression
Maintain strength	Physical therapy; regular exercise program
Prevent obesity	Diet and exercise; offset drugs that cause hyperphagia
Maintain peer contact	School, church, community
Make home more accessible	Wheelchair ramps, move downstairs, make bathrooms handicap accessible
Prevent loneliness	Companion dog
Prevent pulmonary infections	Immunize
Reduce myoclonus when patient most needs to	Re-arrange dosing schedule
Reduce stress	Modify school schedule
Set practical goals	Educational and vocational counseling

immune system, which involves both T-cells and B-cells. All of these different patterns emphasize the need to press for an etiologic diagnosis even in the most complex presentations of myoclonus and tailor the therapy to the etiology.

SUMMARY

The approach to a patient with myoclonus should focus on identifying the underlying etiology in the hope that the disorder can be reversed. The context in which myoclonus occurs is the single most useful clinical clue to etiology, often narrowing the scope of otherwise extensive diagnostic investigations. Neurophysiologic tests are the cornerstone of myoclonic classification and may indicate productive avenues of therapy. Restoring activities of everyday living should be a fundamental therapeutic goal. A regimen of multiple drugs is the rule. Responses to an agent are sometimes dramatic, but more often the improvements are incremental. In patients with substantial myoclonus, the combination of pharmacologic and nonpharmacologic measures can be effective. Therapeutic failure should prompt re-evaluation of the diagnosis and treatment plan and a search for exacerbating factors. In the end, sensitivity to quality of life issues can be the most important contribution a clinician can make.

SUGGESTED READINGS

1. Hallett M. Myoclonus: relation to epilepsy. Epilepsia 1985; 26:567–577.
2. Marsden CD, Hallett M, Fahn S. The nosology and pathophysiology of myoclonus. In: Marsden CD, Fahn S, eds. Movement Disorders. London: Butterworths, 1982:196–248.

3. Minassian BA, Sainz J, Delgado-Escueta AV. Genetics of myoclonus and myoclonus epilepsies. Clin Neurosci 1995; 3:223–235.
4. Pranzatelli MR. Paraneoplastic syndromes: an unsolved murder. Semin Pediatr Neurol 2000; 7:118–130.
5. Shibasaki H, Ikeda A, Nagamino T, et al: Cortical reflex negative myoclonus. Brain 1994; 117:477–486.

25
Combined Muscle and Brain Diseases

Ronald D. Cohn
Johns Hopkins Hospital, Children's Center, McKusick-Nathans Institute of Genetic Medicine, Baltimore, Maryland, U.S.A.

A number of clinically distinct disorders of muscle manifest abnormalities in other organs, most often the brain. The most common of these, Duchenne muscular dystrophy, is discussed in a separate chapter. The disorders that predominantly affect muscle, but manifest with distinctive abnormalities of brain as well, likely do so because of widespread gene expression and other commonalities of brain and muscle. Other than their shared tissue vulnerabilities, there is a wide range of apparent gene function between these disorders. This is a rapidly expanding area of clinical and fundamental neuroscience, and more disorders and a better understanding of those disorders already described is virtually certain in the next few years.

DISORDERS OF PROTEIN GLYCOSYLATION, "DYSTROGLYCANOPATHIES"

There has been a recent explosion in the identification of neuromuscular diseases caused by mutations in genes that affect carbohydrate metabolism or protein glycosylation. A number of these findings relate to defects in the *O*-glycosylation of α-dystroglycan.

Alpha dystroglycan plays a pivotal role within the dystrophin–glycoprotein complex (DGC), which represents a major factor for muscle fiber stability upon contraction. Identification of gene mutations within the DGC and the association with Duchenne/Becker muscular dystrophy and other forms of limb–girdle and congenital muscular dystrophy have dominated the clinical and research field for years.

Recently, the focus has shifted to post-translational modifications of proteins, as genes encoding proteins involved in glycosylation have defined a new area of attention in muscular dystrophy. Although the function of most glycosylation is poorly understood, many vertebrate proteins are post-translationally modified by carbohydrates and it has been estimated that 1% of human genes encode enzymes involved in oligosaccharide synthesis and function. A deficiency in post-translational modification of α-dystroglycan has now been characterized as a common feature in several forms of muscular dystrophy associated with central nervous system abnormalities. It needs to be emphasized that these types of muscular dystrophies appear to be distinct from the congenital disorders of glycosylation (CDG syndromes), a group of diseases that often leads to multisystem disease caused by defects in the well-characterized *N*-glycosylation pathways as opposed to the less defined *O*-glycosylation pathways.

The majority of patients with muscular dystrophy and associated structural brain morphology present with fairly nonspecific symptoms such as profound hypotonia usually at the time of birth suggesting that abnormalities of skeletal muscle and the central nervous system have occurred in utero during early development. Thus, a fairly extensive initial diagnostic workup of the hypotonic infant is generally needed to distinguish this patient group from patients with other causes of neonatal hypotonia such as central nervous system hemorrhage, infection, or neurometabolic diseases.

Abnormalities of serum creatine kinase, a myopathic pattern of electromyography (even in the presence of a normal serum creatine kinase) and any abnormal structural abnormalities detected on CT scan or preferably on MRI should prompt the clinician to perform a skeletal muscle biopsy and consider the above mentioned group of dystroglycanopathies as a potential differential diagnosis (Table 1). The skeletal muscle biopsy generally reveals classic signs of muscular dystrophy involving signs of degeneration and regeneration with centrally located nuclei, fibrosis and fat

Table 1 Overview of Clinical and Molecular Forms of Dystroglycanopathies Associated with Central Nervous System Disease

Dystroglycanopathy	Inheritance	Gene/ protein	Clinical findings
Muscle eye brain disease (MEB)	AR	POMGnT1	Severe muscle weakness, mental retardation, epilepsy, neuronal migration disorder, ocular abnormalities[a]
Walker Warburg syndrome (WWS)	AR	POMT1	Severe muscle weakness, death usually in infancy, severe psychomotor developmental delay, mental retardation epilepsy, neuronal migration disorder, ocular abnormalities[a]
Fukuyama congenital muscular dystrophy (FCMD)	AR	Fukutin	Severe axial and proximal muscle weakness, mental retardation, epilepsy, neuronal migration disorder
Congenital muscular dystrophy 1C (MDC1C)	AR	FKRP	Variable muscle weakness, cerebellar abnormalities cardiomyopathy
Congenital muscular dystrophy 1D (MDC1D)	AR	LARGE	Variable muscle weakness, profound mental retardation, white matter changes, subtle neuronal migration disorder

[a] Ocular abnormalities may include congenital myopia, glaucoma, pallor of optic discs, retinal hypoplasia.
Abbreviations: AR, autosomal recessive; POMGnT1, protein *O*-mannose β-1,2-*N*-acetylglucosaminyltransferase; POMT1, protein *O*-mannosyltransferase; FKRP, fukutin-related protein; LARGE, putative glycosyltransferase.

tissue deposition. In addition, immunohistochemical analysis with antibodies directed towards α-dystroglycan exhibits loss or significantly reduced expression of α-dystroglycan at the sarcolemma of the muscle fibers. Currently, enzymatic tests and mutational screening are being developed for clinical use in order to confirm the clinical/immunohistological diagnosis of dystroglycanopathies.

The prognosis for dystroglycanopathies is extremely variable. All the patients within this disease spectrum who also have structural abnormalities of the brain show mild to severe mental retardation. Patients diagnosed with Walker Warburg syndrome are most severely affected and usually die within the first few years of life. In contrast, patients within the MDC1C and 1D group (Table 1) can have milder phenotypes particularly in respect to their muscle power. At present, there is no specific therapy for any of these disorders. Clinical care is thus directed to supportive and preventative therapy, aiming to prevent secondary sequalae from significant muscle weakness such as joint contractures and chronic respiratory hypoventilation. Therefore, close collaboration with physical therapists, orthopedic surgeons, and pulmonologists is a significant part of management for these patients.Current research is directed towards enzyme therapy in an effort to potentially modify the aberrant glycosylation of α-dystroglycan.

CONGENITAL MUSCULAR DYSTROPHY DUE TO LAMININ α2 DEFICIENCY

This form of congenital muscular dystrophy is associated with early onset of weakness, often very severe, that is thereafter largely stable with good supportive care. A distinctive abnormality of white matter on MRI and CT imaging first suggests profound leukodystrophy, but there is no intellectual or other detectable consistent abnormality in CNS function. Laminin α2 is an extracellular protein that appears to be important in the organization of free water within white matter around charged residues; the result of its absence is that extracellular water thus has magnetic properties similar to that of free water within the ventricles. There is often an associated mild neuropathy, though the importance is lost given the severe end-stage myopathy that is usually present.

MYOTONIC DYSTROPHY, STEINERT'S DISEASE, DM1

The nosology of myotonic dystrophies (DM) is in a state of flux. The DM can be regarded as a clinical syndrome that includes subtypes designated myotonic dystrophy type I (DM1), myotonic dystrophy type 2 (DM2) and so forth, each of which is a single-gene entity. The originally described monogenic disorder by Steinert (DM1) is by far the most common form. This condition, inherited as an autosomal dominant trait, is the most common form of muscular dystrophy of adult life with a worldwide prevalence of 2.1–14.3 per 100,000. While affecting predominantly adults, it also occurs in childhood and early infancy with an estimated incidence of 1 in 8000 births. It is characterized by myotonia in association with muscle weakness and wasting plus a whole syndrome complex with additional features such as frontal balding (males), cataracts, cardiomyopathy with conduction defects, gonadal atrophy possible associated with infertility and low intelligence or dementia (Table 2). The genetic basis for DM1 is an expansion of CTG repeats on chromosome 19.

Table 2 Systemic Involvement in Myotonic Dystrophy Type 1

Eye	Cataract
Endocrine system	Diabetes Thyroid dysfunction Hypogonadism
Gastrointestinal system	Dysphagia Constipation Gallbladder stones Pseudo-obstruction
Central nervous system	Cognitive impairment Mental retardation Attentive disorders
Heart	Cardiomyopathy Conduction defects Mitral valve prolaps Ischemic heart disease

Approximately 10% of patients with DM1 present in infancy with severe neonatal hypotonia, feeding and respiratory difficulties, and mental retardation in those who survive into childhood. Interestingly, infants with congenital DM1 have very large repeat expansions (>1000 CTG repeats). Almost invariably, these infants have inherited the condition from their mother. The maternal bias in transmitting DM1 is due to increased likelihood of generating very large repeat expansions during oogenesis as compared to spermatogenesis. DM1 is also characterized by extreme anticipation generally associated with an intergenerational increase in CTG expansion corresponding to increase in disease severity in the offspring.

The diagnosis of DM1 can be made by clinical findings supported by genetic analysis of CTG repeats of chromosome 19. Serum creatine kinase activity can be elevated in adults but is usually within normal range in infants and mildly affected adults. In case of a significant hypotonic infant, the mother (who may not be aware of their condition) should be clinically examined. The examination should include evaluation for facial weakness (inability to close eyes tightly, bury the eyelashes), myotonia of the hands and percussion myotonia of the tongue. Electromyography studies in adult patients and in minimally affected mothers of infants with the congenital form of DM1 show the pathognomonic spontaneous myotonic bursts of activity with gradual decrement, giving the typical "dive bomber" or "departing motor cycle" sound on acoustic amplification.

DM2 manifests with many of the same features as does DM1. A critical difference, however, is the absence of a congenital form. In general, symptoms and signs first emerge in adult years.

Cardiac arrhythmia, especially heart block caused by progressive degeneration of the conduction system, is the second leading cause of mortality in DM1. Genetic analysis has revealed that patients with larger expansions of CTG repeats are at increased risk of intraventricular conduction delay at baseline and show more rapid progression of the conduction defect. Therefore, cardiac evaluation including basal ECG, 24 hr Holter monitoring and echocardiogram should be routinely performed (once per year) in all patients presenting with DM1. Often, implanting of a pacemaker or a cardioverter-defibrillator is required.

Supportive management of muscle weakness, constipation, endocrine problems, eye abnormalities, and mental impairment comprises a major part of the management of patients with DM1. In addition, it is of utmost importance to emphasize the risk for generalized anesthesia, sedation, and analgesia (especially thiopentane should be avoided) because of sudden death reported in several cases. The risk is independent of the clinical severity of DM1 and clinical catastrophies can occur even in subclinical cases.

CONGENITAL FIBER TYPE DISPROPORTION

Congenital fiber type disproportion (CFTD) is a congenital myopathy initially described by Brooke in 1973 purely on the basis of consistent abnormalities detected on muscle biopsy associated with relatively good clinical prognosis. The type 1 skeletal muscle fibers were found to be smaller than type 2 fibers by a margin of more than 25% of the diameter of the type 2 fibers. These findings are in contrast to normal skeletal muscle in children where type 1 and type 2 fibers are of approximately equal size.

The CFTD is suspected to be inherited as an autosomal recessive trait with some rare exceptions. The clinical picture is characterized by congenital hypotonia and delayed motor milestones. The disease is often associated with congenital dislocation of the hip, high arched palate, kyphoscoliosis, and contractures. Serum creatine kinase may be slightly elevated and infrequently, a myopathic pattern on electromyography can be detected. The diagnosis is finally made after thorough histological analysis of a skeletal muscle biopsy revealing the above described inbalance of type1 and type 2 skeletal muscle fibers. The degree of muscle weakness varies quite considerably involving usually all muscle types. In some rare cases, little voluntary movement of arms and legs can be detected until 2 year of age. In other cases, weakness can be mild enough to cause only a delay in development of the motor milestones, rather than any obvious paralysis. Although the weakness may slightly progress during the first year of life, it is highly significant for CFTD to see no further progression of symptoms past 2 years of age. Instead, as the children grow older, the disease becomes static and often, significant improvement of muscle weakness can be observed. Taken together, the diagnosis of CFTD can be difficult to make and should not be made in the face of obvious clinical pictures such as myotonic dystrophy, Prader Willi syndrome, or congenital muscular dystrophy.

SUGGESTED READINGS

1. Grewal PK, Hewitt JE. Glycosylation defects: a new mechanism for muscular dystrophy? Hum Mol Genet 2003; 12:R259–R264.
2. Mankodi A, Thornton CA. Myotonic syndromes. Curr Opin Neurol 2002; 15:545–552.
3. Dubowitz V. Muscle Disorders in Childhood. 2d ed. Saunders, 1995.

26

Inflammatory Neuropathies: Guillan-Barré Syndrome (GBS) and Chronic Inflammatory Demyelinating Polyradiculoneuropathy (CIDP)

Charlotte J. Sumner
National Institute of Neurological Disorders and Stroke, National Institutes of Health, Bethesda, Maryland, U.S.A.

INTRODUCTION

Inflammatory neuropathies are uncommon in children but critical to diagnose because they are treatable. They are caused by a direct autoimmune attack against peripheral nerve resulting in progressive motor weakness and/or sensory loss. According to the time from symptom onset until maximal severity of disease, these neuropathies can be divided into acute (<4 weeks) and chronic forms (>8 weeks).

GUILLAN-BARRÉ SYNDROME (GBS)

Since the decline in the incidence of polio, GBS has become the most common cause of acute neuromuscular paralysis. GBS has an incidence of 0.5–1.5 cases per 100,000 in the population less than 18 years of age. In recent years, it has been recognized that GBS encompasses a heterogeneous group of disorders that can be distinguished based on clinical, electrophysiologic, and pathologic criteria (Table 1). In some forms, the immune attack is directed primarily against constituents of the myelinating Schwann cell and in other forms, against components of the axon. Acute inflammatory demyelinating neuropathy (AIDP) is the most common form of GBS in North America and Europe, whereas acute motor axonal neuropathy (AMAN) is the most common form of GBS in China.

Diagnosis/Clinical Features

The classical clinical picture of GBS is a previously healthy child who develops ascending symmetrical paralysis evolving over days with loss of tendon reflexes. In

Table 1 Types of GBS

	AIDP	AMAN	AMSAN	MFS
Ages affected	All	Mainly children and young adults	Mainly adults	Adults more than children
Clinical involvement	Motor and sensory	Motor	Motor and sensory	Ataxia and ophthalmoplegia
Electrodiagnosis	Demyelinating	Axonal	Axonal	Demyelinating
Pathology	Attack at Schwann cell surface with vesicular myelin damage; lymphocytic infiltration and macrophage activation	Attack at nodes of Ranvier with frequent periaxonal macrophages and few lymphocytes	Same as AMAN, but also affects sensory nerves and dorsal roots with severe axonal damage	
Recovery	Rapid (most)	Rapid (most)	Slow	Variable

AIDP = acute inflammatory demyelinating polyradiculoneuropahty; AMAN = actue motor axonal neuropathy; AMSAN = acute motor sensory axonal neuropathy; MFS = Miller Fischer syndrome. Adapted from Ref. 1.

approximately half of children, there is a history of symptoms of recent antecedent infectious illness (*Campylobacter* gastroenteritis, *Mycoplasma* pneumonia, or viral illness due to Epstein–Barr virus or cytomegalovirus) or other event such as trauma or surgery. Early in the clinical course, back or leg pain may be the most prominent symptom in children making the early diagnosis somewhat confusing. The three forms of GBS in which weakness predominates are AIDP, acute motor axonal sensory neuropathy (AMSAN), and AMAN. In AIDP and AMSAN, sensory loss also occurs. In other forms of GBS, signs other than weakness predominate, such as ataxia and ophthalmoplegia in Miller Fisher syndrome (MFS) and dysautonomia in acute panautonomic neuropathy. All syndromes are characterized by a limited, monophasic course with eventual recovery.

When evaluating patients with suspected GBS, other causes of acute weakness must be excluded (Table 2). Fever at the outset of neurologic symptoms should raise the possibility of alternative diagnoses. GBS is rare in children less than 1 year of age, increasing the possibility of other diagnoses such as botulism or poliomyelitis syndrome due to poliovirus or other enteroviruses. Spinal cord compression should always be considered and excluded, particularly in patients without cranial nerve palsies or when there is bowel or bladder sphincter involvement. Laboratory investigations should include cerebrospinal fluid (CSF) examination to exclude infectious or lymphomatous polyradiculitis. Elevated CSF protein in the absence of cellular pleocytosis (albumino-cytologic dissociation) reinforces the clinical diagnosis of GBS, although CSF protein can be normal within the first week. Nerve conduction studies and electromyography can also help to exclude other diagnoses (such as myopathy and neuromuscular junction disease) and are useful in the classification of the type of GBS. In demyelinating forms of GBS, the earliest electrophysiologic findings are prolongation of distal motor latencies and loss or prolongation of F wave latencies. Focal conduction block also occurs early, but is often technically difficult to detect because it typically occurs at the proximal nerve roots. It takes several days before reduction of conduction velocity develops. Severe decrease in compound

Table 2 Differential Diagnosis in GBS

Pseudoencephalopathy
Meningitis
Meningoencephalitis
Cerebellar syndrome
Postinfectious cerebellar ataxia
Structural lesion
Myelopathy
Spinal cord compression
Transverse myelitis
Acute disseminated encephalomyelitis
Anterior spinal artery distribution infarction
Anterior horn cells
Enteroviral infection
Poliomyelitis
Peripheral nerve
Tick paralysis
Diptheria
Lyme disease
Toxins/drugs
Acute intermittent porphyria
Critical illness polyneuropathy
Mitochondrial disease
Neuromuscular junction
Botulism
Myasthenia gravis
Neuromuscular blockade
Pseudocholinesterase deficiency
Muscle disorders
Acute myositis
Infectious
Autoimmune
Metabolic myopathy
Glycogen storage disorders, etc.
Periodic paralysis
Critical care myopathy

From Ref. 2.

motor action potential amplitude is more commonly seen in children than it is in adults with demyelinating polyneuropathy, and is associated with incomplete recovery presumably due to axon degeneration. The relative prognostic importance of diminished compound motor action potential amplitude in children is not known. Although serum antibodies to many peripheral nerve antigens have been found in GBS, their role in the pathogenesis of the disease remains unclear.

Therapy

Mortality rates from GBS have fallen dramatically in recent decades mainly because of improvements in nursing and critical care measures. Any child suspected of having GBS should be hospitalized until the maximum degree of clinical disability is established. In the early stages of the disease, respiratory status should be monitored carefully with frequent measurement of vital capacity. Endotrachial intubation and mechanical ventilation should be initiated early, when proper intensive care specialists can be assembled in a careful and controlled manner, rather than waiting for a respiratory crisis. Generally, any sign of compromised airway during the progressive phase of GBS, or vital capacity below 15 cm^3/kg, is an indication for intubation. In older, larger children preventive measures for deep venous thrombosis and pulmonary embolus should include use of leg stockings (TEDS) and subcutaneous heparin. It is essential to monitor patients for autonomic nervous system dysfunction such as blood pressure fluctuations, cardiac arrythmias, gastrointestinal pseudoobstruction, and urinary retention. Nutritional issues should be considered and addressed early. Patients also require frequent turning to prevent skin breakdown. Physical therapy with passive range of motion exercises should be started immediately to avoid contractures. Pain is common in children with GBS, and should be aggressively treated, sometimes with opiates. In profoundly weak children who are unable to communicate, sinus tachycardia and other features of sympathetic activation may represent primary autonomic involvement, pain, or both.

In several large clinical trials in adults, plasma exchange and intravenous immunoglobulin (IVIg) have each been shown to be equally effective in reducing the time to recovery in patients with GBS, if initiated within the first two weeks (Table 3). Observational studies suggest similar benefit in children, although the potential for complications due to plasma exchange increases with smaller body size. On balance, these therapies are recommended only for the minority of children who manifest more severe forms GBS: those that have lost the ability to ambulate or have bulbar weakness causing dysphagia or aspiration. Because of the difficulty with vascular access and potential problems with fluid shifts given smaller blood volume, of the two therapies, treatment with IVIg has become the accepted therapy for GBS in children. The recommended schedule is 2 g/kg of body weight divided into five consecutive daily doses of 400 mg/kg each. Side effects are generally minor, but severe side effects can include chemical meningitis, acute tubular necrosis, and renal failure (particularly in patients with pre-existing renal disease), thomboembolic events, and rarely anaphylaxis.

Table 3 Treatment Options for GBS

Therapy	Regimen	Side effects
Plasma exchange	Remove 200–250 mL/kg of plasma over 7–10 days	Catheter placement may cause pneumothorax, bleeding, deep vein thrombosis, pulmonary emboli, or sepsis. Blood removal may cause hypotension, anemia, thrombocytopenia, or electrolyte derangements
Intravenous immunoglobulin	0.4 g/kg/day × 5 days	Fever, chills, myalgia, fluid overload, hypertension, nausea, vomiting, skin rash, headaches, chemical meningitis, acute tubular necrosis, thromboembolic events, anaphylactic reaction associated IgA deficiency

Administration of plasma exchange requires a central line or large peripheral line. In centers with appropriate experience, this may be safely done in children who weigh more than 10 kg. The usual protocol, derived from experience with adults, involves exchanges on the 1st, 3rd, 5th, and 7th days targeting a total exchange volume of 250 mL/kg. Problems with plasma exchange include difficulty with placement and maintenance of central lines and hypotension during exchanges. If patients experience a relapse within approximately 10 days of the first treatment, retreatment with the same initial agent at half the dose is recommended.

Prognosis

Overall prognosis in GBS is good with approximately 90–95% of affected children making a complete functional recovery within 6–12 months. Those who do not recover completely are often ambulating independently with only minor neurologic residua. Since the advent of modern critical care, mortality from GBS in children is rare.

CHRONIC INFLAMMATORY DEMYELINATING POLYRADICULOPATHY (CIDP)

CIDP is a form of inflammatory motor and sensory neuropathy that evolves over a protracted time of more than 4–8 weeks. CIDP is less common than GBS and occurs less frequently in children than in adults. Nonetheless, CIDP represents approximately 10% of all chronic childhood neuropathies.

Diagnosis/Clinical Features

The classic symptoms and signs of CIDP include largely symmetric weakness in proximal and distal limb muscles, reduced or absent tendon reflexes, and, sometimes, sensory deficits and paresthesias. Most often children present with abnormal gait and frequent falls secondary to weakness of the legs. Rarely CIDP may present with arm weakness. CIDP may manifest with a chronic progressive, monophasic, or relapsing–remitting clinical course. Weakness is primarily a consequence of conduction block resulting from focal demyelination; as such it often responds well to treatment. After years of disease, there can be accumulating axonal degeneration, clinically evident by wasted muscles, which may be irreverisible.

There are many causes of symmetrical weakness in children ranging from central nervous system disorders to muscle disease. In patients without sensory symptoms and signs, anterior horn cell disease (spinal muscular atrophy), neuromuscular junction disease, and muscle disease are important considerations. Neuropathy in children is often due to inherited disorders such as Charcot-Marie-Tooth disease (CMT type 1–4 and X) or less commonly due to inborn errors of metabolism such as Krabbe's disease, metachromatic leukodystrophy, Refsum's disease, adrenomyeloleukodystrophy, or acute intermittent porphyria. A diagnosis of CIDP is made primarily on the basis of nerve conduction studies (Table 4). Although decreased conduction velocities and prolonged distal motor latencies can be seen in both CIDP and hereditary demyelinating neuropathy, CIDP is distinguished by the presence of

Table 4 Clinical and Electrophysiologic Criteria for Childhood CIDP

Mandatory clinical criteria

Progression of muscle weakness in proximal and distal muscles of upper and lower extremities over at least 4 weeks, or rapid progression (GBS-like presentation) followed by a relapsing or protracted course (>1 year)

Major laboratory features

Electrophysiologic criteria

Must demonstrate at least three of the following four major abnormalities in motor nerves (or two of the major plus two of the supportive criteria)

A. Major
   1. Conduction block or abnormal temporal dispersion in one or more motor nerves at sites not prone to compression:
      a. Conduction block: at least 50% drop in negative peak area or peak-to-peak amplitude of proximal compound action potential (CMAP) if duration of negative peak of proximal CMAP is < 130% of distal CMAP duration.
      b. Temporal dispersion: abnormal if duration of negative peak of proximal CMAP is > 130% of distal CMAP duration.
   2. Reduction in conduction velocity (CV) in two or more nerves: <75% mean of mean CV value for age minus 2 standard deviations (SD).
   3. Prolonged distal latency (DL) in two or more nerves: >130% of mean DL value for age +2SD.
   4. Absent F-waves or prolonged F-wave minimal latency (ML) in two or more nerves: >130% of mean F-wave ML for age + 2SD.

B. Supportive

When conduction block is absent, the following abnormal electrophysiological parameters are indicative of nonuniform slowing and thus of acquired neuropathy:
   1. Abnormal median sensory nerve action potential (SNAP) while sural nerve SNAP is normal.
   2. Abnormally low terminal latency index: distal conduction distance (mm)/(conduction velocity [m/sec]) × distal motor latency [msec]).
   3. Side-to-side comparison of motor CVs showing a difference of >10 m/sec between nerves.

Cerebrospinal fluid (CSF) criteria

Protein > 45mg/dL

Cell count <10 cells/mm^3

Nerve biopsy features

Predominant features of demyelination

Exclusion criteria

A. Clinical features of history of a hereditary neuropathy, other disease, or exposure to drugs or toxins known to cause peripheral neuropathy.

B. Laboratory findings (including nerve biopsy or genetic testing) that show evidence of a cause other than CIDP.

C. Electrodiagnostic features of abnormal neuromuscular transmission, myopathy, or anterior horn cell disease.

Diagnostic criteria

A. Confirmed CIDP
   1. Mandatory clinical features
   2. Electrodiagnostic and CSF features

B. Possible CIDP
   1. Mandatory clinical features
   2. One of the three laboratory findings

From Ref. 4.

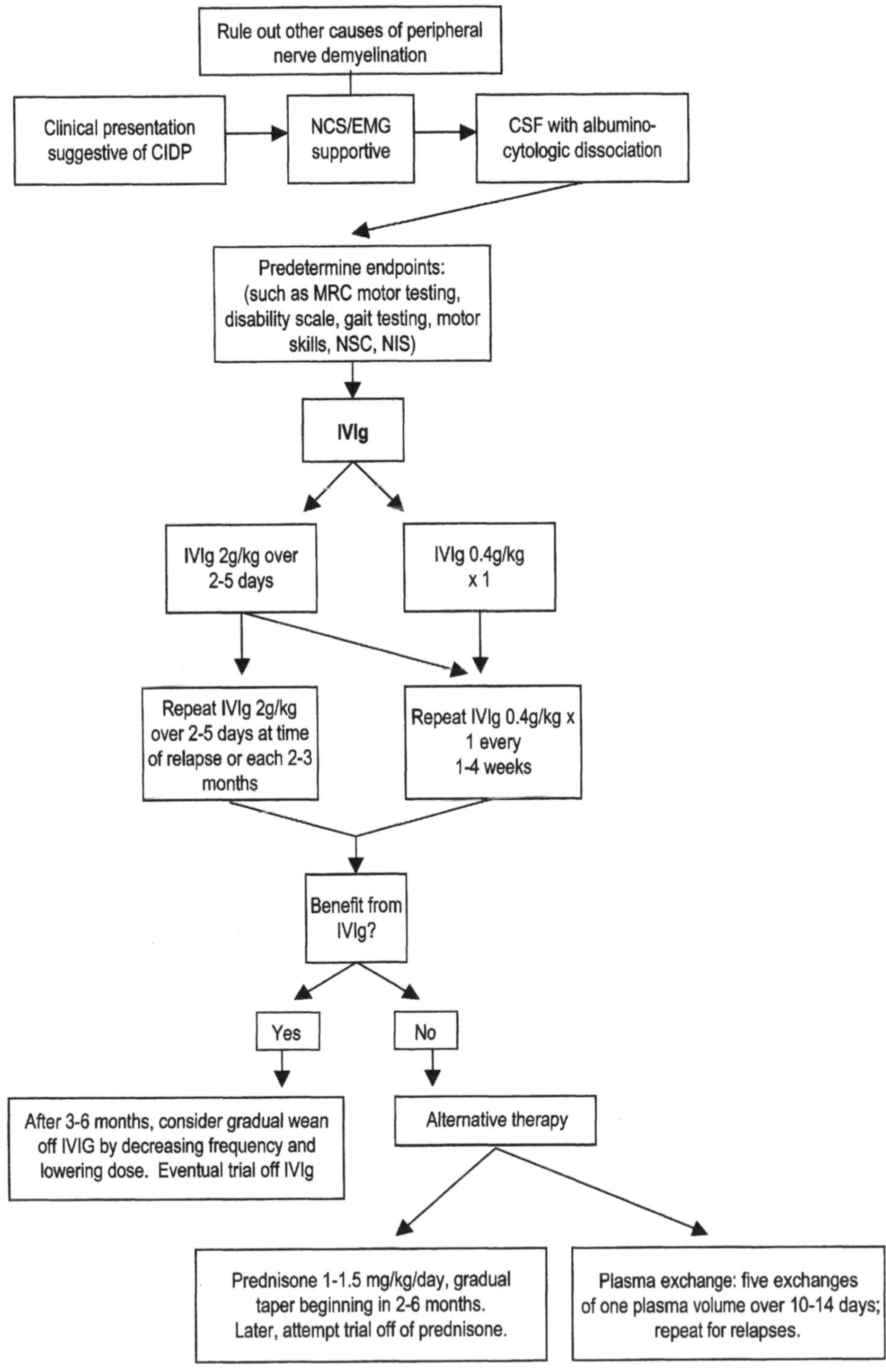

Figure 1 Proposed treatment algorithm for childhood chronic inflammatory demyelinating polyradiculoneuropathy (CIDP). (CSF = cerebrospinal fluid; EMG = electromyogram; IVIg = intravenous immunoglobulin; MRC = Medical Research Council; NCS = nerve conduction study; NIS = neuropathy impairment score; NSC = neuropathy symptoms and change score). (From Ref 4.)

features indicating acquired demyelination, such as motor conduction block, temporal dispersion, and asymmetric involvement. A nerve biopsy is sometimes diagnostic, but not necessary and now not routinely done. An elevated CSF protein without pleocytosis is evident in at least 90% of children with CIDP. Magnetic resonance imaging can show gadolinium enhancement of nerve roots that favors a diagnosis of CIDP over CMT.

Therapy

The two most commonly used immunomodulatory therapies for children with CIDP are oral corticosteroids and IVIg. Treatment should be reserved for children with significant disability. A detailed discussion needs to be undertaken with the patient and family to explain the rationale for treatment and the potential short- and long-term side effects. IVIg has been shown to be effective in clinical trials in adult patients. The reported experience in small case series of children also supports its use in this age group. Prednisone has been used for many years in childhood CIDP and reported to be effective in several case series. Unfortunately, there are many potential side effects of prednisone including weight gain, hyperglycemia, neuropsychiatric disturbance, impaired wound healing, avascular hip necrosis, hyperlipproteinemia, accelerated atherosclerosis, osteoporosis, myopathy, peptic ulcer disease, and cataracts. In some cases intermittent high dose solumedrol infusions, weaning on interval rather than dose, may have enhanced efficacy without the same degree of Cushingoid side effects. There is little published experience with plasma exchange in the children with CIDP, likely due to the significant problems associated with maintaining vascular access. Other treatment options include azathioprine, methotrexate, cyclosporine A, cyclophosphamide, and interferon beta. Because of the limited experience and adverse effects of these drugs, IVIg and prednisone should be first line therapy. A treatment algorithm for childhood CIDP proposed by Burns et al. (3) is detailed in Fig. 1.

Prognosis

The long-term prognosis for children treated for CIDP is favorable. Most patients return to normal strength after treatment and may be asymptomatic for extended periods (months to years) of immunotherapy. Relapses may occur after years of therapy, but are usually not as severe as the original illness. A minority of patients have severe residual weakness.

SUMMARY

When acute and chronic forms of inflammatory neuropathy are accurately diagnosed, supportive and immune modulating therapy can be instituted. This often leads to complete recovery of function. In addition to these treatment measures, however, it is critical to focus time on patient and family communication, and education. From the earliest stages, the patient should understand the risk of progression, the prognosis for recovery, and that the disease process is limited to the peripheral nervous system.

SUGGESTED READINGS

1. Asbury AK. New concepts of Guillan-Barré syndrome. J Child Neurol 2000; 15:183–191.
2. Sladky JT. Guillan-Barré syndrome. In: Jones HR, De Vivo DC, Darras BT, eds. Neuromuscular Disorders of Infancy, Childhood, and Adolescence: A Clinicians Approach. Woburn, MA: Butterworth Heinemann, 2003:407–424.
3. Burns TM, Dyck PJ, Darras BT, Jones HR. Chronic inflammatory demyelinating polyradiculoneuropathy. In: Jones HR, De Vivo DC, Darras BT, eds. Neuromuscular Disorders of Infancy, Childhood, and Adolescence: A Clinicians Approach. Woburn, MA: Butterworth Heinemann, 2003:445–468.
4. Nevo Y, Topalogle H 88th ENMC International Workshop: Childbood chronic Inflammatory Demyelinating Polyneuropathy (including revised diagnostic criteria), Naarden, the Netherlands, Dec 8–10, 2002. Neuromuscul Disord 2002; 12:195–200.
5. Hadden RDM, Hughes RAC. Management of inflammatory neuropathies. J Neurol Neurosurg Psychiatry 2003; 74:ii9–ii14.
6. Lu JL, Sheikh, KA, Wu HS, et al. Physiologic–pathologic correlation in Guillan-Barré syndrome in children. Neurology 2000; 54:33–39.

27
Treatment of Peripheral Neuropathies

Robert Ouvrier
TY Nelson Department of Neurology and Neurosurgery, Children's Hospital at Westmead, Sydney, Australia

Monique M. Ryan
Discipline of Paediatrics and Child Health, Children's Hospital at Westmead, Sydney, Australia

Anthony Redmond
Academic Unit of Musculoskletal Disease, University of Leeds, Leeds, U.K.

INTRODUCTION

Therapeutic measures available for the specific underlying cause of most neuropathies that affect children are few or not very effective. Notable exceptions are the inflammatory and some metabolic neuropathies, where treatment can be remarkably effective. For most of the hereditary neuropathies, the basic mechanisms are poorly understood and progression is irreversible. Even in the absence of a treatment for the primary pathology, however, there are many ways in which function can be enhanced and symptoms minimized. As reviewed by Hallett et al. (1): "Three kinds of therapy are possible. If the etiology of the neuropathy is identified, then therapy directed to the underlying illness may be beneficial to the neuropathy. Regardless of whether the etiology of the neuropathy is known or unknown, it may be possible to improve nerve function with therapy directed to improving nerve metabolism itself. If it is impossible to reverse the neuropathy, it still maybe possible to be helpful with symptomatic therapy." Especially in children, where the additional dimension of growth adds layers of both complexity and opportunity, judicious use of orthotics and surgery may often prevent the contractures and deformities that may occur in those whose primary condition resists treatment.

The following chapter discusses these general aspects of diagnosis and therapy. Those treatments directed to the underlying cause of specific disorders are listed in Tables 1 and 2.

DIAGNOSIS

Peripheral neuropathies are those conditions in which the pathological process primarily affects the peripheral nerves between the brainstem or spinal cord at one

Table 1 Treatment of Inflammatory Neuropathies in Childhood

Disorder	Neuropathy	Therapy
Guillain–Barré syndrome	Demyelinating	IVIG 1 g/kg daily for 2 days or IVIG 0.4 g/kg daily for 5 days
Guillain–Barré syndrome	Axonal (acute motor axonal neuropathy: AMAN)	IVIG 1 g/kg daily for 2 days or IVIG 0.4 g/kg daily for 5 days
Diphtheria	Demyelinating	Diphtheria antitoxin
Chronic inflammatory demyelinating neuropathy	Mostly demyelinating	IVIG 1 g/kg daily for 2 days or IVIG 0.4 g/kg daily for 5 days Repeat at 3–4 week intervals until remission. If response poor, prednisolone 0.5–1.0 mg/kg per day with gradual tapering over months. If response is poor, consider immunosuppression with azathioprine, methotrexate, or cyclosporine A

end and the peripheral terminus at sensory receptors or neuromuscular junctions at the other. In some cases the pathology also extends into the neuronal cell body in the spinal cord, dorsal root ganglion, or sympathetic chain. The major clinical hallmarks of the peripheral neuropathies are weakness, diminished tendon reflexes, and sensory loss. Recognition of one of several characteristic patterns of distribution (Table 3) is a useful first step in diagnosis.

GENERAL MANAGEMENT

Acute Polyneuropathies (Guillain–Barré Syndrome and Others)

Meticulous supportive care is the mainstay of therapy in the acute polyneuropathies, such as the Guillain–Barré syndrome and those associated with a toxic or metabolic cause. Children with rapidly progressive weakness or sensory loss should be closely monitored in the hospital, ideally in an intensive care setting, until their clinical state stabilizes. This is particularly important in younger children in whom objective assessment of respiratory function is difficult. In the older, cooperative child regular measurement of vital capacity is important as long as the overall condition is worsening or if there is any suggestion of respiratory compromise. Ventilatory support should be considered when vital capacity falls below 30% of predicted values and instituted if there is evidence of respiratory insufficiency. Simple bedside observations of the child's ability to count as far as possible with one breath can be very useful. Most children over the age of five years can count to more than 30. Progressive decline in this capacity may warn of impending respiratory insufficiency.

Although relatively rare in childhood Guillain–Barré syndrome, autonomic complications such as hypertension and cardiac arrhythmias need to be watched for and treated appropriately. Because of denervation supersensitivity, treatment should begin with more conservative measures, and be initiated only when vital functions are compromised. For example, sinus tachycardia is relatively common but in

Table 2 Treatment of Neuropathies Associated with Inborn Errors of Metabolism in Childhood

Disorder	Neuropathy	Treatment
Mitochondrial cytopathies	Large fiber demyelination and axon loss	Putative role dichloroacetate, co-enzyme Q, carnitine
Globoid cell leukodystrophy	Large fiber demyelinating	Hematopoietic stem cell transplantation
Metachromatic leukodystrophy	Large fiber demyelinating	Bone marrow transplantation
Fabry disease	Small fiber axonal	Recombinant alpha-galactosidase A therapy
Refsum disease	Large fiber demyelinating	Dietary restriction of phytanic acid and phytol
Adrenomyeloneuropathy	Large fiber demyelination and axon loss	Treatment of adrenocortical insufficiency, dietary supplementation with Lorenzo's oil, restricted dietary intake of very long chain fatty acids, possible role of lovastatin
Type 1 primary hyperoxaluria	Large fiber segmental demyelination and axon loss	Combined liver–kidney transplantation
Cerebrotendinous xanthomatosis	Large fiber demyelination, secondary axon loss	Oral chenodeoxycholic acid, cholic acid, HMG-CoA reductase inhibitors
Abetalipoproteinemia, hypolipoproteinemia	Large fiber demyelination and axon loss	High-dose supplementation vitamins A,D,E, and K
Ataxia with vitamin E deficiency	Large fiber axonal	High-dose supplementation vitamin E
Tyrosinemia type 1	Large fiber axonal	Dietary restriction of tyrosine and phenylalanine, oral hematin, 2-nitro-4-trifluoro-methyl-benzoyl-1,3-cyclohexanedione (NTBC)
Acute intermittent porphyria	Large fiber axonal loss	Intravenous heme and heme arginate

the otherwise healthy child usually does not require treatment. Serum sodium levels are frequently disturbed by the presence of "inappropriate" ADH (vasopressin) secretion, but usually conservative treatment with fluid restriction is sufficient.

Dysphagia or bulbar paresis may necessitate temporary withdrawal of oral feeding, followed if necessary by parenteral, nasogastric, or gastrostomy feeding. Constipation is common and should be anticipated and treated aggressively. Pain is frequent in childhood Guillain–Barré syndrome and may go unrecognized in small children. It is managed with nonsteroidal or narcotic analgesia, gabapentin, and sometimes with intravenous immunoglobulin or corticosteroids.

Chest and limb physical therapy is important to clear secretions and maintain limb mobility. Attention to pain control during therapy sessions often

Table 3 Categories of Peripheral Neuropathies in Children

	Site	Distribution	Most common or important causes
Polyneuropathy	Mixed (motor and sensory) peripheral nerves	Distal predominant, symmetric	Chronic: genetic, toxic, metabolic, nutritional, inflammatory Acute: inflammatory, toxic, metabolic
Mononeuropathy	Single mixed peripheral nerve	Single nerve territory	Trauma, entrapment, neoplastic
Mononeuritis multiplex	Multiple peripheral nerves	Multiple specific nerve territories	Collagen vascular
Radiculopathy	Single spinal root	Single root territory	Structural, tumor, collagen vascular
Polyradiculopathy	Multiple adjacent spinal roots	Multiple adjacent dermatomes/myotomes	Inflammatory, infectious, neoplastic
Plexopathy	Brachial or lumbar plexus	Complex distribution of selected plexus elements	Inflammatory, structural, traumatic

assists mobilization. Splints may be required to prevent contractures due to chronic foot- and wrist drop. Frequent turning of the patient is essential to avoid pressure sores.

Acute neuropathies caused by iatrogenic, inadvertent, or deliberate exposure to medicines, chemotherapeutic agents, environmental toxins and agents of abuse are, fortunately, relatively rare in childhood. In such cases the mainstay of therapy is cessation of exposure to the toxic agent, with or without more specific treatment.

Hereditary Neuropathies

The genetic polyneuropathies of children are divided into several groups, the most prominent of which are the *hereditary motor and sensory neuropathies,* and the *hereditary sensory and autonomic neuropathies.* None of these has a specific treatment for the primary pathophysiology. All are characterized by genetically mediated defects in peripheral nerve structure or metabolism. Very rarely such patients develop a second pathology, in the form of an acquired (inflammatory) demyelinating neuropathy, which may be steroid responsive. Most patients with these disorders, however, derive no long-term benefit from corticosteroids or other immunosuppressive medications. Management of chronic genetically determined pediatric neuropathies mostly consists largely of anticipation and treatment of secondary complications. In addition to these primary genetic neuropathies, there are a number of other disorders in which chronic peripheral neuropathy contributes significantly to functional loss, including Friedreich's ataxia, some inborn errors of metabolism, and neuropathies that arise as a complication of systemic disease.

Children with chronic neuromuscular disorders are best followed in a multidisciplinary clinic in which they can undergo regular review by a multiple specialty team that includes specialists in rehabilitation, physical and occupation therapy, orthopedics, and neurology. As a group, certain complications of chronic peripheral neuropathy can be anticipated, and with foresight sometimes mitigated. These generally involve the hands, feet, and spine. In certain disorders, some more specific complications can be anticipated as discussed below.

Hereditary Sensory and Motor Neuropathies

The Foot

The foot is involved in the majority of cases of peripheral neuropathy. Both cavus contractures and "flail" type planovalgus feet are encountered. Palliative management of problematic feet is largely based on approaches adapted from other areas of practice and can be very helpful. More curative approaches are attractive in principle, especially in younger patients, but often meet with only limited success.

Adequate footwear and appropriate orthoses to improve posture and support foot drop are effective in reducing discomfort and/or minimizing the functional impact of peripheral neuropathy. Ankle/foot orthoses (AFOs) limit foot drop during walking but are cosmetically unattractive and can be unpopular, especially with older children. Strengthening exercises have been shown to result in short-term gains in proximal muscles, but there are no studies evaluating the short- or long-term effect of exercise on the distal musculature, which is most often preferentially denervated in peripheral neuropathy. Passive stretching is thought to prevent contractures in the calf and feet, but a recent controlled trial of night splints in Australian adults and children with Charcot–Marie–Tooth disease type lA revealed no significant gains in ankle joint motion, even after three months of treatment. Compliance with night splinting regimens is a major problem, and especially so in children.

Many children with peripheral neuropathy will ultimately require surgery to correct structural changes in the feet. If contractures are severe and fixed, hindfoot or forefoot reconstruction with selective arthrodesis will stabilize the foot and give adequate function. In younger, flexible, or more dynamic cases there is some controversy over the best surgical approach. Some surgeons advocate early arthrodesis on the premise that the chronic nature of the neuropathy makes further degeneration inevitable. A second school of thought advocates a more dynamic approach, attempting to restore muscle balance through tendon transfer and maintaining joint function as far as possible. There are no good data to support the superiority of either approach. Arthrodesis yields moderately good results in the short and medium term, making this a relatively predictable approach; however, the few studies that have followed cases for 15–20 years suggest that ongoing functional degeneration in neighboring joints often results in reduced patient satisfaction. The joint preserving techniques are conceptually attractive but largely unproven, and many patients will eventually require arthrodesis. Quality data on the outcomes of the surgical approaches would be of great benefit to patients and doctors, but in the meantime patients and parents facing decisions about surgery should be informed that there is little consensus.

The Hand

Many children with peripheral neuropathy will experience difficulties resulting from weakness in the hands. Problems with clothing fasteners such as buttons and zips are common but may be overcome with dressing aids. Many children find that reduced writing speed and increased fatigue hamper their schoolwork. As typing is generally less problematic than writing with a pen, assistance with access to typing, word processing, and special computer equipment or software that speed input from the physically impaired can be very helpful. Night splints may help slow the development of clawing of the hands in children with severe distal weakness.

The Spine

Scoliosis occurs in about 10% of children with hereditary neuropathies. It is more frequent in patients with the more severe forms of hereditary motor sensory neuropathy, (e.g., those with the Déjerine–Sottas syndrome). In most cases, scoliosis is mild (less than 20 degrees) and nonprogressive or only slowly progressive. Only a minority of patients will require surgery because of significant deformity. Careful preoperative assessment of respiratory function is essential in such cases.

Hereditary Sensory and Autonomic Neuropathies

Treatment of dysautonomia is palliative. Impaired swallowing in infancy is dealt with by special nipples, feeding bottles and thickened feeds, but gavage feeding is often required. Gastrostomy and fundoplication should be considered early. Vomiting and hypertensive crises may respond to treatment with oral diazepam. Hypotensive episodes may be alleviated by wearing elastic stockings, lower limb exercises, fludrocortisone and other drugs.

Infants with severe sensory loss require protection from self-mutilation by protective gloves, special footwear and sometimes restraints. Dental prostheses or judicious extractions may be required to prevent tongue biting and lip lacerations in extreme cases. Early education of the patient and family to avoid potentially damaging activities is paramount. Daily inspection of the feet for abrasions and cuts, and of the footwear for roughened areas or protruding tacks, is essential. If sensory deficit is combined with structural deformity of the feet there may be an increased risk of foot ulceration. Foot ulcers should be managed aggressively with offloading (casting, or an "aircast" type boot and elbow crutches) and prophylactic antibiotic cover. Where there is a patent arterial supply, and as long as offloading is adequate, neuropathic ulcers will usually resolve within two weeks.

In some forms of hereditary and sensory neuropathy anhidrosis predisposes to episodic hyperthermia, which may result in febrile convulsions. Hyperthermia should be avoided by avoidance of raised ambient temperatures and the use of air conditioning.

Friedreich's Ataxia

This autosomal recessive disorder is the most common spinocerebellar ataxia of childhood. As no curative treatment is as yet available, treatment of Friedreich's ataxia has traditionally focussed on management of its complications, particularly cardiomyopathy, impaired glucose tolerance, and scoliosis. Friedreich's ataxia is caused by a GAA trinucleotide expansion in the gene for frataxin, a protein implicated in mitochondrial iron metabolism. This finding has prompted therapeutic trials with idebenone, a non-FDA-approved antioxidant and short-chain analog of coenzyme Q. Idebenone (5 mg/kg/day) has shown promise for treatment of the cardiomyopathy associated with Friedreich's ataxia in early trials, but did not demonstrate any benefit to the neurologic features of this disorder. Further trials of this and related treatments are being carried out.

Neuropathies Secondary to Inborn Errors of Metabolism

In recent years advances in treatment of a number of genetic conditions have enabled symptomatic or curative treatment of a range of neuropathies associated with inborn errors of metabolism (Table 2). Important recent advances include the licensing in the United States of recombinant alpha-galactosidase A enzyme for the treatment of Fabry disease, where it has been shown to minimize neuropathic pain and to stabilize renal function. Outcome of adrenoleukodystrophy (ALD) and adrenomyeloneuropathy (AMN) has been improved with treatment of adrenocortical insufficiency, dietary supplementation with Lorenzo's oil, and restricted dietary intake of very long chain fatty acids. Bone marrow transplantation has demonstrated efficacy in early symptomatic cases of childhood-onset cerebral ALD, but is not indicated in primary AMN and has not been shown to affect the neuropathy sometimes associated with AMN.

Peripheral neuropathy is a prominent feature of some mitochondrial disorders such as Leigh syndrome and neuropathy, ataxia and retinitis pigmentosa (NARP). Nonspecific treatment for these disorders is reviewed in Chapter.

Neuropathies Secondary to Chronic Systemic Disease

The neuropathies secondary to chronic renal failure and diabetes are often subclinical during childhood and may improve with improved metabolic control of the underlying condition. In end-stage renal failure, transplantation is the only really effective treatment. Compared to adults, when children suffer from serious systemic illness a secondary polyneuropathy is relatively infrequent.

PROGNOSIS

Most children with genetic polyneuropathies have a normal lifespan marked by very slow progression of debility, the severity of which can be fairly well predicted by the teenage years. Life-threatening complications are generally a consequence of associated conditions or other organ involvement, and only rarely are the genetic neuropathies associated with respiratory compromise. Treatment should thus be offered with the expectation of a long life encumbered to a variable degree by the orthopedic and neurologic problems in the feet and hands. Most can look forward to the fulfilment of schooling, career, and family.

REFERENCE

1. Hallett M, Tandon D, Berardelli A. Treatment of peripheral neuropathies. J Neurol Neurosurg Psych 1985; 48:1193–1207.

SUGGESTED READINGS

1. Burns TM, Ryan MM, Darras BT, Jones HR Jr. Therapeutic options for neuropathies associated with inborn errors of metabolism in childhood: an update. Mayo Clin Proc 2003; 78:858–868.
2. Durr A. Friedreich's ataxia: treatment within reach. Lancet Neurol 2002; 1:370–374.
3. Ouvrier RA, McLeod JG, Pollard JD. Peripheral Neuropathy in Childhood. 2nd ed. London: MacKeith Press, 1999.
4. Westmore RS, Drennan JC. Long-term results of triple arthrodesis in Charcot–Marie–Tooth disease. J Bone Joint Surg 1989; 71:417–422.

28
Congenital Myopathies

Monique M. Ryan and Kathryn N. North
Institute for Neuromuscular Research, Children's Hospital at Westmead, Sydney, Australia

INTRODUCTION

The congenital myopathies are a heterogeneous group of neuromuscular disorders defined by distinctive histochemical or ultrastructural changes in muscle. Most of these disorders present in infancy or early childhood with hypotonia, muscle weakness, and delayed achievement of motor milestones.

DIAGNOSIS AND CLINICAL FEATURES

The congenital myopathies have a number of common features: early-onset generalized weakness, hypotonia and hyporeflexia, and a characteristic body habitus with thin elongated facies, high arched palate, slender build, poor muscle bulk, scoliosis, and pectus carinatum. Each is defined by a single distinguishing, but not specific, morphologic abnormality in muscle fibers. Clinical clues to the specific diagnosis may include the pattern of inheritance and associated features such as ophthalmoplegia and cardiomyopathy (Table 1).

Certain congenital myopathies are well defined clinically, morphologically, and genetically (Table 2). A number of other conditions with specific structural abnormalities remain that have not, as yet, been associated with a demonstrable genetic abnormality. Other myopathies seen in childhood include infantile and juvenile-onset acid maltase deficiency, the inflammatory and metabolic myopathies.

THERAPEUTIC CONCERNS

There are no curative therapies for the congenital myopathies. A multidisciplinary approach to the treatment of individual patients will, however, greatly improve their quality of life and may influence survival. Management of individuals with a congenital myopathy should include the following considerations: prevention; monitoring; risk management; and symptomatic therapy and rehabilitation.

Table 1 Common Clinical Features of the Congenital Myopathies

	Facial weakness	Ptosis	External ophthalmo-plegia	Respiratory involvement	Skeletal deformities	Cardiac involvement
Nemaline myopathy	+++	+++	–	+++	++	+
Central core disease	++	+	–	+	+++	+
Myotubular myopathy	+++	+++	+++	+++	++	–
Centronuclear myopathy	++	++	++	+++	+++	–
Multiminicore disease	+++	+	+	+++	+++	++
Congenital fiber-type disproportion	++	–	–	++	+++	–

Key: +++, common association; ++, occurs occasionally; +, occurs rarely; –, no reported association.

PREVENTION

Genetic counseling for families with congenital myopathies can be challenging, even for those disorders in which disease genes have been identified and molecular genetic testing is available. Causative mutations are identified in only a minority of cases, and in many cases genetic heterogeneity and clinical variability limit the extent to which definitive genetic counseling is possible. Clinical evaluation (and even muscle biopsy) of other family members may identify very mildly affected relatives.

Table 2 Congenital Myopathies with Identified Gene Loci

Disorder	Protein and gene (symbol)	Inheritance	Chromosome localization
Nemaline myopathy	Nebulin (NEB)	AR	2q 21.2–2q22
	Skeletal alpha actin (ACTA1)	AR, AD	1q42.1
	Alpha tropomyosin (TPM3)	AR, AD	1q21–q23
	Beta tropomyosin (TPM2)	AD	9p13.2
	Slow skeletal troponin T (TNNT1)	AR	19q13.4
Actin myopathy	Skeletal alpha actin (ACTA1)	AD	1q42.1
Core-rod myopathy	Ryanodine receptor (RYR1)	AD	19q13.1
	Unidentified	AD	15q21–q24
Central core disease	Ryanodine receptor (RYR1)	AD, AR	19q13.1
Myotubular myopathy	Myotubularin (MTM1)	X	Xq28
Multi-minicore disease	Selenoprotein N1 (SEPN1)	AR	1p36
	Ryanodine receptor (RYR1)	AD, AR	19q13.1

Key: AR, autosomal recessive; AD, autosomal dominant.

MONITORING AND PROSPECTIVE DETECTION OF MEDICAL COMPLICATIONS

The mainstay of therapy for patients with congenital myopathy is early detection of disease manifestations and complications. Particularly important to management of these children are regular monitoring of pulmonary function and sleep, early identification of cardiac involvement, nutritional care, maintenance of mobility, and screening for scoliosis (Table 3).

RISK MANAGEMENT

Surgical Procedures and Anesthetic Risks

Malignant hyperthermia (MH) is characterized by uncontrolled hyperthermia in response to certain anesthetic agents and depolarizing muscle relaxants. Central core disease and multiminicore disease are the only congenital myopathies clearly associated with an increased risk of malignant hyperthermia. Because the diagnosis is unknown in most patients undergoing muscle biopsy, however, MH precautions should be taken in all cases prior to definitive diagnosis. The first exposure to triggering substances elicits an event in only 50% of MH susceptible patients, so previous tolerance to halothane, succinylcholine, or other depolarizing neuromuscular blockade medications does not guarantee safe future use of these agents.

In general, patients with congenital myopathy tolerate surgical procedures and general anesthetics well, but it should be recognized that they have an enhanced risk for respiratory decompensation postoperatively. Preoperative assessment of respiratory status is important in determining the timing of surgical intervention. Prolonged postoperative immobility may exacerbate or worsen muscle weakness. Patients should be mobilized as soon as possible after a surgical procedure.

SYMPTOMATIC THERAPY AND REHABILITATION

Respiratory Care

Respiratory muscle weakness is common to many of the congenital myopathies and is the primary cause of death from these disorders at all ages. It important to be aware that the degree of skeletal muscle weakness does not necessarily reflect that of respiratory muscle involvement. Respiratory compromise occurs secondary to involvement of the intercostal muscles and diaphragm and may be exacerbated by scoliosis. Bulbar weakness increases the risk of aspiration, and poor nutritional status may increase susceptibility to respiratory infection. Respiratory failure can occur at any age and may be of very sudden onset. Most patients, even those with no symptoms of pulmonary disease, will show restriction of their respiratory capacity on formal testing. Patients with congenital myopathy also run a great risk of insidious nocturnal hypoventilation, symptoms of which include sleep disturbance, nightmares, morning headache, daytime fatigue, and weight loss. Nocturnal hypoventilation may occur even in the absence of diurnal symptoms.

All patients with congenital myopathy should have a baseline evaluation of their respiratory status. Children with a vital capacity of less than 50% of their predicted value should be evaluated at least annually. Evaluations include lung function testing (vital capacity, FEV1, and maximal inspiratory and expiratory pressures), waking and sleep oximetry and capnography, and an assessment of bulbar function.

Table 3 Management of Patients with Congenital Myopathies

Compromised function	Clinical problem	Possible therapeutic interventions
Skeletal muscle weakness	Hypotonia	Regular exercise
	Weakness	Stretching, active and passive
	Contractures	Standing frame
		Orthotics/splinting
		Serial plaster casting
		Enhance mobility with walking frames or wheelchair
Respiratory muscle weakness	Reduced vital capacity	Breathing exercises
	Pneumonia	Chest physiotherapy
	Aspiration	Influenza vaccination
	Hypoventilation	Aggressive management of acute infections
	Respiratory failure	Nocturnal or assisted ventilation
Bulbar muscle weakness	Dysarthria	Speech therapy
	Excessive drooling	Anticholinergic medications
		Botulinum toxin injection to salivary glands
		Pharyngoplasty, salivary duct surgery
Cardiac muscle involvement	Conduction defects	Careful anticipatory monitoring
	Cardiomyopathy	Cardiac medication
	Cor pulmonale	
Gastrointestinal function	Constipation	High fiber diet
		Glycerin suppository
		Bowel training
		Laxatives, enemas
Functional activities	Restricted mobility	Wheelchair
	Restricted access	Other mobility aids
		Modifications to car
	Written communication	Assistive technology
		Writing assists
		School visit and modifications
Developmental delay		Formal psychometric assessment
		Early intervention services
Scoliosis		Careful anticipatory follow up
		External bracing
		Surgical fusion
Self-care and feeding		Nursing assistance
Insufficient sports, leisure, social activities		Liaison with school
		Hydrotherapy
		Contact with special sporting organizations
		Contact with community disease-specific organizations
Psychiatric disorders		Individual or family therapy
		Medication

(*Continued*)

Table 3 Management of Patients with Congenital Myopathies (*Continued*)

Compromised function	Clinical problem	Possible therapeutic interventions
Financial distress		Disability eligibility Other community resources
Family planning		Genetic counseling Prenatal diagnosis Anticipation of potential obstetric complcations
Enhanced surgical risk		Malignant hyperthermia precautions Preoperative pulmonary function testing Anticipatory pulmonary physiotherapy Postoperative weaning to noninvasive ventilation
Employment		Anticipatory vocational assessment and training Support in the workplace

Postural drainage, regular chest physiotherapy, and a manually assisted cough may improve respiratory toilet in patients with bulbar weakness, reduced vital capacity, and recurrent aspiration. Respiratory infections should be treated early and aggressively, including antibiotics where indicated. Some children will require short-term assisted ventilation during intercurrent illness. The patient and their family should be educated with respect to the possibility of ultimate respiratory insufficiency and options for home mechanical ventilation.

Indications for ventilatory support include CO_2 retention ($pCO_2 > 50$ mmHg), chronic hypoxia ($pO_2 < 90$ mmHg), very restricted vital capacity for size (less than 1 L in adults), and recurrent pneumonia. The preferred method of home mechanical ventilation will depend on the clinical status of the patient, the rate of progression and the natural history of the underlying disorder, and should be determined in conjunction with an experienced physician, the patient and their family. Options include bilevel positive airway pressure (BiPAP) by nasal or facial mask and tracheostomal ventilation if noninvasive means are not feasible. The institution of home ventilation may not be appropriate in all cases. Aggressive management is commonly more appropriate for the older child, for whom assisted ventilation will often result in marked improvement in quality of life.

Feeding Difficulties

Inability to feed sufficiently to sustain weight and growth, necessitating gavage feeding, is common in newborn infants with congenital myopathy. Many infants will eventually be able to tolerate oral feeds. In others persisting feeding difficulties eventually necessitate insertion of a gastrostomy tube, with or without fundoplication. In older patients bulbar dysfunction can cause chewing and swallowing difficulties and recurrent aspiration, and in combination with facial weakness may cause dysarthria and poor control of secretions.

Joint Contractures and Scoliosis

A regular program of muscle stretches and exercise helps prevent or minimize joint contractures in children with congenital myopathy. Ideally, such a program should become integrated into the child's day-to-day activities. Orthotics, splinting and serial casting may be necessary for mild joint contractures. Surgical release may be indicated for contractures that do not respond to aggressive physiotherapy.

All patients with congenital myopathy should be monitored for the development of scoliosis and kyphosis. Progressive spinal deformity can cause pain, impede motor function and independence, and further compromise respiratory function. Treatment options include bracing and spinal fusion. Spinal bracing does not correct, prevent or reverse spinal curvature but may improve sitting stability and is an option in nonambulatory children. Surgery is indicated if the curve is progressing, pulmonary function is impaired, and spinal fusion is unlikely to impair motor function. The most important factors related to the timing of surgery are a persisting degree of flexibility of the spine and a stable pulmonary forced vital capacity that is more than 30% predicted value.

PROGNOSIS

Most of the congenital myopathies are static or slowly progressive disorders. Management of these conditions is predicated on prediction and prevention of disease complications. Over the next few years, it is likely that genetic loci for the majority of congenital myopathies will be identified, in the first step towards a better understanding of the pathogenesis of these disorders, and the development of curative rather than symptomatic therapies.

SUGGESTED READINGS

1. Bushby K, Mellies U, Wallgren-Pettersson C. Ventilatory support in congenital neuromuscular disorders. 117th ENMC Workshop, Naarden, The Netherlands 4–6th April 2003. Neuromusc Disord 2004; 14:56–69.
2. Goebel HH. Congenital myopathies at their molecular dawning. Muscle Nerve 2003; 27:527–548.
3. North KN. Congenital myopathies. In: Engel A, Franzini-Armstrong C, eds. McGraw-Hill, New York Myology. 2003.

29

Therapy for Spinal Muscular Atrophy

Thomas O. Crawford
Johns Hopkins Hospital, Baltimore, Maryland, U.S.A.

INTRODUCTION

Spinal muscular atrophy is a term applied to both a specific and common disorder, and to a group of related but individually rare disorders. The specific, common disorder is also known as childhood spinal muscular atrophy, proximal spinal muscular atrophy, and historically has been broken up into several subgroups labeled SMA 1 (Werdnig Hoffmann disease), SMA 2 (intermediate childhood SMA), and SMA 3 (Kugelberg Welander disease). All of these labels refer to a recessively inherited genetic disorder caused by mutation of the survival motor neuron gene, *SMN*. The group of disorders collectively known as the spinal muscular atrophies (Table 1) is diverse in many respects. Some are well characterized genetically by defined mutations in known genes, some are clearly genetic from their inheritance pattern but as yet involve unknown genes, and others affect single patients in a manner that suggests a genetic etiology that yet remains unproven. Both the specific SMN-related SMA and the broad range of SMA disorders share in common certain clinical features including slow progressive, symmetric and often diffuse weakness caused by degeneration of the primary motor neurons. Symmetric dysfunction and degeneration of spinal and bulbar motor neurons may be a feature of other disorders (Table 2).

SMN-RELATED SMA

Clinical Appearance and Diagnosis

Affected individuals initially manifest weakness over a range of ages beginning prenatally to young adult years or possibly later. Infants with the common, and well recognized, type 1 SMA (Werdnig–Hoffmann disease) typically are normal at birth but develop weakness of limbs, trunk and neck in the first few months of life. The arbitrary division of type 1 from type II SMA involves the inability to maintain, at any point in the course, an independent sitting position. Infants with type I SMA often have a bright and intelligent appearing face, particularly of the eyes, a strong diaphragm, and normal tone of the anal sphincter but weakness diffusely elsewhere. A "frog leg" recumbent posture with the legs fully externally rotated, knees and hips partially flexed, arms internally rotated at the shoulder and often extended

Table 1 Potential Mimics of Spinal Muscular Atrophy

Brain	Degenerative disease
	Hypotonic cerebral palsy
	Congenital Myotonic Dystrophy
	Prader Willi syndrome, other genetic disorders
Spinal cord/column	Trauma[a]
	Structural disorders: *e.g.* syringomyelia, tethered cord[a]
	Inflammatory or structural vascular disorders[a]
	Tumor[a]
	Acute transverse myelitis[a]
	Epidermal abscess[a]
	Monomelic Amyotrophy
Other motor neuron disorders	Poliomyelitis syndrome due to Polio Virus, other enterovirus, or West Nile Virus[a]
	Following severe acute asthma attack (Hopkins syndrome)
Root	Polyradiculitis[a]
	Leukemia/Lymphoma[a]
Plexus	Chronic lumbar or brachial plexitis[a]
Nerve	Progressive axonal polyneuropathy
	Multifocal motor neuropathy[a]
	Chronic inflammatory demyelinating polyneuropathy[a]
	Toxic polyneuropathy[a]
Neuromuscular junction	Myasthenia gravis[a]
	Botulism[a]
	Tic paralysis[a]
	Drug induced NM blockade or AChE inhibitor[a]
Muscle	Myopathy[a]

[a] Denotes entities with potential specific therapy.

at the elbow is characteristic and strongly suggests the diagnosis. In this form of SMA tongue "fasciculations" are common, but by itself this is a nonspecific feature that often leads to diagnostic error. Infants and children with type II SMA typically manifest weakness at a later age, usually prior to 18 months of age. While able to sit, they cannot maintain a standing position sufficiently well as to take a step—the arbitrary dividing line that distinguishes type 2 from type 3 (Kugelberg Welander) SMA. Individuals with type 2 or 3 SMA often manifest a characteristic tremor, very fine and irregular tremor, termed "minipolymyoclonus," in the fingers when held outstretched. Those with type 3 SMA may manifest weakness at any time in childhood or even as young adults—in which case some investigators apply the term SMA type 4. Weakness is of widely varying severity, but again has the caudal-to-cranial symmetric distribution.

In infants, the diagnosis can be strongly suggested by the appearance alone. In some of the more mildly affected, the clinical features are generally less distinctive. If the clinical suspicion is high, diagnosis is possible with a DNA test alone, looking for the homozygous absence of the SMN1 gene. Because there is a near-homologous copy of the SMN1 gene, termed SMN2, absence of the pathogenic SMN1 gene must be determined by the major distinguishing features within exons 7 and 8, thus the reports generally describe "homozygous absence (or deletion) of SMN exon 7 and 8," which is diagnostic. Specificity of the DNA test in this setting is 100%, and specificity is well over 90% in all cases, and even better in those more severely affected. If the initial clinical suspicion is less striking, nerve conduction and EMG studies can be very useful to raise clinical suspicion to the threshold necessary for genetic testing. The major differential diagnoses include various genetic and acquired myopathies, which should demonstrate myopathic features on EMG, severe neuropathies which should show either slowing or reduced amplitude motor and sensory responses on nerve conduction studies, or severe central hypotonia, which will have normal EMG and NCV studies. Because SMA is a symmetric disorder, a limited study, evaluating only a few nerves and muscles is often sufficient to justify DNA studies. If the DNA studies then obtained are not informative, more extensive testing may then be carried out. Care in limiting the extent of uncomfortable studies to only that which is necessary is much appreciated by parents and children alike.

In most cases, muscle biopsy is unnecessary. The sole exception will be those unusual individuals in whom the SMA gene test is falsely reassuring. In those with true SMN-related SMA, this occurs when there is a rare point mutation in some other portion of the SMN 1 gene than that ascertained by the exon 7 and 8 test. In most such cases, diagnosis will need to be done in centers with access to more sophisticated genetic testing.

As a recessive disease, the risk to future siblings is 25%. Although SMA exists across a spectrum of weakness, siblings are usually similarly affected so the older healthy sibling of all but the mildest affected newly diagnosed patient need not be concerned. The risk to cousins is equal to 1:2 (the probability that the uncle or aunt is a carrier) × 1:40 (the average rate of asymptomatic carriers in the normal population) × 1:4 (recessive risk), or 1:320. Because this involves another allele, however, affected cousins need not have the same degree of weakness. A high-quality (though not perfect) test for the carrier state is available: often the cheapest means of reassuring family member is to test the in-law uncle or aunt since there is a 39/40 chance that the test will demonstrate a noncarrier state and the blood-related aunt or uncle will then not need to be tested.

Across the range of disease severity, the clinical course for children with SMA is unusual for a "degenerative" disorder. The rate of degeneration declines with the passage of time, so that most children enter a very slow "plateau" phase with little or no change in strength over long durations. For those with SMA 1 this level of strength may be very low, and by itself insufficient to prevent respiratory failure due to trivial intercurrent upper respiratory illness or even slowly progressive atelectasis. For those with SMA 2 and SMA 3, the slow rate of change can be complicated by various secondary complications, which then have the effect of dragging function down. Many of these secondary complications can be anticipated and prevented. Thus, fastidious prospective care can have a major influence on function and life span. In older textbooks, children with SMA 2 are said on average to live to early school years but with modern supportive care many in this group are now doing well in high school and beyond.

Special Concerns Regarding Care for Infants with SMA 1

In infants with SMA 1, very complex levels of medical care are mixed with difficult ethical and resource issues. At issue in many of these most severely affected infants is the question of treatment goals. While it is virtually always possible to maintain life with tracheostomy, assisted ventilation and assisted tube feedings, most will never emerge from a state of complete dependence. For some, even yes/no binary forms of communication are difficult or impossible. The burdens of care include

Table 2 Spinal Muscular Atrophy Disorders and Syndromes

Confirmed Monogenic Disorders

MIM#	Inheritance	Title (synonyms)	Gene	Onset, course	Distinguishing features, comments
253300 253550 253400 271150	AR	SMA (SMA 1, 2, 3, 4; Werdnig Hoffmann disease, Juvenile muscular atrophy, Kugelberg-Welander disease)	*SMN1*	Infant to adult	Caudal to cranial distribution, wide range of severity
313200	X	X linked spinal and bulbar muscular atrophy (Kennedy Disease)	Androgen receptor	Adult, progressive	Gynecomastia cramping, fasciculations, pain neuropathy, elevated CK (CAG trinucleotide expansion)
604320	AR	SMA with Respiratory Distress (SMARD1)	(*IGHMBP2*)	Infantile, progressive	Prominent early diaphragm weakness, foot deformity
600794	AD	Distal SMA with upper limb predominance	*GARS*, *BSCL2*	Late teens, slowly progressive	Radial aspect of hand

Presumed Monogenic Disorders (With Distinctive Semiology)

MIM#	Inheritance	Title (synonyms)	Linkage	Onset, course	Distinguishing features, comments
301830	X	Distal X-linked arthrogryposis (infantile X-linked SMA)	Xp11.3–q11.2	Congenital, progressive	Frequent congenital joint deformity, frequent fractures
158580	AD	Distal SMA with vocal cord paralysis	2q14	Juvenile to adult, progressive	Clinically very similar to CMT 2C

Syndromes with characteristic features

MIM#	Inheritance	Title (synonyms)	Onset, course	Distinguishing features, comments
158600	AD	Dominant proximal SMA (Juvenile SMA)	Childhood, slowly progressive	AD otherwise similar to *SMN*-associated SMA
271120 182960 158590	AR	Distal SMA	Any age	Distally predominant denervation and weakness
600175	AD	Congenital nonprogressive SMA of lower limbs	Congenital, nonprogressive	Lower extremities only, nonprogressive arthrogryposis with neurogenic features
	AR	Cervical spinal muscular atrophy	Infancy, progressive	Cranial to caudal distribution, prominent head ptosis, respiratory insufficiency

Note: For Entries with a MIM Designation Number, Extensive Reference Listing can be obtained at http://www3.ncbi.nlm.nih.gov/omim/.

continuous high stress to other family members, limited interest or ability of some medical communities, very high financial costs borne by private and governmental third parties and families, and inevitable patient discomforts associated with the high levels of intervention necessary. For many dedicated and caring parents, these burdens easily surpass the benefit of extending life in the state of complete or near complete immobility for their children. As SMA manifests across a continuous spectrum of severity, and because every family and community will value elements of burden and benefit differently in making decisions about the goals of care, there will inevitably be many difficult cases. In recent years, advancements in "noninvasive" chronic ventilation have made life somewhat less burdensome for many patients and their families, increasing the number of very weak infants for whom a decision to extend life, rather than enter into a program of palliative care, may be a reasonable choice.

Caring physicians have an important role in identifying the probable consequences of each choice, and to help shoulder the inevitable guilt that accompanies any choice made. A choice for pure palliative care for infants with type 1 SMA is extraordinarily difficult for parents. This can be made easier by understanding that most or all of the discomforts associated with SMA 1 can be effectively minimized. Referral to hospice services, when available, is often very useful. Many infants develop difficulty with sucking and swallowing, particularly when during respiratory illness. In anticipation of this time, it is reasonable to place G tubes prospectively at a time when anesthesia concerns can be minimized. Local institutions favor endoscopic or surgical approaches, and general vs. spinal anesthesia; neither is inherently better and local experience and comfort of specialists dictate the best approach. Nissen fundiplication is rarely indicated for patients receiving palliative care. Infants also tolerate thin flexible NG tubes well, which can be placed for days or a few weeks at a time in those infants who cannot tolerate G tube placement. Placement of these artificial means for alimentation do not preclude bottle or even breast feeding for those infants who are able to do so, but alleviate the difficulties with maintaining minimum caloric support that frequently develop over time.

Many infants with SMA 1 eventually develop noisy breathing. This is partially related to an increased risk of aspiration, but is less frequent than might be expected. Oral suctioning is uncomfortable for the infant; with time parents can learn to distinguish noisy breathing from distressed states that are relieved with suctioning by a portable suction machine or bulb syringes. Postural drainage with a small percussive cup, or vibration, placing the most atelectatic lung segments upward can be helpful. Glycopyrrolate (Robinul) is difficult to use well; often the benefit of drying secretions is undermined by increased thickness of secretion that makes the overall situation worse. Infants often benefit from aerosolized bronchodilator treatments during times of increased respiratory distress. Many infants with SMA 1 are more comfortable and breath more slowly and effectively in a Trendelenberg position and on their side or even prone. This position is advantageous given the relative imbalance between chest wall weakness and diaphragmatic strength: in the upright position the increase in thoracic volume created by diaphragmatic contraction is undermined by chest wall collapse, but in the Trendelenberg position the forces to collapse the chest wall are diminished.

Finally, the distress of severe dyspnea can be blunted by use of aerosolized narcotics. This includes the risk of suppression of respiratory drive, but in my experience there is little evidence that delivered in the following manner that induced respiratory depression is a major concern. Instead, the delivered dose appears to be partially adjusted by the diminished respiratory volumes. A dose of 0.5 mg morphine or 0.25 mg Dilaudid in 2 mL normal saline in a 5–10 kg child is appropriate. This is placed in a standard nebulizer and directed to the mouth and nose with enough airflow to last approximately 10 min (usually about 6 L/m). Repeated dosing is possible every 30–60 min observing for effect and the absence of apparent respiratory depression. This does not have to be used only in the terminal stages, though I tend to confine its use to more severe episodes. Parents do not have to be worried that use of this commits the infant to an immediately terminal course, as I have frequently had the experience with infants recovering from severe dyspnea to their prior level of compromised respiratory function.

Care for Children Not in Palliative Care

Those with different levels of weakness due to SMA have varying treatment concerns. Those with the mildest forms of SMA have chiefly orthopedic problems, with deformities of feet and spine of paramount concern. With increasing levels of weakness, respiratory care assumes proportionately greater importance. At all levels there are nutritional, therapy, and parenting issues to be followed.

The principal orthopedic concern is the spine. In children who sit only with effort, the development of scoliosis is virtually inevitable; for those stronger it remains a high risk. The driving force for scoliosis is gravity. In contrast to orthopedic scoliosis, children with SMA develop scoliosis with a broad curve that initially appears slowly, but once established can progress rapidly as the deforming force of gravity increases with the degree of curvature. Use of a light weight rigid jacket brace (thoraco-lumbo-sacral orthosis or TLSO) can be very useful to slow the rate of progression, particularly when begun relatively early in the course. Thus, children with SMA at risk for scoliosis need to have careful and frequent assessment for the development of mild degrees of curvature. Unfortunately TLSO braces are uncomfortable, expensive, and need to be adjusted frequently, but the alternative of catastrophic scoliosis is life threatening or life limiting. The TLSO is fashioned to maintain supportive pressure on the pelvic rim and must below the axilla (which supports at about T7) on the concave side and broadly over the trunk on the convex side of the curve; some looseness of fit can be afforded in the anterior–posterior dimension to maximize room for thoracic expansion. It should be worn full time whenever the child is upright; since it is intended to counter the deforming force of gravity it can be removed when the child is recumbent or in water. The overall goal of TLSO support is to maintain as straight and flexible a spine a possible for as long as possible to improve the outcome with operative spinal fusion. This operation (discussed in Chapter x) is more successful in the long run if done as close as possible to, or after, the onset of skeletal maturity.

Other orthopedic concerns involve the limbs. Dislocation of the hips is common in the nonambulatory or limited ambulatory patient. This rarely limits function more than does the underlying weakness. As surgical "correction" often increases pain and immobility in the long term, thus operative approaches should be approached with caution.

Muscle biopsy specimens show sometimes extensive denervation, but the residual innervated muscle fibers are usually hypertrophied, sometimes to an extraordinary degree exceeding the caliber seen in any other condition, including extremes of training. Thus, the advisability of strength training is unclear. With use-hypertrophy the potential for disuse atrophy is enhanced, so that during illness or enforced immobility there often appears to be a rapid loss of strength and function. Therapy should be designed to enhance routine functions, and in general pure strength exercises in the young child do not easily translate into functional changes. Particular attention to the prevention of hip and knee contractures in the child who requires long-term wheelchair seating is important to preserve the ability to roll easily in bed. Particular attention to maintaining the ability for self-transfers is important, as this is the single most important gross motor task necessary for independent living. I am enthusiastic about providing mobility devices relatively early for children who have restricted range, but restricting their use within the normal perimeter within which independent mobility is possible. For example, it is reasonable to acquire a motorized chair for the child who can walk independently within the confines of the house, but use it only for trips outside the house. For those who can walk around the school, such a chair can be used only for longer trips. The chair is an important tool to extend range, and is a "liberator." I am concerned that the expression "confined to a wheelchair" is internalized by many patients, who reject the assistance that a wheelchair may offer, thus allowing their disease to confine them to an artificially small world.

Children with severe muscular atrophy are vulnerable to metabolic derangements with intercurrent illness. Potassium losses in diarrheal fluids are not easily made up from diminished reserves in skeletal muscle beds, and thus symptomatic hypokalemia may result early. Similarly symptomatic hypoglycemia may result relatively early in catabolic illness because of the absence of substrate from muscle to fuel gluconeogenesis. Thus, individuals with more severe weakness should be evaluated during intercurrent illness relatively early, and if significant supported with intravenous fluid, glucose, and solute supplementation.

Parenting a child with SMA is not easy. Because of the unusual slowing of degeneration, long-term survival into adulthood is a reasonable expectation for all but the most feeble. Whether independent living will be possible as an adult depends in large part on two factors: the level of residual power, and the level of self-confidence and independence. These two are only partially related. The natural tendency of children to grow up and away from their parents, resisted by the natural tendency of parents to resist the evolving separation, is undermined by the child's weakness. Children with SMA should be given as much as possible normal responsibilities, tasks, and should be expected to accomplish for themselves as much as is physically possible—even when this is a slow and labored process. Many children with SMA are very bright and creative; their ability to develop novel solutions to the challenges of weakness is one of their chief assets that serves well for a lifetime if allowed to develop.

Specific Therapies for SMN-Related SMA

Because there is a second, partially functioning, copy of the *SMN* gene in all individuals with SMA, there is now substantial interest in the development of specific therapies. This is an area of substantial interest, and the prospect for agents that will increase *SMN2* gene expression appears good. However, no trials evaluating the potential benefit and burden of such agents have yet been performed.

A pes planus foot, with valgus deformity of the heel, is common. For those with potential for walking long term, associated foot and ankle pain that arises over time from this deformity can be limiting. A UCBl (University of California, Berkeley) brace, supporting the lateral 5th metatarsal distally, medial navicular prominence, and lateral calcaneus can be useful but is a finicky brace that is expensive and requires frequent adjustment during growth years. As a wholly in-shoe orthosis, many insurance companies' policy for durable medial equipment will not cover this brace. The goal is to fix only a part of the deformity, just sufficient to counter the forces that produce additional ligamentous laxity over time.

Respiratory compromise is a persistent concern. For those at the lower end of respiratory function, the ongoing assistance of pulmonary medicine is essential. Important concerns include potential compromise of the airway, particularly at night, and diminished lung expansion leading in the short term to resting hypeercarbia and in the long term to underdevelopment of the lung led many to benefit from night-time noninvasive ventilatory assistance with (Bi-level positive airway pressure) (BiPAP) device fitted through a mask. Many toddlers develop symptomatic night airway obstruction from normal amounts of developmental tonsilar and adenoidal hyperplasia that is relieved with surgery. Aggressive treatment of lower tract disease with bronchodilators, antibiotics, and percussive pulmonary therapy is warranted.

Prospective respiratory care includes immunization with pneumoccal conjugate vaccine, as indicated for persons with high risk, at all ages. Use of the 25 valent Pneuovax every 5 years is also appropriate.

OTHER SPINAL MUSCULAR ATROPHY SYNDROMES

The spinal muscular atrophy label has been applied to a number of other genetic or presumably genetic conditions (Table 2). Many of these non-SMN SMA disorders are identified by the specific regions of weakness and family history. Unfortunately, with the exception of two disorders, the diagnosis by semiologic characteristics alone in isolated cases is insufficiently specific to be useful in genetic counseling. It can be expected that an increasing number of specific genes and gene tests will be found and developed soon. With these findings comes the potential for specific diagnosis, improved prognosis, and perhaps specific therapy.

X-linked spinobulbar atrophy, also known as Kennedy's syndrome, is the first of these two specific non-*SMN* SMA disorders. This affects men mostly as adults, but sometimes manifests in boys during school years. Early symptoms and signs include diffuse cramping and myalgia, fasciculations, and gynecomastia. The CK is often modestly elevated. Diagnosis is furthered by the electrophysiologic evidence of denervation and confirmed by genetic testing of the androgen receptor gene. The second disorder, spinal muscular atrophy with respiratory distress, or SMARD, generally affects infants postnatally with progressive foot deformity and diffuse weakness, especially involving the diaphragm. In contrast to babies with SMA 1, affected infants thus have prominent chest expansion with descent of the abdomen during inspiration. Testing for missense mutations within the causative *IGHMBP2* gene is likely to be commercially available soon.

An infantile form of spinal muscular atrophy, often associated with arthrogryposis, has been linked to the X chromosome and exclusively affects males. Without an X-linked family history there is presently no means of making this diagnosis, though prospect for successful conclusion to the search for the causative gene is good. This is similar to the other named forms of spinal muscular atrophy, for which a positive family history is necessary to make the diagnosis.

SUGGESTED READINGS

1. Bach JR, Rajaraman R, Ballanger F, et al. Neuromuscular ventilatory insufficiency: effect of home mechanical ventilator use vs. oxygen therapy on pneumonia and hospitalization rates. Am J Phys Med Rehabil 1998; 77:8–19.
2. Bentley G, Haddad F, Bull TM, Seingry D. The treatment of scoliosis in muscular dystrophy using modified Luque and Harrington–Luque instrumentation. J Bone Joint Surg Br 2001; 83B:22–28.
3. Crawford TO. Spinal muscular atrophies. In: Jones HR, De Vivo DC, Darras BT, eds. Neuromuscular Disorders of Infancy, Childhood and Adolescence: A Clinician's Approach. Chapter 8. Philadephia, PA: Butterworth Heinemann, 2003:145–166.

30
Therapy for Neuromuscular Junction Disorders

Thomas O. Crawford
Johns Hopkins Hospital, Baltimore, Maryland, U.S.A.

INTRODUCTION

The neuromuscular junction (NMJ) is the remarkable structure at the interface of the motor axon and its innervated muscle fiber that is responsible for neuromuscular transmission. It is a synapse, but a highly specialized synapse because of its both critical and unique physiologic task. The NMJ is designed to transfer the motor axon potential to a muscle fiber action potential with 100% fidelity. In this respect, it is unlike all other synapses in the brain where various excitatory and inhibitory influences engage in a competition with one another to influence postsynaptic firing. That the NMJ normally functions without failure is remarkable given the size difference: the terminal motor axon within the synapse is tiny and the innervated muscle fiber is massive. The infusion current required in order to bring the muscle cell membrane to its depolarization threshold is correspondingly large. Neuromuscular transmission is critical to viability: it is not an accident that the various steps in the process of neuromuscular transmission are the biologic target of choice for evolved toxins injected by many different predators, or that a wide array of rare genetic and acquired disorders of the neuromuscular junction manifest with obvious and often life-threatening symptoms. The complexity of neuromuscular transmission, and the early and obvious manifestation of its dysfunction, is expressed in the array of disorders that affect children. Fortunately, the sophistication of diagnosis rivals that in any other area of molecular, genetic, immunologic, or physiologic branch of neuroscience, and many of the various disorders of neuromuscular transmission are associated with specific and successful treatment.

The process of neuromuscular transmission involves a series of physiologic steps. First, arrival of a sodium channel-mediated conducted action potential to the terminal motor axon opens voltage-gated calcium channels on the presynaptic surface. The influx of calcium triggers a series of proteins to bind and fuse acetylcholine (ACh) containing vesicles to the inner presynaptic membrane, releasing their contents into the synaptic cleft. The ACh then diffuses across the 70 μm space of the synapse, through a loose basal lamina, to bind reversibly to acetylcholine receptors (AChR) on the surface of the muscle cell. This in turn opens a cation channel, permitting the in rush of sodium ion. The membrane depolarization produced by release of a single presynaptic vesicle of ACh into the synaptic cleft is in the range of 1 mV. With each motor axon action potential, approximately 100 vesicles are released, resulting in a summed muscle depolarization of approximately 40 mV, more than enough to meet the 10–20 mV threshold necessary to open adjacent voltage-gated sodium channels surrounding the NMJ. The process of neuromuscular transmission is enhanced by the presence of multiple pleated folds in the postsynaptic muscle membrane that are densely lined with voltage-gated sodium channels. Depolarization of the voltage-gated sodium channels within each of these electrically isolated folds acts as an amplifier, multiplying the current influx and membrane potential difference within the region of the junction. Small cation currents at the AChR thus lead to substantial currents around the NMJ, sufficient to trigger an action potential across the muscle fiber surface that leads to muscle cell contraction through an equally remarkable downstream series of steps. The excess of current beyond that necessary to trigger the muscle cell action potential is called the safety factor.

In one way or another, all symptomatic disorders of neuromuscular junction ultimately act by diminishing the safety factor. The result is that some, or many, of the conducted motor action potentials fail to trigger a muscle fiber action potential, and the muscle fiber fails to contract. This can be by disturbing any step of the process, from decreasing the number of ACh molecules per vesicle, decreasing the number of vesicles that fuse with each motor axon potential, abnormal ACh binding or the associated binding of cation channels, diminished amplification by simplification of the postjunctional clefts, or diminished acetylcholinesterase activity. Infants tend to have less of a physiologic safety factor compared to older children and adults. Junctional failure at a single synapse is an all-or-nothing process, but at the level of the motor neuron it is graded, as some muscle fibers may fail to contract while others respond normally. The specifics of physiologic testing for neuromuscular junction failure are complex and beyond the scope of this chapter, but excellent reviews exist. General features of enhancing the diagnosis of specific disorders of neuromuscular disorders in children are discussed below.

SPECIFIC DISORDERS

Autoimmune Myasthenia Gravis

Autoimmune myasthenia gravis (MG) is by far the single most common disorder of the NMJ in children. This disorder is more common in adults, but can affect children as early as late infancy. In children, the general incidence correlates with age; MG is rarest in the youngest. It tends to affect orbital and bulbar-innervated muscles more than appendicular muscles, but there is wide individual variation. The clinical hallmark of MG is *fatigue*. Muscle power may be normal after a period of rest, but with repeated activation available power drops quickly. Both the intensity and the course of MG are highly variable. The MG can manifest over a range from trivial to catastrophic; the course can be stable and predictable or extraordinarily capricious. In general, the severity and course of any one individual with MG will declare itself relatively early in the course. For example, more than half of affected children have symptomatic weakness restricted to orbital muscles; if early eye muscle involvement does not spread more widely for 6 months it is unlikely to do so thereafter. Similarly, the tendency for minor intercurrent illness to trigger a sudden exacerbation that requires urgent medical intervention usually manifests within the first year.

Diagnosis

The diagnosis of MG is sometimes simple, sometimes extraordinarily difficult. Fortunately, however, the general difficulty of establishing a definitive diagnosis is inversely related to the need for that diagnosis. In those with severe illness the diagnosis is usually straightforward, while the diagnosis in those with subtle transient symptoms may never be established with certainty. Clinical suspicion of MG should be increased whenever weakness is variable from time to time or with fatiguing effort. A frequent clinical test is to examine for decreasing range of extraocular mobility or ptosis with sustained up gaze. Another test is to look for early fatigue while sustaining a horizontal anteverted posture of the arms. In addition, four lines of evidence can contribute to the diagnosis:

- A positive test for antibodies against the acetylcholine receptor (anti-AChR antibodies) has the best predictive value of any single test. Unfortunately, anti-AChR antibodies are less often found in children than adults with MG, and much less often found in those with weakness restricted to the orbital muscles. In the practice of pediatrics, the antibody test thus often operates as does a "one way ratchet"—useful if positive but not if negative.
- Electrodiagnostic testing, demonstrating a characteristic decremental response of muscle action potential amplitude—generally considered as anything greater than 10–15%—decreases from the first to the fourth or fifth response at 2–5 Hz stimulation, can be very useful, particularly if it can be shown to improve following rest or anticholinesterase treatment. Unfortunately this is an insensitive test, particularly in children and when weakness is transient. It is absolutely necessary to obtain a stable baseline and repeated testing, which are difficult to obtain in a less than fully cooperative child. When done poorly, false interpretation of testing to be abnormal is a risk. Sedating the child will improve the sensitivity of the test somewhat and substantially improve test specificity, but sedation of the child with enhanced potential for bulbar muscle weakness must be done in a controlled environment and carefully followed, increasing the morbidity and emotional and financial costs of the test. Very specialized electrodiagnostic testing with a stimulated single fiber technique, looking for abnormal jitter and block, is occasionally useful.
- Evaluation of the clinical response to short-term anticholinesterase inhibitor medications can be very useful, but care must be taken to insure a quality test. To be useful as a test for mysathenia, the child must manifest partial and easily testable weakness in a muscle at the time of treatment. A positive test is one where dramatic improvement can be demonstrated within seconds of infusion and the improvement then lapses back to baseline over a period of minutes. Because edriphonium clearly produces autonomic symptoms, care must be taken not to interpret as positive responses that could be attributable more simply to vigorous stimulation—such as the resolution of ptosis in a sleepy infant.
- In very subtle cases of transient symptoms—such as in children with variable ptosis, the sensitivity of each of the above methods may be limited. Use of a randomized paired on/off trial testing standard oral anticholinesterase medications with a blinded observer can be useful in some such circumstances. One parent can give the medication, while the other is instructed to score whether or not the symptom of concern is improved.

The MG is more likely if the observer reliably identifies the medication day correctly in multiple medication/no medication paired trials, each arm of a trial assigned to a separate day. The observer should also be asked to identify what were the most distinctive features—with post hoc reporting of observed anticholinergic features diminishing the power of the test.

Treatment

Treatment for children with confirmed MG should be tailored to clinical need. The range of required therapy is vast, with some requiring no therapy and some necessitating substantial intervention and tolerance for its associated morbidity (Table 1). Therapeutic modalities include short-term treatment of symptoms with acetylcholinesterase inhibiting agents, intermediate term treatment of the antibody response with plasmapheresis and IVIG, and long-term modifiers of the disorder with corticosteroids, other immunosuppressives, and thymectomy.

Oral acetylcholinesterase inhibitor therapy with *pyridostigminine bromide* can minimize weakness transiently. The onset of action is rapid, and duration of action is approximately 3–4 hr. Dosage can be increased slowly, titrating for benefit and the absence of side effects, usually abdominal cramping and diarrhea. The standard dose for children is xx. Too high a dose may increase weakness, so the dose should not be increased too rapidly. Dosing is best at 4 hr intervals, with 3, 4, or 5 doses daily with meals to minimize GI side effects. If the child wakes strong, night-time dosing is unnecessary. An extended form is available for those who have symptoms in the morning before taking their dose. This come at only 180 mg doses, however, which is generally useful for the adult or child taking 60 mg or more with each dose. Use of the timespan form of pyridostigmine other than at night is contraindicated because of wide variation in daytime absorption and elimination pharmacokinetics. Intravenous neostigmine by continuous infusion can be substituted for oral mestinon in an ICU setting during crises, to tailor dosage and effect, and when oral medications cannot be tolerated. The dose equivalence is 1 mg neostigmine = 60 mg pyridostigimine; thus, an individual receiving 60 mg pyridostigmine every 4 hr should have approximately equal response to 0.25 mg hourly (i.e., 60 mg/4 hr/60). Generally the initial dose is less than this, with escallation to the equivalent dose over a period of hours depending upon response.

Table 1 Treatments for MG

Rapid diagnostic	AChE inhibition	i.v. edrophonium (Tensilon)
Rapid diagnostic/sustained therapeutic in ICU		i.v. or i.m. neostigmine (Prostigmin)
Rapid therapeutic		p.o. pyridostigmine bromide (Mestinon)
Rapid therapeutic		p.o. ephedrine
Short term (days)	Immunomodulation	Plasmapheresis
Short term (days)		IVIg
Long term (weeks)	Immunomodulation	corticosteroids
Long term (months)	Immunomodulation	Azathioprine (Imuran)
Long term (months)		Cyclosporine (Sandimmune)
Long term (months)		Mycophenolate mofetil (CellCept)
Long term (months)	Immunomodulation	Thymectomy

Ephedrine has been reported to help in some cases of MG, probably as a result of presynaptic adrenergic receptors that may increase calcium influx and the number of quanta released with each depolarization. At best the effect is modest, however. This, rapid drug tolerance, and withdrawal of ephedrine from the United States over the counter market all decrease interest in this form of therapy. Anecdotal reports of improvement in weakness following treatment with pseudoephedrine or other over-the-counter cold preparations may be partially explained by this mechanism, however, no dosing recommendations are available.

Thymectomy was first offered for patients in whom MG coexisted with thymoma. The observation that patients' myasthenic symptoms improved led to ever decreasing threshold for the diagnosis of thymoma. Thymectomy has, without benefit of a controlled trial, become generally accepted as an effective long-term therapy based upon the perception among experienced clinicians that there is an associated diminished need for immunosuppressive therapy. This, plus the occurrence of cases of dramatic change in the clinical course of myasthenia following thymectomy further fuel the enthusiasm for its use. An accepted and accepted without controversy about the relative efficacy and safety of thymectomy nonetheless persist around the edges. For example, the minimum severity of myasthenic symptoms necessary to justify operative thymectomy, the minimum and maximum ages for which the relative benefits outweigh the risks, and the effect of duration of myasthenia prior to thymectomy on the efficacy of thymectomy remain controversial in the absence of data. Of importance to children is that no abnormality of immune function appears to be seen in patients who have had thymectomy even in early school years. On the other hand, spontaneous remissions of myasthenic symptoms may be more common among affected children, making the interpretation of improvement in any one child more difficult to interpret.

Fastidious preoperative preparation for thymectomy is an essential element of its success. Reduction of the severity of symptoms with preoperative *plasmapheresis* can substantially increase respiratory function and reserve, diminishing perioperative respiratory insufficiency. Establishment of the dose for optimum anticholineresterase inhibition with continuous neostigmine infusions preoperatively can improve respiratory function in a steady state postoperatively. Fastidious treatment of infection and other catabolic stresses is equally important.

Corticosteroid treatment is the mainstay for long-term therapy of children with symptomatic generalized myasthenia. Initiation of corticosteroid therapy may be associated with transient worsening, so that patients with incipient respiratory compromise should be watched in the hospital. In those who have not experienced worsening with the initiation of steroids, treatment with high-dose pulse IV methylprednisolone may be beneficial. Patients receiving chronic prednisone should have weaning dosing adjustments slowly, because the tendency for relapse can build over time and rapid weaning frequently tends to lead to the need for a significant increase in dosage—hence increasing disease morbidity. In those patients with new onset generalized myasthenia in whom thymectomy is anticipated, it is better if possible to withhold corticosteroid therapy until after surgery, given its impact on perioperative infection risk and wound healing.

IVIG has been associated with short-term improvement of myasthenic weakness. Onset of action is over days, and duration of expected benefit generally measures in weeks. Though expensive, it can be useful to tide over difficult patients until other immunosuppressives can begin to have an effect, and may be useful for the care of patients in crisis when plasmapheresis is not an option.

Plasmapheresis is the most consistent means for improving myasthenic weakness in the short term. The duration of benefit extends from a week or two to longer periods. The amount of benefit is related to the number and extent of exchanges. Pheresis can be useful to prepare a patient for surgery, or in response to a myasthenic crisis. Longer term therapy is limited by the expense and morbidity associated with large caliber catheters necessary for the exchange. The risk associated with these catheters increases substantially with the smaller size of young children.

Other immunosuppressive medications can clearly be useful in the treatment of myasthenia. Because these agents will be needed for years, however, there are real concerns about potentiating later malignancy and other serious side effects. The most common treatment is with azathioprine (Imuran), which is generally best used as a steroid sparing agent after attempts to slowly withdraw daily prednisone is met with disease worsening, or when daily steroid therapy is helpful but not sufficient to maintain sufficient control of symptoms. New to the treatment of myasthenia is the use of mycophenolate mofetil (CellCept), which has shown promise in the treatment of adults with myasthenia.

Passive Transfer Myasthenia (Neonatal MG)

Infants born to a mother with autoimmune MG are at risk for developing weakness that may be more dramatic than that seen in the mother due to the passive transfer of AChR antibodies into the baby. This is a transient disorder, which will improve as the infant replaces this acquired immunoglobulin with that synthesized endogenously. Most affected infants are only mildly weak, manifesting with ptosis or diminished feeding. Treatment is usually not necessary, but use of acetylcholinesterase inhibitors would generally be the mainstay if necessary.

A rare disorder, caused by maternal antibody directed exclusively against a fetal isoform of the AChR, manifests with fetal akinesia that manifests after birth with lethal weakness and arthrogryposis. Once this antibody develops, subsequent pregnancies would be expected to have similar difficulty. Treatment with maternal plasmapheresis throughout pregnancy was shown in one case to result in a normal infant after a series of 4 affected infants with lethal weakness and deformity.

Genetic (Congenital) Myasthenia Syndromes (CMS)

An array of different genetic defects (Table 2) have been described that lead to failure of neuromuscular transmission. Like autoimmune MG, these can have widely varying presentation and course. The possibility of a CMS should be considered in any child with a fatiguable neuromuscular disorder, or unexplained static weakness with prominent bulbar, facial, and extraocular signs and symptoms, that is long standing. No AChR antibody titer should be detected in those with a CMS. Diagnosis with careful electrophysiologic studies, sometimes with stimulated single fiber EMG, or with in vitro studies of neuromuscular transmission, in tertiary centers with special interest in the CMS disorders may be necessary. A "double hump" CMAP response to single shocks of the innervating motor nerve in multiple different nerve–muscle combinations suggests a disorder with increased, rather than decreased, neuromuscular conductance, generally caused by either abnormally sustained open channel time of the acetylcholine receptor-gated sodium channel, or abnormality of the junctional acetylcholineresterase. Genetic testing for the CMS is likely to become increasingly important in the diagnosis.

Table 2 Selected CMS Syndromes

Location	Name (defect)	Inheritance pattern	Features
Presynaptic	Congenital myasthenic syndrome with episodic apnea: (choline acetyltransferase, CHAT)	AR	Severe respiratory and bulbar weakness with illness, onset in infancy
Synaptic	Acetylcholinesterase deficiency	AR	Onset infancy to childhood. Worsens or nonresponsive to AChE inhibitors. "Double hump" CMAP response to single shock of motor nerve
Postsynaptic	Slow channel (AChR subunits ∀, ∃, or ,)	AD	Highly variable onset age, nonresponsive to AChE inhibitors. "Double hump" CMAP response to single shock of motor nerve may respond to Quinidine sulfate
	AChR deficiency (any AChR subunit, most common)	AR	Most common form of CMS. Highly variable phenotype responds to AChE inhibitors

One important form of CMS requires additional suspicion and additional special testing to diagnosis. Congenital myasthenic syndrome with episodic apnea, due to mutation of choline acteyltransferase, is the manifestation of a disorder in which sustained depolarization, either due to fever, illness, prolonged work (as with crying) leads to decreasing concentration of ACh within individual quanta. The disorder presents with intermittent and sometimes severe respiratory failure precipitated by infection. Conventional repetitive nerve conduction studies are normal. During healthy times, sustained stimulation at 10 Hz for 5–10 min is necessary to demonstrate a decremental response. This will obviously require anesthesia to perform, and hence diagnosis requires vigilance and a high degree of suspicion on the part of caring physicians.

Unlike autoimmune MG, therapies directed toward an immune pathogenesis will have no effect. The mainstay of pharmacologic therapy is oral pyridostigmine, with occasional patients also benefitting from ephedrine. Much attention should be directed to safety concerns in the newly diagnosed baby or toddler with a CMS, since some patients develop unexpected airway and respiratory compromise swiftly in times of new upper respiratory infections or other intercurrent illness.

Infant Botulism

Enteric colonization with toxin-forming *Clostridium botulinum* species is responsible for nonepidemic acquired weakness in babies, chiefly in the first 6 months of life, nationwide. Affected infants are often breast fed in transition to formula feeds, and have a history of constipation prior to the onset of weakness. Weakness of bulbar and extraocular muscles often precedes appendicular weakness, leading to a soft cry, diminished oral intake, and ptotic, impassive face. If present, pupilary dilation

Table 3 Complications of Infant Botulism

Complication	Treatment
Hypoventilation/respiratory failure	Assisted ventilation
Constipation/malnutrition	Increasing rate of gavage feeds
Low serum Na^+, SIADH	Transient fluid restriction
Autonomic instability	Monitoring, minimal symptomatic treatments
Family and social stresses with extended hospital stay	Encourage long-term planning for family visitation and social work consultation beginning at time of diagnosis; contact with other families previously affected

and sluggish responsiveness to light is a significant physical sign. The most important factor to prognosis is an enhanced diagnostic suspicion: the most dangerous time for airway and vital support is before the diagnosis is made. Sedation for radiologic procedures, or prolonged trunk flexion for a diagnostic lumbar puncture, can be of special risk. Immediate diagnosis can be suggested by electrophysiologic testing. Analysis of the toxin from stool specimens is definitive.

Once the diagnosis is made, the mainstay of therapy is careful supportive care. The prognosis for full return of muscle power is excellent, although the course may be prolonged. Intubation for airway and respiratory muscle support should be instituted early when the course is clearly progressive. Although endotrachial intubation is frequently prolonged, side effects such as subglottic stenosis is rare as long as uncuffed tubes with some leak are used; immobility of the infant likely reduces physical irritation of the tube against the trachial lining. Relapses of respiratory failure after weaning have been reported; prolonging the period of careful observation after successful weaning of support is prudent. Although the infant is frequently constipated at the outset, re-initiation of feeds by gavage is usually successful and important to sustained health during the period of immobility. Tachyarrhythmias and other autonomic abnormalities are generally mild and respond best to conservative treatment. In the first days after intubation some infants manifest low serum sodium levels likely due to an acquired syndrome of inappropriate antidiuritic hormone excess; this can be treated with volume restriction and rarely persists for more than a few days.(3).

Human-derived botulinum immune globulin (BIG) was recently licensed for treatment of infant botulism due to botulinum toxins A and B, these two being responsible for the vast majority of cases. It has been shown to reduce the time of hospitalization and duration of requirement for assisted ventilation. Its effectiveness is highly related to speed of administration, so that with high probability cases treatment should be initiated before toxicologic confirmation. Information about obtaining human-derived BIG is available at www.infantbotulism.org.

SUGGESTED READINGS

1. Crawford TO. Infant botulism. In: Jones HR, De Vivo DC, Darras BT, eds. Neuromuscular Disorders of Infancy, Childhood and Adolescence: A Clinician's Approach. Chapter 32. Philadelphia, PA: Butterworth Heinemann, 2003:547–554.
2. Harper CM. Congenital myasthenic syndromes. In: Brown WF, Bolton CF, Aminoff MJ, eds. Neuromuscular Function and Disease; Basic, Clinical and Electrodiagnostic Aspects. Chapter 93. Philadelphia: W.B. Saunders, 2002:1687–1695.

31
Therapy for Muscular Dystrophies

Richard T. Moxley, III and Michael E. Yurcheshen
Department of Neurology, University of Rochester Medical Center, Rochester, New York, U.S.A.

The muscular dystrophies represent a group of slowly progressive inherited diseases that usually have a very specific pattern of muscle wasting and weakness. Because of better physical therapy, surgical, and ventilatory techniques, the lifespan of those patiets with these often progressive illnesses has grown in the last 50 years. With a few notable exceptions, however, current therapy for muscular dystrophies remains largely supportive and rarely targeted. Because of major advances in the diagnosis and treatment of Duchenne dystrophy, this chapter will focus primarily on this dystrophinopathy. Briefer sections, as well as information contained in Table 1 address systemic treatment of some of the other muscular dystrophies that occur in childhood.

DUCHENNE DYSTROPHY

Duchenne dystrophy is a slowly progressive muscle-wasting disease marked by symptoms that develop before age 5. Early in its course, Duchenne dystrophy affects the proximal hip and shoulder girdle muscles as well as the anterior neck and abdominal muscles. The pathology is caused by absence or extreme deficiency of a large cytoskeletal protein, dystrophin, encoded in the Xp21 region. This protein attaches to the inner surface of the muscle fiber membrane as a part of a complex of glycoproteins. Dystrophin also is part of the inner membrane structure of smooth and cardiac muscle and of certain cells in the central nervous system and in specialized connective tissues, such as the myotendinous junctions. This distribution of dystrophin corresponds closely to those tissues with major damage in Duchenne dystrophy.

Duchenne dystrophy typically manifests between 2 and 4 years of age. Parents notice weakness of forward head flexion that persists beyond infancy, accompanied by slowed motor development. Patients have difficulty keeping up with their peers, both physically and sometimes cognitively. Diagnosis hinges on careful history and physical, as well as laboratory testing (i.e., serum creatine kinase levels, leukocyte DNA testing for the Duchenne dystrophy mutation), occasionally electrodiagnostic testing, and in situations in which DNA testing is not informative in obtaining a muscle biopsy. Muscle biopsy also helps distinguish many of the recently described autosomal dominant and autosomal recessive forms of limb girdle

Table 1 Muscular Dystrophies in Childhood: Complications and Treatment

	Duchenne dystrophy	Becker dystrophy	Myotonic dystrophy	Limb girdle muscular dystrophy
Muscle weakness	Treatment with prednisone slows or stabilizes muscle strength; lightweight long-leg bracing maintains ambulation in later stages	No controlled studies of prednisone treatment; bracing is helpful in late stages	No specific therapy; braces for foot drop; children usually can participate in gym in school	No specific therapy; braces for foot drop; children usually can participate in gym in school
Respiratory problems	Forced vital capacity is monitored (in later stages, atelectatic pneumonitis is common); colds are treated aggressively; if signs of respiratory failure develop, nasal/oral ventilation should be considered	Uncommon until late stages; management then is as with Duchenne dystrophy	For congenital cases, ventilary care often is needed; the prognosis for survival is very poor if the patient is ventilator dependent >4 weeks; other management is as for Duchenne dystrophy	Uncommon until late stages; management then is as with Duchenne dystrophy
Cardiac problems	Occasionally cardiomyopathy leads to congestive heart failure—afterload-reducing therapy often helps; the role of digoxin is uncertain; patient should be monitored for intracardiac clots	Occasionally, severe cardiomyopathy develops; treatment is the same as for Duchenne dystrophy	Occasionally, tachyarrhythmias or heart block develop in childhood forms, and pace maker treatment is indicated	Occasionally, severe cardiomyopathy develops; treatment is the same as for Duchenne dystrophy
Orthopedic problems	Achilles tendon contractures respond to stretching in early stages, later tendon release surgery often is necessary; contractures at the hips, knees, elbows, and wrists usually develop after the patient becomes wheelchair bound; scoliosis often develops when patients stop ambulating, and spinal stabilization surgery helps maintain use of the arms and preserves pulmonary reserve	Uncommon; contractures are much less common than in Duchenne dystrophy	Talipes deformity requires treatment with stretching and orthotic support; occasionally surgery is necessary	Uncommon; contractures are much less common than in Duchenne dystrophy
Nervous system symptoms	Increased incidence of cognitive and behavioral problems; some patients improve with small doses of methyl-phenidate	Uncommon	Mental retardation is common, especially in congenital cases, and special classroom care is needed; hearing deficits are common and may require hearing aids; facial weakness, dysarthria, and hearing problems exaggerate the impression of mental retardation	Uncommon

Facioscapulohumeral dystrophy	Fukuyama-type congenital muscular dystrophy	Congenital muscular dystrophy: primary deficiency of merosin	Emery–Dreifuss muscular dystrophy
No specific treatment; patients should avoid lifting with arms fully extended and abducted; braces are sometimes needed	No specific treatment; bracing and physical therapy are useful in some patients	Same as Fukuyoma-type congenital muscular atrophy	No specific treatment; skeletal muscle weakness often is relatively mild compared with cardiac problems and does not limit function
Uncommon	As with Duchenne dystrophy; patients often succomb to respiratory failure late in childhood or in early teens	Same as Fukuyoma-type congenital muscular atrophy	Mild other than symptoms related to cardiac dysfunction
Uncommon	Uncommon	Uncommon	Frequent cardiac conduction defects; atrial paralysis, cardiac arrest, and sudden death are common; pacemaker treatment and preventive therapy for cardiac emboli often are necessary
Occasionally, knee effusion and low back pain develop secondary to weakness; conservative care measures are effective; in late stages some surgeons have reported good results with procedures to stabilize the scapula; surgery is uncommon	Contractures develop in 70% of patients by 3 months of age at the ankles, knees, and hips	Contractures, especially feet and hips	Contractures, especially in the elbows and ankles, occur early and respond somewhat to physical therapy; surgical release of achilles tendon may be necessary; some patients develop a rigid spine syndrome, for which there is no effective therapy
Uncommon; in rare cases, the infant onset form of the disease occurs in association with hearing loss and/or retinal disease	Generalized or focal seizures occur in most patients; anticonvulsant therapy is necessary; mental retardation is common; most patients have microcephaly,as well as polymicrogyria, pachygyria, and heterotopias, in the brain on postmortem examination	Mental retardation common; MR of head shows increased signal from white matter on T2 weighted images; occipital agyria	Due only to stroke from heart block or cardiac emboli

muscular dystrophy (LGMD) that sometimes have a close clinical similarity to Duchenne dystrophy.

Treatment

The overall goals in managing patients who have Duchenne dystrophy are to maintain ambulation for as long as possible, to optimize the development of the patient's cognitive abilities, and to anticipate the occurrence of complications, such as excessive weight gain, joint contractures (especially of the Achilles tendons), respiratory insufficiency, scoliosis, gastrointestinal hypomotility, and occasionally cardiomyopathy. Table 1 summarizes the principal problems and treatment options. The patient and his family need to work closely with the physicians, schoolteachers, physical educators, and physical and occupational therapists to develop an individualized care plan for each stage of Duchenne dystrophy. Early in the illness the patient usually can play with his peers in most activities, but by the first or second grade some adaptation of physical education requirements becomes necessary.

Orthopedic Concerns

The natural history of Duchenne dystrophy predicts that the patient will become wheelchair bound between 10 and 12 years of age. Often, lightweight long-leg bracing is helpful at this stage to prolong weight bearing and ambulation, both of which delay the development of joint contractures and scoliosis. Contractures and scoliosis develop primarily after the patient becomes wheelchair bound. They do not appear at a specific age but depend largely on the functional ability of the patient. Once contractures begin to develop, usually at the ankles and elbows (flexion and pronation), it is important to obtain physical therapy (PT) and occupational therapy (OT) consultations. Once significant heel cord contractures develop, it also is useful to obtain an orthopedic consultation. The orthopedist can help guide the timing of the use of long-leg bracing and can discuss the possible need for surgery to lengthen the Achilles tendons.

Scoliosis develops in the middle (wheelchair dependent) and late (respiratory insufficiency) stages of Duchenne dystrophy. Orthopedic consultation and serial follow-up to monitor contractures and degree of spinal curvature are part of optimal care. Most spine surgeons recommend preventive stabilization surgery in Duchenne dystrophy once the patient is nonambulatory and clearly progressive curvature exceeds 20 degrees. Other surgical approaches, such as more limited spinal surgery with lumbar fixation at L5, are also undergoing evaluation. Prior to spinal stabilization surgery and prior to any major surgery in patients with Duchenne dystrophy, it is necessary for the neurologist and primary care physician to obtain what will likely be ongoing consultative assistance from pulmonary medicine and cardiology.

Treatment of Systematic Complications

An involved pediatrician is critical in the early, middle, and late stages of Duchenne dystrophy. Minor medical problems can sometimes provoke major complications. In the later stages, a mild cold may lead to atelectatic pneumonitis and acute respiratory insufficiency. Even chronic constipation can produce respiratory compromise in the later stages of Duchenne dystrophy due to abdominal distention and upward pressure on the diaphragm. Respiratory insufficiency is common in the late stages of

Duchenne dystrophy. Forced vital capacity declines, usually into the range of 600–1000 mL. Recent reports describe the management options, which include nasal ventilation rather than positive pressure ventilation via tracheostomy. Considerable discussion is necessary to educate the patient and his family at this stage and to help to decide which options are most appropriate for them. Often neuromuscular physicians and nurses are the individuals who educate the family, and the roles of the pediatric pulmonologist and pediatrician have to be tailored to each medical care setting. The function of other organ systems may be compromised later in the course of Duchenne dystrophy, either as a direct consequence of the absence of dystrophin within vascular and gastrointestinal smooth muscle, within cardiac muscle, or as a downstream consequence of reduced skeletal muscle mass. Acute gastric dilation is one such infrequent complication in the late stages of Duchenne dystrophy. This typically occurs in association with an idiopathic metabolic acidosis and responds rapidly to nasogastric tube decompression of the stomach and intravenous hydration. Caution must be used with intravenous repletion of potassium because in the late stages of the disease the muscle mass of the patient is considerably diminished and is not available to buffer an acute rise of extracellular potassium. Chronic intestinal hypomotility (constipation) is also a recognized problem. Good hydration, a balanced dietary intake, and regular bowel habits are the mainstays of treatment for these problems.

Occasionally, in the late stages of Duchenne dystrophy, patients develop symptomatic cardiomyopathy. Clinical expression of more common mild cardiomyopathy is masked by the diminished capacity for exercise due to skeletal muscle weakness. Symptomatic cardiomyopathy is associated with cardiomegaly with a reduced cardiac ejection fraction to 10–20% of normal. Heart failure often is exacerbated by coexisting respiratory insufficiency. In all these cases simultaneous ventilatory support must be considered, provided the patient and his family have decided to pursue a vigorous course of treatment of his illness. Heart failure in its advanced stage is difficult to manage, and anticipaton of this complication by treatment with afterload reduction therapy often is more effective than later treatment with digoxin. Typically, initial treatment is with an angiotensin converting enzyme inhibitor, titrating diastolic blood pressure to 60–70 mmHg. If left ventricular dysfunction persists or worsens, beta-blocker therapy is necessary with the goal of keeping heart rate between 55 and 70 beats per minute. Cardiology consultation needs to guide the care plan. Occasionally, ventricular and/or atrial clots are present, and long-term anticoagulant therapy is necessary.

Specific Treatments

The only effective therapy for Duchenne dystrophy is prednisone. Double-blind, randomized, controlled studies have shown that prednisone in a daily dose of 0.75 mg/kg maintains muscle strength and functions for at least 18–36 months. These studies also have demonstrated that daily treatment is more effective than alternate-day therapy. Some benefit occurs at doses as low as 0.3 mg/kg/day and prolonged improvement of strength has occurred at doses ranging from 0.5 to 0.6 mg/kg/day. Trials of deflazacort have shown efficacy equal to prednisone with fewer complications, but this agent is unavailable in the United States.

How corticosteroids produce their beneficial effects in Duchenne dystrophy is unknown. The answer may lead to new, more effective, therapy with fewer side effects. However, there are several clues about the time course related to the benefit.

The increase in strength begins to develop after only 10 days of treatment and reaches a maximum response after 3 months of therapy. Muscle mass increases 10% after 3 months of prednisone treatment, and by 6–8 weeks the rate of muscle breakdown declines in association with maintenance of a normal rate of muscle protein synthesis. One investigation compared the efficacy of 12 months of azathioprine immunosuppressive therapy with that of prednisone; and, no beneficial effect occurred with azathioprine. This result argues against the possibility that an immunosuppressive effect accounts for the improvement in muscle strength with the use of prednisone.

Patients have received long-term prednisone at only a small number of specialized neuromuscular centers. Prednisone treatment preferably is monitored by or coordinated with the guidance of one of these centers. The protocol for monitoring side effects and for assessing muscle strength and function has been published previously. The most common side effects are excessive weight gain, mood disturbances (more aggressive, more tearful), and cushingoid facial appearance. More serious side effects (high blood pressure, GI bleeding, severe infections, or diabetes) are uncommon. Some patients have developed small, dot-shaped cataracts; others, as expected, have had decreased linear growth, which probably has helped maintain ambulation.

To allow monitoring for the development of side effects, patients are seen every 3 months for weight, blood pressure, pulse, forced vital capacity, urinalysis, and an assessment of neuromuscular functioning. At each visit the patient undergoes timed function tests (time needed to travel 30 feet, to arise from supine to standing position, and to climb four standard steps) and a muscle strength evaluation (shoulder abductors, elbow flexors and extensors, knee extensors, hip flexors and extensors). These measures along with assessment of side effects help guide the physicians in adjusting the dosage of prednisone. The blood count and serum electrolyte levels are measured at 6-month intervals. With close follow-up, patients have been kept stable or showed only very mild progression of muscle weakness for periods exceeding 5 years. Even in the late stages, prednisone appears to maintain respiratory muscle power and has reduced the number of patients who develop respiratory failure.

Other agents are in various stages of study for DMD and include oxandrolone, growth hormone, creatine, glutamine, oxatomide, co-enzyme Q10, albuterol, and gentamicin. Advances in gene therapy coupled with successes in manufacturing small segments of DNA containing the normal gene for dystrophin have raised hopes that direct gene therapy, either by local injection or by viral vector, will be useful. Stem cell therapy is being planned, but gene transfer and stem cell therapy are probably years away in terms of routine treatment.

MYOTONIC DYSTROPHIES

The myotonic dystrophies are a group of diseases that share an autosomal dominant inheritance and have the core features of myotonia, early onset cataracts, and weakness. Classical myotonic dystrophy of Steinert, termed myotonic dystrophy type 1 (DM1), is the most common form of myotonic dystrophy, and it is due to an abnormal enlargement of an unstable trinucleotide repeat expansion in the 3 prime nontranslated region of the DM gene on chromosome 19. Discovery of the gene defect has led to the development of gene probes to identify both symptomatic and asymptomatic carriers. Genetic counseling and prenatal testing can now be performed with a high degree of accuracy, an important advance in preventive therapy. Another form of myotonic dystrophy, myotonic dystrophy type 2 (DM2) also results from an unstable nucleotide repeat expansion, a CCTG repeat. A standardized DNA test is available to screen for DM2. At present, it appears that infant or childhood onset cases of DM2 are very rare or do not occur. A recent review discusses management of DM1 in detail. The reader may want to consult that reference for more information on neonatal and childhood manifestations of DM1. It also emphasizes complications that occur when patients receive anesthetics and describes the problems involved in pregnancy and delivery.

The mainstays of treatment for DM1 in infancy and childhood are largely supportive. In infants with congenital DM1 aggressive pulmonary toilet, ventilator support (if needed), feeding tube, and orthotic care for talipes are often necessary. In cases with childhood onset careful monitoring of learning disability, hearing problems, and gastrointestinal dysfunction often lead to placement of these patients in special classes and tutoring. Occasionally, antimyotonia therapy is helpful for the intestinal dysfunction. Myotonia of the grip, swallowing, and speech usually do not develop until late childhood or the teens. This is also the case for early onset cataracts. During the late teens and early adulthood, the complications typical for adult onset DM1 occur. Close observation for complications, like cataracts, cholecystitis, cardiac conduction abnormalities, and endocrine dysfunction is integral to providing good care. These complications can be mitigated with appropriate surgical procedures, hormone replacement, and occasionally pacemaker placement. Encouraging responses to certain medical treatments in DM1 have occurred. For example, mexiletine and tocainide show promise in lessening myotonia. Modafinil has reduced hypersomnolence, Coenzyme Q10 may ameliorate cardiac dysfunction. Troglitazone and possibly the currently available thiozolidine diones can reduce the insulin resistance, and dehydroepiandosterone (DHEA) may be useful for cognitive problems and for myotonia relief. Controlled, randomized studies are necessary to evaluate these new potential treatments.

LIMB–GIRDLE MUSCULAR DYSTROPHIES

At the moment there are 10 autosomal recessive forms and 5 autosomal dominant forms of LGMD. Because of their pattern of weakness, the LGMDs are often confused with Duchenne dystrophy. However, most forms of LGMD are more slowly progressive than Duchenne dystrophy and have fewer complications. Only some forms have cardiomyopathy. It is important to avoid making a prognosis for survival, the development of complications, or for the rate of progression for different types of LGMD based upon the natural history of Duchenne dystrophy. It is also important not to assume that corticosteroid therapy will be effective in the different forms of LGMD.

For all of the LGMDs care relies on early orthopedic, respiratory, and physical conditioning measures. Cardiomyopathies and conduction defects are particularly prevalent in some forms of LGMD, for example, two autosomal recessive forms of LGMD, alpha and gamma sarcoglycanopathies, and two dominant forms, LGMD1B and LGMD1D. Close monitoring of cardiac status is crucial. Specific therapy to reverse muscle wasting and weakness is not currently available.

OTHER MUSCULAR DYSTROPHIES

Facioscapulohumeral dystrophy (FSHD) is not common in childhood and usually does not pose significant management problems. DNA diagnosis is possible by detection of a reduced number of repeats of a large repetitive sequence at the end of chromosome 4, yet curiously the causal gene has not yet been identified. A more detailed review of FSHD is given in a recent text.

The infant-onset congenital muscular dystrophies are rare disorders and are not usually confused with Duchenne dystrophy, LGMD, Becker dystrophy, or FSHD. For more detailed discussion, the reader should refer to the recent reviews.

Emery–Dreifuss muscular dystrophy (EDMD) is a rare x-linked and more rarely an autosomal recessive or dominantly inherited disorder. The EDMD is clinically and genetically distinct from x-lined Duchenne and Becker muscular dystrophies. Occasionally, there may be confusion with Becker muscular dystrophy. The EDMD can result from mutations either in emerin (x-linked form) or in A-type lamin (autosomal dominant form). It can have severe cardiac complications that require urgent treatment, typically pacemaker implantation. Cardiac symptoms may prompt medical evaluation in EDMD before complaints about muscle weakness or contractures.

SUGGESTED READINGS

1. Darras BT, Menache CC, Kunkel LM. Dystrophinopathies. In: Jones HR, DeVivo DC, Darras BT, eds. Neuromuscular Disorders of Infancy, Childhood, and Adolescence—A Clinicians Approach. Amsterdam: Butterworth Heinemann, 2003:649–700.
2. Finsterer J, Stollberger C. The heart in human dystrophinopathies. Cardiology 2003; 99(1):1–19.
3. Gozal D. Pulmonary manifestations of neuromuscular disease with special reference to Duchenne muscular dystrophy and spinal muscular atrophy. Pediatr Pulmonol 2000; 29(2):141–150.
4. Heller KD, Wirtz DC, Siebert CH, Forst R. Spinal stabilization in Duchenne muscular dystrophy: principles of treatment and record of 31 operative treated cases. J Pediatr Orthop B 2001; 10(1):18–24.
5. Moxley R. Corticosteroid and anabolic hormone treatment of Duchenne muscular dystrophy. In: Jones HR, DeVivo DC, Darras BT, eds. Neuromuscular Disorders of Infancy, Childhood, and Adolescence. Amsterdam: Butterworth Heinemann, 2003:1209–1226.
6. Moxley R, Meola G. The myotonic dystrophies. In: Rosenberg RN, Pruisiner SB, D.Mauro S, Barchi RL, Nestler EJ, eds. The Molecular and Genetic Basis of Neurologic and Psychiatric Disease. Philadelphia: Butterworth Heinemann, 2003:511–518.
7. Tawil R. Facioscapulohumeral dystrophy. In: Rosenberg RN, Pruisiner SB, D.Mauro S, Barchi RL, Nestler EJ, eds. The Molecular and Genetic Basis of Neurologic and Psychiatric Disease. Philadelphia: Butterworth Heinemann, 2003:519–526.
8. Zatz M, de Paula F, Starling A, Vainzof M. The 10 autosomal recessive limb girdle muscular dystrophies. Neuromuscul Disord 2003; 13(7–8):532–544.

32
Dysphagia

Maureen A. Lefton-Greif
Johns Hopkins University School of Medicine, Baltimore, Maryland, U.S.A.

INTRODUCTION

Dysphagia (swallowing difficulty) in the pediatric population is generally one component of a broad continuum of complex medical, health, and developmental problems and is common in infants and children with histories of prematurity, genetic syndromes, and neurologic disorders. Swallowing dysfunction may result in respiratory problems, stunted growth or nutritional compromise, and disruptions in the relationships between children and their caregivers. Early identification and appropriate treatment improve outcomes for these children and their caregivers.

NORMAL SWALLOWING

The primary functions of swallowing are to direct materials from the mouth to the stomach while keeping the airway protected, and to provide the right types of liquids and foods for children to grow and develop optimally. For discussion purposes, the act of swallowing is divided into three highly integrated and partially overlapping phases—the *oral, pharyngeal,* and *esophageal* phases of swallowing. During the *oral* phase, food is processed into a "swallow-ready ball" (bolus), which is then transported to the back of the mouth. In the infant, this phase is limited to sucking fluid from a nipple. For solid foods, bolus formation is dependent upon the consistency of food and may require chewing skills in older children. The *pharyngeal* phase is comprised of a series of complex and interrelated motor events that direct and propel a bolus through the pharynx and into the esophagus while keeping the airway protected. During the pharyngeal phase of swallow, breathing stops, the larynx elevates, the vocal folds adduct, the palate elevates and approximates the posterior pharyngeal wall, and the pharyngeal muscles contract to propel the bolus through a relaxed upper esophageal sphincter. The *esophageal* phase begins when the bolus enters the esophagus and ends when it passes into the stomach.

CONDITIONS AND CLINICAL PRESENTATIONS ASSOCIATED WITH NEUROGENIC DYSPHAGIA

Dysphagia is not a disease. It is a symptom of any disruption in the passage of secretions or nutrients from the mouth to the stomach. Structural or anatomic abnormalities or neurologic conditions, which obstruct the passage or interfere with the coordination of bolus movement, may cause dysphagia. Children with syndromes, sequences, or associations (e.g., Velocardiofacial syndrome, Pierre Robin sequence, Charge association) may experience dysphagia caused by a combination of structural anomalies and coordination problems.

Neurogenic dysphagia may be characterized by difficulties in any or all phases of swallowing. Factors that influence the nature and progression of the swallowing dysfunction include site of pathologic process (e.g., central nervous system, peripheral nervous system, or neuromuscular disease), the extent of the insult, and the course of the underlying condition. Neurogenic dysphagia may result from acute or chronic conditions; in turn, chronic conditions may be linked to static or progressive processes. Some conditions associated with an acute onset of dysphagia are encephalopathies, intracranial hemorrhages, cerebral infarctions, and infections. In the pediatric population, cerebral palsy (CP) is the most common chronic static condition associated with neurogenic dysphagia. Many children with CP or other static conditions improve with time and the initiation of appropriate therapeutic interventions. Others may regress in feeding and swallowing skills when they are challenged with increased nutrition or hydration requirements, or foods which require the use of more developmentally mature oral-motor skills (e.g., chewing), or intercurrent illnesses (e.g., respiratory syncytial virus). With progressive disease processes, feeding and swallowing skills usually worsen. These children may present when "home remedies" fail to facilitate compensations that were previously effective. The treatment implications for progressive neurogenic dysphagia are significant and family counseling is critical. For children with undiagnosed conditions, swallowing dysfunction may be the first indicator of an underlying medical or health disorder.

Dysphagia should be part of the differential diagnosis for all children with feeding or swallowing problems, or signs and symptoms suggestive of these probelms. Although clinical presentations of pediatric dysphagia are variable, manifestations may include:

- Respiratory problems
  - Chronic (e.g., pneumonia, frequent or long lasting chest infections)
  - Episodic (e.g., coughing, choking, congestion, or respiratory changes with feeding)
- Poor weight gain, growth compromise, or failure to thrive
- Lengthy feeding times (>30 min on a regular basis)
- Sudden onset of swallowing difficulties or regression in feeding and swallowing skills
- Negative behavioral responses to feeding (e.g., irritability, refusal to feed, lethargy)

EVALUATION

History

Establishing a diagnosis and developing a treatment plan for pediatric patients with swallowing dysfunction generally require input from multiple medical, health, and developmental disciplines including a feeding/swallowing specialist, who is usually a speech-language pathologist (SLP). The feeding/swallowing specialist completes a comprehensive bedside or clinic evaluation that includes a detailed history, physical examination, oral-motor/feeding observation, and instrumental assessment, if appropriate. A carefully tailored feeding history is critical and includes some of the questions listed below.

- *What is the nature of the problem and when did it start*? Manifestations of the problem, the age of onset, and whether the problem has stabilized or is continuing to worsen will guide further evaluation and management efforts.
- *Does the child cough, choke, become congested, or change breathing patterns during or after feeding*? Responses to these questions may enable the examiner to distinguish between symptoms of oropharyngeal dysphagia vs. gastroesophageal reflux (GER). Of note, the absence of coughing or choking during feeding does not preclude the possibility of dysphagia with concomitant aspiration. Silent aspiration (i.e., aspiration without cough) is common in individuals with neurogenic dysphagia, and reported to occur in 70 97% of pediatric patients with radiologic evidence of aspiration. Silent aspiration is problematic because the protective cough mechanism is absent, and caregivers and clinicians may underestimate the presence of swallowing dysfunction because "silent aspiration," by definition, does not provide overt evidence of airway contamination.
- *Is there evidence of gastroesophageal reflux disease (GERD)*? GERD is common in children with neurologic conditions, with pathologic GER reported in approximately 75% in children with CP. Manifestations of GERD are variable and may include emesis or regurgitation, fussiness, irritability, arching or posturing during or between feeds, or limited food intake despite the appearance of being hungry. A patient's response to past conservative (e.g., thickened feeds, small frequent feedings), pharmacologic (e.g., ranitidine, metoclopramide), or surgical (e.g, fundoplication) therapies for GERD, will guide further evaluation and management efforts. For children on tube feedings, the ability to tolerate bolus feedings is a prerequisite for successful oral feeding.
- *Are problems greater with liquids or solids, or are they equally difficult*? Although children with neurogenic disorders usually have the most difficulties swallowing thin liquids, some have problems regardless of texture. Difficulties with higher textured foods may be related to oral-motor skill development, texture sensitivity, or anecdotally to GERD.
- *What is the duration of mealtimes and are there changes as the meal progresses*? Mealtimes in excess of 30–40 min on a regular basis may be indicative of inefficient oral-motor skills or dysphagia involving any of the phases of swallowing. In addition, lengthy meals may adversely affect the relationship between the child and caregivers. Clinicians should ask whether the child improves or has more problems as the meal progresses. Children who are responsive to oral-motor or sensory stimulation may

improve over the course of a meal. Children with oropharyngeal dysphagia, cardiopulmonary problems, or those who fatigue may have more problems as the meal continues.

- *What medications are being administered*? Is the child taking drugs that may influence feeding or swallowing function? For example, common side effects of baclofen (frequently used to treat spasticity) include fatigue, increased drooling, and fatigue. Other medications (e.g., benzodiazepines) have sedative side effects and may influence the brainstem centers that regulate swallowing.
- *How is the family coping with feeding and swallowing problems*? Some families are relieved when professionals are able to alleviate concerns about swallowing dysfunction, and the associated respiratory or nutritional problems, or lengthy mealtimes. Others may be more cautious or anxious because dysphagia may be "another" problem to address. Attention to the caregiver's concerns is critical because family involvement is necessary for obtaining optimal outcomes.

Diagnostic Testing

The clinical evaluation provides information that enables clinicians to identify appropriate diagnostic tests, and ascertain whether a child is medically stable, ready, and able to participate in a specific procedure. Specific diagnostic tests are frequently needed to define the underlying pathophysiology because infants and children with neurogenic dysphagia are at increased risk for pharyngeal phase deficits, and clinical observations, including assessment of a gag reflex or pulse oximetry, do not define pharyngeal phase function (Fig. 1). The Videofluoroscopic Swallow Study (VFSS) is gold standard for determining the presence and extent of pharyngeal phase deficits, elucidating the underlying pathophysiology, and identifying potential therapeutic interventions.

Other diagnostic tests may be indicated for patients with specific diagnostic concerns. The Flexible Endoscopic Evaluation of Feeding (FEES) is a modification of the otolaryngologic examination and may help delineate the anatomic and structural integrity of the pharyngeal and laryngeal structures, and the coordination of respiration with swallowing of secretions, liquid, or food boluses. The FEES may be particularly helpful for children who are nonoral feeders. Other common diagnostic tests include the upper gastrointestinal series for assessing the anatomic and structural integrity of the gastrointestinal tract, the pH probe for determining the frequency of GER, and scintigraphy for quantifying the volume and fate of aspirated materials (e.g., secretions).

TREATMENT

Unfortunately, there is no tool or algorithm to predict the best treatment modalities for pediatric patients with dysphagia. Given that balance between severity of the dysphagia and the child's compensatory mechanisms determines the impact of the dysfunction, the primary goals of dysphagia interventions are to correct or control treatable etiologies, and avoid or minimize the consequences of the swallowing

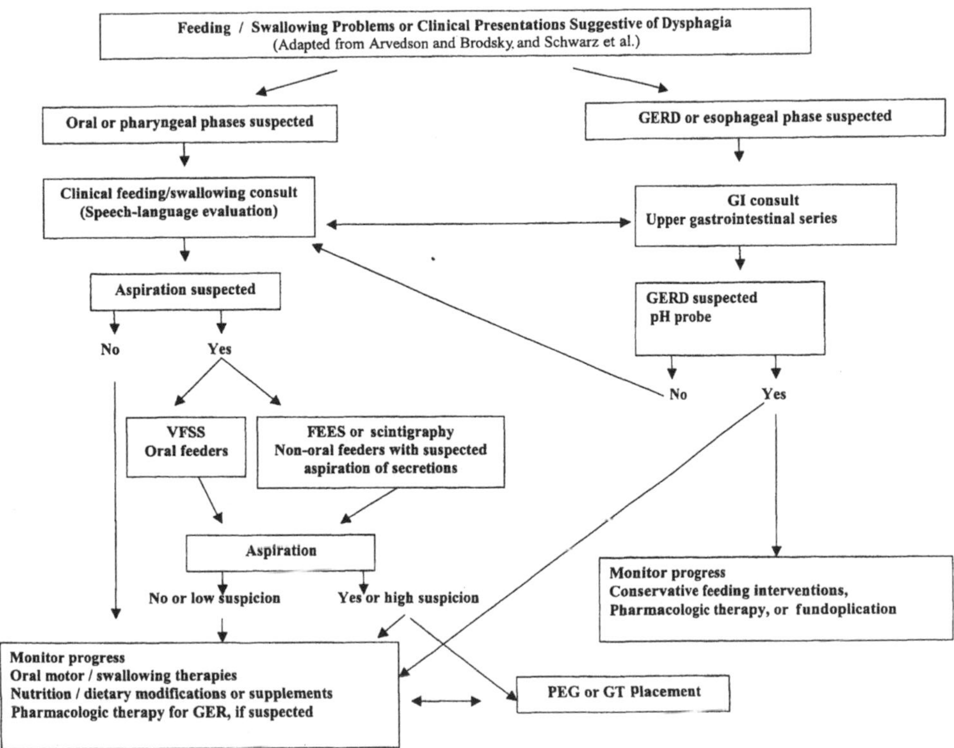

Figure 1 Feeding/swallowing problems or clinical presentations suggestive of dysphagia.

deficits. Medical or surgical management may be appropriate for some inflammatory conditions (e.g., esophagitis) or anatomic anomalies (e.g., laryngeal cleft, vascular rings). For some children, management approaches may lessen the impact of the swallowing dysfunction by focussing on nutrition, GER, behavioral, or oral-motor and swallowing therapies. (Fig. 1). Interventions may include modifications in feeding routine or diet, and the introduction or adjustment of medications (e.g., anticonvulsants, antireflux medications, or respiratory agents). Early initiation of nutritional support is critical and results in the greatest reversal of nutritional deficits in children with central nervous system insults and poor growth.

Oral-motor and swallowing therapies may include changes in texture, utensils, position, posture, or pacing of feeding, and the introduction of activities that strengthen swallowing musculature or support developmentally appropriate movement patterns for feeding and swallowing. Older children may benefit from direct therapies and the use of compensatory techniques to increase the safety and efficiency of swallowing. Adjustments in therapeutic goals and interventions need to parallel improvement or regression in the underlying condition.

Although some children are unable to feed orally because it is unsafe or too difficult, current evidence indicates swallowing is the best exercise for swallowing. Consequently, regardless of whether children are oral or nonoral feeders, oral-motor and swallowing therapies may facilitate the production of swallows, which in turn may promote handling of secretions. Additionally, since oral/dental disease appears to contribute to lung infections in older individuals with dysphagia, it is reasonable to incorporate oral hygiene into intervention programs for all children with feeding and swallowing problems.

The progression or anticipated course of the underlying etiology will influence decisions for nutritional management. For example, neurogenic dysphagia secondary to an acute condition with anticipated recovery (e.g., traumatic brain injury, cerebral vascular accident) is managed differently from dysphagia caused by chronic static (e.g., CP with profound mental retardation) or progressive (e.g., Ataxia-Telangiectasia) condition. Whereas a nasogastric tube may be appropriate for short-term nutritional and aspiration concerns, a gastrostomy tube (GT) (or percutaneous gastrostomy [PEG]) may be more appropriate for long-term issues. Objective markers to distinguish between short- and long-term supplemental nutritional needs are not available; however, three or more months of anticipated supplemental feeding needs may constitute an appropriate time interval for making recommendations for GT placement in children without medical contraindications. When clinicians counsel caregivers about placement of long-term feeding tubes, families frequently want to know how long GTs will be needed. Families need to be told that feeding tubes will be removed when underlying conditions have been corrected or resolved, or when children are able to compensate for swallowing dysfunction without compromising their general health and overall well being. Clinical experience indicates that many infants and young children with acute or static conditions improve with prompt initiation of appropriate interventions and time, and thereby, lessen or eliminate the need for tube feedings. Caregivers should be reassured that although many families struggle with initial decisions about whether to place GTs, following GT placement, 90% of caregivers report that tube feedings have improved the quality of life for their children and the family.

SUMMARY

Oropharyngeal dysphagia is common in children with neurologic diseases. The underlying condition determines the nature and extent of the swallowing dysfunction, and governs the prognosis for recovery. Early detection of the problem and prompt initiation of appropriate interventions are necessary for improving outcomes for these children and their caregivers.

SUGGESTED READINGS

1. Arvedson JC, Brodsky L. Aspiration. In: Arvedson JC, Brodsky L, eds. Pediatric Swallowing and Feeding: Assessment and Management. 2nd ed. Pacific Grove, CA: Global Rights Grp, 2002:480.
2. Lefton-Greif MA, Loughlin GM. Specialized studies in pediatric dysphagia. Semin Speech Lang 1996; 14(4):311–329.
3. Mackay LE, Morgan AS, Bernstein BA. Swallowing disorders in severe brain injury: risk factors affecting return to oral intake. Arch Phys Med Rehabil 1999; 80(4):365–371.
4. Rogers, B. Neurodevelopmental presentation of dysphagia. Semin Speech Lang 1996; 17(4):269–280.
5. Sanders KD, Cox K, Cannon R, Blanchard D, Pitcher J, Papathakis P, Varella L, Maughan R. Growth response to enteral feeding by children with cerebral palsy. J Parenter Enteral Nutr 1990; 14(1):23–26.

6. Schwarz SM, Corredor J, Fisher-Medina J, Cohen J, Rabinowitz S. Diagnosis and treatment of feeding disorders in children with developmental disabilities. Pediatrics 2001; 108(3):671–676.
7. Smith SW, Camfield C, Camfield P. Living with cerebral palsy and tube feeding: a population-based follow-up study. J Pediatr 1999; 135(3):307–310.

33
Migraine Prevention

Donna J. Stephenson
Wilmington, Delaware, U.S.A.

Migraine is a common childhood disorder characterized by recurrent headaches. Most children with migraine are symptom free between episodic headache attacks. Headache frequency and severity increase over time for a subset of pediatric migraneurs. Chronic migraine headache, transformed migraine, chronic nonprogressive headache, and chronic daily headache probably represent a spectrum of migraine headache syndromes. As headaches increase in severity and/or frequency, patients and their families are likely to experience significant disability. The burden of chronic migraine not only includes severe head pain but also missed school and extracurricular activities, academic underachievement, depressed mood, and anxiety. This chapter will focus on therapeutic approaches to chronic headache syndromes; acute therapies are covered.

The goal of preventative treatment should be to decrease significantly the frequency and severity of migraine headache, improve quality of life, and increase the effectiveness of abortive therapy. There is no fixed number of headaches per month that requires prophylaxis. Pharmacologic therapy is usually started when headache begins to interfere with a patient's activities, or when abortive therapy becomes less effective because of overuse (Table 1).

Physicians should help patients develop realistic expectations about the limits of treatment for this chronic disorder. Responsibility for headache control should be shared among patient, family, and physician. Patients and physicians often find that a headache diary recording both frequency and severity of attacks as well as possible trigger factors is useful in monitoring the efficacy of treatment.

Table 1 When to Consider Preventative Medication

Recurrent headaches that interfere significantly with daily activities
Ineffectiveness or contraindications to abortive medication
Analgesic overuse
Very frequent headaches
Patient preference
Headaches with significant neurologic threat (i.e., hemiplegic migraine)

Table 2 Frequently Used Preventative Medications

Medication	Common side effects	Most effective for cases involving
Cyproheptadine	Sedation, weight gain	Young children
Amitriptyline, nortriptyline	Drowsiness, dry mouth, orthostatic hypotension	Insomnia, depression
Propranolol	Bronchospasm, bradycardia, hypotension, dizziness, fatigue	Contraindicated in asthmatics
Valproic acid	Nausea, weight gain, fatigue, tremor, alopecia	Epilepsy, bipolar disorder
Topiramate	Paresthesias, fatigue, weight loss, concentration difficulty	Epilepsy, obesity

Common triggers for migraine include diet, sleep and exercise patterns, dehydration, stress, hormonal change, and analgesic overuse. Caffeine, chocolate, monosodium glutamate, processed and smoked meat and fish, nuts, vinegar and red wine, citrus fruits, cheeses (especially aged), and aspartame tend to precipitate headache in susceptible individuals. Foods like hotdogs, some corn and potato chips, pizza, soda, and peanut butter must be included on any list for children. Skipping meals, especially during the school day, can lead to headache. Irregular, decreased, or increased sleeping hours can lead to headache. Lack of exercise can also increase the likelihood of headache. Dehydration, especially in the summer and during sports, is an under recognized trigger in many children. Stress, good or bad, is a trigger in most children with migraine. The hormonal changes of puberty may trigger an increase in headaches several months to years before menarche or obvious external signs are present. The cyclical nature of many girls' headaches suggests a hormonal component. Use of over-the-counter or prescription medication for acute migraine (NSAIDS, acetaminophen, triptans) more than three times a week can lead to an increase in headaches and poor response to abortive medication. A timely (or rather untimely)

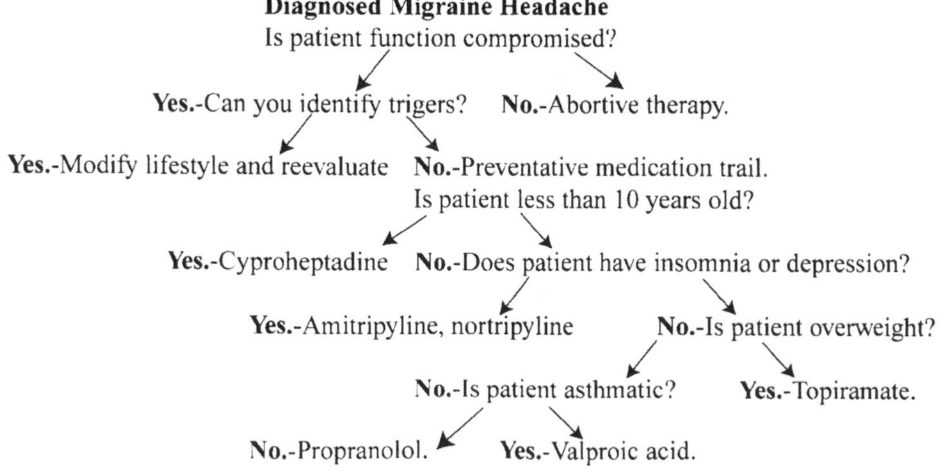

Figure 1 A strategy for headache prevention.

combination of trigger factors often culminates in a migraine attack in susceptible individuals. Identification of triggers and modification of lifestyle often result in a decrease in headaches.

In general, a preventative medication is chosen for its efficacy as well as side effect profile (Table 2). Consideration should be given to comorbid conditions and concurrent medication use (Fig. 1). A single medication should be started at low doses and titrated gradually upward to the effective or maximum dose. A full therapeutic trial will often take up to six months. Patients must be advised that most prophylactics take two to four weeks to begin working. If a first choice medication is not effective, a medication from another class should be considered as an alternative choice.

FIRST LINE THERAPIES

Antihistamines

Cyproheptadine is an antihistaminergic and antiserotonergic drug most useful in young children (less than 10 years old). Starting dose is 0.25 mg/kg divided BID or TID, or 2 mg BID, and is increased slowly to an effective maximum tolerated dose. Maximum recommended dose per day is 16 mg. Common and dose-limiting side effects include increased appetite, weight gain, and sedation.

Tricyclic Antidepressants

Tricyclic antidepressants are especially effective in those patients with comorbid insomnia, anxiety, or depression. Both nortriptyline and amitriptyline are effective. Starting dose is 0.1–0.2 mg/kg qhs (usually 10–25 mg) and is increased slowly in weekly increments to 0.5–1 mg/kg qhs (usually 50–75 mg). Above this range, the likelihood of side effects limits dosage increases. Side effects are common and include dry mouth, increased appetite, drowsiness, urinary retention, constipation, tachycardia, hypotension, reduced seizure threshold, and triggering of a manic episode in bipolar patients. EKG monitoring rather than blood levels is a more effective way or monitoring the potential arrhythmogenic effects with doses above 50 mg/day.

Beta-Blockers

Of the beta-blockers, propranolol is generally the best tolerated. The effective dose range is usually 0.6–1.5 mg/kg/day divided BID or TID. The maximum dose should not exceed 4 mg/kg/day. There is an extended release preparation available (twice daily dosing). The tendency of beta-blockers to produce bronchospasm in asthmatics limits its use in many children. Side effects are common and include bradycardia, hypotension, dizziness, fatigue, depression, and weight gain.

Anticonvulsants

Divalproex has been approved by the FDA for migraine prophylaxis in adults. It is generally well tolerated in children. Starting dose is 5–10 mg/kg/day divided BID, and is increased to a dose of 15–20 mg/kg/day. It is available as an extended release preparation that can be used once daily. Common side effects include nausea, fatigue, weight gain, tremor, and alopecia. Rare side effects include thrombocytopenia, hepatic dysfunction, and pancreatitis.

Topiramate is a good choice for overweight patients with headache because of the often-coveted side effect of decreased appetite. Starting dose is 1–2 mg/kg (15 or 25 mg) qhs, and is increased by 15 or 25 mg increments weekly to the target dose, not usually to exceed 200 mg. Common side effects include digital and perioral parethesias, fatigue, concentration problems, word-finding difficulties, and weight loss. The incidence of kidney stones due to carbonic anhydrase inhibition is approximately 1%, and is increased in those with a family history of kidney stones. There is an increased risk of oligohydrosis and heat stroke in patients taking topiramate. Zonisamide may be a suitable alternative to topiramate in those using oral contraceptive medications as topiramate can interfere with the efficacy of estrogen containing contraceptive medications.

ALTERNATIVES

Other agents effective in migraine prophylaxis include calcium channel blockers, selective serotonin reuptake inhibitors, gabapentin, zonisamide, and tizanidine. Botulinum toxin injections to the frontal and posterior neck muscles have been well studied in adult migraine, and have an extremely low risk of adverse effects. Nevertheless, it remains a relatively unappealing option for both pediatric patients and families. Feverfew is a popular herbal remedy for fever and inflammation and more recently for headache prevention. There are little data on its use in pediatric patients and its safety profile is not well established. Riboflavin has also been popularized for headache prophylaxis. The dose for young patients (up to 6 years) is 100 mg daily, 6–8 years 200 mg daily, 8–13 years 300 mg, and 13 years and up 400 mg. It tends to have a strong odor and taste and produces bright yellow urine. Magnesium at doses of 200–400 mg daily usually produces no side effects. Stress reduction techniques such as biofeedback yoga, counseling for stress management techniques, and exercise are complimentary to pharmacologic therapy.

LONG-TERM CONTROL

Although prophylactic medication is often necessary to break the cycle of chronic headache, optimal management of most chronic headache syndromes will rely on identification and avoidance of trigger factors. Once headaches are well controlled on preventative medication, the dose should be slowly tapered off. Often headaches remain under reasonable control, especially if patients begin to adopt lifestyle changes to avoid headache triggers.

SUMMARY

Chronic migraine headache can produce significant disability. A comprehensive treatment plan including realistic patient expectations, patient education, and judicious use of abortive and preventative medications is necessary for successful long-term control of migraines.

SUGGESTED READINGS

1. Caruso JM, Brown WD, Exil G, Gascon GG. The efficacy of divalproex sodium in the prophylactic treatment of children with migraine. Headache 2000; 40:672–676.
2. Hershey AD, Powers SW, Bentti A, de Grauw TJ. Effectiveness of amitriptyline in the prophylactic management of childhood headaches. Headache 2000; 40:539–549.
3. Hershey AD, Powers SW, Vockell AB, LeCates S, Kabbouche M. Effectiveness of topiramate in the prevention of childhood headaches. Headache 2002; 42:810–818.
4. Millichap JG, Yee MM. The diet factor in pediatric and adolescent migraine. Pediatr Neurol 2003; 28(1):9–15.
5. Buchholz D. Heal Your Headache the 1-2-3 Program for Taking Charge of Your Pain. New York, NY: Workman Publishing Company, Inc., 2002.

34
Abortive (Acute)Treatment of Migraine

Eric M. Pearlman
Mercer University School of Medicine,
Savannah, Georgia, U.S.A.

INTRODUCTION

While migraine is a well-recognized phenomenon in adults, it is often overlooked or minimized in children and adolescents. Headache is quite a common complaint in children, and migraine often has its onset in the first two decades of life. Recognition and appropriate treatment can have a significant impact on the quality of life for young sufferers as well as their caregivers, and may ultimately impact the course of the illness.

The diagnostic criteria differ slightly between children and adults. The criteria in children less than 15 years requires headaches of 1–48 hr in duration instead of the 4–72 hr in individuals greater than 15 years of age. The remainder of the criteria is similar to the adult diagnostic criteria including: at least five attacks with photophobia and phonophobia, nausea or vomiting; and two symptoms out of unilateral pain, throbbing or pulsatile pain, moderate or severe pain intensity, or exacerbation by routine activity.

The treatment of migraine in children and adolescents follows the same general principle as for adults, including lifestyle modification, trigger avoidance, nonpharmacologic treatments, acute treatment, rescue treatment and, where appropriate, preventive treatment. It is very important to establish the diagnosis of migraine and convey this clearly to the patient and parents. Many parents are concerned that there is an underlying organic cause for their child's headache, and unless these fears are dispelled, treatment plans are often unsuccessful. Patients and parents are much more likely to accept a treatment plan if they believe the diagnosis. Therefore, it is important to spend time with the patient and the parents explaining the diagnosis and the disorder. This needs to be done at a level that the child and parents can understand. Reading materials, booklets, brochures, diaries, and videos can help teach the patient and their families about what to expect from their disorder, how to recognize an attack and management goals. Ongoing education should be part of every office visit with emphasis on lifestyle modification, trigger avoidance, and treatment strategies. Expectation management is also important, so that patients and families will recognize treatment success and failure. Patient participation is instrumental in treatment plan success, especially regarding teenagers who may not comply with a treatment plan that they do not agree with. Adolescents and teenagers often need to feel like they are part of the decision-making process. This can include dosage formulations, routes of administration, or types of medication. For the purposes of this chapter, I will limit my discussion to the abortive therapy of migraine rather than prevention.

Nonpharmacological Therapies and Lifestyle Modification

Nonpharmacologic therapies may be well received in younger patients, including adolescents. Resting in a dark room, using an ice pack, and playing quiet music can be beneficial. Basic lifestyle modifications may be reinforced in adolescents such as implementing regular sleeping patterns. Sleep patterns are often disrupted with changes in weekly schedules vs. weekend schedules—often triggering or exacerbating migraine. Sleep deprivation is a common trigger in children and adolescents. Regular sleep routines can often reduce attack frequency. Regular meals, consistent sleep patterns, and routine exercise may be simple life-style changes that can improve adolescent and childhood headaches. Stress is often a factor in children and adolescents with migraine; however, stress factors differ in children vs. adults. School stress can include anxiety about workload, grades, and relationships with peers. Many children are overextended with extracurricular activities, and they may not have time to complete their schoolwork or time to relax and enjoy a little social or leisure activity. For some children, reducing the number and frequency of after-school activities allows them to focus on schoolwork, perform well, sleep regularly, and participate in leisure activities.

Pharmacological Treatment

Medications used in the acute treatment of migraine attacks can be divided into two major categories: migraine specific and migraine nonspecific therapies. Studies are available supporting use of several of these medications for treatment of migraine. However, further study is warranted for all medications, with specific attention needed for dosing strategies. Common nonspecific acute medications are listed in Table 1 and available migraine-specific therapies with their formulations and available doses are detailed in Table 2.

Scientific Evidence

There is limited clinical evidence for nonspecific acute therapies for treatment of migraine in children and adolescents. Hamalainen and colleagues compared

Table 1 Nonspecific Medications for Acute Migraine Therapy

Medication	Suggested dose
Acetaminophen	15 mg/kg up to 1000 mg
Nonsteroidal anti-inflammatory drugs (NSAIDs)	
Ibuprofen	10 mg/kg up to 800 mg
Naproxen sodium	10 mg/kg up to 400 mg
Narcotics	
Codeine	0.5–1 mg/kg up to 60 mg

Table 2 Migraine-Specific Acute Therapies

Triptan	Dosage strengths
Sumatriptan	Injection 6 mg Nasal spray 5 mg, 20 mg Tablet 25 mg, 50 mg, 100 mg
Zolmitriptan	Tablet 2.5 mg, 5 mg ODT 2.5 mg, 5 mg Nasal spray 5 mg
Rizatriptan	Tablet 5 mg, 10 mg ODT 5 mg, 10 mg
Naratriptan	Tablet 1.25 mg, 2.5 mg
Almotriptan	Tablet 6.25 mg, 12.5 mg
Frovatriptan	Tablet 2.5 mg
Eletriptan	Tablet 20 mg, 40 mg
Ergotamine	Injection
(DHE 45)	Nasal spray

acetaminophen, ibuprofen, and placebo in a double-blind crossover study. Eighty-eight children aged 4–15 years were enrolled. Each child headaches was treated with acetaminophen (15 mg/kg/dose), ibuprofen (10 mg/kg/dose), and placebo. Acetaminophen and ibuprofen were statistically significantly more efficacious than placebo, and ibuprofen was more efficacious than acetaminophen. In another single center study, Lewis compared ibuprofen suspension (7.5 mg/kg/dose) to placebo, in a double-blind, parallel group trial in children aged 6–12 years. There were 45 children in the ibuprofen arm and 39 children in the placebo arm. Headache response at 2 hr was significantly higher in the ibuprofen arm (76% of attacks) compared to placebo (53% of attacks, $p = 0.006$). Pain-free response was 44% compared to 25% for placebo ($p < 0.07$). Only one child in the ibuprofen arm needed rescue medication compared to 15 in the placebo arm ($p < 0.001$). These studies suggest that ibuprofen in doses 7.5–10 mg/kg/dose is effective as an acute therapy for children. However, caution must be used in the use of nonsteroidal anti-inflammatory drugs (NSAIDs) due to the risk of rebound headache (otherwise known as transformed migraine), which can occur with perhaps as little as two to three doses of medication per week.

There are several studies examining the efficacy and tolerability of sumatriptan in children under 12 years of age. A total of 67 children have been reported in open-label trials utilizing sumatriptan subcutaneous injection. In both studies, sumatriptan injection was fairly well tolerated and effective. Sumatriptan nasal spray has also been investigated in children and adolescents. An open-label, retrospective study of 10 children aged 5–12 years found sumatriptan nasal spray well tolerated and effective. A randomized, double-blind, placebo-controlled crossover trial of 14 children aged 6–9 years demonstrated that sumatriptan nasal spray 20 mg/dose was effective and well tolerated. Collectively, these studies suggest that sumatriptan given subcutaneously (0.06 mg/kg) or intranasally (20 mg) is effective in treating migraine in children aged 6–12 years.

There is a building collection of clinical evidence from large multicenter, randomized, double-blind, placebo-controlled, parallel group trials that assess the efficacy of triptans specifically in adolescents over 12 years of age. In a study of

302 patients comparing sumatriptan 25, 50, and 100 mg tablets to placebo, the primary endpoint of 2 hr headache response failed to reach significant differences from placebo (49%, 50%, 51% compared to placebo 42%). All three doses of sumatriptan were statistically significant compared to placebo at 3 (65%, 64%, 69% compared to 45%) and 4 hr (73%, 73%, 74% compared to 53%), however. The 50 mg dose was significant compared to placebo at 90 min (47% compared to 30%), while the 25 mg (38%) and 100 mg (38%) doses were not. Two things to note about this trial are that the placebo rate was quite high compared to those normally observed (30–40%) in most adult triptan trials. Also, this study failed to report a dose–response curve.

In a large randomized, double-blind, placebo-controlled study of sumatriptan nasal spray, 5, 10, and 20 mg vs. placebo, subjects were required to have headaches lasting longer than 4 hr in addition to meeting IHS criteria for migraine with or without aura. Subjects were required to self-administer study medication at home under the supervision of their parents. Five hundred and seven patients were enrolled. The primary endpoint was headache response at 2 hr. Only the 5-mg dose was found to be statistically significantly superior to placebo ($p < 0.05$). The 10- and 20-mg doses did not statistically differ from placebo, although there is a numerical trend favoring active treatment. This study differs from adult trials in that there was no apparent dose–response curve noted.

A large study of rizatriptan used similar inclusion criteria as the sumatriptan nasal spray study reviewed previously. In addition, patients were instructed to take study medication within 30 min of onset of a moderate/severe attack. The primary endpoint of 2-hr pain relief was achieved in 66% of subjects treated with rizatriptan 5 mg compared to 56% for placebo, which was not statistically significant. Posthoc analysis found that for those attacks treated on weekdays, the response rates were 66% for rizatriptan and 61% for placebo. However, for those attacks treated on weekends, the response rates were 65% and 36%, respectively. The response rates were essentially the same for rizatriptan, but the placebo response rate for weekends was much lower than during the week. To sum, there have been over 1650 subjects between 12 and 18 years involved in clinical trials published so far with an excellent tolerability and safety record. The evidence regarding efficacy has been marred by very high placebo response rates. This does not imply that the medications are not effective but demonstrates the difficulty in studying pain in this population. Further studies are ongoing with efforts to correct the shortcomings of prior studies.

Treatment Algorithm

The use of migraine-specific medications should be considered early in the course of treatment so as not to deny significant treatment benefits. Triptans are beneficial and have been studied in children as described. The goal of the therapy is to achieve effective headache relief without paying any significant penalty in terms of tolerability and safety. It is quite reasonable to use nonspecific medications, such as acetaminophen and ibuprofen, as first-line acute therapy, as long as they are used in appropriate doses (15 mg/kg/dose up to 1000 mg maximum for acetaminophen; 10 mg/kg/dose up to 800 mg for ibuprofen). It is then important to have adequate follow-up arranged so that the treatment plan can be modified appropriately without a long delay. The decision to use preventive medications in children should be considered after an adequate trial of acute treatment if frequent or disabling attacks persist.

The goal of rescue therapy is to terminate a migraine attack when typical acute medications such as NSAIDs and triptans have been unsuccessful. At this point the attack has persisted long enough so that there is less concern over medication-induced sleep. In fact, this is one of the goals of rescue medication, along with relief of pain and associated symptoms such as nausea. The choices of rescue medication thus include medications with sedation as a common side effect. If a child is taking a NSAID for acute therapy, then appropriate rescue medications include antiemetics and oral narcotics. If a migraine-specific medication is used for acute treatment, then a combination of a NSAID with an antiemetic or narcotic is appropriate. Commonly used antiemetics are metoclopramide (0.1 mg/kg/dose, 10 mg max), prochlorperazine (0.1 mg/kg/dose, 10 mg max), and promethazine (0.5 mg/kg/dose, 50 mg max). If vomiting is prominent then rectal administration may be most appropriate. The most commonly used narcotics in children is codeine. For adolescents, other narcotics such as hydrocodone or oxycodone may be used. Sometimes, antihistamines such as diphenhydramine, hydroxyzine, or cyproheptidine can be used to help induce sleep.

If home rescue fails, then treatment in the office or emergency room may be required. This in general involves parenteral interventions and should begin with rehydration intravenously, typically with normal saline. There are several options for rescue medication. None have been adequately studied in the pediatric population. Ketoralac given IV or IM (15–60 mg) is a potent analgesic and can be given in combination with an antiemetic and a narcotic if necessary. Other non-narcotic options include serotonin 1B/1D agonists, steroids, dopaminergic agents, and anticonvulsants. Sumatriptan and dihygroergotamine can be given subcutaneously if the patient has not been previously treated with a serotonin agonist in the past 24 hr. Dopaminergic agents include the antiemetics. There is also some evidence that parenteral atypical antipsychotics can abort an acute migraine. For status migrainosus, intravenous dihydroergotamine and/or steroids such as methyprednisolone or dexamethasone can be effective.

SUMMARY

For acute medications, there is a large body of evidence supporting the safety and tolerability of several migraine-specific medications. Treating children and adolescents with migraine can follow many of the same principles used in adults with important consideration to the differences between adult patients and pediatric patients. It is important not to underestimate the impact of headache in the child or adolescent and their family and friends. Recognizing migraine and instituting appropriate treatment will lead to greater patient and physician satisfaction.

SUGGESTED READINGS

1. Hamalainen ML, Hoppu K, Valkeila E, Santavuori P. Ibuprofen or acetaminophen for the acute treatment of migraine in children: a double-blind, randomized, placebo-controlled, crossover study. Neurology 1977; 48:102–107.
2. Hershey AD, Powers SW, LeCates S, Bentti AL. Effectiveness of nasal sumatriptan in 5- to 12-year-old children. Headache 2001; 41:693–697.
3. Lewis DW, Kellstein D, Dahl G, et al. Children's ibuprofen suspension for the acute treatment of pediatric migraine. Headache 2002; 42:780–786.

4. Rothner AD, Winner P, Nett R, Asgharnejad M, et al. One-year tolerability and efficacy of sumatriptan nasal spray in adolescents with migraine: results of a multicenter, open-label study. Clin Ther 2000; 22:1533–1546.
5. The International Classification of Headache Disorders, Part 1: the primary headaches. Cephalalgia 2004; 24(suppl 1);1–59.
6. Ueberall MA, Wenzel D. Intranasal sumatriptan for the acute treatment of migraine in children. Neurology 1999; 52:1507.
7. Winner P, Rothner AD, Saper J, Nett R, Asgharnejad M, Laurenza A, Austin R, Peykamian M. A randomized, double-blind, placebo-controlled study of sumatriptan nasal spray in the treatment of acute migraine in adolescents. Pediatrics 2000; 106(5):989–997.

35
Pseudotumor Cerebri

Michael X. Repka
Johns Hopkins Hospital, Baltimore, Maryland, U.S.A.

INTRODUCTION

Although a number of terms have been used to describe the typical clinical picture, I prefer the term pediatric pseudotumor cerebri (PPTC), rather than the alternative: idiopathic intracranial hypertension. The diagnosis of PPTC allows inclusion of individuals who fit the typical clinical picture, yet have a putative cause identified, to be classified as a case of associated PPTC. Another older name, benign intracranial hypertension, should be avoided because it minimizes the potential for serious ocular morbidity from this condition.

DIAGNOSIS/CLINICAL FEATURES

Definition

Pseudotumor cerebri is defined as elevated intracranial pressure (>200 mm water), normal brain on imaging, normal or small sized ventricles, and normal CSF composition. The neurological examination is usually normal, though some patients may have ocular motor problems or other minor neurological symptoms.

Epidemiology

Pediatric pseudotumor cerebri may develop throughout the first two decades of life. It is relatively rare in childhood, but increases after puberty. Prior to puberty the gender ratio is 1:1, while after puberty girls outnumber boys by 2 to 1. Obesity is noted in patients with PPTC, but only in about 25% prior to puberty and 50% after puberty.

Symptoms

The most common symptom is headache, often posterior, which occurs in up to 86% of cases. In young children and infants, irritability and apathy have been noted, rather than headache. Other common symptoms are nausea, visual loss, vomiting, and fatigue. Fatigue is frequent in younger children. Less frequent symptoms include ataxia, dizziness, neck pain, paresthesias, facial and limb numbness, and tinnitus. An occasional child will be asymptomatic. The most common ocular symptom is decreased vision, followed by horizontal double vision. This may be intermittent or constant. Transient visual obscurations and visual loss are rarely presenting symptoms in children.

Signs

The key physical finding is papilledema. This will be found in nearly every patient, though it can be unilateral or markedly asymmetric. Papilledema is manifested by elevation of the optic disc tissue, blurring of the disc margin, and obscuration of the retinal blood vessels as they cross the disc margin. The optic nerve swelling should be assessed not only for the elevation, but also the presence of nerve fiber layer infarcts, hemorrhages, exudates, and macular edema. The latter findings are evidence of chronicity and a greater likelihood of permanent damage to the visual pathways. Papilledema is occasionally seen in infants with PPTC, even among those who have open fontanelles.

Visual acuity is typically normal, though about 1/3 of the children able to complete optotype acuity testing will present with reduced acuity in their better eye. Decreased vision should be considered a sign both of chronicity and of high pressure and often signals irreparable visual loss.

An additional ophthalmological finding is the presence of an esotropia. This may be from paresis of one or both lateral rectus muscles from abducens nerve damage, but may also occur without clinical evidence of an ocular motor neuropathy. Esotropia occurs in about 1/3 of pediatric patients. Other ocular motor findings include trochlear nerve paresis, oculomotor nerve paresis, internuclear ophthalmoplegia, and hypertropias, all of which produce diplopia or torticollis in an attempt to fuse a vertical misalignment. Neurological signs, other than the ocular motor abnormalities, are unusual, except for a facial nerve palsy, which has been reported in a number of series.

Etiologies (Table 1)

Cerebral venous drainage impairment is the most often cited association with PPTC. Venous sinus thrombosis is a common cause, usually of the lateral sinus, frequently with a history of otitis media. Thromboses of the superior sagittal sinus or cavernous sinus have also been implicated. Sinus thrombosis may also be the final pathway for some of the other associations. Corticosteroid use or withdrawal may be associated. The use of some antibiotics may cause a nondose related rise in intracranial pressure. In my experience, this is most commonly seen with doxycycline and minocycline, two tetracycline class antibiotics used for the management of acne.

EVALUATION

A history is performed specifically evaluating the patient for symptoms as well as any potential precipitating associations. The laboratory evaluation includes neuroimaging of the brain and orbits looking for evidence of a mass lesion or hydrocephalus. For the diagnosis of PPTC, the scan should be normal with either small or normal ventricles. Enlarged optic nerve sheaths may be seen on orbital sections. Lumbar

Table 1 Etiologies of Pediatric Pseudotumor Cerebri

Cerebral venous drainage impairment
Transverse sinus obstruction
Sagittal sinus obstruction
Coagulopathy
Trauma
Drugs
Corticosteroid use or withdrawal
Tetracycline type drugs (including minocycline and doxycycline)
Cyclosorin
Medroxy-progesterone
Nalidixic acid
Vitamin A
Endocrinological conditions
Hypoparathyroidism
Menarche
Thyroid replacement
Nutritional
Weight loss or gain
Vitamin D deficiency
Vitamin A deficiency
Metabolic
Renal disease
Infectious
Lyme

puncture is necessary to examine the composition of the spinal fluid, which must have normal cell count, cytology, and chemistry. The opening pressure should be measured with a manometer prior to removing any spinal fluid. The patient needs to be calm and in a recumbent position, occasionally requiring sedation. Intracranial pressures greater than 200 mm of water support the diagnosis. A neurological exam should be performed, but is most often unremarkable (Fig. 1).

A complete ophthalmological evaluation should be performed as soon as possible. This examination should include careful measurement of best-corrected visual acuity using age appropriate test charts, color vision, pupillary light responses, visual fields, and ophthalmoscopy. Color photographs of the optic discs should also be obtained for comparison at subsequent visits. Visual fields should be measured with a perimeter whenever possible. Quantitative perimetry is preferred because it seems to be the most sensitive test of optic nerve dysfunction. In addition, such studies can be electronically compared from one visit to the next, improving the clinicians ability to detect improvement or deterioration. Recently, computerized scanning using light or ultrasound has become widely available. These instruments make three-dimensional maps of the optic nerve. Such electronic images can be compared both visually and electronically from visit to visit enhancing the physician's ability to detect improvement or progression of the disc swelling. Ophthalmoscopy should include an evaluation of the optic disc for swelling, hemorrhage, exudates, as well as the presence or absence of venous pulsations. Normal pulsations are usually compatible with normal intracranial pressure, though the absence of pulsations occurs in both normal and high intracranial pressure states. If there is evidence of an optic neuropathy on any of the tests of acuity, color vision, pupils or field, the pace of treatment

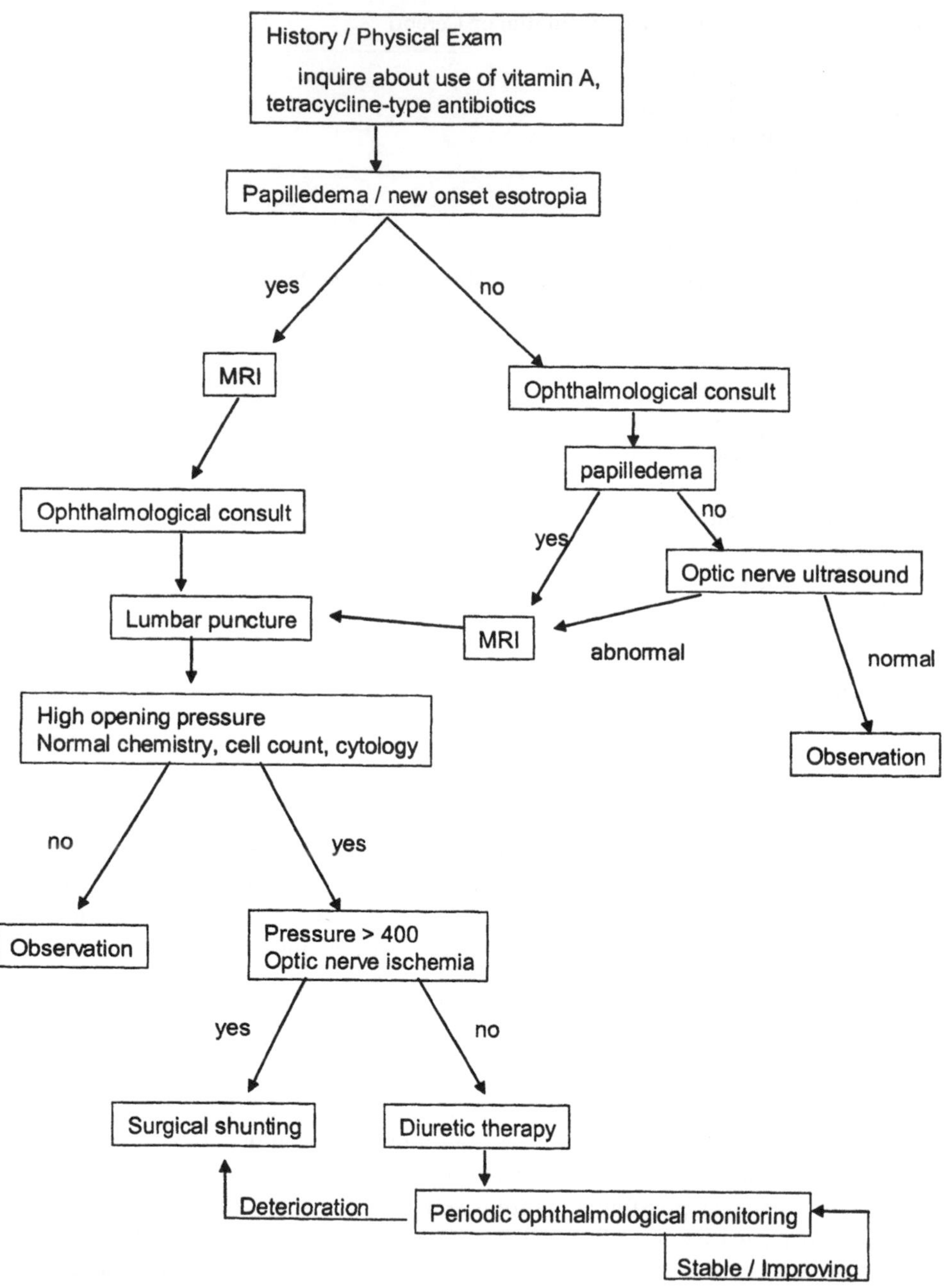

Figure 1 Treatment algorithm.

is accelerated to avoid additional and potentially permanent visual loss. Evidence of progression during follow-up examinations of any test should also cause the clinician to consider intensifying the therapy.

Papilledema requires a few days to develop in patients with increased intracranial pressure and will take several weeks to disappear after correction of the increased pressure. In patients with symptoms, but optic discs that are difficult to be certain of the presence of papilledema, hospitalization and placement of an intracranial pressure monitoring device may be essential in making the diagnosis of PPTC.

THERAPY

The initial therapy depends on the state of the visual system and possible associations discovered during the history. For asymptomatic patients with no visual loss and moderate pressure elevation, no therapy need be started immediately. If an association can be identified, it is reasonable in cases with no or a mild optic neuropathy to just stop the putative agent or correct the underlying medical problem. Typically this is enough to allow resolution of the symptoms. For patients who are obese, weight management is the best initial treatment.

Pharmacotherapy

The mainstay of pharmacotherapy is oral acetazolamide, though there are no clinical trials proving efficacy. For children, the initial dose is 30 mg/kg/day orally divided into four doses, whereas for teens the dose is 1 g divided into four doses per day. Higher doses have been used, with the most frequent side effect being paresthesias. Systemic corticosteroids have been found in some patients to be helpful, especially when the PPTC is associated with systemic inflammatory disease, like sarcoidosis. Some patients have been found to be responsive to other diuretics, especially furosemide.

Lumbar Puncture

Serial lumbar punctures are performed to lower the pressure. This approach may work by creating a number of holes in the dura of the spinal canal allowing enough cerebrospinal fluid egress to normalize the intracranial pressure. This method is difficult to accomplish in children over a long period of time for practical reasons, but can be used over a short period of time until more definitive therapies can be arranged.

Surgical Treatment of PPTC

Surgical treatment is not often needed for PPTC, possibly because there are frequent associations, which can be corrected with rapid normalization of the pressure. However, the physician must be prepared to intervene when there is optic neuropathy, very high pressure, or documented progression of optic nerve damage. Unfortunately, there is insufficient published evidence to clearly recommend one over the other procedure. Repeat eye examinations are required to monitor the outcome of either surgical drainage procedure.

Lumboperitoneal Shunt

Lumboperitoneal shunting involves the placement of a silicone tube from the lumbar subarachnoid space to the peritoneal cavity. These have long been used by neurosurgeons for PPTC, though not always successfully. This approach leads to a rapid resolution of the PPTC, but the tubes can obstruct, become infected, and are associated with the development of a Chiari malformation. Failure to drain is common and blockage leads to a rapid increase in pressure, which can cause catastrophic damage to the optic nerve. Ongoing ophthalmologic observation is recommended especially when there is a recurrence of symptoms.

Optic Nerve Sheath Fenestration

This treatment has been reported in many adults for the relief of pseudotumor cerebri, but has only been performed in a small number of children. An incision in the dural sheath of optic nerve is made from an orbital approach under general anesthesia. Fenestration has been shown to relieve papilledema of the operated nerve and sometimes even the contralateral nerve. If the contralateral eye does not show evidence of improvement, a second procedure will be needed for this eye. Most patients do not experience much relief from their headache.

PROGNOSIS

Most children with PPTC have a self-limited course, resolving once the causative problem has been corrected. However, the clinician should be vigilant for older children and teens, who may have more chronic elevation of intracranial pressure or lack an obvious association. Permanent damage to the optic nerves is found in about one-fourth of affected pediatric patients. There does not seem to be any age difference in the occurrence of this unfavorable outcome.

SUMMARY

Pediatric pseudotumor cerebri is an uncommon neurologic disease of childhood. Obesity is less common in the childhood form of the disease and there is often an associated condition. Management requires collaboration of neurology, ophthalmology, and pediatrics in evaluating and monitoring the patients. The sooner the increased pressure is reduced, the less likely there will be permanent visual impairment.

SUGGESTED READINGS

1. Baker RS, Baumann RJ, Buncic JR. Idiopathic intracranial hypertension (pseudotumor cerebri) in pediatric patients. Pediatr Neurol 1989; 5:5–11.
2. Chumas PD, Kulkarni AV, Drake JM, et al. Lumboperitoneal shunting: a retrospective study in the pediatric population. Neurosurgery 1993; 32:376–383.
3. Cinciripini GS, Donahue S, Borchert MS. Idiopathic intracranial hypertension in prepubertal pediatric patients: characteristics, treatment, and outcome. Am J Ophthalmol 1999; 127:178–182.
4. Kesler A, Fattal-Valeski A. Idiopathic intracranial hypertension in the pediatric population. J Child Neurol 2002; 17:745–748.
5. Lee AG, Patrinely JR, Edmond JC. Optic nerve sheath decompression in pediatric pseudotumor cerebri. Ophthalmic Surg Lasers 1998; 29:514–517.
6. Phillips PH, Repka MX, Lambert SR. Pseudotumor cerebri in children. J AAPOS 1998; 2:33–38.
7. Rekate HL, Wallace D. Lumboperitoneal shunts in children. Pediatr Neurosurg 2003; 38:41–46.

36

The Management of Pediatric Pain

Benjamin H. Lee and Myson Yaster
Departments of Anesthesiology, Critical Care Medicine, and Pediatrics, The Johns Hopkins Hospital, Baltimore, Maryland, U.S.A.

INTRODUCTION

The International Association for the Study of Pain defines pain as "an unpleasant sensory and emotional experience connected with actual or potential tissue damage, or described in terms of such damage." Operationally, pain can be defined as "what the patient says hurts" and exists "when the patient says it does." Infants, preverbal children, developmentally handicapped, and critically ill children may be unable to describe their pain or their subjective experiences. This has led many to conclude incorrectly that children do not experience pain in the same way as adults do.

Unfortunately, even when their pain is obvious, children frequently receive no treatment or inadequate treatment for pain and for painful procedures. There are many reasons for this. There is a lack of knowledge of pain assessment, pain syndromes, and the use of powerful analgesics, particularly the opioids, in the treatment of pain by many health-care professionals. There is in an unwarranted fear of producing opioid-induced respiratory depression and of inducing opioid addiction. Health-care providers are often focused on the treatment of underlying disease pathology and not on symptom management. Finally, there is an under appreciation by physicians and nurses of the consequences of the failure to treat pain adequately.

Infants have the capacity to perceive pain at birth. The structures necessary for nociception are present and functional between the first and second trimesters. Maturation of the fetal cerebral cortex has been confirmed by various studies. Newborn infants have a functionally mature hypothalamic-pituitary axis and can mount a fight-or-flight response.

MEASUREMENT OF PAIN IN CHILDREN

Ongoing assessment is essential to adequate pain treatment. Reliable, valid, and clinically sensitive tools exist to assess pain in children from neonates to adolescents. Pain and response to treatment, including adverse effects, should be routinely monitored by caregivers ("the fifth vital sign") and recorded on the patient's record to facilitate communication between caregivers. Pain can be assessed by a variety of measures, including self-report (visual analogs scales, Oucher scale), physiological (heart rate, vagal tone, respiratory rate, and oxygen saturation), behavioral (facial activity, cry, and body movements), and composite measures [Neonatal Infant Pain Scale (NIPS), Premature Infant Pain Profile (PIPP)], depending on the age and cognitive ability of the child and his communication skills. Rating scales have been validated to assess pain in cognitively impaired patients and young children.

Accurate pain assessment requires consideration of the plasticity of pain perception and the developmental and psychological state of the child. Self-report of pain is the preferred method of assessment. Pain expression reflects the physical and emotional state, coping style, and family and cultural expectations and can be misinterpreted by the health-care provider. Cultural and language differences may make assessment difficult. Careful and thorough assessment is required in children with severe developmental disabilities, as well as severely emotionally disturbed children. Proxy report from a parent, guardian, or caregiver is often used in young children, but the proxy will often underestimate the pain experience.

DEVELOPMENTAL PHARMACOLOGY

It is well known that the pharmacokinetics and pharmacodynamics of analgesics change during the child's development. These changes are most pronounced during the first year of life. Whereas neonates have reduced clearance of many drugs, children 2–6 years of age have greater weight-normalized clearance than adults for many drugs. This greater clearance in young children is attributed to the larger liver mass/kilogram of body weight, resulting in higher rates of metabolism of drugs by the cytochrome P-450 mechanism. More rapid clearance by the liver usually means that more frequent dosing intervals are required in young children.

NOCICEPTIVE PAIN

General Principles

Nociceptive pain is pain that is associated with tissue injury or inflammation and serves a protective role in preventing further injury. Common examples of nociceptive pain include pain due to trauma, surgery, or obstruction of a viscus. This pain may be acute and self-limiting or chronic (e.g., arthritis). Chronic nociceptive pain is common in children, and recurrent pain (headaches, abdominal, and musculoskeletal pain) occurs in as many as 30–40% of children on a weekly basis. Pain assessment and management in children with a significant neurologic impairment present many challenges, and factors to consider include the patient's baseline behavioral and health condition, developmental level, and communicative ability. General principles of pain management include regular pain assessments, appropriate analgesics with regular dosing intervals, and adjunctive therapy to treat side effects. Acetaminophen and non-steroidal anti-inflammatory drugs NSAIDs are useful for relieving milder forms of nociceptive pain. Severe pain can usually be controlled with opioid analgesics. Guiding principles of analgesic administration include the following: "by the clock"—regular analgesic administration with fixed doing intervals and "rescue" doses for "breakthrough" pain, "by the child"—regular assessment for clinical effectiveness and individualized dosing, and "by the mouth"—analgesics given by the simplest and most effective route.

Classes of Medications

Antipyretics with Weak Analgesic Properties

The "weaker" or "milder" analgesics, of which acetaminophen, salicylate, ibuprofen, naproxen, and diclofenac are the classic examples, comprise a heterogeneous group of NSAIDs and nonopioid analgesics with antipyretic properties. These analgesic agents are usually administered enterally and are particularly useful for inflammatory, bony, or rheumatic pain. Parenterally administered NSAIDs, such as ketorolac, are now available for use in children in whom the oral or rectal routes of administration are not possible. Unfortunately, regardless of dose, the nonopioid analgesics reach a "ceiling effect" above which pain cannot be relieved by these drugs alone.

The most commonly used nonopioid analgesic in pediatric practice remains acetaminophen. Unlike aspirin and the NSAIDs, acetaminophen has minimal, if any, anti-inflammatory activity. When administered in normal doses (10–15 mg/kg, PO or PR), acetaminophen has very few serious side effects. It is an antipyretic and like all enterally administered NSAIDs takes about 40–60 min to provide effective analgesia. Dosage guidelines for the most commonly used non-opioid analgesics are listed in Table 1. Recent studies have recommended acetaminophen doses as high as 30–40 mg/kg when administered rectally as a single (loading) dose. Follow-up rectal doses are 15–25 mg/kg every 6 hr.

The discovery of at least 2 cyclo-oxygenase (COX) isoenzymes, COX-1 and COX-2, has updated our knowledge of NSAIDs. In addition to the induction of COX-2 in inflammatory lesions, it is present constitutively in the brain and spinal cord, where it may be involved in nerve transmission, particularly that for pain and fever. The discovery of COX-2 has made possible the design of drugs that reduce inflammation without removing the protective prostaglandins in the stomach and kidney made by COX-1.

Table 1 Dosage Guidelines for Commonly Used NSAIDs

Generic name	Dose (mg/kg) frequency	Maximum adult daily dose (mg)	Comments
Salicylates (aspirin)	10–15 q 4 hr	4000	Inhibits platelet aggregation, GI irritability, Reye syndrome
Choline magnesium trisalicylate	7.5–15 q 6 hr	4000	Aspirin compound that does not affect platelets
Acetaminophen	10–15 PO q 4 hr 25–40 PR q 6 hr	4000	Lacks anti-inflammatory activity
Ibuprofen	4–10 q 6–8 hr	2400	Available as an oral suspension
Naproxen	5–10 q 12 hr	1500	Available as an oral suspension
Indomethacin	0.3–1 q 6 hr	150	Commonly used IV in NICU to close PDA
Ketorolac	IV or IM Load 0.5 Maintenance 0.2–0.5q 6 hr	120	May be given orally Maximum dose 30 mg Causes GI upset and ulcer, discontinue after 5 days

Opioids

Opioid receptors are primarily located in the brain and spinal cord, but also exist peripherally. The most commonly used agonists of the mu receptor include morphine, meperidine, methadone, and the fentanyls. Mixed agonist–antagonist drugs (pentazocine, butorphanol, buprenorphine, and nalbuphine) act as agonists or partial agonists at one opioid receptor (e.g., mu) and antagonists at another receptor (e.g., kappa or sigma).

Many factors are considered including pain intensity, patient age, co-existing disease, potential drug interactions, prior treatment history, physician preference, patient preference, and route of administration when deciding which is the appropriate opioid analgesic to administer. At equipotent doses most opioids have similar effects and side effects (Table 2).

Codeine, oxycodone, and hydrocodone are opiates frequently used to treat pain in children and adults, particularly for less severe pain. In equipotent doses, they are equal both as analgesics and respiratory depressants (Table 2). These drugs have a bioavailability of approximately 60% following oral ingestion. Their analgesic effects occur as early as 20 min following ingestion and reach a maximum at 60–120 min; their plasma half-lives of elimination are 2.5–4 hr. Sustained-release oxycodone is for use only in opioid-tolerant patients with chronic pain, and not for routine postoperative pain.

Morphine is also very effective when given orally, but only about 20–30% of an oral dose reaches the systemic circulation. Oral morphine is available as a liquid, tablet, and sustained-release preparation. The liquid is particularly easy to administer to children and severely debilitated patients. Indeed, in terminal patients who cannot swallow, liquid morphine will provide analgesia when simply dropped into the patient's mouth.

Patient (Parent and Nurse) Controlled Analgesia

In order to give patients, and, in some cases, parents and nurses, some measure of control over their, or their children's, pain therapy demand analgesia or patient-controlled analgesia (PCA) devices have been developed. These are microprocessor-driven pumps with a button that the patient presses to self-administer a small dose of opioid.

The PCA devices allow patients to administer small amounts of an analgesic whenever they feel a need for more pain relief. The opioid, usually morphine, hydromorphone, or fentanyl is administered either intravenously or subcutaneously. The dosage of opioid, number of boluses per hour, and the time interval between boluses (the "lock-out period") are programmed to allow maximum patient flexibility and sense of control with minimal risk of overdosage (Table 3). Typically, we initially prescribe morphine, 20 mcg/kg per bolus, at a rate of 5 boluses/hr, with a 6–8 min lock-out interval between each bolus. Variations include larger boluses (30–50 mcg/kg) and shorter time intervals (5 min). Hydromorphone may have fewer side effects than morphine and is often used when pruritus and nausea complicate morphine PCA therapy. Because it is 5–7 times more potent than morphine, the size of the hydromorphone bolus dose is reduced to 3–4 mcg/kg. The fentanyl equivalent is less clear. Although fentanyl is considered 50–100 times more potent than morphine when given as a single bolus, a conversion of 40:1 was used in a study in which parents and nurses controlled the PCA pump. In that study, fentanyl 0.5 mcg/kg was administered by continuous infusion, and bolus doses were 0.5 mcg/kg.

Table 2 Commonly Used Mu Agonist Drugs

Agonist	Equipotent IV dose (mg/kg)	Duration (hr)	Bioavailability (%)	Comments
Morphine	0.1	3–4	20–40	• "Gold Standard," very inexpensive • Can cause seizures in newborns • Histamine release, vasodilation (avoid in asthmatics and in circulatory compromise) • MS-Contin® 8–12 hr duration (pill), cannot be crushed or given via a gastric tube • Liquid morphine 2–20 mg/mL
Meperidine	1	3–4	40–60	• Catastrophic interactions with MAO inhibitors • Tachycardia; negative inotrope • Metabolite produces seizures • 0.25 mg/kg effectively treats shivering • Not recommended for routine use
Hydromorphone (Dilaudid)	0.015	3–4	50–70	• Less itching and nausea than morphine, commonly used when morphine produces too many of these systemic side effects
Fentanyl	0.001	0.5–1		• Very effective for short painful procedures • Bradycardia; minimal hemodynamic alterations • Chest wall rigidity (>5-mcg/kg rapid IV bolus). R_x naloxone or succinylcholine or pancuronium • Oral transmucosal dose 10–15 mcg/kg
Methadone	0.1	4–24	70–100	• Liquid preparation available • Long duration of action makes it ideal for cancer pain, weaning dependent patients, etc., weaning
Codeine	1.2	3–4	40–70	• PO only • Prescribe with acetaminophen
Hydrocodone	0.1	3–4	60–80	• PO only • Usually prescribed with acetaminophen • Less nausea than codeine
Oxycodone	0.1	3–4	60–80	• PO only • Sustained-release tablet available • Usually prescribed with acetaminophen • Less nausea than codeine

Table 3 Intravenous PCA Treatment Guidelines

Drug (concentration mg/mL)	Basal rate range (mg/kg/hr)	Bolus rate range (mg/kg)	Lock out interval range (min)	Number of boluses/hr range
Morphine (1.0) (in older patients or dependent patients, concentrations can be increased to 10 mg/mL)	0.01–0.03 (10–30 mcg) (usually 0.02) (20 mcg)	0.01–0.03 (usually 0.02) (20 mcg)	5–10 (usually 8 min)	2–6 (usually 5)
Fentanyl (0.01 in children < 20 kg, 0.05 in children > 20 kg)	0.0005 (0.5 mcg)	0.0005–0.001 (0.5–1 mcg)	5–10	1–6
Hydromorphone (0.2 in children < 50 kg 0.5–1.0 in children > 50 kg)	0.003–0.005 (3–5 mcg) (usually 0.004) (4 mcg)	0.003–0.005 (3–5 mcg) (usually 0.004) (4 mcg)	5–10 (usually 8 min)	2–6 (usually 5)

Many PCA units allow low "background" continuous infusions (morphine, 20–30 mcg/kg/hr, hydromorphone 3–4 mcg/kg/hr, fentanyl 0.5 mcg/kg/hr) in addition to self-administered boluses. A continuous background infusion is particularly useful at night and often provides more restful sleep by preventing the patient from awakening in pain but increases the potential for overdosage. The PCA requires a patient with enough intelligence and manual dexterity and strength to operate the pump. In fact, it has been our experience that any child able to play video games can operate a PCA pump (age 5–6). Allowing parents or nurses to initiate a PCA bolus is controversial. We recently demonstrated that nurses and parents can be empowered to initiate PCA boluses and to use this technology safely in children less than even a year of age. Difficulties with PCA include its increased costs, patient age limitations, and the bureaucratic (physician, nursing, and pharmacy) obstacles (protocols, education, storage arrangements) that must be overcome prior to its implementation. Contraindications to the use of PCA include inability to push the bolus button (weakness, arm restraints), inability to understand how to use the machine, and a patient's (or parent's) desire not to assume responsibility for his/her own care.

NEUROPATHIC PAIN

Neuropathic pain is described as pain that is associated with injury, dysfunction, or altered excitability of portions of the peripheral, central, or autonomic nervous system and is not associated with ongoing tissue inflammation or injury (i.e., not nociceptive pain). It is manifested by cutaneous hypesthesia, hyperalgesia, allodynia, and hyperpathia, and is often associated with neurogenic inflammation, autonomic dysregulation, and motor phenomena.

The pathophysiologic mechanisms underlying the development of neuropathic pain are complex and just recently being characterized. Central sensitization is the hallmark of neuropathic pain. After peripheral tissue damage or nerve injury, neuronal plasticity and reorganization within the CNS occur.

It was commonly thought that the prevalence of chronic pain in children was quite low; however, recent studies have shown that chronic pain (nociceptive and neuropathic) is a significant problem in the pediatric population affecting 15–20% of children. The prevalence of neuropathic pain in children is unknown, and it is likely that neuropathic pain is not properly diagnosed in many children. The most common causes of neuropathic pain in children include post-traumatic and postsurgical neuropathic pain, complex regional pain syndromes 1 and 2 (CPRS 1 and 2, formerly known as reflex sympathetic dystrophy and causalgia) and tumor-associated neuropathic pain. Less frequent causes include metabolic and toxic neuropathies, neurodegenerative disorders, and pain after CNS injury.

Treatment of Neuropathic Pain

Neuropathic pain is notoriously difficult to treat and often does not respond to conventional analgesic therapy. The management of pain is often frustrating for the patient and the health-care provider. It is rarely possible to predict high success rates for any single therapy and often the patient will receive multimodal therapy. The treatment often involves trial and error, titration of medication as limited by side effects, and weighing of risks and benefits of therapy. The functional rehabilitative approach is often emphasized with return to school and palliation being the goals as often the pain will be persistent.

Most pharmacologic treatment is based on extrapolation from treatment for adults, with opioids, antidepressants, anticonvulsants, and local anesthetic-like drugs demonstrating varying degrees of effectiveness. Many of the medications used are not traditional analgesics, and the safety and pharmacokinetic data for the use of these drugs in children have come from clinical trials for the treatment of depression, epilepsy, and enuresis (Table 4). Generally, a slow titration of these medications is recommended to minimize side effects and detect adverse reactions. There is often a trade-off between moderate analgesia and some side effects.

Classes of Medications

Tricyclic Antidepressants

The effectiveness of tricyclic antidepressants (TCAs) is well established for treatment of a variety of neuropathic pain conditions including diabetic neuropathy, postherpetic neuralgia, and central poststroke pain. Nortriptyline has less anticholinergic side effects than amitriptyline, and is a common first-line agent used in the treatment of neuropathic pain (Table 5). Common side effects include sedation, dry mouth, orthostatic hypotension, constipation, urinary retention, and tachycardia.

A small number of patients who have received TCAs have had sudden death attributed to dysrhythmia. It is unknown whether these children had a pre-existing conduction disturbance, and these drugs have been used safely in children for decades. We recommend a baseline ECG to rule out rhythm disturbances prior to starting a TCA and also when escalated to a full antidepressant dose range. These drugs should be used with extreme caution in patients with pre-existing rhythm disturbances or cardiomyopathy. There is no established correlation between plasma

Table 4 Adjuvant Medications to Treat Neuropathic Pain

Drug	Indications and uses	Pediatric dosing	Toxicity and notes
Lidocaine	Neuropathic pain, refractory visceral pain	150 mcg/kg/hr	Measure plasma level every 8–12 hr and maintain 2–5 μg/mL
Mexiletine	See lidocaine	10–15 mg/kg	Sedation, fatigue, confusion, nausea, hypotension
Carbamazepine	Trigeminal neuralgia, neuropathic pain, migraine prophylaxis	15–30 mg/kg	Blood dyscrasias, monitor plasma level and periodic CBC
Valproate	Neuropathic pain, migraine prophylaxis, mood lability	10–60 mg/kg	Blood dyscrasias, hepatotoxicity, dose divided t.i.d., monitor plasma level periodic CBC and LFTs
Gabapentin	Neuropathic pain, migraine prophylaxis	5–30 mg/kg	Dose divided t.i.d. or q.i.d., escalate dose over several weeks to target dose
Amitriptyline, nortriptyline	Neuropathic pain, migraine prophylaxis	0.05–2 mg/kg	Escalate dose over several weeks to target dose, does given h.s., obtain screening ECG before use, contraindicated in prolonged QTc
Venlafaxine	Chronic pain with depression, neuropathic pain	1–2 mg/kg	Dose divided b.i.d. or t.i.d., caution when used with TCAs or other SSRIs because of reported arrhythmias
Clonidine	Neuropathic pain, visceral pain, postoperative pain	0.05–0.2 mcg/kg/hr	By oral, transdermal, or continuous epidural infusion; may produce hypotension, bradycardia, somnolence

CBC, complete blood count; t.i.d., three times a day; LFTs, liver function tests; q.i.d., four times daily; h.s., at bedtime; ECG (electrocardiogram); b.i.d., twice a day; TCAs, tricyclic antidepressants; SSRIs, selective serotonin reuptake inhibitors.

(From Krane EJ, Leong MS, Golianu, Leong YY. Treatment of pediatric pain with nonconventional analgesics. In: Schechter NL, Berde CB, Yaster M, eds. Pain in Infants, Children, and Adolescents. 2d ed. Philadelphia: Lippincott Williams, and Wilkins, 2003, used with permission.)

Table 5 Sample Dose Titration Regimen for Nortriptyline and Gabapentin for Neuropathic Pain

1. Slow titration (e.g., ambulatory outpatients who are attending school or work)		
	< 50 kg	
a. Nortriptyline or amitriptyline	Obtain baseline ECG	
Days 1–4	0.2 mg/kg q.h.s.	
Days 5–8	0.4 mg/kg q.h.s.	
Increase as tolerated every 4 to 6 days until i. good analgesia ii. Limiting side effects or iii. Dosing reaches 1 mg/kg/day (< 50 kg) or 50 mg (> 50 mg) iv. If condition iii, consider measuring plasma concentration and ECG before further does escalation. Consider twice-daily dosing (25% in morning, 75% in evening).		
	< 50 kg	> 50 mg
b. Gabapentin		
Days 1–2	2 mg/kg q.h.s.	100 mg q.h.s.
Days 3–4	2 mg/kg b.i.d.	100 mg b.i.d.
Days 4–6	2 mg/kg t.i.d.	100 mg t.i.d.
Days 7–9	2, 2, 4 mg/kg (t.i.d. schedule)	100, 100, 200 mg
Increase as tolerated every 3 days (with 50% of daily dose in the evening) until i. Good analgesia ii. Limiting side effects or iii. Dosing reaches 60 mg/kg daily < 50 kg) or 3 g daily (> 50 kg)		
2. Rapid titration (e.g., nonambulatory patients with widely metastatic cancer) a. Tricyclics: begin at 0.2 mg/kg (10 mg for > 50 kg) and titrate up every 1–2 days in steps according to the slow titiation regimen b. Gabapentin: begin at 6 mg/kg b.i.d. (300 mg b.i.d. for > 50 kg) for 1–2 days, 6 mg/kg t.i.d. (300 mg t.i.d. for > 50 kg) for 1 to days, 6 mg/kg morning and midday, 12 mg/kg q.h.s (300, 300, 600 mg for > 50 kg) for 1–2 days, and increase as tolerated to 60 mg/kg daily (3 g/day for > 50 kg) over 5–10 days.		

ECG (electrocardiogram); q.h.s., once daily at bedtime; b.i.d., twice daily; t.i.d., three times daily. (From Berde CB, Lebel AA, Olsson G. Neuropathic pain in children. in: Schechter NL, Berde CB, Yaster M, eds. Pain in Infants, Children, and Adolescents. 2d ed. Philadelphia: Lippincott, Williams, and Wilkins, 2003, used with permission.)

concentration of TCAs and analgesic efficacy; therefore, routine measurement of plasma drug levels is useful only to determine patient compliance, optimization of dose before aborting a therapeutic trial, or to identify patients who need dosing modification based on metabolism of the drug (i.e., those patients who may need b.i.d. dosing). If the drug needs to be discontinued for any reason, the dosing should be tapered over 1–2 weeks to avoid irritability and agitation. Other antidepressants have been used for neuropathic pain without much success, and the selective serotonin reuptake inhibitors (SSRI) such as paroxetine are not as effective as the TCAs for pain control but are helpful with associated depression, sleep disturbance, and anxiety.

Anticonvulsants

Along with the TCAs, anticonvulsants are usually considered as first-line agents for the treatment of neuropathic pain. Gabapentin has emerged as the most common anticonvulsant for the treatment of neuropathic pain. It has been used for neuropathic cancer pain, centrally mediated pain, trigeminal neuralgia, and migraine.

Gabapentin is used as a first-line drug due to effectiveness, low side effect profile, and low frequency of adverse reactions. The drug is also beneficial in the treatment of mood disorders and is commonly used for anxiety. Pediatric use of gabapentin as an anticonvulsant for epilepsy is well documented; however, the use of gabapentin for neuropathic pain in children is largely confined to case reports. Due to the relatively benign side effect profile, it is becoming very commonly used for pediatric neuropathic pain, and a recommended dosing schedule is found in Table 5. Side effects include somnolence, dizziness, ataxia, tremor, and occasional oppositional behavior.

Other agents less commonly used include carbamazepine, valproic acid, and clonazepam. These agents may have significant hematologic, cardiovascular, and CNS adverse effects.

Membrane Stabilizers

Drugs such as intravenous lidocaine and oral mexilitine are useful for the treatment of neuropathic pain by interfering with the conduction of sodium channels in peripheral and central neurons, reducing the spontaneous impulse firing. The pharmacokinetics of these drugs are similar in children and adults. Lidocaine is used as an adjunct treatment for pain and is reportedly predictive of efficacy of mexilitene. Side effects such as nausea, vomiting, sedation, and ataxia limit the usefulness of this drug.

Alpha Agonists

Drugs such as clonidine are effective in the treatment of pain by acting at the dorsal horn to facilitate the descending inhibitory pathways as well as a potential mechanism of action involving increasing secretion of acetylcholine. Efficacy has been demonstrated for epidural use in neuropathic pain associated with cancer. There is less evidence of efficacy with the use of this medication by the oral, intravenous, or transdermal route. Side effects may include sedation, bradycardia, and hypotension.

Nonpharmacologic Treatment of Neuropathic Pain

Many patients with neuropathic pain will benefit from the use of cognitive-behavioral treatments (CBT) for pain management. This treatment often involves relaxation training, biofeedback training, and structured counseling regarding coping strategies and stress management. This therapy is supplemented by supportive individual or family counseling for school avoidance, depression, anxiety, and family dysfunction. An accepted model for treatment is a rehabilitative one which emphasizes full participation in school and other activities when possible.

Physical therapy for CPRS often involves cutaneous desensitization and transcutaneous electric nerve stimulation (TENS) for allodynia as well as aerobic exercise training, strength training, and postural exercises for the deconditioned state. Studies have shown excellent efficacy for the use of physical therapy and CBT in CRPS.

CONCLUSION

The past two decades have witnessed an explosion in research and interest in pediatric pain management. Multidisciplinary pain service teams provide the pain management for acute, postoperative, terminal, neuropathic, and chronic pain. In this chapter we have tried to consolidate in a comprehensive manner the recent advances in the pharmacologic and nonpharmacologic treatment of childhood pain.

SUGGESTED READINGS

1. Berde CB, Sethna NF. Analgesics for the treatment of pain in children. N Engl J Med 2002; 347(14):1094–1103.
2. Monitto CL, Greenberg RS, Kost-Byerly S, Wetzel R, Billett C, Lebet RM, Yaster M. The safety and efficacy of parent-/nurse-controlled analgesia in patients less than six years of age. Anesth Analg 2000; 91(3):573–579.
3. Schechter NL, Berde CB, Yaster M. Pain in Infants, Children, and Adolescents 2d ed. Philadelphia: Lippincott Williams and Wilkins, 2003.
4. Yaster M. Acute pain in children. Pediatr Clin N Am 2000; 47:487–755.
5. Yaster M, Krane EJ, Kaplan RF, Cote' CJ, Lappe DG. Pediatric Pain Management and Sedation Handbook. St. Louis: Mosby Year Book, Inc., 1997.

37
Neurologic Effects of Cancer and Its Therapies

Paul Grahan Fisher
The Beirne Family Director of Neuro-Oncology at Packard Children's Hospital, Stanford University, Stanford, Calefornia, U.S.A.

INTRODUCTION

The incidence of pediatric cancer has climbed now to 16 per 100,000 children every year. In conjunction with this rise, survival for these patients has vastly improved. By the year 2010, 1 in 250 young adults will be survivors of childhood cancer. As treatments have become increasingly intense or novel, the neurologist is consulted more often to assist in the diagnosis and management of problems experienced by either the child recently diagnosed with cancer or the long-term survivor. An exhaustive review of the neurologic difficulties experienced by the patient with cancer is expansive and can consume a textbook (see Suggested Readings). In this chapter, our aim will be to address the clinical features, diagnosis, and management of the most common neurologic complaints, along with their most common causes, encountered by pediatric oncology patients.

ENCEPHALOPATHY

An alteration in level of consciousness can be caused by a variety of "metabolic" (i.e., nonlocalizing or diffuse) and structural processes in the child with cancer. Acutely, chemotherapeutic agents (Table 1), as well as cranial irradiation, weeks, to sometimes years, after delivery are concerns. Post radiotherapy somnolence syndrome is marked by lethargy and anorexia for days to weeks about a month or two after whole-brain irradiation. Nonlocalizing leukemic meningitis and leptomeningeal metastases from other cancers can also lead to mental status changes. Metabolic derangements, neurotoxicity from supportive agents commonly used (e.g., narcotics, benzodiazepines, corticosteroids, antihistamines, or tricyclic antidepressants), or infection such as viral encephalitis—most commonly herpes simplex or varicella zoster—can produce encephalopathy. Depression or behavioral changes masquerading as encephalopathy are diagnoses of exclusion.

Structural lesions can certainly produce encephalopathy, too. Perhaps most worrisome are neoplastic processes, including primary brain tumor, metastasis from

Table 1 Chemotherapeutics Associated with Encephalopathy

BCNU (carmustine) high dose and intra-arterial
Cisplatin intra-arterial
Corticosteroids
Cyclophosphamide (mild symptoms)
Cyclosporine
Cytarabine high dose
5-Fluorouracil high dose
Ifosfamide (worsened symptoms with prior cisplatin $> 300\,mg/m^2$)
Interferons
Interleukin-2 high dose
L-Asparaginase
Methotrexate high-dose intravenous and intrathecal
Procarbazine
Thiotepa high dose
Vinblastine
Vincristine

cancer elsewhere in the body, and secondary malignancy. Cancer metastasizing to the central nervous system (CNS) is rare in children, and occurs most frequently late in the course of rhabdomyosarcoma, Ewing sarcoma, neuroblastoma, or Wilms tumor, or less often, renal rhabdoid tumor, hepatoblastoma, or embryonal carcinoma. Glioblastoma multiforme, sarcomas, and meningioma can occur as secondary malignancies years after cranial irradiation (Table 2). Intracranial abscess (e.g., bacterial, fungal, or mycobacterial, or rarely protozoal), or strokes are other possibilities. Stroke can result from several causes (Table 3).

Cognitive decline or leukoencephalopathy can be notable years after a large field of supratentorial radiotherapy. Methotrexate, particularly high-dose intravenous or intrathecal, can also cause a striking acute to more commonly chronic leukoencephalopathy. Toxicity is potentiated by radiotherapy. Patients may display specific learning disabilities or nonspecific developmental delay. Computed tomography of the head might reveal microcalcifications at the gray–white junction, while magnetic resonance imaging (MRI) shows bilateral frontal greater than posterior subcortical increased white matter signal on T2-weighted or FLAIR MRI. The mechanism of methotrexate neurotoxicity remains unclear, although effects on methylene tetrahydrofolate reductase, homocystine, and NMDA metabolism have been postulated.

In recent years, a syndrome of reversible posterior leukoencephalopathy, characterized by transient headaches, confusion, seizures, or visual impairment, has been reported, particularly during induction therapy for acute lymphoblastic leukemia or non-Hodgkin lymphoma. Magnetic resonance imaging of the brain reveals reversible, bilateral parieto-occipital white matter increased signal abnormalities, with sparing of the occipital cortex, seen best on T2-weighted or FLAIR images. This syndrome may represent hyperfusion breakdown of the blood–brain barrier. Reversible posterior leukoencephalopathy in leukemia may be triggered by methotrexate, steroids, vincristine, and/or high-dose cytarabine, and in other situations has been associated with hypertension or immunosuppression, triggered by renal failure, cyclosporine, or FK506 (tacrolimus). This syndrome tends to resolve spontaneously.

Reversal of encephalopathy in the pediatric oncology patient can be challenging. First, unexplained encephalopathy in the febrile, immunocompromised patient should always prompt initiation of broad-spectrum antibiotics and acyclovir. For chemotherapy-related alterations producing severe or life-threatening encephalopathy, or any other profound neurologic insults, discontinuation of the offending agent is usually the wisest choice. Methylene blue has been reported as an antidote for ifosfamide encephalopathy. Acute dysfunction from elevated methotrexate levels can be treated with increasing leucovorin, although whether this affects long-term sequelae is debatable. For children with leukoencephalopathy or cognitive decline, supportive treatment with stimulants such as methylphenidate may prove helpful. Data on use of atomoxetine in such situations are lacking.

INCREASED INTRACRANIAL PRESSURE

Elevated intracranial pressure (ICP) can be heralded by a change in mental status, lethargy, headache, or vomiting. Increased ICP can arise from the structural lesions mentioned above, as well as hydrocephalus, meningitis, and pseudotumor cerebri. The retinoids *cis*-retinoic acid and fenretinide, used in neuroblastoma, and all-*trans* retinoic acid, utilized in acute promyelocytic leukemia, can cause pseudotumor. The clinician should maintain an orderly approach to the urgent and emergent treatment of increased ICP (Table 4).

SEIZURES

Seizures in children with cancer may arise from primary brain tumors or metastatic disease, leukemic meningitis, stroke, CNS infection, metabolic abnormalities, or treatment sequelae. Antineoplastic therapy may cause seizures too (Table 5). Intrathecal methotrexate can cause seizures 7–10 days after administration, while high-dose intravenous methotrexate can lead to seizures more acutely. Standard neurologic management of status epilepticus and seizures, described elsewhere in this book, should be followed. For the child undergoing chemotherapy, special consideration should be given to the choice of antiepileptic agent. Recent data have shown marked reduction in bioavailability of chemotherapy metabolized by the cytochrome P450 mono-oxygenase system, when patients concurrently receive the enzyme-inducing anticonvulsants phenytoin, phenobarbital, or carbamazepine. For these children, if chronic anticonvulsant therapy is warranted, selection of a non-enzyme-inducing agent, such as gabapentin, levetiracetam, lamotrigine, or topiramate, is preferable to avoid this complication. Furthermore, carbamazepine and valproic acid are avoided owing to their potential bone marrow myelosuppression.

MYELOPATHY

The neurologist should always think beyond cerebral processes and consider myelopathy to explain motor loss, sensory deficit with a dermatomal level, or autonomic (i.e., bowel and bladder) changes, even when findings are asymmetric and particularly when they are accompanied by back pain. Spinal irradiation, months to years after its administration, can lead to myelopathy, often symmetric. Intrathecal agents,

Table 2 Syndromes of Damage Following Cranial Irradiation (XRT)

Syndrome	Timing after XRT	Pathogenesis	Symptoms, signs, and laboratories	Treatment and outcome
Somnolence syndrome	4–8 weeks	Whole-brain or large-field XRT to cerebrum may cause oligodendrocyte dysfunction with secondary inhibition of myelin production	3–7+ days of lethargy, anorexia, nausea, and vomiting; delta activity on electroencephalogram	Usually self-limited; can respond to dexamethasone
Radiation necrosis	Most often 3 months to 3 years	Idiosyncratic; risk increases with higher dose per fraction or total dosage $\geq$55 Gy	Focal neurologic deficits, seizures, increased intracranial pressure, coma; magnetic resonance spectroscopy shows elevated lactate peaks	Focal areas resectable; dexamethasone if unresectable or small
Transient radiation myelopathy	2 weeks to months	Edema and transient suppression of myelin production	Electric-shock sensations from the neck down the spine (Lhermitte sign)	None, resolves spontaneously
Radiation myelitis	6 months to years	Demyelination, edema, and perhaps necrosis from excessive radiotherapy dose per fraction	Paraparesis to quadriparesis, bowel and bladder dysfunction	May be permanent
Mineralizing micrangiopathy/ vasculopathy	9 months to 30 years	Dystrophic calcification to small vessels, inflammation and telangiectasia to larger vessels;	None or possibly headaches, seizures, cognitive decline, strokes	Possibly responds to antiplatelet agents, anticoagulation, or

		endothelial cell damage also present; occurs with ≥20 Gy and potentiated by methotrexate, intrathecal cytarabine		hyperbaric oxygen therapy—efficacy unproven
Moyamoya disease	6 months to 15 years	Fibrous intimal thickening of large arteries leading to occlusion, after ≥40 Gy; associated with neurofibromatosis I	Headaches, seizures, transient ischemic attacks, strokes, progressive cognitive decline; magnetic resonance imaging with narrowing/occlusion of carotid or cerebral arteries with distal telangiectatic collateral vessels—"puff of smoke"	Some cases stabilize from spontaneous collateral vessel formation; arterial bypass surgery may improve outcome
Neurocognitve damage	Increases with time; unclear if plateaus	Any XRT, particularly to cerebrum; increases with larger total dosage or volume, or younger age; may stem from ongoing vascular degeneration; complicated by the effects of tumor mass effect, hydrocephalus, infection, surgical trauma, and chemotherapy	Cognitive deficits, learning disabilities, particularly in short-term memory, visuomotor processing, spatial relations, and calculations	Requires remediation and special education; may continue over time; stimulants can be helpful
Secondary brain tumor	≥5–25 years	≥18 Gy, perhaps potentiated by chemotherapy and genetic predisposition	High-grade astrocytoma, sarcoma, meningioma	Often highly malignant, poor prognosis tumors

Table 3 Differential Diagnosis for Stroke in the Child with Cancer

Acute promyelocytic leukemia
Chemotherapeutics
BCNU (carmustine) intra-arterial
Cisplatin intra-arterial
L-Asparaginase
Hyperleukocytosis, in leukemia
Intratumoral hemorrhage—high-grade astrocytoma, medulloblastoma
Methotrexate-associated stroke-like events days to a week plus after intravenous high dose
Neuroblastoma metastatic to the dura or torcula
Platelet-resistant thrombocytopenia

such as cytarabine, methotrexate, and thiotepa, can cause acute to subacute spine necrosis, specifically when these drugs distribute unevenly in the subarachnoid space because of blockage from tumor. Nuclear medicine studies with technetium or indium can often demonstrate blockage in the presence of leptomengineal disease, even when spine MRI appears to show patent spaces.

SPINAL CORD COMPRESSION

The most alarming cause of myelopathy in the oncology patient is compression of the spinal cord by tumor. Acute compression occurs in 3–5% of children with cancer. Tumor most often infiltrates through intervertebral foramina, unlike in adults where vertebral body involvement is more often found. Epidural tumor spread through the foramina is seen most frequently with Ewing sarcoma, neuroblastoma, osteosarcoma, rhabdomyosarcoma, Hodgkin disease, and non-Hodgkin lymphoma. Tumor can sometimes metastasize along the dura mater in neuroblastoma. Spinal subarachnoid tumor can develop with leukemia and "drop metastases" from the primary brain tumors medulloblastoma, embryonal tumors, ependymoma, and astrocytoma.

In addition to the signs of myelopathy already described, these patients commonly have exquisite back pain and localized tenderness to percussion over the spine. For children suspected to harbor pathology of the inferior cord, spending considerable time distinguishing between localization to the conus medullaris (i.e., upper

Table 4 Management of Increased Intracranial Pressure

Urgent
Place head in midline elevated 30°
Restrict fluids to 3/4 maintenance with isotonic solutions
Dexamethasone 1–2 mg/kg intravenous
Furosemide 1 mg/kg intravenous
Uninterrupted oxygenation
Gentle blood pressure control
Emergent
Mannitol 0.5–1.0 g/kg intravenously
Hyperventilation
Ventriculostomy, surgical decompression
Possible high-dose barbiturates

Table 5 Chemotherapeutics Associated with Seizures

BCNU (carmustine) intra-arterial
Busulfan high dose
Cisplatin (rare)
Cyclosporine
Cytarabine intrathecal
Ifosfamide
Methotrexate high-dose intravenous and intrathecal
Vincristine (rarely)

motor neuron) vs. cauda equina (i.e., lower motor neuron) is not useful, since tumor frequently involves both. Instead, to expedite diagnosis for any child suspected to have spinal cord compression, spine MRI is always the study of choice.

Emergent treatment of spinal cord compression should commence with dexamethasone 1 mg/kg intravenously. In suspected cases of lymphoma, the oncolytic effect of steroids can be so profound that biopsy should be performed immediately to confirm diagnosis. For some tumors, laminectomy and posterior decompression may suffice as initial therapy, along with steroids. Surgery is particularly recommended as initial therapy when the primary tumor is unknown and another easily accessible disease site cannot provide the diagnosis, all or most of the neoplasm can be removed, or relapse occurs during or after maximal radiotherapy. Thrombocytopenia and coagulopathy should be corrected before surgery (or before lumbar puncture, as described above) is attempted. If the diagnosis is known and the tumor radioresponsive, then radiotherapy is the therapy of choice. No controlled comparison of surgery vs. radiotherapy in children with compression has been performed. A few reports of initial chemotherapy for young children with spinal cord compression and newly diagnosed neuroblastoma, Ewing sarcoma, germ cell tumors, and osteosarcoma have shown efficacy, but the symptomatology of these patients is often minimal and the choice of therapy nonrandomized.

ATAXIA

As ataxia connotes simply incoordination, the clinician should exclude cerebral or spinal processes already described before localizing the process to the cerebellum. Nevertheless, a number of agents are known to produce cerebellar ataxia, particularly cyclosporine, cytarabine, 5-fluorouracil, ifosfamide, intrathecal methotrexate, and procarbazine. The ataxia with cytarabine is most often seen when the drug is administered in high dosage, e.g., $3\,g/m^2$ for several consecutive doses, in children with acute myelogenous leukemia (AML). Cytarabine injures Purkinje cells and the ataxia typically but not always resolves spontaneously. Although this chemotherapeutic is key in the treatment of AML, whether a child whose ataxia resolves should be re-challenged with this drug is unclear.

While paraneoplastic syndromes are rare in children, opsoclonus-myoclonus associated with ataxia in a toddler can be the harbinger of thoracic or abdominal neuroblastoma. As opsoclonus-myoclonus is an autoimmune reaction associated with humoral response to neuroblastoma, the syndrome often resolves with just therapy of the tumor. In some instances, the autoimmune response can cause more extensive or persistent neurologic damage. Isolated reports have described improvements to persistent neuroblastoma-associated opsoclonus-myoclonus with use of prednisone, ACTH, or intravenous immunoglobulin.

NEUROPATHY

Neuropathy, in general, is rare in children but in the oncology setting seen most often with vincristine or cisplatin. With vincristine, the neuropathy is a length-dependent, small-fiber axonal neuropathy. Pathologic examination of nerves shows axonal degeneration with regeneration affecting both myelinated and unmyelinated axons. Foot and toe dorsiflexion and foot everters are initially affected, with loss of ankle jerks. Patients can complain of parasthesias in the fingertips. The associated weakness is reversible, with recovery taking months after drug discontinuation, although some patients have persistent minor residual deficits. It is usually best to "dose through" rather than reduce vincristine in the presence of neuropathy while employing ankle–foot orthoses and physical therapy, unless the neuropathy threatens walking. Cranial neuropathies (often unilateral rather than bilateral) are less common, but may result in jaw pain or facial weakness upon infusion early in treatment. Ptosis is seen sometimes, especially in younger children. Vincristine must be avoided in children with Charcot–Marie–Tooth disease, in which there is risk of irreversible paralysis with administration of the drug. It is essential that the clinician inquire about a family history of this disease, pes cavus, or neuropathy before administering this drug.

Cisplatin causes a sensory, dose-related (usually $>200\,\mathrm{mg/m^2}$ cumulatively) large-fiber peripheral neuropathy. Children will show depression of vibratory sensation and loss or proprioception, sometimes with refusal to walk or bear weight. Pain and temperature sensations are spared. Muscle cramps occur more commonly with cisplatin neuropathy than vincristine neuropathy. Cisplatin also produces ototoxicity by damage to cochlear hair cells. This high-frequency hearing loss is irreversible and progresses with increased cumulative dosage. Prior radiotherapy may enhance damage, as the radiotherapy can cause an obliterative cochlear arteritis. Other agents associated with neuropathy in the setting of childhood cancer are listed in Table 6.

Table 6 Chemotherapeutics Associated with Neuropathy

Carboplatin
Cisplatin
Cytarabine (rare)
Doxorubicin (rare)
Etoposide
Paclitaxel
Procarbazine
Teniposide
Thalidomide
Vinblastine
Vincristine

MYOPATHY

In the oncology setting, myopathy is noted commonly with the prolonged administration of dexamethasone in patients with brain tumors or prednisone or other steroids in children with other malignancies. Steroid myopathy is treated by discontinuation of the drug, if possible, after which, the myopathy usually resolves over months. Supportive care and rehabilitation are required. Chemotherapeutics associated with myopathy include 5-azacytidine, doxorubicin, and paclitaxel. Myopathy can occur subacutely following vincristine exposure.

SUGGESTED READINGS

1. Packer RJ, Vezina G. Neurologic complications of chemotherapy and radiotherapy. In: Berg BO, ed. Principles of Child Neurology. New York: McGraw-Hill, 1996:1383–1412.
2. Pizzo PA, Poplack DG, eds. Principles and Practice of Pediatric Oncology. 4th ed. Philadelphia: Lippincott, Williams & Wilkins, 2002.
3. Posner JB. Neurologic Complications of Cancer. Philadelphia: F.A. Davis Company, 1995.
4. Schiff D, Wen PY. Cancer Neurology in Clinical Practice. Totowa, NJ: Humana Press, 2003.

38

Supratentorial Tumors of Childhood

Kaleb Yohay
Department of Neurology, Johns Hopkins Hospital, Baltimore, Maryland, U.S.A.

INTRODUCTION

According to data from the Central Brain Tumor Registry of the United States (CBTRUS), the incidence of childhood brain tumors is 3.9 cases per 100,000 person-years, making brain tumors the most common solid malignancy of childhood. It is estimated that there are 26,000 children diagnosed with a primary brain tumor living in the United States, and over 3000 children are diagnosed with a primary brain tumor every year. Infratentorial tumors are more common in children aged 3–11years, while supratentorial tumors predominate in infants and toddlers, as well as in older children. The distribution of CNS tumors is much more diverse with regard to both histopathological type and grade when compared to adults. Though improvements in therapy have resulted in improved survival of children with brain tumors, mortality remains high, with an overall survival rate of 63% at 5 years following the diagnosis of a primary malignant brain tumor. In addition, morbidity from the tumors and their therapies is extremely high.

OVERALL MANAGEMENT

For most supratentorial tumors, surgical resection is the initial and an essential step of the treatment process. Surgery is useful for obtaining tissue for diagnosis, symptom control, and to improve the efficacy of other therapies. Surgery can result in cure when a gross total resection is achieved and histology is favorable. Improved technology including frameless stereotaxy, intraoperative MRI, and improved endoscopy has improved the extent of resection. However, inherent limitations make surgery in some situations impossible or extremely risky.

Radiation therapy (RT) is another treatment modality used to treat macroscopic tumor and treating local or distant microscopic disease. In some circumstances, RT is used alone, but it is most often utilized as an adjunct to surgery. The use of conformal field radiation has allowed the delivery of higher doses to the tumor while minimizing side effects. Side effects of radiation to normal brain are frequently a limiting factor, particularly in younger children in whom it can result in severe cognitive dysfunction. Stereotactic radiosurgery is likely to become more commonly used in children, and can be very effective in some instances.

The blood–brain barrier (BBB) presents special challenges for the chemotherapeutic treatment of brain tumors. Recent work has shown that chemotherapy may be helpful in treating some primary tumors and metastases by delaying radiation therapy and by decreasing the total radiation dose required. Side effects and morbidities associated with chemotherapy are variable.

Seizures are a frequent complication of supratentorial tumors, occurring in 22% of children under 14 years old and in 68% of children greater than 14 years old, according to data from the Childhood Brain Tumor Consortium. Seizures due to the presence of a supratentorial tumor are most likely to be partial in onset, with or without secondary generalization. The choice of anticonvulsant therapy should take this into account along with the age of the patient, route of administration, and potential interactions with steroids, chemotherapeutic agents, or other medications. Despite the high prevalence of seizures associated with brain tumors, studies in adults have not shown an advantage to prophylactic treatment with anticonvulsants in preventing a first seizure. Some studies have examined the role of perioperative prophylaxis with anticonvulsants such as phenytoin and have shown some benefit of short-term use, while other studies have shown no benefit. After surgical resection of a tumor, the duration of antiepileptic therapy should be based on a number of factors, including the type and severity of seizures and the extent of resection. Typically, patients are treated for a seizure-free interval lasting from several months to two years, though there is no specific data to suggest the most efficacious duration of therapy.

Corticosteroids, especially dexamethasone, can be useful in decreasing edema associated with brain tumors and can significantly improve symptoms related to swelling. Their use should be considered in any patient with symptomatic peritumoral edema. We use a loading dose of dexamethasone of 1–2 mg/kg up to 10 mg followed by 1–1.5 mg/kg/day to a maximum of 16 mg/day divided every 4 hr. Corticosteroids are also frequently used in asymptomatic patients several days prior to surgery. Aside from the common side effects of steroids such as psychosis, GI bleeding, hypertension, and hyperglycemia, steroids can have the unintended effect of decreasing BBB permeability and can interact with chemotherapeutic agents, increasing toxicity and/or decreasing efficacy.

In patients with evidence of raised intracranial pressure, appropriate emergency measures to decrease ICP and maintain cerebral perfusion pressure should be undertaken; as detailed.

SPECIFIC THERAPIES

Gliomas

Astrocytomas are among the most common supratentorial tumors in children, making up over one-third of childhood brain tumors. In contrast to the adult population, low-grade astrocytomas predominate in children and in many instances treatment may not be needed. A tumor with features of a low-grade astrocytoma on neuroimaging may be followed expectantly with serial scans. For low-grade astrocytomas that cause significant symptoms and cannot be adequately managed symptomatically, surgery is the mainstay of treatment. For low-grade astrocytomas in locations conducive to gross total resection (GTR), outcomes are excellent with near 100%

long-term progression-free survival. When GTR is not possible, surgical debulking can prolong survival and improve symptoms, but the incidence of progression is high. Radiation therapy and/or chemotherapy may be used in instances of tumor recurrence. For unresectable low-grade astrocytomas located in the optic pathways, thalamus or hypothalamus, chemotherapy or local radiation therapy may be used as the primary treatment. Stereotactic radiosurgery may prove to be an effective alternative in cases of recurrence or unresectable low-grade astrocytomas.

High-grade astrocytomas (anaplastic astrocytomas and glioblastoma multiforme) have been a treatment challenge and most options have had limited success. Maximal surgical resection provides some survival benefit and adjuvant therapy with RT and/or single or combination chemotherapy may provide the modest benefit. Combination therapy with lomustine, vincristine, and prednisone and single agent therapy with temazolamide have shown some efficacy. Other therapies being tried include interstitial brachytherapy with radioisotope seeds implanted into the tumor bed, high-dose chemotherapy with autologous stem cell rescue, radiosensitizers, and local administration of chemotherapeutic agents with implanted polymers. Gene therapy and other molecular techniques are also being explored.

The management of optic pathway gliomas (OPGs) presents its own set of challenges and controversies. These low-grade astrocytomas have a variable natural history ranging from no progression or even regression to being very aggressive and even deadly. In contrast, OPGs generally have a more benign course in NF-1 patients. Generally, conservative management with serial ophthalmologic examinations and MRI scanning is preferred. Surgery may be considered in instances of significant proptosis or visual loss, and particularly in unilateral, anteriorly located tumors. Shunting may be required if obstructive hydrocephalus develops. Chemotherapeutic agents have been shown to be effective and are often used in symptomatic patients under 5 years old in whom radiation would carry high morbidity. Various combination regimens using vincristine, etoposide, carboplatin, and/or cisplatin are most commonly used. Radiation may be helpful in older children who have had a partial resection or progression after surgery and/or chemotherapy.

Oligodendrogliomas are uncommon in children, making up only about 1% of intracranial tumors. Oligodendrogliomas are more likely to be low grade in children. Gangliogliomas are somewhat more common, accounting for 4–8% of brain tumors in children. Both frequently present with long histories of seizures or other neurologic deficits. For progressive or symptomatic tumors, surgical resection is the mainstay of treatment. The effectiveness of adjuvant treatment with radiation or chemotherapy is unproven.

Ependymomas make up about 10% of childhood brain tumors. Only about one-third of ependymomas are located supratentorially. Ependymomas have a propensity for seeding the neuraxis, with reports of metastatic rates ranging from 5% to 20%. Evaluation should include MR imaging of the entire neuraxis at the time of diagnosis. In contrast to infratentorial ependymomas that are typically located in association with the ventricular system, supratentorial ependymomas tend to be located within the parenchyma. The peak incidence in children is around 4–5 years of age with a moderate male predominance. Survival rates for patients after GTR range from 50% to 70% and 0–30% after subtotal resection (STR). For tumors that are resectable with a wide margin and with no evidence of metastatic disease, adjuvant therapy may not be necessary. Adjuvant radiotherapy is typically used in the settings of STR, anaplasia, or neuraxis dissemination. In younger children where the morbidity from radiation therapy is high, lower doses may be used or even be deferred with the use of adjuvant chemotherapy. Chemotherapeutic regimens have included etoposide, cisplatin, and ICE (ifosfamide, carboplatin, and etoposide). Salvage therapy with oral etoposide in instances of recurrence has shown modest benefit.

Primitive Neuroectodermal Tumors

Supratentorial primitive neuroectodermal tumors (PNETs) tend to occur in infancy and early childhood. They are much less common than infratentorial PNETs (medulloblastoma). Overall, they account for about 3% of brain tumors in children. Five-year survival rates range between 12% and 34%. They are most commonly located in the cerebral hemispheres or in the pineal region. The PNETs have a propensity to spread along the neuraxis. Treatment includes surgical resection, craniospinal irradiation, and chemotherapy. The tendency of this tumor to present in younger children presents additional treatment challenges due to the high morbidity of RT. Treatment regimens in these children have included intensive chemotherapy with stem cell rescue to delay or potentially avoid the need of RT. In this setting younger children may receive focal radiation. Complete resection is often difficult because of the highly invasive nature of the tumor. In children 3 years of age or younger, negative prognostic indicators include the presence of metastatic disease and residual tumor after resection.

Craniopharyngioma

Craniopharyngiomas (low-grade neoplasms that arise from remnants of Rathke's pouch) are the most common nonglial brain tumor of childhood, accounting for about 3% of all intracranial tumors. There are two types of craniopharyngioma, of which the adamantimous type is much more common in childhood, with a peak incidence around age 5–9 years. The squamous papillary type rarely occurs in children. Endocrine dysfunction frequently occurs with about 75% of the children having growth hormone deficiency at time of presentation. Hypothyroidism, diabetes insipidus, adrenal insufficiency, increased intracranial pressure, and/or visual changes are often present. Surgical resection remains the mainstay of therapy, despite the fact that the cystic and adherent nature of these tumors often make surgical resection difficult or impossible. When complete resection is not achieved, adjuvant radiation therapy is used. Intralesional therapy with radioisotopes or infusion of bleomycin has been helpful in recurrent or progressive cystic tumors. Despite therapy, recurrence rates are as high as one-third by 10 years.

Germ Cell Tumors

Germ cell tumors (GCTs) arise from embryonic cell rests located in the midline of the brain. These tumors arise in midline structures, most often in the suprasellar or pineal regions, accounting for 3% of childhood brain tumors. They typically occur in childhood and adolescence, with a peak age of 10–12 years, occurring twice as often in boys. Because of differential response to therapy, GCTs are typically divided into germinomas and nongerminomatous germ cell tumors (NGGCTs). Germinomas are the most common GCT, making up about half. Suprasellar GCTs typically present with visual field defects, diabetes insipidus, early or delayed puberty, or growth arrest. Pineal region tumors more commonly present with signs and symptoms of elevated intracranial pressure. If a GCT is suspected on the basis of neuroimaging, cerebrospinal fluid should be examined for the presence of malignant cells as well as biochemical markers (αFP, β-hCG, PLAP), which may be helpful in establishing a diagnosis, particularly of the NGGCTs. In addition, neuroimaging of the entire neuraxis should be performed because of the propensity for metastasis. Imaging should be performed prior to the lumbar puncture or surgery. In germinomas, surgical resection and histopathological evaluation are necessary for diagnosis though the relative importance of GTR vs. STR is controversial. The mainstay of treatment is radiation therapy with craniospinal radiation for disseminated disease. Adjuvant or neoadjuvant chemotherapy, particularly with platinum-based regimens is sometimes used. Though malignant in character, cure for germinomas is usual. The NGGCTs (except mature teratomas) require maximal surgical resection, with adjuvant radiation therapy and chemotherapy. Chemotherapeutic agents used include combination therapy with etoposide and cisplatin and other combination regimens. High-dose chemotherapy with stem cell rescue has also been used. Mature teratomas can be treated with GTR alone. The prognosis for yolk sac tumors, embryonal carcinomas, and choriocarcinomas is poor with frequent recurrence and dissemination.

SUMMARY

Supratentorial tumors in children are pathologically diverse and clinical course is variable. They present many diagnostic and therapeutic challenges. Therapeutic options are frequently limited and inadequate, and carry with them risk of significant morbidity. New therapeutic modalities for brain tumors are being explored. These include gene therapies and other molecular techniques, localized administration of chemotherapeutic agents (intravascularly or via impregnated polymers), and localized RT using implanted radioisotopes.

SUGGESTED READINGS

1. CBTRUS (2002). Statistical Report: Primary Brain Tumors in the United States, 1995–1999. Published by the Central Brain Tumor Registry of the United States.
2. Packer RJ, Cohen BH, Cooney K. Intracranial germ cell tumors. Oncologist 2000; 5: 312–320.
3. Saran F. Recent advances in paediatric neuro-oncology. Curr Opin Neurol 2002; 15: 671–677.

PATIENT RESOURCES

Children's Brain Tumor Foundation (CBTF) 274 Madison Avenue, Suite 1301, New York, NY 10016, U.S.A. www.cbtf.org

The Childhood Brain Tumor Foundation 20312 Watkins Meadow Drive, Germantown, MD 20876, U.S.A. Tel.:+1-301-515-2900. www.childhoodbraintumor.org

Pediatric Brain Tumor Foundation of the United States, 302 Ridgefield Court, Asheville, NC 28806, U.S.A. Tel.: +1-828-665-6891 www.pbtfus.org

39

Posterior Fossa Tumors of Childhood

Roger J. Packer
Neuroscience and Behavioral Medicine, Division of Child Neurology, Children's National Medical Center, The George Washington University, Washington, D.C., U.S.A.

INTRODUCTION

Childhood brain tumors constitute nearly 20% of all childhood cancers and are the most common form of solid tumor of childhood. The reported incidence of childhood brain tumors is approximately 3.5 cases per 100,000 children per year. The incidence is inversely proportional to age, as most tumors occur in younger children.

One-half of all childhood brain tumors occur in the posterior fossa and are comprised of three major subtypes: medulloblastoma, gliomas, and ependymomas. Posterior fossa tumors are also commonly separated by anatomic site of origin; as an example, cerebellar astrocytomas (which are histologically pilocytic and relatively well localized in 80% of cases) are conventionally separated from brainstem gliomas (which are usually diffuse infiltrating fibrillary tumors arising in the pons). Another histological subtype, the atypical teratoid/rhabdoid tumor, has been described recently and comprises 10–20% of all primitive tumors of the posterior fossa arising in children less than two years of age.

DIAGNOSIS AND EVALUATION

Signs and symptoms of posterior fossa lesions are dependent on the location of the tumor and the age of the patient. In very young children, especially those less than one year of age, symptomatology is notoriously nonspecific. Presentations include lethargy, failure to thrive, and a slowing or retardation of developmental milestones until specific neurologic signs are appreciated. Hydrocephalus associated with downward deviation of the eyes is a frequent presentation for infants with large posterior fossa masses. Obstructive hydrocephalus is present in the majority of children with medulloblastoma, as the tumor fills the fourth ventricle early in the course of illness, whereas patients with brainstem gliomas and laterally placed cerebellar astrocytomas more commonly present with lateralizing or focal neurologic deficits prior to the onset of signs and symptoms of increased intracranial pressure.

With current means of neuroradiographic diagnosis, identification of a posterior fossa tumor is not difficult. Except for diffuse intrinsic brainstem gliomas, surgical conformation is required to determine the exact type of tumor. Surgery also is a critical component of management for most posterior fossa tumors.

Staging has become a mandatory component of the management of medulloblastoma and atypical teratoid tumors and is performed for children with other types of posterior fossa tumors. Appropriate disease staging usually requires MR imaging of the entire brain and spine, (preferably done prior to surgery to avoid postoperative artifact) and postoperative cerebrospinal fluid cytological examination. Molecular genetic changes in the tumor have recently been shown to be predictive of outcome, especially for medulloblastoma, and are presently being prospectively assessed to determine if their incorporation into staging/risk-based stratification will alter management.

TREATMENT

General Considerations

The treatment for childhood brain tumors has not changed dramatically over the past two decades. For most tumors, therapy consists of a combination of surgery, radiation, and chemotherapy. Aggressiveness of treatment is usually based on disease-risk stratification. There is significant reluctance to utilize radiotherapy in very young children with posterior fossa tumors, especially in those less than three years of age; however, with advances in the delivery of radiotherapy, there has been a recent reassessment of the use of focal radiotherapy in young children with relatively localized disease. Surgery followed by chemotherapy is the most common approach for children less than three years if adjuvant therapy is required.

Medulloblastoma

Medulloblastoma comprises approximately 40% of all posterior fossa brain tumors. It is an embryonal small cell tumor that peaks in incidence between the ages of three and five years. Treatment is complicated by the proclivity of medulloblastoma to disseminate within the nervous system early in the course of illness. Approximately one-third of patients have disease spread to other central nervous system sites at the time of diagnosis, most commonly the spine. This incidence is even higher in younger children. Staging is critical for medulloblastoma. A tumor size/metastases (or TM) staging system is most commonly employed based on the impressions of the surgeon at the time of surgery, imaging of the entire neuroaxis (preferably performed before surgery), and postoperative cerebrospinal fluid cytological examination. A variety of molecular markers have also been related to outcome, but they have not yet been prospectively assessed and are not currently a component of stratification schemas. Patients are conventionally stratified into two major risk categories: average risk—those with totally and near-totally resected, nondisseminated tumors; or poor risk—those with disseminated tumors or those with tumors that are only partially resected. Another factor utilized in the staging system with medulloblastoma has been age, as younger children have poorer outcomes.

For children greater than three years of age at diagnosis with average-risk medulloblastoma, treatment consists of postoperative craniospinal and local boost radiotherapy followed by chemotherapy (Fig. 1). The radiotherapy required includes

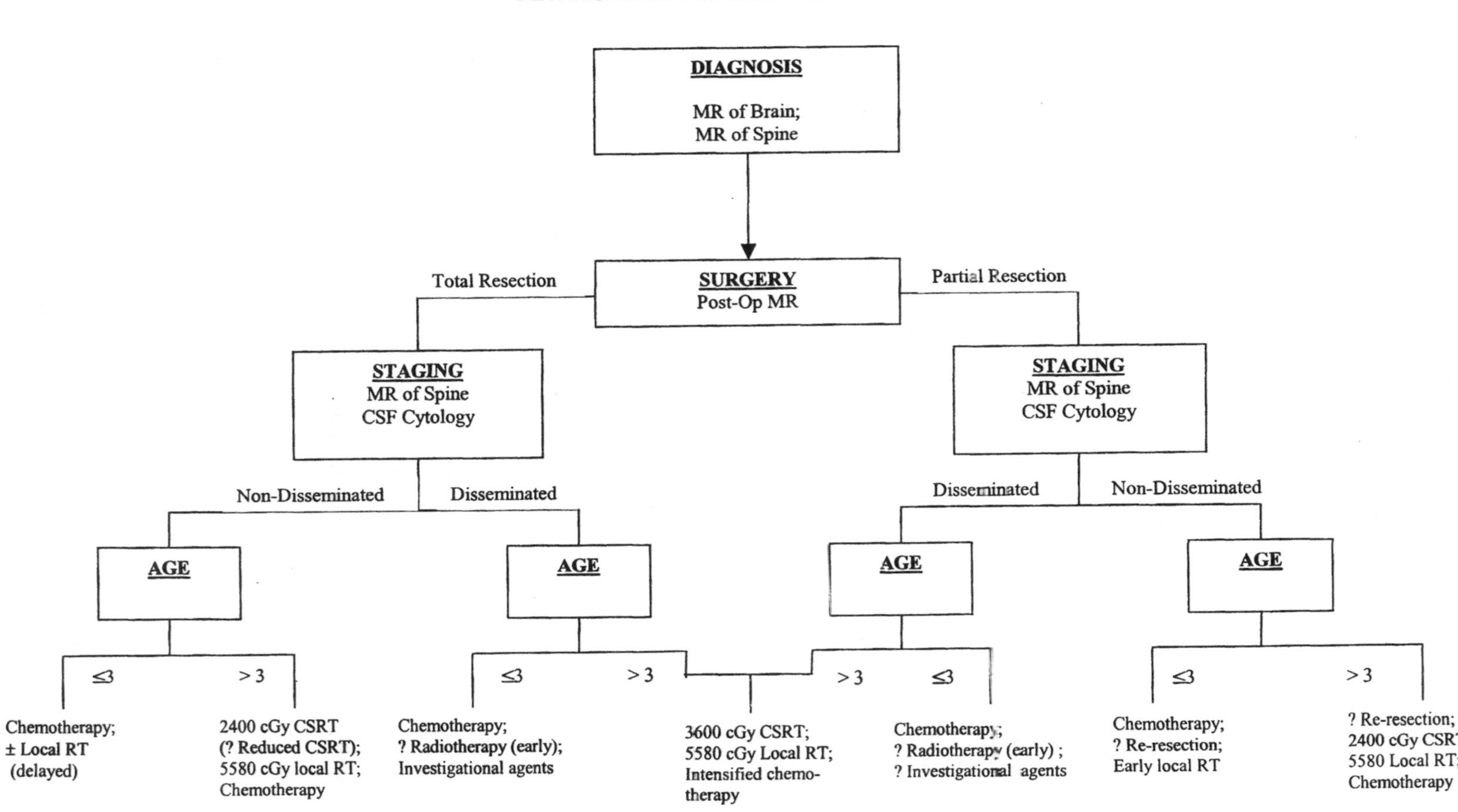

Figure 1 Management of medulloblastoma.

craniospinal radiation therapy to prevent leptomeningeal disease relapse with additional local boost radiotherapy. In the past, conventional doses of craniospinal radiotherapy were 3600 cGy with a local boost of 5400–5600 cGy. After such treatment, without chemotherapy, 50–60% of children with average-risk disease were free of progressive disease five years from diagnosis. The addition of chemotherapy, given during and after radiotherapy, has improved the progression-free survival rate to 80% at five years. Due to concerns over the deleterious effects of cranial irradiation, especially intellectual function, recent studies have decreased the dose of craniospinal radiation therapy to 2400 cGy in children with nondisseminated disease. Preliminary evidence suggests that this will reduce sequelae and result in an equivalent disease control rate as long as chemotherapy is also employed.

The optimal chemotherapeutic regimen to be used with radiotherapy is still under study. The best results have been with vincristine during radiotherapy and a combination of CCNU, vincristine, and cisplatinum after radiotherapy.

For children with poor-risk medulloblastoma, treatment with full-dose craniospinal radiotherapy and chemotherapy results in long-term disease control in between 50% and 65% of patients (Fig. 1). Studies are presently underway evaluating the utility of chemotherapy as a radiosensitizer and the use of higher doses of chemotherapy after radiotherapy, supported by peripheral stem cell rescue.

Children less than three years of age with medulloblastoma remain an extremely challenging subgroup of patients to treat (Fig. 1). There is significant reluctance to utilize craniospinal irradiation therapy due to the risk of long-term sequelae. Treatment approaches have focused on the use of high-dose chemotherapy following surgery in attempts to delay the need for cranial irradiation. Such therapy results in long-term disease control in 20–40% of children with localized disease at the time of diagnosis. High-dose chemotherapy with peripheral stem cell rescue has also been used. Other approaches under study include the use of intrathecal chemotherapy and the earlier introduction of focused radiation therapy to the primary tumor site after chemotherapy.

Long-term sequelae of therapy are a major issue in the treatment of children with medulloblastoma. Complications of surgical therapy of medulloblastoma include the posterior fossa mutism syndrome, which is being increasingly recognized in children following surgery for medulloblastomas. Patients develop the delayed onset (usually 6–24 hr after surgery) of mutism associated with severe cerebellar deficits, hypotonia, supranuclear cranial nerve palsies, and emotional lability. The etiology is unclear. It occurs in up to 20% of children after posterior fossa surgery and one-half of affected children will have permanent sequelae.

Neurocognitive sequelae are common after treatment of medulloblastoma and are related to a variety of factors, including the presence of hydrocephalus at the time of diagnosis and postoperative complications. A primary cause of intellectual compromise is radiotherapy. Studies are underway attempting to reduce the dose of craniospinal radiation therapy in patients without disseminated disease at diagnosis. Radiotherapy also causes delayed permanent endocrine deficts, especially growth hormone deficiency. Decreased linear growth is exacerbated by the effects of radiotherapy on the spine. Growth hormone replacement therapy partially ameliorates this sequela without an increase in tumor relapse. Other long-term problems include acute and delayed ototoxicity secondary to cisplatinum (intensified by the use of concomitant radiotherapy), potential mutagenesis, and sterility.

Treatment for medulloblastoma is a balance between the need to control disease in a tumor that is both sensitive to radiotherapy and chemotherapy and the long-term deleterious effects of treatment. The incorporation of new biologic approaches, especially molecularly targeted therapy based on advances on the understanding of medulloblastoma, promises to dramatically change treatment approaches in the years ahead.

Cerebellar Astrocytomas

Approximately 40% of all posterior fossa tumors in childhood are cerebellar astrocytomas. They usually arise in the cerebellar hemispheres and most commonly present with unilateral cerebellar deficits followed by headaches, nausea, and vomiting as the mass extends to obstruct the fourth ventricle.

The majority of childhood cerebellar astrocytomas are pilocytic astrocytomas. The typical pilocytic cerebellar astrocytoma is characterized as a solid nodule (the so-called "mural nodule") with a large surrounding cyst arising in one cerebellar hemisphere. Treatment with surgery alone is curative in up to 95%. After gross total resections, no adjuvant therapy is required. The majority of recurrences are due to remnants of tumor left after the original surgery and the treatment is resection.

A subgroup of cerebellar astrocytomas tends to be more solid and arises in the midline. They are often more difficult to totally resect, as they may be attached to the brainstem or cerebellar peduncles. Solid cerebellar astrocytomas are also more histologically diverse, with fibrillary tumors as common as pilocytic lesions. Surgery remains the treatment of choice but because of tumor location, other forms of treatment including focal radiotherapy and chemotherapy (in very young children) may be required for disease control.

Brainstem Gliomas

The most common form of childhood brainstem gliomas is a diffuse infiltrating lesion, which usually involves the pons but may also contiguously involve the midbrain and medulla (Table 1). Such lesions may also extend rostrally and caudally. The management of diffuse intrinsic brainstem gliomas has not changed radically over the past 40 years. Surgery has never been shown to be of benefit and most patients are now treated without histological confirmation. MRI is diagnostic in the majority of cases, as findings on biopsy may be misleading and are not helpful in guiding therapy.

Treatment with radiation therapy alone, in doses ranging between 5500 and 6000 cGy, results in transient clinical improvement in majority of patients. However, over 90% of children will develop progressive disease despite radiotherapy and die within 18 months of diagnosis. Alterations in the dose and dose schedule of radiation therapy and the addition of chemotherapy have not altered prognosis. Current studies are evaluating the efficacy of a variety of different drugs, including antineoplastic agents during radiotherapy to act as radiosensitizers.

Approximately 20% of brainstem gliomas may be more focal, with two main subvarieties (Table 1). One subtype occurs in the tectum, usually presenting with hydrocephalus. Patients with tectal tumors have indolent courses and 75% require no treatment for many years other than cerebrospinal fluid diversion. At time of progression, management usually includes biopsy to confirm the type of tumor and either focal radiotherapy or, in young children, chemotherapy.

The second subtype occurs at the cervicomedullary junction and is usually exophytic. It tends to enhance on MR or CT and may be partially cystic. Histologically,

Table 1 Brainstem Gliomas

Tumor type	Location	Symptoms/signs	Treatment	Outcome
Diffuse pontine; intrinsic	Pons; may extend rostral and caudal	Cranial nerve palsies, long tract signs, ataxia; sensory loss	No surgery indicated; local radiotherapy; investigational approaches	90–95% deceased within 18 months of diagnosis
Cervicomedullary	Exophytic from dorsum of medulla	Vomiting, dizziness, nonspecific headaches, ±ataxia	"Gross-total resection" or partial resection plus local radiotherapy or chemotherapy	80% alive 3–5 years after treatment
Tectal	Tectal plate	Headaches, vomiting, long-standing hydrocephalus	± biopsy; local radiotherapy; chemotherapy	Indolent; after ventricular spinal fluid diversion, >75% need no treatment 3–5 years
Focal	Usually pons; cyst with mural nodule	Isolated 6th or 7th nerve palsy	Surgery; radiotherapy or chemotherapy	Majority alive 3–5 years after diagnosis

the majority are pilocytic astrocytomas. Patients commonly present with relatively long histories of nonspecific headaches and vomiting. Later, children may develop lower cranial nerve findings or cerebellar deficits. Long-term disease control has been noted after surgery alone, although extensive resections can result in significant permanent neurologic morbidity. Alternatively, these patients have been treated with partial resection followed by local radiotherapy or chemotherapy. The combination of carboplatin and vincristine chemotherapy has been shown to be effective for patients with partially resected tumors.

Ependymomas

Posterior fossa ependymomas outnumber cortical ependymomas by a ratio of 4:1. Although these tumors may occur in the midline, they often arise in or involve the cerebellopontine angle. Because of this, they are often intertwined with multiple cranial nerves, especially the sixth and seventh cranial nerve, making surgical resection difficult.

Outcomes are primarily dependent on the degree of surgical resection. After gross total resection and focal radiotherapy, five year disease-free survival is 70%, while disease-free survival is between 20% and 40% for children after partial resections. Histology has been related in some studies to outcome, as patients with anaplastic ependymomas do not fare as well as those with benign or cellular ependymomas.

Postoperative focal radiotherapy, ranging in doses between 5500 and 6000 cGy, has been a conventional component of therapy for patients with ependymomas. Patients who undergo total resections may fare well after total resection without any other form of adjuvant therapy. However, the majority of such reports have been in patients with cortical, as opposed to posterior fossa, ependymomas. Local radiotherapy is as effective as craniospinal plus local radiotherapy. Until recently, chemotherapy has not been shown to improve survival for patients with ependymomas. Preliminary data suggest that the addition of chemotherapy prior to radiotherapy improves disease control in patients with partially resected lesions.

Atypical Teratoid/Rhabdoid Tumors

Atypical teratoid/rhabdoid tumors of the central nervous system have been increasingly recognized over the past decade. They most frequently arise in children less than three years of age. Approximately one-half to two-thirds of these tumors arise in the posterior fossa. Dissemination at the time of diagnosis is noted in 30–50% of patients.

These tumors cannot be reliably separated from other tumors on imaging. Since they exhibit histological features consistent with other forms of primitive neuroectodermal tumors and have a population of rhabdoid cells, diagnosis is often difficult. Immunohistochemical analysis is critical, as the rhabdoid regions of the tumor can express epidermal membrane antigen, vimentin, and smooth muscle actin in the majority of cases. Molecular genetic analysis documenting a mutation on chromosome 22 is critical in separating atypical teratoid/rhabdoid tumors from other primitive neuroectodermal tumors of the posterior fossa.

The management of atypical teratoid/rhabdoid tumors is quite challenging. In the majority of patients less than two years of age, treatment with chemotherapy alone or chemotherapy plus local radiotherapy has resulted in disease control in less than 10% of patients. Treatment with chemotherapy followed by early craniospinal and local boost radiotherapy in older patients has been shown to result in a better rate of long-term disease control. The management approaches utilized for patients with poor-risk medulloblastoma are often utilized for children with atypical teratoid/rhabdoid tumors, although recent studies have suggested that an intensification of therapy may be necessary to improve disease control.

PROGNOSIS

Over 75% of children with posterior fossa tumors can be expected to be alive five years from diagnosis, many cured of their disease. Therapy is rapidly evolving and biologic-based treatment is beginning to be incorporated into management. The tumors or their treatment may result in significant long-term sequelae in children with posterior fossa tumors, especially in those requiring radiotherapy.

SUMMARY

Childhood posterior fossa tumors are comprised of five major subtypes—medulloblastoma, cerebellar astrocytoma, ependymoma, brainstem glioma, and atypical teratoid/rhabdoid tumors. Presentation, diagnosis, management, and outcome are dependent on tumor type, age, disease, extent at diagnosis, tumor biology, and treatment.

SUGGESTED READINGS

1. Duffner PK, Horowitz ME, Krischer JP, et al. Postoperative chemotherapy and delayed radiation in children less than three years of age with malignant brain tumors. N Engl J Med 1993; 328:1725–1731.
2. Packer RJ, Ater J, Allen J, et al. Carboplatin and vincristine chemotherapy for children with newly diagnosed progressive low-grade gliomas. J Neurosurg 1997; 86:747–754.
3. Packer RJ, Goldwein J, Nicholson HS, et al. Treatment of children with medulloblastomas with reduced-dose craniospinal radiation therapy and adjuvant chemotherapy: a Children's Cancer Group study. J Clin Oncol 1999; 17:2127–2136.
4. Pollack IF, Polinko P, Albright AL, et al. Mutism and pseudobulbar symptoms after resection of posterior fossa tumors in children: incidence and pathophysiology. Neurosurgery 1995; 37:885–893.
5. Pomeroy SL, Tamayo P, Gaasenbeck M, et al. Prediction of central nervous system embryonal tumour outcome based on gene expression. Nature 2002; 415:436–442.
6. Robertson PL, Zeltzer PM, Boyett JM, et al. Survival and prognostic factors following radiation and chemotherapy for ependymomas in children: a report of the Children's Cancer Group. J Neurosurg 1998; 88:685–694.
7. Rorke LB, Packer RJ, Biegel JA. Central nervous system atypical teratoid/rhabdoid tumors of infancy and childhood: definition of an entity. J Neurosurg 1996; 85:56–65.

40
Congenital Infections and the Nervous System

Lonnie J. Minerand and James F. Bale
Division of Neurology, Department of Pediatrics, The University of Utah School of Medicine, Salt Lake City, U.S.A.

INTRODUCTION

This chapter describes the epidemiology, clinical features, diagnosis, and treatment of congenital infections affecting the central nervous system. In the early 1970s physician scientists at Emory University and the Centers for Disease Control and Prevention introduced the unifying concept of TORCH–an acronym that refers to *Toxoplasma gondii*, Rubella, Cytomegalovirus, and Herpes simplex virus, potential causes of human congenital infection. Although improved laboratory methods have supplanted the original TORCH titers and new pathogens have been added to the list of causes, TORCH remains a useful paradigm, emphasizing that these agents, when acquired in utero, produce similar clinical manifestations in infected infants.

EPIDEMIOLOGY

Viruses

Cytomegalovirus. Cytomegalovirus (CMV), the most common cause of congenital viral infection in developed countries, infects approximately 1% of newborns, usually asymptomatically. Adults and children acquire CMV by direct contact with infected humans. Fetuses become infected during 40% of primary maternal CMV infections.

Rubella. After licensure of the rubella vaccine in 1969 and effective immunization programs, the incidence of the congenital rubella syndrome (CRS) in nations with compulsory rubella immunization declined substantially. Rubella is transmitted by contact with infected aerosols.

Herpes simplex viruses. Herpes simplex virus (HSV) types 1 and 2 affect approximately 1000 infants annually, causing mucocutaneous or invasive disease of neonates and rarely congenital infections. Approximately 5% of neonatal HSV infections represent congenital infections. The HSVs are acquired by direct human contact with infected mucosal surfaces.

Varicella zoster virus. Varicella zoster virus (VZV), the agent of chickenpox (varicella) and shingles (zoster), occasionally causes congenital infection, the fetal varicella syndrome. Women who have chickenpox during the first or second trimester have a 2% risk of delivering an infant with the fetal varicella syndrome. Humans acquire VZV by contact with infected persons or virus-infected aerosols.

Other viral causes. Venezuelan equine encephalitis (VEE) virus, West Nile virus (WNV), lymphocytic choriomeningitis (LCM) virus, and parvovirus B19, the cause of erythema infectiosum (fifth disease), are rare causes of the TORCH syndrome.

Parasites

Toxoplasma gondii. *T. gondii*, an obligate, intracellular protozoan, infects birds and many mammals, especially members of the cat family, worldwide. Humans acquire infection by ingesting meat, fruits, vegetables, and other foodstuffs contaminated by the organism. Approximately 0.1–2% of the adult population acquire *T. gondii* annually, and like CMV, fetal infections complicate approximately 40% of the infections in pregnant women.

Trypanosoma cruzi. The protozoan cause of Chagas' disease, *T. cruzi*, exists endemically throughout Latin America. Congenital infection occurs during maternal parasitemia, but many aspects of the epidemiology and pathogenesis of congenital *T. cruzi* infection have not been determined.

Spirochetes

Treponema pallidum. The overall incidence of congenital syphilis, the consequence of intrauterine infection with *T. pallidum*, is low in the United States, but syphilis remains a threat in urban areas or the rural South. In virtually all other developed countries, congenital syphilis rarely occurs. Untreated maternal infections cause perinatal death, stillbirth, miscarriage, or congenital infection.

CLINICAL MANIFESTATIONS

Viruses

Cytomegalovirus. Approximately 90% of the CMV-excreting newborns have no signs of infection at birth. Infants with symptomatic CMV infections exhibit intrauterine growth retardation, jaundice, hepatosplenomegaly, microcephaly, chorioretinitis, and petechial or purpuric rash.

Rubella. Symptomatic infants with CRS have cataracts, retinopathy, microophthalmia, microcephaly or sensorineural hearing loss, as well as meningoencephalitis, osteopathy, pneumonitis, hepatitis, hepatosplenomegaly, thrombocytopenia, jaundice, myocarditis, patent ductus arteriosus, valvular stenosis, or ventricular or atrial septal defects.

Herpes simplex viruses. Infants with congenital HSV infections have skin lesions at birth, chorioretinitis or cataracts, microphthalmia, and microcephaly or hydranencephaly, and closely resemble neonates with the fetal varicella syndrome.

Varicella zoster virus. Infants with the fetal varicella syndrome have skin lesions, chorioretinitis, microphthalmia, cataracts, paralysis, microcephaly or hydrocephalus, congenital Horner syndrome, and limb hypoplasia. The cicatrix, a characteristic feature of congenital varicella infection, consists of skin scarring and new skin formations that conform to a dermatomal distribution.

Lymphocytic choriomeningitis virus. The clinical features of congenital LCM virus infection mimic those of intrauterine CMV or *T. gondii* infections and include chorioretinopathy, macrocephaly, microcephaly, and vesicular or bullous skin lesions.

Arboviruses (VEE and WNV). Infants infected in utero with VEE virus can be stillborn or have microcephaly, microphthalmia, hydranencephaly, or hemorrhagic lesions of the CNS. Offspring of women infected with WNV during pregnancy can have chorioretinitis and cystic encephalomalacia.

Parvovirus B19. Human parvovirus B19 can infect the fetus and cause red blood cell aplasia, anemia, and cardiac failure. Severe infections are associated with hydrops fetalis, which can cause cerebral hypoperfusion and CNS sequelae.

Parasites

T. gondii. Symptomatic neonates commonly exhibit jaundice, splenomegaly, hepatomegaly, fever, anemia, chorioretinitis, hydrocephalus or microcephaly, and petechiae, secondary to thrombocytopenia.

T. cruzi. Infants with congenital Chagas' disease have hepatosplenomegaly, jaundice, anemia, respiratory distress, seizures, and bony lesions resembling congenital syphilis or CRS.

Spirochetes

T. pallidum. Early signs of congenital syphilis consist of intrauterine growth retardation, rash, hepatosplenomegaly, jaundice, lymphadenopathy, pseudoparalysis, and bony abnormalities such as osteochondritis. Late signs of congenital syphilis include sensorineural deafness, dental abnormalities, saddle nose, saber shins, hydrocephalus, and developmental delay.

DIAGNOSIS

Congenital infections should be suspected in newborn infants with jaundice, hepatosplenomegaly, rash, seizures, macrocephaly, microcephaly, chorioretinitis or cataracts. Certain clinical features, such as head size at birth, skin lesions, and the presence of congenital heart disease, provide useful clues to the specific infectious agent. These features enable construction of diagnostic algorithms (Fig. 1). However, because the agents display considerable overlap in the clinical manifestations, recapitulating the TORCH paradigm, infants with suspected congenital infections require thorough microbiologic evaluations. These infants require ophthalmologic examinations, audiometry, neuroimaging (beginning with CT in the perinatal period), and when CRS is possible, a cardiac evaluation to determine the spectrum and severity of neurologic, ophthalmologic, audiologic, and systemic complications.

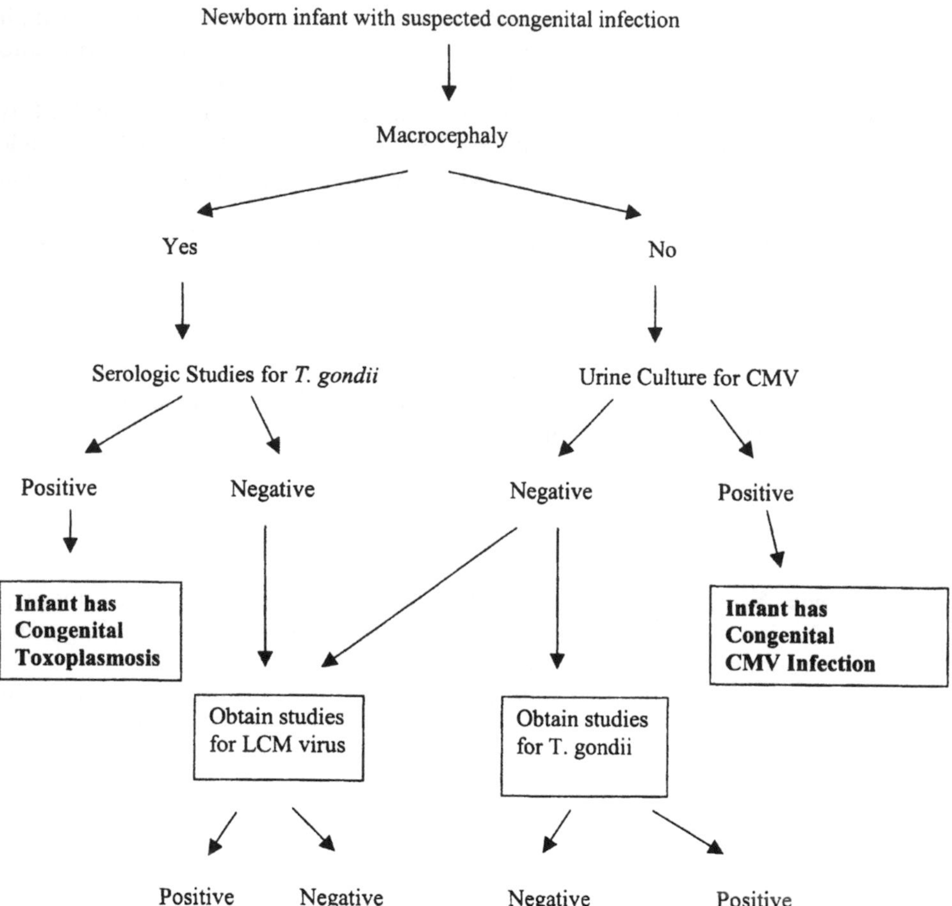

Figure 1 Diagnosis of congenital infections.

Laboratory Features

Laboratory abnormalities compatible with congenital infection include thrombocytopenia, anemia, leukopenia, direct hyperbilirubinemia, and elevations of serum hepatic transaminases. The cerebrospinal fluid can be normal or show a mixed pleocytosis, modestly depressed glucose content, and elevated protein content. Skeletal radiographs during the perinatal period may show osteochondritis in infants with congenital infections due to *T. cruzi*, *T. pallidum*, or rubella virus, and chest radiographs can detect pneumonitis during infections with several agents, including rubella, HSVs, CMV, and *T. cruzi*.

Neuroimaging Features

Intracranial calcifications are the hallmark of intrauterine infections, occurring in infants with congenital infections with CMV, rubella virus, LCM virus, HSV, VZV, *T. gondii*, and *T. cruzi*. Calcifications tend to be periventricular in infants with CMV, rubella, and LCM virus, but can be diffuse in congenital toxoplasmosis or involve the thalamus or basal ganglia symmetrically in congenital HSV and VZV infections. Periventricular leukomalacia commonly accompanies intracranial calcifications in infants with congenital CMV infection and CRS.

Cortical dysplasias, including polymicrogyria or focal dysplasia, and developmental defects, such as lissencephaly-pachygyria, schizencephaly, and agenesis of the corpus callosum, have been reported as a consequence of congenital infections, especially with CMV. These abnormalities reflect the timing of intrauterine infection. Additional abnormalities linked to congenital infection include subependymal (germinal matrix) cysts, cystic encephalomalacia, intraparenchymal hemorrhage, and cerebellar hypoplasia.

Obstructive hydrocephalus occurs commonly in infants with congenital infections with *T. gondii* or LCM virus. Infants infected with the latter virus can have microcephaly in the neonatal period but later show progressive macrocephaly and hydrocephalus requiring shunt placement. Infants with congenital HSV, VZV, VEE virus, and WNV infections can have hydranencephaly or cystic encephalomalacia.

Microbiologic Studies

The diagnosis of intrauterine CMV infection (Table 1) is made by detecting the virus in urine or saliva samples collected during the first three weeks of life. The diagnosis of CRS can be confirmed by detecting infectious virus in body fluids (nasal secretions, urine, or CSF) or rubella virus-specific IgM in the infant's serum. Congenital and neonatal infection with the HSVs can be confirmed by isolating HSV-1 or 2 from the conjunctiva, throat, rectum, circulating leukocytes, CSF, or skin lesions.

Infections with several agents, including VZV, LCM virus, *T. gondii*, *T. cruzi*, and *T. pallidum*, and parvovirus B19, are established by detecting pathogen-specific IgM in the infant's serum. When LCM virus is suspected, serum samples should be sent to the Centers for Disease Control and Prevention for analysis. When *T. gondii* infection is suspected, samples can be sent to Palo Alto Laboratories, Stanford, CA [(650)-853-4828] for a comprehensive panel of serologic markers, including toxoplasma-specific IgG, IgM, IgA, and IgE. Certain pathogens including CMV, *T. gondii*, and VZV can be detected prenatally by sampling the amniotic fluid or fetal cord blood, but such methods may not distinguish symptomatic from asymptomatic fetal infections.

THERAPY AND PROGNOSIS

Infants with congenital infections have variable prognoses that reflect the agent, the timing of infection, the severity of brain involvement, and the availability and efficacy of postnatal therapy. Infants with intracranial calcifications or other neuroimaging abnormalities are more likely to have permanent neurologic sequelae. Because infants and children with several different congenital infections can experience sensorineural hearing loss, audiometry should be obtained in the perinatal period and periodically thereafter into the school years.

Cytomegalovirus. In a prospective, controlled clinical trial of symptomatic newborns with CNS disease or chorioretinitis, ganciclovir given at doses of 8 or 12 mg/kg/day intravenously for 6 weeks reduced viral shedding and had modest beneficial effects on hearing outcomes. The effect of postnatal ganciclovir therapy on long-term neurologic outcomes of CMV-infected infants is unknown,

Table 1 Organisms Causing Congenital Infections and Their Associated Clinical Manifestations

Organism	Clinical manifestations
Cytomegalovirus	Hepatosplenomegaly, jaundice, petechial rash, microcephaly, chorioretintitis, sensorineural hearing loss
Rubella	Hepatosplenomegaly, jaundice, petechial rash, microcephaly, osteopathy, chorioretinopathy, cataracts, sensorineural hearing loss, congenital heart defects
Herpes simplex viruses	Microcephaly, cataracts, vesicular skin rash, cystic encephalomalacia, microphthalmia
Varicella zoster virus	Hydranencephaly, cataracts, microphthalmia, cicatrix, limb hypoplasia, congenital Horner syndrome
LCM[a] virus	Hydrocephalus, microcephaly, chorioretinitis
Arboviruses	Chorioretinitis, hydranencephaly, cystic encephalomalacia
Toxoplasma gondii	Hepatosplenomegaly, jaundice, hydrocephalus, chorioretinitis
Trypanosoma cruzi	Hepatosplenomegaly, jaundice, seizures, osteopathy
Treponema pallidum	*Early:* intrauterine growth retardation, rash, hepatosplenomegaly, jaundice, lymphadenopathy, pseudoparalysis, osteochondritis *Late:* sensorineural deafness, dental abnormalities, saddle nose, saber shins, hydrocephalus
Parvovirus B19	anemia, hydrops fetalis

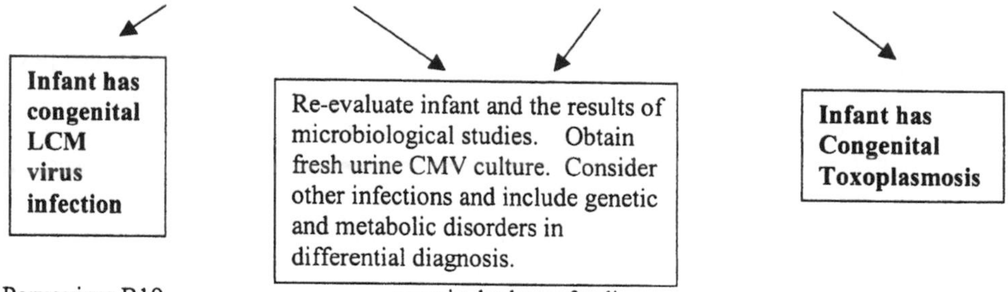

Infant has congenital LCM virus infection

Re-evaluate infant and the results of microbiological studies. Obtain fresh urine CMV culture. Consider other infections and include genetic and metabolic disorders in differential diagnosis.

Infant has Congenital Toxoplasmosis

although one report suggested more favorable outcomes in a small number of treated infants.

Approximately 90% of the infants with symptomatic CMV infections have long-term sequelae affecting development, behavior, intelligence, or hearing. By contrast, infants with asymptomatic congenital CMV infections have low rates of sequelae except for sensorineural hearing loss, a complication affecting approximately 10% of such infants. Although CMV is not highly contagious, pregnant women should not have direct, intimate contact with CMV-infected infants.

Congenital rubella syndrome. Because CRS cannot be treated effectively by postnatal antiviral therapy, prevention through vaccination is essential. All children require rubella virus immunization during early childhood (12–15 months of age) and again at school entry (4–6 years of age). Infants with suspected rubella require standard and droplet precautions (private room; masks, gowns, and gloves for persons having patient contact). Infants with confirmed infections should be considered contagious for at least 12 months, unless nasopharyngeal and urine cultures are negative on serial samples obtained after 3 months of age. Nonimmune pregnant women must not have contact with infants with CRS.

Neurologic sequelae of CRS include microcephaly, language delay, autism, and developmental delays or mental retardation. Progressive sensorineural hearing loss can develop in children who survive CRS. Children with CRS also have increased risks of growth failure or diabetes mellitus beginning in the second or third decades.

Herpes simplex viruses. Infants with suspected HSV infections should receive acyclovir at 60 mg/kg/day intravenously in evenly divided doses every 8 hr. For maximum sensitivity, cultures should be obtained prior to acyclovir treatment, but HSV CSF PCR can remain positive for 24–48 hr or longer after initiation of acyclovir therapy. Although treatment of congenital HSV infections seems prudent, especially when there is uncertainty regarding the timing of infection, there are no data to suggest that acyclovir therapy improves the outcome of infants with congenital HSV infections. Infants with perinatal HSV infections require 21 days of acyclovir therapy. Infants who survive congenital HSV infections have high rates of cerebral palsy, vision loss, epilepsy, and developmental delays. Additional information regarding ongoing trials of antiviral therapy for HSV infections can be obtained from the Collaborative Antiviral Study Group, Birmingham, Alabama [(205) 934-5316].

Varicella zoster virus. There is no effective postnatal therapy for congenital varicella syndrome. By contrast, VZV infections acquired in the perinatal period should be treated with acyclovir using 60 mg/kg/day intravenously in divided doses every 8 hr for 7–14 days. Because of the damaging effects of VZV on the developing brain, infants who survive congenital varicella syndrome commonly have cerebral palsy, developmental delays, vision loss, and epilepsy.

Lymphocytic choriomeningitis virus. There is no effective therapy for congenital LCM virus infection. Infants with congenital LCM virus infection often have severe neurology sequelae consisting of cerebral palsy, vision loss, epilepsy, and developmental delay. Progressive hydrocephalus requires placement of ventriculoperitoneal shunts.

Arboviruses (*VEE and WNV*). None of the currently available antiviral agents has proven efficacy against these viruses, especially when acquired in utero. Although infants with these infections can have severe outcomes with fetal or neonatal death, developmental delay, and cerebral palsy, the numbers of infants with these disorders are too few to determine the precise spectra of outcomes. Public health officials should be consulted when these infections are suspected.

Parvovirus B19. No specific antiviral therapies exist for intrauterine parvovirus infections.

Congenital toxoplasmosis. Infants with proven, symptomatic congenital toxoplasmosis should be treated with prolonged courses of pyrimethamine and sulfadiazine. Although opinions differ regarding the duration of therapy, an appropriate regimen consists of one year of pyrimethamine, 1 mg/kg/day orally every 2–3 days, and sulfadiazine, 100–200 mg/kg/day orally every day. Folinic acid, 5–10 mg orally three times per week, should be provided concurrently. Prenatal diagnosis allows maternal antitoxoplasma therapy, using agents such as spiramycin, an antitoxoplasma drug available from the manufacturer, Rhône-Poulenc Rorer.

Aggressive antitoxoplasma therapy and neurosurgical intervention appear to reduce the likelihood of permanent neurodevelopmental sequelae of intrauterine toxoplasmosis. In one trial, 79% of treated infants had mental development within the normal range, and children with hydrocephalus responded favorably to shunt placement. Infants with high CSF protein and venticulomegaly ("hydrocephalus ex vacuo") have less favorable prognoses.

Trypanosoma cruzi. Nifurtimox or benznidazole is used to treat active Chagas' disease in children or adults, and benznidazole has been used to treat infants infected in utero. In one report infants received benznidazole 7 mg/kg BID for 60 days. Infants who survive congenital Chagas' disease can have cerebral palsy, epilepsy, and developmental delay.

Treponema pallidum. Neonates with proven or highly suspected, symptomatic congenital syphilis require aqueous crystalline penicillin G 50,000 U/kg intravenously every 12 hr during the first week of life and every 8 hr thereafter for a total of 10 days. Alternatively, procaine penicillin G can be given intramuscularly at a dose of 50,000 U/kg once a day for 10 days. Infectious disease experts should be consulted regarding current treatment strategies for infants whose mothers received inadequate treatment, infants with asymptomatic infections, or infants older than 4 weeks with possible syphilis and neurologic involvement. Should penicillin G not be available, alternative treatment recommendations can be found at www.cdc.gov/nchstp/dstd/penicillinG.htm/.

SUGGESTED READINGS

1. Bale JF Jr. Congenital infections. Neuro Clin 2002; 20:1039–1060.
2. Committee on Infectious Diseases. 2003 Red Book: Report of the Committee on Infectious Disease. 25th ed. American Academy of Pediatrics, 2003.
3. Gregg NM. Congenital cataract following German measles in the mother. Trans Ophthal Soc Aust 1941; 3:35–41.
4. Grose C. Congenital infections caused by varicella zoster virus and herpes simplex virus. Semin Pediatr Neurol 1994; 1:43–49.
5. Hollier LM, Cox SM. Syphilis. Semin Perinatol 1998; 22:323–331.
6. Reef SE, Plotkin S, Cordero JF, et al. Preparing for elimination of congenital rubella syndrome (CRS). Summary of a workshop on CRS elimination in the United States. Clin Infect Dis 2000; 31:85–95.
7. www.cdc.gov/ncidod/dvbid/westnile/clinical_guidance.htm.

41
Meningitis

Charlotte Jones
Joan C. Edwards School of Medicine, Marshall University, Huntington, West Virginia, U.S.A.

INTRODUCTION

Meningitis, specifically bacterial meningitis, remains a major concern for physicians treating children because of the high mortality if untreated, as well as the significant morbidity even when diagnosed and treated early. With the development of the *Haemophilus influenzae* vaccine, there has been a striking decrease in the number of pediatric meningitis victims. Meningitis is defined as the occurrence of inflammation of the meninges, evidenced by increased cells in the cerebrospinal fluid (CSF), and the simultaneous identification of infection from CSF or blood culture. It is worth remembering that bacteria, particularly *Neisseria meningitidis*, may be isolated from CSF even though it appears normal.

ETIOLOGY

In neonates, there has been a decrease in Group B *Streptococcal* early infections as a result of maternal pretreatment. However, the late infection (defined as over 7 days postpartum), usually associated with meningitis, continues to occur and is unaffected by maternal pretreatment with ampicillin since the organism is not transmitted vertically during delivery as is the early infection. Gram-negative bacteria and *Listeria* are the other frequent causative agents in this age group.

Beyond the neonatal age, *Streptococcus pneumoniae* and *N. meningitidis* are the most common causative agents of bacterial meningitis. Although bacterial meningitis is the greatest concern, most cases of meningitis are due to viral infections, with enteroviruses causing up to 95% of aseptic meningitis. The majority of other viral agents (excluding the nonpolio enteroviruses but including the arboviruses), herpes viruses, measles, mumps, rubella, and West Nile are more likely to present as meningoencephalitis rather then meningitis. *Borrelia burgdorferi*, Rickettsiae, and *Ehrlichia* species may cause a pure meningitis and should be considered in the setting of tick bite, summer and fall infection, and appropriate geographic location. Fungal infections are more common in the immunocompromised patient, but even normal children should be evaluated for such in the case of an uncharacteristic meningitis picture, especially of a chronic nature. *Mycobacteria tuberculosis* meningitis remains a rare but serious disease in both developing and developed countries. Children are infected by adolescents and adults with disease and may present with meningeal disease as the predominant symptom.

PATHOGENESIS

The pathogenesis of typical childhood bacterial meningitis follows a predictable pattern. Initially, invasion occurs across the respiratory tract with bacteria entering the blood stream, then entry into the central nervous system (CNS) across the blood–brain barrier. The presence of bacteria in the brain results in alteration in blood flow secondary to cerebral edema, vasospasm, and thrombosis, all of which can lead to brain injury. Additional brain injury occurs from inflammatory mediators, free radicals, and the toxic effects of excessive excitatory amino acid production.

Children with immunodeficiencies, shunts, recent neurosurgical procedures, CSF leaks, and congenital heart disease may have a different initiating event than that described above. In these children there is an increased risk of meningitis; aggressive evaluation and treatment are mandated.

DIAGNOSIS

The classic triad for meningitis of fever, headache, and neck stiffness is frequently absent in children. Even in adults it has been found that, in patients with less then 1000 cells/mm^3 in CSF, the sensitivity and specificity of Kernig's and Brudzinski's signs and nuchal rigidity are quite low. For neonates, a suspicion of meningitis should be raised if the infant demonstrates temperature instability, apnea, irritability, poor feeding, respiratory distress, diarrhea, or a bulging fontanelle. The American Academy of Pediatrics (AAP) recommends lumbar punctures (LPs) after febrile seizures in children less than 12 months of age, due to the nonspecific findings of meningitis in this age group. In the older child, headache, fever, neck stiffness or pain, alteration in consciousness, vomiting, focal neurological findings, and seizures (often focal) are the most frequent signs and symptoms of meningitis. Bacterial meningitis may progress rapidly within hours, proceed at a more moderate pace, or insidiously worsen over days. A positive LP is the gold standard for confirming meningitis, as it allows identification of the organisms involved and may allow early customizing of treatment based on Gram stain results. Early treatment of meningitis should be the primary goal. However, if the LP is to be delayed while awaiting a CT scan or postponed altogether, antibiotic treatment should be initiated immediately. The CT scans are indicated in the setting of focal neurologic signs or insignificantly depressed consciousness. In the absence of these signs, it is not required before proceeding to LP. A normal CT scan does not guarantee that intracranial pressure (ICP) is not increased. An LP should not be performed in the presence of worsening levels of consciousness, posturing, papilledema, pupillary changes, or any other sign of incipient herniation. Seizure and fever are rarely the only signs of meningitis; however, if additional indications point towards meningitis, the LP should at least be delayed 30 min after short seizures and postponed or deferred after longer seizures. This is to decrease the risk of herniation resulting from increased blood flow and ICP during seizures.

Table 1 CSF Findings in Meningits

	Bacterial	Viral	Mycobaterial
CSFcell count	500–10,000	>6–500	>6–1000
Predominant WBC cell type	PMNs[a]	Lymphocytes[b]	Lymphocytes
Protein	Elevated	Normal-Mildly Elevated	Elevated
CSF:Serum Glucose ratio	Decreased	Normal	Decreased

[a] PMNs = polymorphonuclear cells.
[b] Polymorphonuclear cells may predominate initially in viral infections.
Adapted data from Kaplan (1), Rotbart (2), and Starke (3).

The LP is contraindicated in the setting of an uncorrected bleeding disorder or if infection is present that could be introduced into deeper locations with the procedure.

Antibiotics can result in sterilization of CSF, a negative Gram stain, and normalization of glucose within minutes to hours but the pleocytosis and protein changes will remain evident for at least 48 hr. The advantages of early treatment cannot be overstressed; however, if suspicion is low or an LP can be performed safely and expeditiously, the value of a positive culture with the ability to determine antibiotic susceptibility outweighs immediate treatment.

While culture is the gold standard for identifying the etiology of meningitis, the initial CSF may help distinguish between bacterial and viral meningitis. Bacterial meningitis is usually associated with a significant (>1000 cells/mm^3) pleocytosis with a polymorphonuclear predominance, elevated protein (>80 mm/dL in the non-neonate), and decreased CSF serum glucose ratio (< 0.6 and often as low as 0.2). Viral meningitis is usually associated with a cell count of less then 300 cells/mm^3, normal protein and normal glucose, and a lymphocytic predominance. Early results may show polymorphonuclear cell predominance. However, while predictive models to distinguish between bacterial and viral infections are being developed, the most common practice in the United States is for a 48–72 hr course of antibiotics in the presence of meningitis (defined as more than 6 cells/mm^3 in the CSF in non-neonates or 22 cells/mm^3 in the neonate) until bacterial cultures become negative. Enterovirus PCR may shorten hospitalizations in those institutions that can provide test results in a rapid manner by confirming a nonbacterial source of the meningitis and allowing earlier discharge before bacterial cultures are final. Tubercular meningitis usually presents with a clinical course progressing over weeks, a CSF WBC count in the range of 500 cells/mm^3, very low glucose, and elevated protein with a lymphocytic predominance. The article by Starke provides a thorough review on TB meningitis. Table 1 summarizes the CSF findings in various forms of meningitis.

TREATMENT

Empiric therapy for bacterial meningitis should not be delayed for diagnostic studies. Appropriate empiric treatment should be started based on the age of the patient and the patterns of resistance in the area from which the patient acquired the infection. As an example, *S. pneumoniae* can have resistance rates as high as 40% to penicillins; in that case, vancomycin would be the first choice for coverage, rather than cephalosporins alone. This information is readily available from local microbiology labs or Departments of Health in respective cities, counties, and states. For the neonatal age group, I use ampicillin and either and aminoglycoside such as gentamicin or a third generation cephalosporin, such as cefotaxime. Doses are dictated by the infant's gestational age, chronologic age, and weight. They can be found in a variety of neonatal texts. For children over the age of 3 months, I recommend coverage with vancomycin (15 mg/kg every 6 hr, up to a maximum dose of 2 g per day) and a third generation cephalosporin, such as ceftriaxone (50 mg/kg every 12 hr, up to a maximum of 4 g per day). Later adjustment of antibiotic choices should be made based on Gram stains and, ultimately, isolation of the organism and its antibiotic susceptibility. To decrease the risk of drug resistance, vancomycin should be discontinued promptly if bacterial susceptibilities allow it.

Dexamethasone use has been shown to be beneficial in reducing hearing loss in children with *H. influenzae* meningitis. It may also prevent hearing loss in *S. pneumoniae* meningitis if given prior to antibiotic administration. A recent Cochrane review concluded that steroids are beneficial for children with acute meningitis. Other analyses focusing on the most recent studies have been less emphatic in their conclusion of benefit. Experts remain divided on treatment, as noted by the AAP's Red Book statements on dexamethasone use. Theoretical concerns based on animal studies suggest that steroid use may decrease vancomycin entry into the CSF, although this has not been seen clinically. If steroids are to be used, they should be used at least 30 min prior to or at least concurrently with the first dose of antibiotics so that the benefit of decreasing inflammation triggered by bacterial death can be gained. A reasonable course of treatment would be a dose of 0.6 mg/kg/day of dexamethasone for 2 days. As a neurologist, I am rarely consulted until long after the effectiveness of steroids is gone.

Coverage for other causes of meningitis, such as herpes simplex, Lyme, and tuberculosis, is covered in the chapter on Encephalitis.

PROGNOSIS

Mortality in neonates is reported as 10% in developed countries with up to 1/3 of survivors suffering long-term sequelae including hearing loss, cortical blindness, cerebral palsy, and mental retardation. In older children, mortality is between 2% and 5% in developed countries while morbidity is 10–20%. Increased risk of poor outcome is associated with infection with *S. pneumoniae*, presence of coma, focal seizures or seizures continuing more then 72 hr after treatment, or CSF glucose less then 20. Major morbidity includes severe mental retardation, hydrocephalus, blindness, and the most common serious side effect, deafness.

With continuing research and clinical work, we hope the next version of this book will be able to recommend agents to treat viral meningitis and further eradication of bacterial meningitis with broadly effective vaccines against *S. pneumoniae* and *N. meningitidis*.

SUMMARY

The management of meningitis is continuously evolving due to advances in immunization and emerging changes in resistance patterns for various organisms. The signs of meningitis may be subtle, depending on both the patient and the organism.

Lumbar puncture remains the gold standard for diagnosis but should not be delayed for effective therapy. Initial selection of antibiotics should be based on local resistance patterns and then narrowed based on the organism's sensitivity pattern.

REFERENCES

1. Kaplan SL. Clinical presentations, diagnosis, and prognostic factors of bacterial meningitis. Infect Dis Clin North Am 1999; 13:579–594.
2. Rotbart H. Viral meningitis. Semin Neurol 2000; 20:277–292.
3. Starke J. Tuberculosis of the central nervous system in children. Semin Pediatr Neurol 1999; 6:318–331.

SUGGESTED READINGS

1. Kanegaye JT, Soliemandzadeh P, Bradley JS. Lumbar puncture in pediatric bacterial meningitis: defining the time interval for recovery of cerebrospinal fluid pathogens after parenteral antibiotic pretreatment. Pediatrics 2001; 108:1169–1174.
2. Oostenbrink R, Moons, KGM, Donders ART, Grobbee DE, Moll HA. Prediction of bacterial meningitis in children with meningeal signs: reduction of lumbar punctures. Acta Paediatr 2001; 90:611–617.
3. Pickering LK, ed. Red Book 2003: Report of the Committee on Infectious Diseases. 26th ed. Elk Grove Village, IL: American Academy of Pediatrics, 2003.
4. Polin RA, Harris MC. Neonatal bacterial meningitis. Semin Neonatol 2001; 6:157–172.

42

Treatment of Pediatric Neurological Disorders: Encephalitis

Fiona Goodwin and Colin Kennedy
Department of Pediatric Neurology, Child Health, University of Southampton and Southampton University Hospitals, Southampton, U.K.

INTRODUCTION

Encephalitis is inflammation of the brain parenchyma. Its cardinal clinical manifestations, occurring singly or in combination, are headache, fever, altered consciousness, and focal neurological deficits. The inflammatory process may be generalized throughout the brain or restricted to focal involvement. It may also involve the meninges. The diversity of clinical features reflects these patterns of involvement and a particular clinical picture is seldom specific to an individual infectious agent. Encephalitis is often an unusual manifestation of a common infection. This leads to variation in the relationship between the systemic infection and the neurological illness because individual agents vary in their propensity for CNS involvement and the prognosis of the neurological illness. The pathogenesis of encephalitis is heterogeneous even for a single infectious agent and may follow an acute, subacute, or chronic course. This chapter will be limited to discussing infective causes. Prion disease, metabolic or toxic encephalitides, postinfectious demyelinating disease, and encephalitis in immunodeficiency, including that caused by HIV infection, are not discussed in this chapter.

DIAGNOSIS

Encephalitis is a generic term associated with numerous infective etiologies. A specific infectious agent may be suggested by geographical, environmental, and seasonal factors in the history or clinical features on examination. Rarely, however, can a specific causative infection be identified on clinical grounds alone. The diagnosis of encephalitis is, strictly speaking, histological but with the exception of HSV1 infection, has usually been based only upon assessment of clinical features and exclusion of other possibilities leaving the pathogenesis and even the diagnosis in doubt.

The importance of antibody serology as a diagnostic tool in this context is often underestimated. Furthermore, its diagnostic potential is frequently not realized because of failure to collect convalescent samples. Acute phase samples are required to detect elevated concentration of specific IgM and both acute and convalescent samples for detection of a fourfold rise in serum IgG titers. Its value in guiding treatment is limited by the delay, until convalescence in most cases, of definitive diagnostic information.

CSF analysis is central to diagnosis but may be contraindicated by clinical or imaging evidence of raised intracranial pressure. CSF pleocytosis has been reported in between one-third and two-thirds of reported series of consecutive cases of encephalitis. A nonspecific increase in CSF protein level may be seen in an additional percentage but the etiological agent can only be established with certainty by additional laboratory investigations. Meticulous collection of appropriate samples (CSF, throat swab, blood, stool, and urine) for viral and bacterial culture and serology enabled a diagnosis of a specific infectious agent to be made in around 80% of a large reported series cases of encephalitis of presumed viral etiology. In clinical practice, less than half of this yield of diagnoses would be typical.

Viral culture of CSF is rarely positive but techniques to identify specific viral amino-acid sequences, such as polymerase chain reaction (PCR), are highly sensitive and specific, with the possibility of simultaneous screening for multiple infectious agents now available. As with serological testing, CSF antibody analysis is most sensitive in the convalescent period (peaking around 6 weeks after infection). It is most reliably interpreted in relation to serum antibody levels using the specific antibody ratio, which is a comparison of the CSF-to-serum ratio of specific antiviral IgG antibody with that of total IgG. If the fraction of specific antiviral IgG in the CSF exceeds the fraction of total IgG in the CSF by more than 1.4 to 1, intrathecal antibody synthesis is probable. This test has proved both sensitive and specific in the diagnosis of HSV-1 encephalitis applied to CSF obtained more than 10 days after the onset of the illness. The CSF IgG index, another measure of intrathecal IgG synthesis, is a comparison of the CSF-to-serum ratios of total IgG and albumin. Elevation of the ratio supports intrathecal IgG synthesis, but, unlike the specific IgG ratio, cannot be used to confirm the relevance of a specific agent to the neurological illness.

EEG changes will corroborate evidence of an encephalopathic process but with the exception of subaute sclerosing panencephalitis (SSPE) and herpes encephalitis are not usually helpful in identifying a specific aetiology. Cranial imaging with CT is often normal in encephalitis but usually performed as an integral part of assessing a patient with acute encephalopathy. MR imaging may show diffuse or focal edema; focal changes in specific brain areas can be suggestive of particular infections (see below).

BRIEF DESCRIPTION OF DISEASE AND TREATMENT

Supportive Care

The initial treatment of a patient with acute encephalitis involves supportive measures and symptomatic treatment with intensive care management if necessary. Seizure and temperature control, avoidance of electrolyte imbalance, maintenance of cerebral perfusion pressure, and treatment of systemic dysfunction are common issues in clinical management.

Compared to other acute encephalopathies, the pathologic process in encephalitis is often temporary or reversible so that an excellent recovery is possible in some cases despite an illness that is very acute and severe. Attention to the details of supportive care of patients at their nadir is therefore critical. The value of steroid treatment has not been subjected to systematic scientific evaluation but has a clear rationale for use in parainfectious, as opposed to invasive, viral disease.

Prompt initiation of intravenous acyclovir is mandatory once a diagnosis of encephalitis is suspected, with empirical treatment continued until a diagnosis of herpes infection is excluded. HSV encephalitis is the only example of viral encephalitis in which there is a well-established evidence that neurological outcome is improved by specific antiviral treatment after the onset of neurological symptoms.

Herpes Viruses

HSV-1 and -2 are common infections but only rarely do they involve the CNS. HSV-1 is nevertheless the commonest cause of nonepidemic focal infective encephalitis in the USA and untreated has a high mortality and morbidity. It causes focal encephalitis with a predilection for temporal structures, which is often but not always reflected in clinical features, EEG (periodic sharp waves in the temporal leads in the later stages), and MR imaging abnormalities in the temporal lobes. CSF PCR and/or convalescent CSF antibodies are important since serum antibody concentrations can be unhelpful. Viral DNA studies have shown HSV encephalitis occurring due to HSV strains other than the original infection in HSV seropositive individuals.

Early initiation of treatment with acyclovir has been shown to reduce greatly the mortality and morbidity of HSV encephalitis. Delays beyond 4 days from the onset of neurological symptoms decrease its effectiveness. Recommended regimes for HSV-1 encephalitis are $500\,mg/m^2$ or $10\,mg/kg$ 8 hourly for 14 days intravenously in immunocompetent patients. Relapse following completion of acyclovir treatment has been reported as more likely to occur with lower dose regimes of shorter duration. Some studies recommend continuing treatment for 21 days to minimize risk of relapse, but the evidence for this is not yet strong.

Neonatal HSV encephalitis is usually due to HSV-2 acquired during delivery from a mother with genital herpes. After 3 months of age, HSV encephalitis is almost exclusively due to HSV-1. Treatment of neonatal infection is covered in Chapter 40 (Congenital Infections and the Nervous System).

New antiherpetic agents, such as ganciclovir, vidarabine, cidofovir, valaciclovir, and famciclovir, have an established role in the treatment of non-CNS herpes infection but not in the treatment of immunocompetent patients with encephalitis and acyclovir remains the treatment of choice. Acyclovir resistance is emerging in HIV-positive patients. This may impact on future treatment of the general population. Special considerations apply in the treatment of HSV encephalitis in immunocompromised patients but are beyond the scope of this chapter.

Other herpes encephalitides caused by varicella, cytomegalovirus, human herpes virus 6 (the infective agent in roseola infantum), and Epstein–Barr virus are usually benign and do not require antiviral therapy for an immunocompetent host. Herpes B encephalitis is a severe and often rapidly fatal infection transmitted from the Macaque monkey. Management guidelines by the Herpes B 1994 working group include advice regarding wound cleaning, appropriate investigation, prophylaxis, and treatment with acyclovir or ganciclovir.

Measles Virus

Measles infection is said to be responsible for 1% of deaths from all causes worldwide. Although the majority of these deaths are attributable to other complications, neurologic involvement is common. Encephalomyelitis affects 1 in 1000 cases of measles and is not always accompanied by a rash. Acute inclusion body encephalitis, in which viral replication is prominent, and demyelinating postinfectious encephalitis can be clinically indistinguishable.

Subacute sclerosing panencephalitis is due to latent persistence of a mutant measles virus infection. No adequate therapy is currently available for SSPE, which is usually fatal within 3 years. Several agents have been suggested to modify the disease course. Isinoprine and interferon alpha are immune modulators that have been reported to stabilize or improve clinical symptoms but are not yet an established treatment. Combination therapies with ribavarin and triexyphenidyl may be beneficial. Immunoglobulins, plasmapharesis, steroids, and cimetidine have been tried in clinical practice with limited success.

Arboviruses

These enveloped RNA viruses cause a variety of geographically specific encephalitides transmitted by mosquitoes, sandflies, or ticks. Worldwide, Japanese B encephalitis is the greatest cause of death with 30,000 to 50,000 cases, mostly in young healthy children. It is rare in the USA, where Eastern Equine encephalitis is the least benign of the arboviruses commonly seen.

Rabies

Rabies, a rhabdovirus, is transmitted following an infected animal bite or exposure to respiratory aerosols of the virus in caves housing bat colonies. Domestic animals rarely carry the virus in Western Europe and the USA but in parts of South America, Africa and Asia, dogs remain a common vector of the disease. If clinical disease develops following exposure, it is almost invariably fatal. Vaccination is available for high-risk individuals and a combination of human immunoglobulin and rabies vaccine given after exposure can decrease the incidence of clinical disease. The diagnosis is made by PCR examination of saliva or tissue biopsy of brain, cornea, or nuchal skin to detect viral proteins. Lyssavirus causes a rabies-like infection and is transmitted to humans from bats.

Bacterial, Rickettsial, Parasitic, and Fungal Encephalitis

These agents can all cause acute encephalitis, whose treatment is summarized in Table 1. Regional variations in antimicrobial resistance may alter recommended first line treatments from those listed.

PUBLIC HEALTH MEASURES AND PREVENTION

Globally, mosquitoes and tics are important vectors of viral encephalitides, such as Japanese B and West Nile Encephalitis. In the absence of new developments in antiviral therapies, the control of host reservoirs and intermediate vectors has become

Table 1 Bacterial, Rickettsial, Fungal, and Parasitic Infections Causing Encephalitis

Bacterial infection	Specific features	Treatment
Brucella	Transmitted primarily from cattle and goats or unpasteurized milk. Fever and systemic illness, CNS involvement rare. Meningoencephalitis, cerebellar syndrome, neuritis. Diagnosis by classical serum agglutination test or specific CSF antibodies	< 6 years: rifampin + streptomycin or gentamicin or + cotrimoxazole > 7 years: doxycycline + streptomycin or gent Immunization of cattle and milk pasteruization important
Bartonella (Rochalimaea) Henselae. Cat scratch fever	Lymphadenopathy and granuloma formation. CNS involvement uncommon	Ciprofloxacin, cotrimoxazole, rifampicin, or erythromycin
Mycoplasma pneumoniae	Agitation, respiratory infection, ADEM	Azithromycin or tetracycline
Legionella	Pneumonia. Seizures, confusion	Azithromycin/rifampin
Salmonella typhi	"Typhoid fever" with acute diarrheal illness. Confusion, hallucination, and psychosis	Cefotaxime or ceftriaxone
Nocarida—actinomycetes	Acute or chronic suppurative disease. Respiratory disease, disseminated infection One third have CNS involvement, meningoencephalitic illness/multiple abscesses	Sulfonamides/amikacin
Campylobacter	Enteritis/acute colitis. Subdural collections; hemorrhagic stroke	Ciprofloxacin or erythromycin
Listeria monocytogenes	Encephalitis common. Brainstem involvement and abscess formation. Neonates, pregnant women, and immunosuppressed patients most susceptible to infection	Ampicillin +/− gentamicin. Cotrimoxazole if penicillin allergic
Mycobacterium tuberculosis	Meningoencephalitis/tuberculomas. Risk of paradoxical inflammatory response after starting treatment	Quadruple therapy; local guidelines. Steroid adjunct therapy
Borrelia burgdorferi Lyme disease	Tick-borne spirochete infection. Erythema migrans rash. Bilateral VII palsies common. Peripheral neuritis	Doxycycline, amoxicillin or ceftriaxone
Tropheryma whippeli. Whipples disease	Cognitive deterioration with cerebellar syndrome and hypersomnolence. CNS symptoms predominate;	Trimethoprim, ceftriaxone, or penicillin and streptomycin. May need adjunct steroids

(Continued)

Table 1 Bacterial, Rickettsial, Fungal, and Parasitic Infections Causing Encephalitis (*Continued*)

Bacterial infection	Specific features	Treatment
	joint or GI involvement. Rare in children	Long-term antibiotic therapy used to prevent relapse
Rickettsial infection	Includes Mountain spotted fever, endemic typhus, epidemic typhus, Q fever, human monocytic ehrlichiosis	Doxycycline, chloramphenicol, or fluoroquinolone
	Mite, louse, and tick vectors. Invade and multiply in vascular endothelium, vasculitic disease. Myalgia common; rash characteristic in Rocky mountain fever	
Parasitic infection	Associated with eosinophilia/eosinophilic meningitis	
Malaria. *Plasmodium falciparum*	Diagnostic criteria for cerebral malaria: altered consciousness, unable to localize pain; parasitaemia with *P. Falciparum;* exclusion of other causes. Seizures common; hypoglycemia in 30%. Twenty percent residual disability, 40% mortality	IV Quinine if suspected chloroquine resistance. Combination with pyrimethamine and sulphadoxine may improve parasitic clearance
Echinococcus granulosa. Hydatid disease	Common in hill sheep farming areas. Slow growing cysts; symptoms of raised ICP	Surgical resection, albendazole or mebendazole
Neurocystercercosis	Characteristic ring lesions on CT. Serum antibodies useful. Seizures common	See chapter on neurocystercercosis
Human African trypanosomiasis. "Sleeping Sickness"	Transmitted by tsetse flies. Anemia, lymphadenopathy, endocarditis, and vasculitis followed by stage II CNS spread Progressive somnolence, agitation, and movement disorder	Eflornithine, pentamidine, tryparsamide, and suramine. Melarsoprol also used but may need adjunct steroid therapy to prevent drug-induced encephalopathy
Naegleria fowleri	Rare. Freshwater organism. Nasal inoculation and spread along olfactory mucosa. Purulent leptomeningitis;	Amphotericin B

	severe haemorrhage/ oedema in cortical grey matter. Altered taste/smell precedes neurological deterioration	
Schistosomiasis	Encephalitis with spinal cord involvement-granulomas, transverse myelitis, radiculitis	Niridazole, praziquantel
Mycotic Infection	Usually opportunistic, following prolonged antibiotic use, immunosuppression or shunt in situ. Granulomas and abscess formation common	Amphotericin B
Cryptococcosis	Acute or insidious onset. Malaise, confusion and headache; cranial nerve palsies, hydrocephalus common; fever uncommon	Amphotericin B, flucytosine. Risk of raised ICP may need surgical intervention
	Granulomatous arachnoiditis. Difficult to culture; CSF antigen useful. High mortality; blindness and deafness common in survivors	
Histoplasmosis	Usually disseminated from respiratory disease. Insidious onset, confusion and cognitive decline. Antibody serology for diagnosis	Amphotericin B
Candida Albicans	Microabscesses, granulomas and vasculitis	Amphotericin B and 5-Fluorocytosine
Coccidiomycosis	Associated with disseminated systemic infection. Antibody serology for diagnosis	Amphotericin B, fluconazole
Blastomycosis	Multiple pyogranulomas. Pulmonary disease, skin lesions, arthritis. CNS involved as complication of late disease	Amphotericin B

Readers should be mindful of the need to discuss therapies with microbiologists before starting treatment since all of these infections are uncommon and first line therapies could change.

increasingly important. Epidemiological surveillance of birds, mosquitoes, and other vectors enables activation of specific public health interventions, such as mosquito control programs, during anticipated high-risk periods. Public awareness is also important in encouraging risk-avoiding behaviors. Vaccination is available against several viruses responsible for encephalitis, either on population vaccination programs or for individuals at high exposure risk. Measles vaccination has been reported not to be associated with a risk of encephalitis, vaccinated populations having a "background rate" of encephalitis of 1.8 per million. Rabies vaccine is used only for high-risk contacts. Vaccination against HSV-2 is under trial and results are encouraging but not yet available for widespread use.

PROGNOSIS

The morbidity and mortality associated with encephalitis is determined primarily by the underlying infective cause. Some infections have a notoriously poor outcome with high mortality and neurological morbidity of survivors, including rabies, Japanese B, untreated HSV, and Eastern Equine encephalitis. Mumps and chickenpox encephalitis are usually benign infections with few sequelae. Acyclovir has significantly reduced both mortality and severe neurological disability following HSV encephalitis. Mortality is now 28% overall for treated HSV encephalitis with the greatest benefit seen in those treated early. Long-term follow up for acyclovir treated patients suggests that although the majority of survivors live independently, rigorous testing identifies cognitive deficits and behavioral changes in most. Memory impairment, consistent with bilateral temporal lobe involvement, is often under-recognized as a clinical problem.

Clinical factors at presentation can be used to predict poor outcome, even if the underlying infection is not identified. Age less than 3 years, a modified Glasgow Coma Score of less than 9, abnormal oculocephalic responses, and abnormal CSF findings with evidence of infection or high CSF:serum albumin ratio are all predictors of poor outcome.

SUMMARY

The treatment available for infectious encephalitis remains largely supportive except for HSV and nonviral encephalitis. The prognosis is often good but with important exceptions. Specific sequelae, especially those affecting cognition, memory, and behavior are under-recognized. Significant advances have been made in diagnostic techniques and these have facilitated public health measures of vaccination, vector control, and other disease prevention strategies that remain the most important factors in limiting the morbidity of the diverse spectrum of infectious encephalitis.

SUGGESTED READINGS

1. Chaudhuri A, Kennedy PGE. Diagnosis and treatment of viral encephalitis. Postgrad Med J 2002; 78:575–583.
2. Garg RK. Subacute sclerosing panencephalitis. Postgrad Med J 2002; 78:63–70.

3. Holmes GB, Chapman LE, Stewart JA, et al with the B Virus Working group. Guidelines for the prevention and treatment of B-virus infections in exposed persons. Clin Infect Dis 1995; 20:421–437.
4. Kennedy CR. Viral infections excluding herpes simplex, rabies, and HIV. In: Lambert, ed. Infections of the Central Nervous System. Philadelphia: Decker, 1991:300–316.
5. McGrath N, Anderson NE, Croxson MC, Powell KF. Herpes simplex encephalitis treated with acyclovir: diagnosis and long term outcome. J Neurol Neurosurg Psychiat 1997; 63:321–326.
6. Solomon T. Exotic and emerging viral encephalitides. Curr Opin Neurol 2003; 16: 411–418.
7. Whitley RJ, Gnann JW. Viral encephalitis: familiar infections and emerging pathogens. Lancet 2002; 359:507–514.

43

Neurocysticercosis

Constance Smith-Hicks and Eric H. Kossoff
The Johns Hopkins Hospital, Baltimore, Maryland, U.S.A.

INTRODUCTION

Neurocysticercosis is the most prevalent parasitic disease that affects the nervous system and the most common cause of epilepsy in the world. The causative parasite is actually the larva (*Cysticercus cellulosae*) of the pork tapeworm *Taenia solium*. Although found worldwide, cysticercosis has particularly high prevalence rates in areas with poor sanitation and where human fecal material is used for fertilizer. It is most common in Central and South America, Mexico, Spain, Portugal, Sub-Saharan Africa, and East Asia—including India, Indonesia, and China. In the United States, it is mainly a disease of immigrants; however, because of the increase in travel to endemic areas, the incidence has increased, primarily in the southwestern states, California, and Chicago.

Taenia solium has a two-host biological cycle with the pig as the intermediate host carrying the larvae (cysticerci). Humans become the definitive host, harboring the intestinal tapeworm by ingesting poorly cooked infected pork. Cysticercosis, infection not with the tapeworm but its larva, is acquired by fecal-oral transmission. The ova liberate oncospheres in the intestines that migrate to the central nervous system where they form cysts.

Neurocysticercosis is a pleomorphic disease; its manifestation depends on the number and location of tapeworm cysts and the host response. Cases of neurocysticercosis are rarely seen in infants because of its prolonged incubation period of 3–5 years. Children with only a single exposure tend to have a solitary cyst and a more benign course, experiencing vague symptoms (e.g., headache or dizziness) with the lesion resolving spontaneously in 2–9 months. Those living in endemic areas may have a less favorable prognosis marked by a more complicated disease process as a result of multiple lesions. Cysts in the brain commonly cause focal seizures in children.

Most children have normal physical and neurologic examinations, although some may present with hemiparesis due to Todd's paralysis after a focal seizure. Less common presentations are focal neurologic disturbances, movement disorders, neuropsychiatric disturbances, communicating and non-communicating hydrocephalus, gait disturbance, and meningitis.

Table 1 Diagnostic Criteria for Neurocysticercosis

Absolute
- (a) Biopsy-positive lesion from the brain or spinal cord demonstrating the parasite
- (b) Cystic lesion showing the scolex on CT or MRI
- (c) Direct visualization of subretinal parasites by fundoscopic exam

Major
- (d) Lesions on neuroimaging highly suggestive of neurocysticercosis
- (e) Positive immunoblot for detection of anticysticercal antibodies
- (f) Resolution of intracranial lesion after treatment with abendazole or praziquantel
- (g) Spontaneous resolution of small single enhancing lesion

Minor
- (h) Lesions on imaging study compatible with neurocysticercosis
- (i) Clinical manifestations suggestive of neurocysticercosis
- (j) Cysticercosis outside of the central nervous system

Epidemiological
- (k) Household contact with *T. solium* infection
- (l) Contact with individuals from cysticercosis
- (m) History of frequent travel to disease-endemic area

DIAGNOSIS

The diagnosis is made primarily by non-contrast head CT. Features seen on CT include the cyst (with or without a calcified center) possibly with edema surrounding it. MRI with gadolinium is complementary and is more sensitive in identifying non-inflamed and intraventricular cysts. The lesions may be ring-enhancing and calcified, which indicates the death of the larva and its resulting inflammatory reaction. Visualization of an eccentric nodule within the ring lesion is suggestive of neurocysticercosis and represents the scolex. The cysts are usually located in the cortex at the gray-white junction, but the deep ganglia, white matter, ventricles, and meninges are not exempt. The enzyme-linked immunotransfer blot assay (EITB) is the test of choice for detecting the antibody of *T. solium* in serum and is available through the CDC. It has 100% specificity and 90% sensitivity with more than two lesions, and 50–70% sensitivity with one lesion. When the parasites are located in the brain parenchyma, results of the CSF analysis may be normal or may reveal either a lymphocytic or eosinophilic pleocytosis. Although the stool test for *T. solium* is rarely positive, the presence of ova may be the only diagnostic confirmation in some children.

Diagnostic criteria were proposed in 1996, and recently modified based on clinical, imaging, immunologic, and epidemiological data (Table 1). Definitive diagnosis requires one absolute or two major, one minor, and one epidemiological criterion. Probable diagnosis requires one major and two minor criteria, one major, one minor, and one epidemiological criteria, or three minor and one epidemiological criteria.

TREATMENT

The introduction of praziquantel and albendazole in the treatment of neurocysticercosis has led to intense controversy and confusion as to their role. A team of experts at a meeting in Lima, Peru created consensus guidelines for the treatment of neurocysticercosis. The guidelines were individualized based on the viability of the lesions within the nervous system, and the location and number of the lesions. An algorithm based on these recommendations is presented in Fig. 1.

Parenchymal Neurocysticercosis

Details of antihelminthic and corticosteroid therapy are described in Table 2. Whereas several case series have shown that single parenchymal lesions resolve without antiparasitic drugs, others have suggested that treatment results in a faster disappearance of cysts. Thus, the decision to treat children with single lesions is still controversial. It is believed that patients who are at risk for cyst growth with resulting ventricular invasion and hydrocephalus should be treated with antiparasitic agents. Carpio prospectively evaluated the evolution of viable cysts in patients with single or multiple cysts, with or without antihelminthic therapy, and suggested that patients with moderate infection burden (more than five cysts) benefit from treatment. These patients are thought to be at a higher risk for cyst growth and aggressive treatment is recommended. In cases of heavy infection with widespread inflammation and cerebral edema, the current practice is to treat with corticosteroids

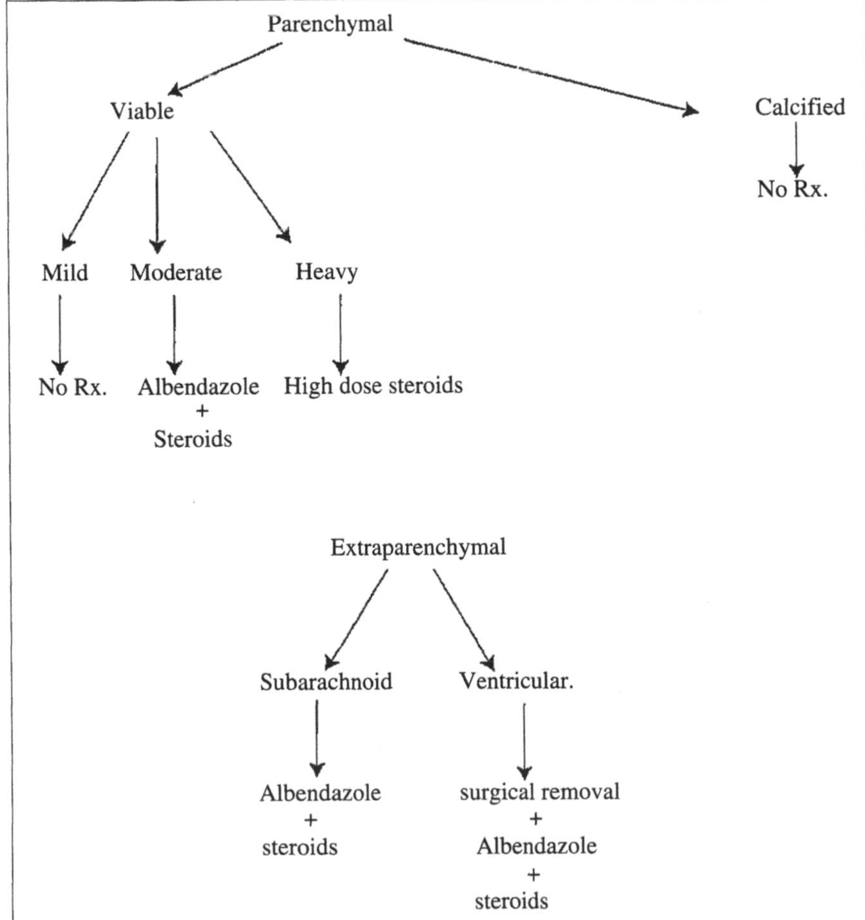

Figure 1 Algorithm for treatment of neurocysticercosis.

Table 2 Drug Therapy for Neurocysticercosis

Therapy	Doses	Advantages	Disadvantages
Albendazole	15 mg/kg/day	High cysticidal effect Low cost Good CSF penetration One-week course just as effective as four weeks	Possible hypersensitivity Risk of increased ICP with cyst death
Praziquantel	50 mg/kg/day	Fifteen-day course	Possible hypersensitivity Higher cost
Prednisone	1–2 mg/kg/day	Effective in children to reduce local inflammation secondary to death of larvae	

to minimize worsening cerebral edema. There is no consensus on the use of antihelminthics after the cerebral edema is resolved.

Seizures are managed in a manner similar to that used in other causes of secondary seizure disorders, with carbamazepine and phenytoin reported as first-line drugs. After resolution of infection, patients who remain seizure-free for 1–2 years can be taken off antiepileptic agents.

Extraparenchymal Neurocysticercosis

The management of intracranial hypertension and hydrocephalus in patients with extraparenchymal neurocysticercosis takes first priority, as it is associated with a worse prognosis. Treatment may require neuroendoscopic resection for cysts located within the ventricles, the use of shunts, and antiparasitic agents for infections involving the basal cisterns. There is general agreement that subarachnoid cysticercosis should be managed with both antihelminthics and corticosteroids.

PROGNOSIS

The mortality and morbidity associated with neurocysticercosis depends highly on whether the disease process is simple or complicated. Patients with mild disease burden tend to have fewer complications and a favorable prognosis. Treatment with antihelminthics results in significant regression or complete resolution in 80–90% of cases, and patients can be weaned from their anticonvulsants within 1–2 years. Depending on the location of the cysts, patients in endemic areas are at risk for major complications, for example increased intracranial pressure, recalcitrant seizures, and focal neurologic deficits.

SUGGESTED READINGS

1. Davis LE, Kornfeld M. Neurocysticercosis: neurologic, pathogenic, diagnostic and therapeutic aspects. Eur J Neurol 1991; 31:229–240.
2. Garcia HH, et al. Current consensus guidelines for treatment of neurocysticercosis. Clin Microbiol Rev 2002; 15:747–756.

3. Kossoff E. "Neurocysticercosis" Pediatrics. An On-line Medical Reference. Ist Edition St. Petersburg Emedicine Online Textbooks. Ed.Steven Altschuler et. al. 1999. Emedicine.com, Inc.http://www.emedicine.com/PED/topic1573.htm.
4. Singhi P, et al. Clinical spectrum of 500 children with neurocysticercosis and response to albendazole therapy. J Child Neurol 2000; 15:207–213.

44

Neurologic Complications of HIV Infection in Infants and Children

George K. Siberry
The Johns Hopkins Hospital, Department of Pediatrics, Baltimore, Maryland, U.S.A.

Robert M. Gray
Kennedy Krieger Institute, Department of Neuropsychology, Baltimore, Maryland, U.S.A.

INTRODUCTION

Perinatal infection is the most common route of HIV infection among children living with HIV infection in the United States. Currently, adolescents are the pediatric age group at highest risk of new infection through sexual and drug-using behaviors (readers are referred to other references for diagnosis and management of neurologic disease in adolescent-acquired HIV infection).

Neurologic manifestations of HIV infections vary in type and frequency across the wide range of ages, developmental stages, comorbidities, immunologic status, and medication regimens of HIV-infected infants, children, and adolescents. As in adults, progressive decline in immune function is the major risk factor for opportunistic infections, malignancies, and vascular events of the central nervous system. Peripheral neuropathy, whether due to medication toxicity or HIV infection itself, can also occur in children but less often than in adults. Diagnosis and management of infants and children with HIV presents unique demands on the health care practitioner, as immunological, medical, neurological, and neuropsychological complications must be considered within a neurodevelopmental framework.

DIAGNOSIS AND EVALUATION BY CLINICAL PRESENTATION

HIV Encephalopathy

HIV encephalopathy in children (usually in those not receiving effective highly active antiretroviral therapy (HAART)) produces global deficits but the pattern and severity may vary. The diagnosis is suspected by clinical history and exam, and there is no specific diagnostic test to confirm HIV encephalopathy, although neuropsychological examination results over time can aid in identifying encephalopathic progression. Infants can present with developmental regression and, ultimately apathy and withdrawal, in a severe, progressive course (without HAART). Less severely affected infants will show delayed but continued acquisition of developmental milestones with ultimately below average functioning in all areas of development. Motor and tone abnormalities most commonly are of the spastic diplegia type though other cerebral palsy-type patterns occur. Examination of CSF, if undertaken, may reveal mild elevations of protein and/or mononuclear cells, but is neither sensitive nor specific. CSF viral loads are not of proven diagnostic or prognostic utility in this setting. The purpose of CSF exam, neuroimaging, and other testing is generally to evaluate for other conditions rather than to confirm the diagnosis of HIV encephalopathy. Opportunistic infections are more likely considerations in the child with seizures, stroke, or focal neurologic abnormalities, altered mental status, fever, or rapid onset or progression of findings.

Progressive Multifocal Leukoencephalopathy

Progressive multifocal leukoencephalopathy (PML) occurs mostly in severely immunocompromised patients (occasionally with lesser degree of immunosuppression) as a result of reactivation of JC virus. It occurs far less frequently in children than in adults. The typical presentation is progression of motor, visual, auditory, cranial nerve, and cognitive deficits over a period of weeks to months in the absence of headache or fever. CSF exam is usually normal. MRI demonstrates increased T2 signal without mass effect, reflecting the JCV-mediated destruction of oligodendroglia. Positive CSF JCV PCR confirms the diagnosis but is not positive in all cases.

Meningoencephalitis

In general, the more common causes of meningoencephalitis tend to be predominant in children, even with HIV. However, some specific pathogens need to be considered in the differential diagnosis when symptoms occur.

Cryptococcal

Cryptococcal meningitis is much less common in children than adults and occurs with severe immunosuppression. Presentation is often subacute (over weeks) headache and fever; meningismus, seizures, altered mental status or focal signs can also occur at presentation. CSF exam may show elevated opening pressure, mononuclear pleocytosis, elevation of protein and low glucose, but these abnormalities may be minimal or absent. Neuroimaging may show evidence of increased intracranial pressure (ICP) or other nonspecific abnormalities. Diagnosis is confirmed by positive culture, positive fungal stain or positive capsular antigen test on CSF. Serum cryptococcal antigen tests are positive in most cases of cryptococcal meningitis.

Tuberculous

Tuberculous (TB) meningitis should be considered in any child presenting with meningitis. Risk factors for increased likelihood of *acquiring* tuberculosis infection should be sought (suspected or confirmed TB contact, children/family who immigrated from or traveled to TB endemic countries, homelessness, incarcerated contacts, illicit drug use). Risk of developing TB disease in those who have acquired TB infection is increased even in infants and young children without HIV infection; HIV infection only increases this risk further, particularly with progressive immunosuppression. Tuberculous meningitis may present with rapid progression of fever, headache, seizures, and increased ICP (more common in infants and young children) or may present subacutely, with 1–2 weeks of headache, fever, and irritability followed by more abrupt onset of lethargy, depressed mental status, meningismus, seizures, and cranial nerve abnormalities. CSF exam routinely shows elevated protein (often extremely elevated, 400–1000) and low glucose; pleocytosis can be neutrophilic early on but typically is mononuclear with variable counts (10–500). AFB stain of CSF stain is typically negative; larger volume CSF samples (minimum 5 mL, preferably 10 mL or more) are more likely to yield positive AFB cultures, but cultures are often negative. PPDs should be placed on child but are frequently negative; investigation and PPD testing of family and other contacts may help determine the likely source of TB infection for the child. Chest x-ray should be performed for evidence of TB infection and (if abnormal chest x-ray) three early morning gastric aspirates should be sent for AFB culture. Supportive head CT findings include basilar enhancement, hydrocephalus, and focal areas of ischemia.

CMV

CMV encephalitis is uncommon in adult AIDS patients and rare in children with AIDS. Patients have extremely low CD4 counts (<50 cell/mm^3) and present with rapid onset, progressive delirium, headache, fever, cranial nerve deficits, and ataxia. CSF is highly variable and may be normal, though low glucose, elevated protein, and *neutrophilic* pleocytosis are common. MRI shows confluent lesions in brainstem and periventricular distribution, often with enhancement. CMV PCR from CSF is more useful than culture for diagnosis, though definitive diagnosis requires brain biopsy for pathology and culture. Patients should have a dilated retinal exam for concomitant CMV retinitis.

Varicella Zoster Virus (VZV)

Varicella zoster virus (VZV) encephalitis can occur coincident with primary varicella (as it occasionally can in normal children). However, in AIDS patients, VZV can also present subacutely with headache, behavior changes, fever, altered mentation, seizures, and focal deficits. The illness can occur with or following a zoster eruption but may also occur in the absence of skin lesions. CSF exam usually shows mild mononuclear pleocytosis and protein can be mildly elevated. MRI may show patchy demyelination. CSF VZV DNA PCR is used to confirm the diagnosis.

Cerebral Toxoplasmosis

Cerebral toxoplasmosis occurs much less commonly in children than adults and is associated with severe immunosuppression. Since most cases are due to reactivation of latent infection, toxoplasma seropositivity is the main risk factor for disease and toxoplasmosis prophylaxis (e.g., bactrim) is indicated in severely immunosuppressed, toxoplasma IgG positive patients. Illness onset is subacute or acute; altered mentation, headache, and fever are typically accompanied by focal neurologic findings and/or seizures. Typical findings on CT include multifocal ring-enhancing cerebral lesions with a predilection for basal ganglia and corticomedullary junction. CSF may show mild mononuclear pleocytosis and protein elevation but often is normal. Negative CSF EBV PCR helps exclude lymphoma and CSF Toxoplasma PCR, where available, may help confirm the diagnosis. Empiric therapy is indicated for typical presentation and neuroimaging findings in a severely immunocompromised patient who is seropositive for *Toyoplasma gondii*, but lesion biopsy may be necessary to prove the diagnosis and exclude other diagnoses (especially lymphoma) in seronegative cases, cases that do not respond to therapy and cases of lesser diagnostic certainty (e.g., solitary lesions). Infants with suspected congenital toxoplasmosis should have a dilated retinal exam for concomitant chorioretinitis, but chorioretinitis is otherwise uncommon in HIV-infected patients with toxoplasmosis.

Primary Lymphoma

Primary lymphoma of the central nervous system occurs with increased frequency in children with AIDS, often after years of very low CD4 counts. Headache and personality changes in the absence of fever developing over a several-week period would be typical. Focal neurologic deficits are common; seizures also occur. CSF is often normal and elevated protein and mononuclear cells are nonspecific. Contrast CT or MRI shows single or multiple large (>2 cm) irregularly enhancing lesions usually with edema and mass effect. CSF EBV PCR is highly specific (somewhat less sensitive) for confirming the diagnosis, though biopsy is required for definitive diagnosis.

Stroke

Though uncommon in HIV-infected children, stroke is much more common than in children overall. HIV-infected children presenting with focal deficits should undergo urgent neuroimaging, usually with CT, then MRI and often MRA or conventional angiography if the process remains unclear. Differential includes stroke due to hemorrhage (usually with thrombocytopenia), thromboembolic disease (protein C & S deficiency may be more common), or ischemic infarction (primary or secondary vasculitis, vasculopathy), as well as toxoplasmososis, lymphoma, and PML. CSF exam is indicated in most cases to evaluate for evidence of an infectious or malignant process, and directed testing for VZV, HSV, JCV, EBV, and malignant cells can be helpful.

Seizure

As emphasized throughout this chapter, consideration to all of the usual causes of seizure should be given to seizure in an HIV-infected child. Etiologies of particular importance in the context of HIV infection include bacterial meningitis and tuberculous meningitis, and, in those with more advanced immunosuppression, cryptococcal meninigitis, cerebral toxoplasmosis, varicella zoster encephalitis, and lymphoma. Neuroimaging and lumbar puncture are indicated in most cases of seizure; see prior descriptions of individual entities for diagnostic evaluation. Since protease inhibitors (ritonavir, indinavir) prolong the action of diazepam and midazolam, lorazepam may be preferable for gaining initial control of seizures. If ongoing anticonvulsant treatment is needed, the interactions of many anticonvulsants (e.g., carbamezipime, phenobarbitol, phenytoin) with antiretrovirals should first be reviewed.

CNS Vasculitis/Vasculopathy

When neuroimaging and/or angiography is undertaken for HIV-infected children, usually in the setting of a suspected stroke, multiple areas of stenosis and aneurysmal dilatation of the vessels in and emanating from the Circle of Willis may be identified. These cerebral large vessel abnormalities occur predominantly in children with advanced immunodeficiency. It is not clear if these vasculopathic changes are due to active vasculitis of the involved vessels, damage from past vasculitis that is no longer active or other nonvasculitic processes. HIV vasculopathy/vasculitis becomes a diagnosis of exclusion, and complete evaluation for causes of secondary vasculitides (e.g., VZV, other infections), other primary vasculitis syndromes, and thrombophilias are warranted.

Gait Disturbance and Extremity Complaints

Distal Neuropathy

As in adults, children with AIDS may complain of chronic, bilateral, distal pain, and paresthesias in the lower extremities, interfering with walking. Distal vibration sense and ankle jerks are often diminished and weakness may be present. Upper extremities may also be involved. Bowel and bladder function are not affected. This distal neuropathy may be due to advanced HIV infection itself or may be due to certain NRTIs (ddI, d4t, ddc), especially ddI in combination with d4t. It is important to consider other nonantiretroviral neuropathy-inducing drugs (e.g., dapsone, INH), B12 deficiency, and other conditions (e.g., diabetes) associated with neuropathy. If there is diagnostic uncertainty, skin biopsy showing epidermal denervation and nerve-conduction studies showing axonal neuropathy can be used to confirm the diagnosis.

Guillain-Barré Syndrome

Guillain-Barré syndrome can present early or late in HIV infection, can improve with HAART or can appear during HAART-mediated immune reconstitution. In most cases, no specific opportunistic pathogen can be identified, but CMV has been implicated in some cases with severe immunosuppression. Clinical presentation may be similar to non-HIV-associated cases. As in non-HIV associated GBS, CSF protein is generally elevated, but in HIV-associated cases, mild pleocytosis may occur more often (though not in all cases) and course is more likely to be chronic. CSF PCR for CMV and perhaps other agents should be considered in patients with CD4 <50–100.

Myelopathy

Myelopathy may be due to an opportunistic pathogen, occur without identifiable pathogen besides HIV (HIV-associated vacuolar myelopathy) or be due to causes seen in HIV-uninfected patients. Leg weakness, gait disturbance, bowel/bladder dysfunction and leg pain and paresthesias in a patient with low CD4 counts would be typical. Spinal MRI is warranted. In addition to cultures for bacteria, fungus, and viruses, CSF should be sent for VDRL, cryptococcal antigen, and PCR testing for CMV, enteroviruses, HSV, and VZV. Serum for RPR and HTLV-1/II should also be sent.

Polyradiculitis

Patients with lumbosacral radicultitis have low CD4 counts and usually present with paraparesis, lower extremity areflexia, and voiding dysfunction. CSF usually reveals a neutrophilic pleocytosis, elevated protein, and positive CMV PCR.

Neuropsychological Deficits

Studies of a variety of pediatric HIV populations have documented impairments in motor skills, visual spatial processing, executive functioning, attention, processing speed, receptive and expressive language, memory and social and emotional functioning. Differential profiles of impairment have been noted among children with vertical vs. transfusion-based transmission, with less severe neuropsychological impairment noted in children infected through transfusion of blood. Children with an onset of HIV related symptoms before age 1 or 2 often demonstrate a much more rapid and progressive course of both neurological and neuropsychological deterioration, while those who remain asymptomatic through school age typically present with more subtle but important neuropsychological impairments.

In addition to cognitive, motor, and language impairments noted in pediatric HIV populations, these children also experience significant difficulties with social and emotional functioning. While some children demonstrate remarkable resilience in the face of multiple stressors, in general, higher rates of depression, anxiety, social withdrawal, and disruptive behavior can be expected in this population. Emotional and behavioral difficulties may be related to primary neurological effects (as HIV impacts cortical and subcortical sites associated with emotional and behavioral regulation), multiple psychosocial stressors experienced in this population, or some combination of neurological and environmental risk factors.

TREATMENT

There are four main aspects of the treatment of HIV-related neurologic problems: (1) initial stabilization and empiric treatment, (2) directed, specific treatment, (3) role of antiretrovirals in causing the problem, and (4) role of effective HAART in ultimately treating and preventing recurrence of the problem. Treatment of psychosocial and neuropsychological problems is an additional critical element in appropriate care for children with HIV.

Cerebral Toxoplasmosis

Pyrimethamine/sulfadiazine/leucovorin is initiated in toxoplasma seropositive patients with suspicious clinical and neuroimaging findings. Pyrimethamine loaded at 1 mg/kg/dose (max 50 mg) BID for 3 days followed by maintenance dosing at 1 mg/kg daily (max dose 25 mg); leucovorin 5–10 mg given with each dose of pyrimethamine. Sulfadiazine dose is 25–50 mg/kg/dose (max 1.5 g) QID. Progression of disease or failure to improve within 2 weeks would require additional diagnostic procedures (e.g., biopsy). After treatment, lifelong suppressive therapy (usually with bactrim) should be given to prevent recurrence; sustained immune reconstitution though HAART may allow discontinuation of this secondary prophylaxis.

CMV

CMV-associated encephalitis and polyradiculitis are treated with antivirals with activity against CMV (ganciclovir or foscarnet), but recovery probably ultimately depends more on the ability to immune reconstitute with effective HAART.

HSV or VZV Meningoencephalitis

Intravenous acyclovir at 10 mg/kg/dose TID (20 mg/kg/dose for neonates) for 2–3 weeks is used for treating HSV or VZV meningoencephalitis. It is often used for CNS vasculopathy/vasculitis syndromes with positive CSF VZV PCR, though it is difficult to prove benefit in this setting.

Cryptococcal Meningitis

This condition should be treated with amphotericin B (0.25–0.5 mg/kg initially then increased to 1.0 mg/kg daily) + flucytosine (50–150 mg/kg per day divided QID with serum levels of 40–60 mg/L measured after 4 days) though fluconazole (400 mg load then 200–400 mg daily) has been successfully used in adult patients with less severe disease. Elevated intracranial pressure may require serial lumbar punctures. Amphotericin/flucytosine should be used for at least 2 weeks and until CSF cultures are negative, though flucytosine toxicity may lead to earlier discontinuance. Total amphotericin therapy lasts 6 weeks followed by lifelong fluconazole suppression. Data for adults, not available for children, show that "lifelong" suppression can be safely discontinued with sustained reconstitution on HAART.

CNS Vasculitis/Vasculopathy

Acyclovir therapy is commonly used until PCRs for HSV and especially VZV are negative. Immune reconstitution may help prevent additional vascular damage, but already damaged vessels may put the child at risk for additional strokes. Active CNS vasculitis has also been suspected in some patients but even meningeal and brain biopsies may fail to reveal a vasculitic process discovered later at autopsy. The approach to these patients is multidisciplinary, involving intensivists, HIV/ID specialists, neurologists, hematologists, and rheumatologists. Most experts agree that immune reconstitution with HAART is important. Low-dose aspirin or other thrombosis prophylaxis is frequently used to try to prevent additional strokes; more intensive anticoagulation may be warranted if a specific thrombophilia is diagnosed. There is no consensus about the role or steroids, cyclophosphamide, or other immunosuppressive agent for presumed CNS vasculitis as a means to prevent additional strokes.

CNS Lymphoma

This condition should be managed by a multidisciplinary team including a pediatric oncologist and pediatric infectious disease specialist and is beyond the scope of this chapter.

Problems Due to Antiretrovirals

In cases of distal neuropathies, lesser acuity allows for outpatient management of change in HAART regimen without an obligatory antiretroviral-free interval. Prompt discontinuation of ddI, d4t and/or ddc may result in improvement within several weeks, but continued use of the offending antiretrovirals may produce a more recalcitrant neuropathy. Failure to improve after stopping these agents may also indicate the neuropathy is HIV-related (not drug induced) or of another etiology.

In all cases, adjunctive supportive measures including limits on walking distances, comfortable footwear, and cold foot soaks can be helpful.

Problems Treated by Effective HAART

Effective HAART may be the only treatment that can arrest the progression or even reverse the abnormalities in HIV encephalopathy, PML, HIV myelopathy, HIV vasculopathy, and HIV neuropathy. In addition, while ganciclovir and foscarnet are used for CMV polyradiculitis and encephalitis, effective HAART is likely the more important aspect of successful treatment. For all of the opportunistic CNS infections, in fact, effective HAART in combination with specific therapy will yield the best outcome and reduce the risk of relapse or recurrence. However, institution or reinstitution of HAART can be safely deferred several days while the patient is stabilized, diagnoses are clarified and other specific therapies are initiated.

Neuropsychological/Psychosocial Issues

Management of developmental, learning, and behavioral problems in HIV-infected children, as for HIV-uninfected children, includes early intervention services, school-based multidisciplinary services using individualized educational plans (IEPs), pharmacotherapy for ADHD and mood disorders, behavioral psychological services, and intense psychosocial support as well. While findings regarding HAART and neuropsychological functioning continue to be debated, there is evidence to suggest that individuals taking HAART may demonstrate less severe neuropsychological impairments and that HAART may potentially yield improvement in many areas of neuropsychological functioning.

SUMMARY

HIV-infected children experience a wide range of central and peripheral neurologic problems due to direct effects of HIV infection, HIV-mediated immunosuppression, and HIV pharmacotherapies. The context of HIV infection should lead the careful clinician to broaden the diagnostic evaluation of neurologic signs and symptoms without neglecting the comprehensive evaluation that would be indicated for such complaints in the absence of HIV infection. Evaluations are more extensive and aggressive and multiple empiric therapies are commonly necessary, particularly in children with more advanced immunosuppression and more serious neurologic illness. In addition to specific, directed therapies (when available), optimization of HAART is often the most important determinant of ultimate recovery. Consideration of neuropsychological status as well as regular neuropsychological monitoring is also recommended.

SUGGESTED READINGS

1. Belman AL. HIV-1 infection and AIDS. Neurol Clin 2002; 20(4):983–1011.
2. Brouwers P, Wolters P, Civitello L. Central nervous system manifestations and assessment [Chapter 18]. In: Pizzo PA, Wilfert CM, eds. Pediatric AIDS: The Challenge of HIV

Infection in Infants, Children and Adolescents. 3rd ed. Baltimore: Lippincott Williams & Wilkins, 1998.
3. Bartlett JG, Gallant JE. Medical Management of HIV Infection. Baltimore, MD: Johns Hopkins University-Division of Infectoius Diseases and AIDS Service, 2003. http://www.hopkins-aids.edu/.
4. Pickering LK, ed. Red Book: 2003 Report of the Committee on Infectious Diseases. 26th ed. Elk Grove Village, IL: American Academy of Pediatrics, 2003.
5. Wachsler-Felder JL, Golden CJ. Neuropsychological consequences of HIV in children: a review of current literature. Clin Psychol Rev 2002; 22(3):441–462.
6. Blanchette N, Smith ML, King S, Fernandes-Penny A, Read S. Cognitive development in school-age children with vertically transmitted HIV infection. Dev Neuropsychol 2002; 21(3):223–241.

45

Neurologic Manifestations of Lyme Disease

David Lieberman and Julia McMillan
Johns Hopkins Hospital, Departments of Pediatric Neurology and Pediatric Infectious Disease, Baltimore, Maryland, U.S.A.

INTRODUCTION

Lyme borreliosis is a multisystem disease resulting from infection by the spirochete *Borrelia burgdorferi* transmitted by the symptomless bite of certain ticks of the *Ixodes* species. Although several genospecies of *B. burgdorferi sensu lato* have been characterized, only *B. burgdorferi sensu stricto* is endemic in North America (Table 1). The differences in the tick vector in Europe, Eastern Europe, Asia, and North America, the proportion of infected ticks in different geographic areas, the virulence differences of the transmitted *Borrelia* genospecies, and possible concurrent infection with babesiosis or ehrlichiosis all contribute to the different clinical syndromes in different parts of the world.

EPIDEMIOLOGY

Lyme borreliosis is the most common arthropod-born disease in the United States. The estimated prevalence of Lyme disease in the United States is 6 per 100,000 with roughly 15,000 new cases per year. In highly endemic areas, the attack rate reaches 2–3% of the population. Roughly 20% of infections are asymptomatic. People with greater occupational, recreational, or residential exposure to either tick-infested

Table 1 Comparison of Lyme Disease by Geography

Geographical site	Spirochete	Organ involvement
North America	*B. burgdorferi sensu stricto*	Joints, nervous system
Europe	*B. garinii*	Nervous system
	B. afzelii	Skin (acrodermatitis chronica atrophans), nervous system

woods or fields near woods in areas of endemic spread are at greater risk of developing Lyme borreliosis.

In the United States, the highest rate of Lyme disease is in children aged 5–10 years. The age-specific incidence rate for Lyme disease in children 5–15 years is 140 per 100,000. Children account for a disproportionate number of Lyme borreliosis cases presumably because of increased exposure and decreased attention to prevention.

In this chapter, we present a brief synopsis of the clinical presentation, clinical course, diagnosis, and treatment of Lyme disease effects on both the central (CNS) and peripheral (PNS) nervous systems, i.e. lyme neuroborreliosis.

CLINICAL PRESENTATION

In 201 consecutive children with a median age of 7 years followed in the state of Connecticut, Lyme borreliosis manifested as erythema chronicum migrans in 89% of cases, musculosketal complaints such as myalgias or arthralgias in 6%, facial nerve palsy in 3%, meningitis in 2%, and carditis/AV block in 0–5%. The clinical manifestations of Lyme borreliosis are believed to be the result of the inflammatory response to infection by *B. burgdorferi.*

CLINICAL SIGNS

The most common finding in patients with Lyme disease is erythema chronicum migrans (ECM) at the site of a recent tick bite, typically located around the knees, axilla, or groin. This lesion is classically described as a nonpruritic expanding, erythematous macule/papule forming a large annular bull's eye with central clearing, but the lesion can also be irregular, raised, vesicular, or pruritic. It typically occurs at day 7–14 (range of incubation period is 3–30 days) and represents early localized infection. Secondary annular, erythematous lesions, smaller than the primary lesion, appearing 3–5 weeks after a tick bite represent an early disseminated form of Lyme disease.

Neurologic manifestations, known as Lyme neuroborreliosis, occur in 5–20% of North American cases (10–40% of infected individuals worldwide), and are more common in children than adults in European studies. Patients may present with aseptic meningitis, encephalopathy, facial nerve palsy, and/or peripheral neuropathy. Headache, photophobia, fever, and meningismus are not always seen. Lyme neuroborreliosis is known as a great mimicker, as its clinical manifestations are variable (Table 2). Neurologic manifestations can occur in either early or late disease.

EARLY DISEASE

Peripheral Nervous System (PNS)

Paresthesias, radicular pain, and hyperesthesia are the most common peripheral nerve complaints. The typical mechanism is thought to involve perivascular inflammation with axonal loss due to an immune response to *B. burgdorferi* epitopes that cross-react with axonal proteins. Peripheral nervous system involvement occurs in 10–15% of infected adults and up to 25% in those with chronic untreated infection.

Table 2 Neurologic Involvement in Lyme Disease

Early local infection (<30 days)
EM with CNS seeding (headache, stiff neck, cognitive difficulties)
Flu-like syndrome with CNS seeding (headache, stiff neck, cognitive difficulties)
Early disseminated infection (<3 months)
Aseptic meningitis
Meningoencephalitis (acute cerebellar ataxia, acute myelitis)
Cranial nerve palsy (facial nerve palsy)
Acute painful radiculoneuritis (Bannwarth's syndrome, lymphocytic meningoradiculitis)
Late persistent infection (>3 months)
Encephalopathy
Chronic axonal polyradiculoneuropathy
Chronic encephalomyelitis

EM erythema migrans; CNS central nervous system

The radicular symptoms may include acute polyradiculopathy, a brachial or lumbosacral plexopathy, or as mononeuropathy multiplex, thus affecting plexus, nerve roots, and nerves either singly, or in combination. EMG/nerve conduction typically shows an axonal sensorimotor neuropathy with diffuse involvement of both proximal and distal nerve segments.

Cranial Nerve Palsy

Cranial neuropathy is seen in up to two-thirds of patients with early disseminated Lyme neuroborreliosis. The facial nerve, cranial nerve VII, is most frequently affected, often with bilateral involvement. Lyme neuroborreliosis is suspected to be the etiology of acute facial palsy more often in children than adults. Children with neuroborreliosis related facial nerve palsy are less likely than adults to experience systemic symptoms such as fatigue, arthralgias, myalgias, headache, lymphadenopathy, fever, and/or chills.

An inflammatory CSF, suggesting actual CNS infection, generally accompanies Bell's palsy secondary to neuroborreliosis. In one European series, a CSF lymphocytic pleocytosis was detected in 26% of children with multiple erythema migrans alone. Cranial nerves III, IV, V, VI and VIII can also be affected, resulting in diplopia, facial numbness and/or pain, vertigo, or hearing impairment.

Meningoencephalitis

Lyme meningitis is the single most common presentation in early-disseminated Lyme neuroborreliosis. Headache is the major complaint in Lyme meningitis, while fever and meningismus are usually mild or absent. CSF findings in Lyme meningitis can be indistinguishable from viral meningitis, with a mild to moderate lymphocytic pleocytosis (usually 100–170 cells/mm^3), a mild elevation of CSF protein (100–300 mg/dL), and a normal to a mildly low CSF glucose. In comparing viral to lyme meningitis, patients with neuroborreliosis tend to have lower body temperatures, longer duration of headache, neck pain, and malaise, more often present with cranial neuropathy, and papilledema, and have fewer white blood cells, but a higher percentage of mononuclear cells in the CSF.

In Europe, 10–20% of cases of early disseminated neuroborreliosis present with an encephalomyelitis, an acute inflammatory process involving brain and spinal cord parenchyma. In the United States, only 0.1% of untreated patients develop an encephalomyelitis. White matter is affected predominantly with spasticity, ataxia, and even seizures being seen. Virtually all these patients have a lymphocytic pleocytosis.

LATE DISEASE

Encephalopathy

Lyme encephalopathy occurs more commonly in North America than in Europe, presenting as cognitive impairment with somnolence or insomnia, irritability, confusion, memory difficulty, depressed mood, and problems with complex tasks. The deficits can be described by the mini-mental exam, but formal neuropsychologic testing is more reliable. The pattern of abnormal findings in Lyme neuroborreliosis is different from that seen in depression, anxiety, or metabolic effects. When the impairments are due to neuroborreliosis, they tend to resolve with antibiotic treatment. Objective neurologic findings tend to be lacking. In Lyme encephalopathy, a CSF pleocytosis may be present in only 5% of patients, while protein content may be increased in 20–45%. In those who are treated, but whose deficits persist, a diagnosis of "post-Lyme syndrome," or chronic Lyme disease, may be made.

There are no formal objective criteria to diagnose chronic Lyme disease syndrome, leading to over-diagnosis and/or over-treatment. Patients complain of headache, arthralgias, fatigue, malaise, mild cognitive abnormalities, and sleep disturbances. These nonspecific phenomena are also seen after influenza, hepatitis, infectious mononucleosis, or in chronic fatigue syndrome.

Post-Lyme syndrome has been described in seronegative individuals with nonspecific symptoms who did not likely have tick exposure. It has also been considered in endemic areas to explain nonspecific symptoms in seronegative and seropositive individuals. We feel the diagnosis should be considered only in those patients with clear-cut Lyme disease (see below) who received recommended adequate treatment, yet continue to note problems that date to their original *B. burgdorferi* infection.

Diagnosis

The diagnosis of Lyme disease usually is based on the recognition of the characteristic clinical findings, a history of exposure in an area where the disease is endemic, and an antibody response to *B. burgdorferi* by enzyme-linked immunosorbent assay (ELISA) and Western blotting. In patients with evidence of erythema migrans on presentation, no serologic laboratory data are required to confirm the diagnosis. In patients without the classic rash, the diagnosis remains ultimately a clinical one, with laboratory data intended to help support the clinical diagnosis (Table 3).

Serologic Diagnosis

Serologic testing involves a two-tier system, according to the criteria of the Centers for Disease Control. The first-tier testing consists of an enzyme-linked immunosorbent assay (ELISA), while the second-tier antibody test by Western blot is performed on specimens that are positive by ELISA. The sensitivity of the two-step ELISA and Western blot was 100%.

Table 3 AAN Practice Guidelines for Neurologic Lyme Disease

Exposure to appropriate ticks in Lyme endemic region
Compatible neurologic abnormality without other cause
One or more of the following criteria:

(1) Skin manifestation (EM or histologically proven lymphocytoma cutis, acrodermatitis chronica atrophicans)
(2) Immunologic evidence of *B. burgdorferi* exposure (seroconversion or fourfold rise in titer of anti-*B. burgdorferi* antibodies in paired serum specimens)
(3) Detectable *B. burgdorferi* (by culture, histology, or PCR)
(4) Intrathecal intrathecal CSF anti-*B. burgdorferi* antibody production
(5) Lymphocytic meningitis ± cranial neuropathy, painful radiculoneuritis, or both
(6) Encephalomyelitis
(7) Peripheral neuropathy
(8) Encephalopathy

(From Ref. 1.)

Most first-tier ELISA tests use a spirochete preparation containing shared and specific antigens, making low titer or inconsistent first titer results likely to be false positive. False positive results can be seen in syphilis, tuberculous meningitis, bacterial endocarditis, rheumatoid arthritis, varicella, Ebstein–Barr virus, Rocky Mountain spotted fever, and AIDS. Second-generation tests using recombinant *B. Borrelia* proteins, or synthetic peptides, in a first-tier ELISA provide better sensitivity and specificity than a sonicate-based assay.

Western blot results can be considered positive only if the consensus criteria are met for positive IgM and/or IgG immunoreactive bands (Table 4). IgM antibodies typically are not detected on Western blot until roughly 2 weeks after spirochete inoculation (peaks at 3–6 weeks). Specific IgG antibody peaks weeks to months later. Antibody testing may therefore be inaccurate if testing is performed too early in the disease course. After the first month of infection, only the IgG response should be used to support the diagnosis, since an IgM response alone is likely to represent a false positive result. Since Western blotting is designed to achieve higher specificity at the price of sensitivity, this test should not be used when the ELISA is negative.

Positive serologic testing at a single time-point can suggest prior exposure to, but not an active infection from, *B, burgdorferi.* Treatment of *B. burgdorferi* may permanently prevent the ability to detect serum antibodies. When treatment is partial, serum antibodies maybe undetectable, but the organism may still exist within the individual, particularly in the CNS, allowing for persistent infection. Nevertheless, antibody detection should not be used to assess the success of treatment, because antibodies may persist for years. Lyme urine antigen testing is grossly unreliable and is not recommended.

Table 4 Consensus Criteria for Positive Western Blots

IgM	IgG
Two out of the following three immunoreactive bands: 23, 39, and/or 41 kDa	Five out of the following 10 immunoreactive bands: 18, 23, 28, 30, 39, 41, 45, 58, 66, and/or 93 kDa

CSF Diagnosis

CSF studies help to document neurologic involvement, but the invasion of the nervous system by *B. burgdorferi* may be difficult to prove. The small bacterial load, the slow reproduction time, and the predominance of spirochetes found tissue-bound rather than free-floating in CSF or blood are some of the reasons given for the difficulty in making a definitive diagnosis of Lyme neuroborreliosis. Culturing *B. Borrelia* in Barbour–Stoenner–Kelly medium permits definitive diagnosis, but positive cultures for the spirochete are obtainable primarily from skin lesions with ECM, less often from plasma and only rarely from CSF. In patients with clinically diagnosed Lyme disease presenting with meningitis, only 10% will have spirochetes cultured from their CSF.

The most helpful specific test to support a diagnosis of Lyme neuroborreliosis is intrathecal anti-*B. burgdorferi* antibody production. If present, this test provides indirect evidence for CNS seeding by the spirochete. Intrathecal antibody without CSF pleocytosis, however, should exclude active neuroborreliosis and points to previous infection or disruption of the blood–brain barrier. CSF anti-*B burgdorferi* antibodies (usually IgG or IgA) and oligoclonal bands may be present in up to 80–90% of patients with Lyme neuroborreliosis. Paired CSF and serum samples must be collected to determine an anti-*B. burgdorferi* antibody index. CSF and serum are normalized to the same total (i.e. not borrelia specific). IgG concentration before ELISA is run. Local CSF antibody production is implied when the CSF antibody to serum antibody index is greater than 1. Absence of CSF antibodies in patients with Lyme neuroborreliosis may occur due to restricted access caused by the immunoprivileged status of the CNS, local production of antibodies which do not reach CSF, a shift in the immune response from B-cell to T-cell mediated, or antibody testing is performed too early, during the so-called diagnostic gap.

TREATMENT

Lyme disease is rarely fatal and is not contagious, but it is not always a mild illness. Untreated Lyme disease is more likely to be associated with arthralgias, sleep difficulties, mild residual cognitive deficits, and physical limitations compared with patients who had received treatment. Lyme borreliosis should be treated early, not only to shorten the course of illness, but also to prevent late manifestations. When treatment is started in the early phase with no evidence of neurologic involvement, oral antibiotics are successful in 90% of patients. In general, intravenous (IV) antibiotics are recommended for neurologic infection with associated CSF abnormalities, except in isolated facial nerve palsy that has an excellent prognosis, with rare late sequelae (Table 5).

The frequency of Lyme disease after a recognized tick bite is roughly 1%. The infected tick must be attached for at least 24 hr for transmission to occur. Thus, if an attached tick is removed quickly, no other treatment is usually necessary. After a tick bite has occurred, the body of the tick should be grasped with medium-tipped tweezers as close to the skin as possible and removed by gently pulling the tick straight out, without twisting motions. If some of the mouth parts remain embedded in the skin, they should be left behind because they are eventually extruded; additional attempts to remove these fragments often result in unnecessary damage to the tissue and may increase the risk of local bacterial infection.

Table 5 Recommended Treatment Guidelines from the Red Book

Stage	Antibiotic
Early infection (local or disseminated)	Doxycycline, 100 mg p.o. bid for 14–21 days
	Amoxicillin, 25–50 mg/kg/day p.o. div tid for 14–21 days
	If allergic: cefuroxime or erythromycin (30 mg/kg/day divided tid)
Neurologic disease	Ceftriaxone, 75–100 mg/kg/days IV or IM qd(maximum 2 g IV qd) for 21–28 days (may extend to 6 weeks for severe parenchymal involvement)
	Cefotaxime, 150 mg/kg/day divided tid or qid for 21–28 days
	Penicillin G, 300,000 U/kg/day IV in six divided doses (maximum 20 million U/d) for 21–28 days
	If allergic: doxycycline 100 mg IV or p.o. tid for 30 days
Facial nerve palsy alone	Oral regimens may be adequate, 21–28 days course

Chemoprophylaxis within 72 hr of a tick bite with a single dose of doxycycline (200 mg) is 87% effective in preventing Lyme disease. Prophylactic antibiotic therapy is not generally recommended, however, because the adverse effects of antibiotics are felt to outweigh the risk that an individual tick was both infected with *B. burgdorferi* and transmittted the infection.

Erythema Chronicum Migrans (ECM)

Doxycycline is the first-line agent for ECM. The oral absorption is 95%, and plasma levels are equivalent whether the drug is given orally or parenterally. It shows good pharmacokinetics, and the concentration of this lipophilic agent in CSF by therapeutic oral administration is higher than the MIC_{90} for *B. burgdorferi.* In addition, it treats *Ehrlichia* infection, which may be transmitted by the same tick species that carries *B. burgdorferi.* Major side effects are photosensitivity and gastrointestinal upset. It should not be used in children younger than age 8 because of the risks of tooth discoloration and retardation of skeletal development. Amoxicillin is an alternative medication in this age group. Erythromycin can be used for treating penicillin allergic children, but it may be less effective. Erythema migrans resolves within several days of treatment, but other signs and symptoms of Lyme disease often persist longer.

Facial Nerve Palsy

In the case of uncomplicated facial nerve palsy without CSF abnormalities, oral antibiotic therapy for 3–4 weeks is adequate to prevent further sequelae. Doxycycline and amoxicillin are first-line drugs, while clarithromycin, azithromycin, and cefuroxime have also been used. Amoxicillin is recommended in children under age 8 (and pregnant women). Ceftriaxone can also be given as a first-line medication for a 2–3 week treatment course, especially when compliance with oral medications is questionable. Antibiotic therapy does not hasten resolution of facial nerve palsy, but it does help prevent late effects. Corticosteroids are not recommended for the treatment of Lyme disease associated Bell's palsy.

Lyme Neuroborreliosis

If the clinical picture of facial nerve palsy is complicated by other neurologic findings, a lumbar puncture and Western blot of CSF should be obtained in a seropositive patient before initiating intravenous antibiotic therapy. When the CNS is involved, such as in cases of headache, meningitis, or encephalopathy, ceftriaxone, cefotaxime, penicillin, or doxycycline should be given IV for 3–4 weeks. Ceftriaxone is preferred to penicillin because better serum levels are achieved, it penetrates the blood–brain barrier better, and it is more effective in vitro against *B. burgdorferi.* In a European study of children with neuroborreliosis, a 10-day course of treatment resulted in 58% of children being symptom free by the end of treatment, 92% after 2 months and 100% by 6 months after treatment. These same good results have not been achieved in adults regardless of time of initiation of therapy, or immune status.

The Jarisch–Herxheimer reaction presenting as fever, headache, myalgias, and worsening constitutional symptoms lasting less than 24 hr can occur with the initiation of antibiotic therapy. This transient reaction is thought to result from the sudden release of bacterial products from injured and/or killed bacteria, as described following treatment for secondary and tertiary syphilis, brucellosis, and enteric fever. Antibiotics should be continued and nonsteroidal anti-inflammatory agents given to reduce symptomatic complaints.

Length of Therapy

Long-term IV antibiotics are not recommended for "resistant" or "dormant" infection. Persistence of symptoms after treatment is due either to slowly resolving Lyme neuroborreliosis, irreversible tissue damage, inadequacy of initial treatment, post-Lyme disease syndrome, or initial misdiagnosis. Post-Lyme borreliosis syndrome is best treated symptomatically rather than with prolonged courses of antibiotic therapy. The use of IV antibiotics for longer than 4–6 weeks is not supported by published studies because *B. burgdorferi* resistance to penicillin and ceftriaxone has not been reported.

Prevention

Protective measures for the prevention of Lyme borreliosis may include the avoidance of tick-infested areas, the use of protective clothing, repellents containing DEET (diethyltoluamide), and acaricides, tick checks, and modifications of landscapes in or near residential areas.

Vaccinations

A vaccine for Lyme disease, consisting of recombinant OspA in adjuvant, was commercially available in the United States. Although efficacious and apparently safe, the vaccine against Lyme disease was withdrawn from the market in February 2002 because of safety concerns and prohibitive expense for widespread use. According to experts in the field, a second-generation vaccine will not likely be marketed in the near future.

Steroids

In addition to antibiotics, Lyme borreliosis patients have been given steroids to treat pain syndromes, hasten the resolution of facial palsy, or treat late neurologic complications of chronic infection, all with various results. Little is known about the effects of steroids on the course of infection with *B. burgdorferi.* Persistence of inflammation with or without residual infection may explain why some patients with Lyme borreliosis remain symptomatic despite treatment with adequate doses of antibiotics. Patients treated with antibiotics and steroids may recover faster than those treated with antibiotics alone. There are concerns, however, that treatment with steroids can reactivate latent infection and impair the host's ability to clear the infection. Therefore, there are no current recommendations for treatment of Lyme neuroborreliosis with steroids.

Prognosis

Residual neurologic symptoms after treatment for Lyme disease may occur in up to 25% of individuals and may include facial palsy, concentration and learning difficulties, vertigo, cerebellitis, arthralgias, weight loss, paresthesia, and neuropathy. Compared to adults, children have favorable long-term outcomes including normal cognitive function 2 years after treatment. Associations with dementia, multiple sclerosis, and movement disorders have been suggested, but not proven.

The recovery rate of children with acute facial palsy due to *Borrelia* infection is roughly 82% after 1 year, higher than the 61% rate for children with facial palsy from other causes (e.g. varicella-zoster virus, herpes simplex virus, Epstein–Barr virus, etc.). Up to one-fifth of children develop permanent nerve dysfunction following Lyme associated facial palsy. Sequelae after facial palsy are not only cosmetic and psychological, but may also include problems with pronunciation and tear secretion. Recovery may be incomplete if significant damage to the neuroaxis has occurred, commonly with gliosis as a residual insult. Actual tissue damage is not only due to the invading organism, but is amplified by the local immune response, perhaps by autoreactive CSF T cells.

CONCLUSIONS

The diagnosis of Lyme neuroborreliosis depends mainly on history and clinical manifestations. Laboratory studies are meaningful only in the setting of a high clinical suspicion and should not be used as a screening tool. The optimal duration of therapy is still controversial, but most treatments with standard antibiotics are generally successful for each of the stages of Lyme disease. As newer diagnostic tools and the results of more clinical trials become available, the management of Lyme disease will continue to be refined and debated.

REFERENCES

1. Halperin JJ, Logigian EL, Finkel MF, Pearl RA. Practice parameters for the diagnosis of patients with nervous system Lyme borreliosis (Lyme disease). Quality Standards Subcommittee of the American Academy of Neurology. Neurology 1996; 46:619–627.

2. American Academy of Pediatrics. Lyme disease. In: Pickering LK, ed. Red Book: 2003 Report of the Committee on Infectious Diseases. 26th ed. Elk Grove Village, IL: American Academy of Pediatrics 2003.

SUGGESTED READINGS

1. Belman AL, Reynolds L, Preston T, et al. Cerebrospinal fluid findings in children with Lyme disease-associated facial nerve palsy. Arch Pediatr Adolesc Med 1997; 151: 1224—1228..
2. Christen HJ, Hanefeld F, Eiffert H, Thomssen R. Epidemiology and clinical manifestations of Lyme borreliosis in childhood. A prospective multicentre study with special regard to neuroborreliosis. Acta Paediatr Suppl 1993; 386:1–75.
3. Coyle PK, Schutzer SE. Neurologic aspects of Lyme disease. Med Clin North Am 2002; 86:261–284.
4. Hengge UR, Tannapfel A, Tyring SK, Erbel R, Arendt G, Ruzicka T. Lyme borreliosis. Lancet Infect Dis 2003; 3:489–500.
5. Huppertz H-I. Lyme disease in children. Curr Opin Rheumat 2001; 13:434–439.
6. Steere AC. Lyme disease. N Engl J Med 2001; 345:115–125.

46

Shaken Baby Syndrome (Shaken-Impact Syndrome)

Richard Kaplan
Southern California Permanente Medical Group, San Diego, California, U.S.A.

INTRODUCTION

Shaken baby syndrome (SBS), also known as nonaccidental or inflicted head injury, are often used to describe craniospinal injuries sustained by infants or children as a result of violent physical actions of adults or teenagers caring for them. Although forceful shaking alone may cause significant injury, in many instances, the head is struck against a surface. Others have proposed the term "shaken-impact syndrome," since it more accurately reflects the age range and different mechanisms of injury. In its classic form, SBS involves an infant less than 6 months of age who presents with subdural and/or subarachnoid hematomas, bilateral retinal hemorrhages, and minimal or absent signs of external trauma. Long bone and/or rib fractures or evidence of other injuries (e.g., abdominal or urogenital) of differing ages are common findings. Regardless of whether shaking occurs alone or is accompanied by impact, the injury to the brain and eye results from sudden angular acceleration–deceleration of the head, which can cause intracranial hemorrhage and wide spread parenchymal axonal injury.

INCIDENCE AND EPIDEMIOLOGY

Prior evidence of abuse is common occurring in up to 50% of cases highlighting the need for increased vigilance by the medical community. The true incidence is unknown but estimates range from 750 to 3750 cases per year in the United States. Two recent British surveys estimated an annual incidence between 21 and 25 per 100,000 children under 1 year. Infants who were premature, or had congenital defects, developmental delays, or difficult temperament are at greater risk for SBS, possibly due to poor parental bonding.

CLINCIAL PRESENTATION AND EVALUATION

The onset of symptoms typically appears hours to weeks before the child is brought to the attention of medical professionals and presenting symptoms are often attributed to a recent mild illness or accidental fall, inconsistent with the physical findings and subsequent evaluation. Common presenting symptoms include: seizures (in one series, 45% of patients presented this way), decreased consciousness (43%), respiratory difficulties (34%), irritability (25%), lethargy (23%), vomiting (22%), apnea (21%), sleepiness, and poor feeding. Rapid head growth noted on routine examination in an otherwise healthy child can also be indicative of nonaccidental trauma. If child abuse is suspected, the appropriate authorities should be contacted immediately to begin an investigation.

Retinal hemorrhage is the most consistent finding on examination occurring between 65% and 90% of cases. A recent large retrospective Canadian study of 364 children reported retinal hemorrhage in 76% of the children of which 83% were bilateral. Retinal hemorrhages can be missed unless both direct and indirect ophthalmoscopy is performed. Retinal injury is usually secondary to the acceleration–deceleration of the eye brought on by shaking. Other possible although less likely causes include tracking of intracranial blood into the orbit (Terson syndrome), increased intracranial pressure, and increased thoracic pressure induced by the perpetrator grabbing the chest or, very rarely, from cardio-respiratory resuscitation by medical personnel. The findings should be well documented and photographed at the earliest possible time. Hemorrhage into superficial retinal layers results in a splinter or flame appearance whereas hemorrhage located in deeper retinal tissue results in a dot or blot appearance. Hemorrhage in front of the retina (preretinal) obscures the underlying retinal vessels whereas vessels are visible if the blood is subretinal. Blood can also extend into the vitreous gel (vitreous hemorrhage). Traumatic retinoschisis in which the retina at the macula is separated, raised, and folded by shearing forces may be highly suggestive of SBS when found in a young child. Retinal hemorrhage is not usually helpful in determining when the injury occurred. Newborn infants can also have retinal hemorrhages within the first week of life, so interpretation in this setting can be a challenge. Retinal vascular abnormalities can be seen very rarely in patients with selected vascular malformations (e.g., cavernomas), endocarditis, hematological disorders, and encephalitis.

Imaging studies are essential in demonstrating the extent of injuries and in establishing the diagnosis. CT scan with bone and soft-tissue windows should be performed emergently since it may demonstrate injuries that require prompt intervention. Subdural hematoma most prominent in the interhemispheric fissure, cerebral edema, and subarachnoid hemorrhage are the most common intracranial abnormalities seen on CT. In more severely affected infants, unilateral or bilateral hypodensities can also be seen along with loss of gray-white matter differentiation.

An MRI of the brain and cervical spine including diffusion-weighted sequences (looking for edema) and gradient echo sequences (looking for old hemorrhages) in at least two planes should be obtained when the child is stable to identify small subdural hematomas (located near the base of the brain and vertex), parenchymal lesions including cerebral contusions and shearing injuries to the white matter, cerebral infarction, and spinal cord trauma (from C1 to C4). Cerebral contusions (ovoid shaped intraparenchymal blood with surrounding edema) are typically located in the anterior temporal, and orbitofrontal regions and are caused by the brain forcefully striking the skull. Shearing injuries commonly occur at the gray-white matter junction, centrum semiovale, and corpus callosum and are caused by the stretching and disruption of axonal fibers. Diffusion-weighted sequences are particularly sensitive early on to axonal injury and cerebral ischemia. Both CT and MRI can be helpful in determining when the injury occurred and documenting prior trauma. In CT

Table 1 Guideline for Evaluating Age of Hemorrhage on MR

Time	Hematoma stage	T1 (short TR)	T2 (long TR)
Few hours (0–4 hr)	Oxyhemoglobin	Slightly hypointense or isointense	Slightly hyperintense
Acute (4 hr–3 days)	Deoxyhemoglobin	Slightly hypointense	Hypointense
Early subacute (3 days–2 weeks)	Intracellular methemoglobin	Hyperintense	Hypointense
Late subacute 1 week–1 year)	Extracelluar methemoglobin	Hyperintense	Hypointense
Chronic (>1 month)	Hemosiderin	Slightly hypointense	Hypointense

imaging, acute bleeding (within the first 7 days) appears hyperdense; subacute bleeding (7–21 days) is isodense, and chronic bleeding (>21 days) is hypodense. Table 1 outlines dating of blood on MRI sequences. It is important to remember that a mixture of old and new blood does not necessarily indicate additional trauma since rebleeding into a chronic subdural can occur without new injury.

Skull films and a skeletal survey are essential since bone fractures are a common in SBS with up to 50% of children affected. Complex or multiple skull fractures are suggestive of nonaccidental injury. Similarly, rib fractures from holding the infant tightly while shaking and old and/or new long bone fractures are suggestive of SBS. Fractures can also involve other areas including the fingers, spine, and scapula.

Laboratory studies including CBC, platelets, PT, PTT, and a metabolic panel, and an arterial blood gas can rule out other causes and identifying abnormalities that require treatment or monitoring. A mild coagulopathy can be seen but significant clotting dysfunction is rare and should suggest other disorders. Mild to moderate anemia may also occur from intracranial bleeding and/or internal bleeding elsewhere. A lumbar puncture, when performed to rule out meningitis, can yield bloody spinal fluid that is often xanthrochromic, suggesting that the intracranial hemorrhage is at least several hours old and not the result of a traumatic tap.

DIFFERENTIAL DIAGNOSIS

Table 2 lists the differential diagnosis of SBS. Rare causes of intracranial hemorrhage include congenital deficiency of coagulation factors, vitamin K deficiency,

Table 2 Differential Diagnosis

Accidental trauma
Congenital deficiency of coagulation factors
Acquired coagulation disorders
Vitamin K deficiency
Congenital arterial aneurysm or AVM
Benign enlargement of the subarachnoid spaces
Gluteric aciduria type I
Menkes
Osteogenesis imperfecta
SIDS/ALTE

acquired coagulation disorders (e.g. from infection or leukemia), congenital arterial aneurysm, and arteriovenous malformations (AVMs). MRI and MRA can rule out congenital vascular malformations. Bleeding diatheses are usually ruled out by the history, physical examination, and coagulation studies. A pediatric hematology consultation should be obtained if a bleeding disorder is suspected.

Rare inborn errors of metabolism can present with features of SBS. Subdural hematomas can be seen in both glutaric acidura type I (GA-1) and Menkes disease (discussed further elsewhere in this text).

GA-1 is autosomal recessive disease caused by a deficiency in glutaryl-CoA dehydrogenase. Patients may present with an acute encephalopathy following an infection or with more gradual neurological deterioration consisting of developmental delay, large head, hypotonia, and movement disorder. Although subdural fluid collections can sometimes be seen, more typical MRI findings include frontal temporal atrophy manifested by widening of the Sylvian fissures and CSF fluid anterior to the temporal lobe, widening of the mesencephalic cistern, and abnormal high T2-weighted signal intensity in the basal ganglia and periventricular white matter. Abnormalities can also be seen in the brainstem and cerebellum. Urine organic acids usually show marked increase in glutaric acid and 3-hydroxy glutaric acid. The diagnosis can be confirmed by fibroblast analysis.

MEDICOLEGAL ISSUES

Child abuse, especially when accompanied by serious or permanent injuries, is a particularly vile crime that always needs societal intervention. Even though the perpetrator may be emotionally disturbed or a substance abuser, it is the responsibility of the legal system, not the medical team, to determine culpability and appropriate punishment. In order that the system works fairly both for the victim and perpetrator, it is essential that the medical team works closely with both social services, child protection investigators, and the police during the initial hours and days of the hospitalization. As soon as is it is medically practical, a physician familiar with child abuse along with appropriate legal authorities should interview the people involved with the child's care and obtain appropriate evidence including photographs, radiological reports, and reports detailing the physical condition of the child when first evaluated. The initial interview with the family and providers is often key and, if possible, should be done with each member separately so that inconsistencies in the history can be documented for later follow up.

Although the suspected perpetrator should face prosecution and punishment according to state law, therapeutic intervention, especially when injuries do not result in death or permanent disability, can be an important means of preventing more severe injuries in the future. Medical, psychiatric, and social service input should be obtained in planning the appropriate intervention. The goal is to prevent further harm and restore physical and emotional well being to both the child and those involved in child's care.

TREATMENT

The initial management of those children with marked impairment of consciousness and/or breathing includes intubation and ventilation, maintaining adequate circulation, and anticonvulsant therapy. Evacuation of large acute subdural hematomas should be considered. Aggressive management of increased intracranial pressure using hyperosmolar therapy, ICP monitoring, hyperventilation, pressors, and pentobarbital coma is controversial due to unproven long-term benefit, although recent guidelines on this subject have been published. Less severely effected children should be observed closely. Neurosurgery, ophthalmology, and neurology consultations should be obtained as soon as possible.

OUTCOME

The outcome depends on the severity of brain injury. Factors suggesting a poor prognosis include: unresponsiveness on admission, poor vision and an absent or diminished pupillary response on presentation, early and intractable posttraumatic seizures, age under 6 months, need for intubation, and bilateral or unilateral diffuse hypodensities on CT scan. Mortality rates are high and range between 15% and 40% with a median of 20–25%. In a limited follow-up study of 14 children contacted on average 9 years after injury, 7 were severely disabled or vegetative, 2 were moderately disabled, and 5 had a good outcome. Other reports similarly suggest that a majority of surviving children suffer some permanent disability which may include visual impairment usually from cortical damage and optic atrophy, mental retardation, learning disabilities, cerebral palsy and other motor deficits, hearing loss, hydrocephalus, and epilepsy. Long-term follow up is required since the deficits may not be apparent until the child enters school.

SUGGESTED READINGS

1. American Academy of Pediatrics—Committee on Child Abuse and Neglect. Shaken baby syndrome: rotational cranial injuries—technical report. Pediatrics 2001; 108:206–210.
2. Barlow KM, Gibson RJ, McPhillips M, Minns RA. Magnetic resonance imaging in acute non-accidental head injury. Acta Paediatr 1999; 88:734–740.
3. Duhaime A, Christian C, Moss E, Seidl T. Long-term outcome in infants with the shaking-impact syndrome. Pediatr Neurosurg 1996; 24:292–298.
4. Duhaime A, Christian CW, Rorke L, Zimmerman RA. Nonaccidental head injury in infants—the "Shaken Baby Syndrome". New Engl J Med 1998; 338:1822–1829.
5. King WJ, MacKay M, Sirnick A. with the Canadian Shaken Baby Study Group. Shaken baby syndrome in Canada: clinical characteristics and outcomes of hospital cases. Can Med Assoc J 2003; 168:155–159.
6. Levin A. Ophthalmology of shaken baby syndrome. Neurosurg Clin N Am 2002; 13: 201–211.

47
Coma

J. Michael Hemphill
Department of Neurology, Medical College of Georgia,
Savannah Neurology, Savannah, Georgia, U.S.A.

INTRODUCTION

Coma is a state where arousal to wakefulness and conscious awareness cannot be achieved despite sufficient stimulation. Depression in level of consciousness may exist at any level between the fully alert state and the unresponsive state and demands urgent evaluation and treatment. The level of consciousness usually determines the degree of urgency with complete unresponsiveness—coma—demanding the most immediate response.

Management of coma usually begins in the emergency room and continues in the intensive care unit. The major challenge for the clinician is in the early management of coma when it first presents. It may be the end-result of any pathological brain insult of sufficient severity. Initial treatment must be aimed at supporting the patient and initiating specific treatment for the responsible etiology. Long-term management consists of maintenance of physiological function and assessing prognosis—a task usually reserved exclusively for the pediatric neurologist. If all brain function is lost, this must be recognized, so that futile care is not given and organ procurement can be considered.

Coma in infants, children, and adolescents will be addressed. The unresponsive neonate represents a special situation best dealt with under the appropriate conditions requiring treatment.

EARLY ASSESSMENT AND INTERVENTION

Gathering of history, physical examination, laboratory testing, and imaging must occur simultaneously with early supportive treatment. Initial assessment should focus both on identifying the etiology and on assessing the level of central nervous system depression. At the same time, emergency resuscitative measures must be initiated.

Assessment and Stabilization

The etiology of coma may be evident from history or circumstances, as in the case of trauma or in-hospital hypoxic–ischemic encephalopathy. Where it is not, rapid assessment of possible etiologies is necessary to insure initiation of appropriate specific treatment. These may be structural, infectious, toxic, metabolic, or hypoxic. In children, structural causes for coma are usually due to trauma and less likely to be due to primary intracerebral hemorrhage, infarction, or a previously unsuspected mass. Trauma may be obvious direct head injury or occult injury, as with a shaken baby. Epidural, subdural, and intraparenchymal hemorrhage will be identified on noncontrast head computed tomography (CT), which should be performed as soon as the child is stable. Occult trauma may be suspected with the finding of retinal hemorrhages in the absence of obvious CT abnormalities. Where trauma is a possibility, cervical spine injury must also be suspected, and immobilization should be performed prior to examination, early treatment, or imaging.

The history from available sources will depend on how apparent the etiology of coma is at presentation. In nontraumatic situations, the physician must determine whether the loss of consciousness was abrupt or gradual, whether there have been any underlying illnesses or other predisposing factors, whether seizure activity was observed, and what preceding symptoms may have been present. The presence of behavior change, headache, vomiting, diarrhea, or rash may point to central nervous system infection. Accessibility of the child to medications, cleaning agents, or other toxins determines the level of suspicion of ingestion. The identity and circumstances of the caregiver prior to the call for help may raise the question of nonaccidental trauma. Sudden onset of coma without obvious explanation, in a previously healthy child, especially a toddler or adolescent, suggests an ingestion, warranting early decontamination. More gradual deterioration suggests infection or metabolic abnormality. Treatable etiologies must be considered first.

Initial supportive care consists of standard emergency resuscitative measures. An adequate airway must be established and maintained. Cervical immobilization should be employed where there is any possibility of cervical spine trauma. Where there is respiratory insufficiency on observation, pulse oximetry, or blood gases, intubation using the rapid sequence induction technique should be performed by an experienced person. This technique involves administration of a short-acting sedative/hypnotic agent followed by a rapidly acting neuromuscular blocker and cricoid pressure to prevent regurgitation. Circulation and perfusion must be maintained with intravenous or intraosseous administration of fluids and pressors.

Physical Examination

General examination may provide useful clues to etiology. Alterations in body temperature may suggest infection or confirm near-drowning. Nuchal rigidity points to meningitis. Petechiae, rash, or purpura may also indicate infection. Red, hot, dry skin may be seen with anticholinergic poisoning. Unusual odors should raise a suspicion of an inborn error of metabolism. Retinal hemorrhages on funduscopic examination indicate occult trauma, especially the shaken baby syndrome. Papilledema would suggest an intracranial mass producing chronic increased intracranial pressure. A cardiac murmur should raise the suspicion of endocarditis or congenital heart disease with its risk of brain abscess or infarction. A rigid abdomen may point to a source for sepsis, and hepatomegaly may go along with hepatic failure with encephalopathy or may indicate a storage disease.

Neurologic assessment of the level of central nervous system depression consists of evaluation of level of consciousness, motor symmetry, and brainstem reflexes. Level of consciousness should be described in the most specific terms possible, so that serial examinations can be compared. General terms, such as obtundation or stupor, may be used differently by different examiners and do not facilitate ready comparison over time. The Glasgow Coma Scale (GCS), an abbreviated, scored list of best eye, verbal, and motor responses, is widely used in adults, especially in cases of trauma, and may be used in children beyond age 5. There are several pediatric coma scales, which represent modifications of the GCS that take into account normal phases of development and can be used for infants and young children. None of these scales assess brainstem reflexes or specific motor function.

The brainstem reflexes that should be assessed are the pupillary light and vestibuloocular reflexes. Corneal reflexes are helpful, if present, but may be absent because of corneal edema, not brainstem injury and, so, are less reliable. Pupillary light reflexes should be assessed with an adequately bright light. Anisocoria suggests an oculomotor nerve palsy and may indicate uncal herniation. Absence of light reflexes, if not pharmacologic, indicates loss of midbrain function and usually is seen with structural or hypoxic–ischemic injury. Miosis may represent opioid or other ingestion. The vestibuloocular reflex, which requires an intact brainstem from the vestibular nuclei in the lower pons up to the oculomotor nuclei in the upper midbrain, can be assessed with the oculocephalic maneuver or with ice water irrigation of the external auditory canals. With the oculocephalic maneuver, the head is turned from side-to-side or up-and-down. In the unconscious patient with no visual fixation present, the eyes should move proportionately to the amount of head movement, degree for degree ("doll's eyes"). If the vestibuloocular pathways are nonfunctional, indicating pontomesencephalic injury, the eyes will not move and will remain in a fixed position. If no "doll's eyes" can be obtained, then 10–30 cm^3 of ice water can be irrigated into the external auditory canal, against the tympanic membrane, to suppress vestibular tone on that side. This may not be needed in the initial examination, when etiology and urgent treatment are still being considered, but it is important in the subsequent serial evaluation of the patient. In the intact brainstem, the eyes will deviate toward the ear being irrigated, being driven to that side by vestibular tone from the contralateral side that is unopposed. There is no point in assessing more than one side at a time, since vestibular tone will remain suppressed in the first ear for a brief period. If both the pupillary light reflexes and vestibuloocular reflexes are absent, then it can be assumed there is no brainstem function down to the medulla, which is likely also impaired and may need to be assessed later with an apnea challenge to determine death by brain criteria.

Motor examination may help identify the brain pathology and its localization. Abnormal posturing of the trunk and extremities may indicate increased intracranial pressure, along with hypertension, widening of the pulse pressure, and bradycardia (Cushing's triad). An asymmetry of limb movement may be seen with cerebral infarction, mass, or trauma and can often be detected by elevating the limbs and observing whether one side drops more freely than the other. An asymmetric withdrawal response may be seen with deep painful stimulation, as well.

Laboratory

Initial evaluation should include measurement of blood sugar, serum electrolytes, BUN/creatinine, liver functions, ammonia, urinalysis/urine drug screen, and complete blood count. Arterial blood gases and EKG should have been included as part of initial and stabilization, if needed. If there is no obvious etiology from the clinical assessment, immediate laboratory values, or CT, then lumbar puncture and blood cultures should be considered, especially if the child is febrile. Empiric antibiotics can then be given, depending on the level of suspicion of meningitis, encephalitis, or sepsis.

Therapy

Specific intervention is diagnosis-specific. Once assessment has determined the most likely cause of the depressed level of consciousness and resuscitative measures have stabilized respiratory and hemodynamic status, further treatment will then be guided by the presumed pathophysiology.

Increased ICP

For cerebral edema due to traumatic head injury, hypoxic–ischemic or metabolic encephalopathy, or infection, nonsurgical treatment is directed toward increased intracranial pressure (ICP) and cerebral perfusion pressure (CPP) to prevent herniation and cerebral ischemia. For cerebral edema due to neoplasms or other space occupying lesions, treatment may also include dexamathasone. Early measures should be aimed at avoiding any further increase in ICP. These include avoiding neck flexion, which may obstruct jugular venous return, and elevating the head of the bed 15–30° to reduce venous outflow pressure. Likewise, sedation or neuromuscular blockade can be initiated to avoid Valsalva maneuvers from coughing, which is common with an endotracheal tube in place. Mechanical ventilation should be set so that there is enough relative hyperventilation to reduce the pCO_2 to 25–35 mm Hg. (This can be accomplished quickly, but the benefits are transient.)

Further management requires an accurate knowledge of the child's fluid balance, frequent monitoring of blood chemistries, and, especially with traumatic brain injury, monitoring of intracranial pressure. If ICP monitoring is undertaken, ICP over 20 mm Hg warrants treatment measures. Intracranial pressure can be measured with one of several monitoring techniques. A ventricular catheter allows the most accurate measurement and also allows therapeutic drainage of CSF to lower ICP, but it may be difficult to place because of small or shifted ventricles. Other devices include transducers placed in extradural, subdural, or subarachnoid spaces, which carry a lower risk of complications but do not allow for fluid drainage.

Fluid restriction should be avoided because there may be accompanying hypovolemia. Somewhat hypertonic solutions that maintain a normal or slightly increased intravascular volume are recommended. Hypertonic saline has been shown to be effective for control of increased ICP after severe head injury. A continuous infusion of 3% saline at a rate between 1 and 2 mL/kg/hr, aiming to raise serum sodium to 145–155 mEq/L, can be used to keep the ICP below 20 mm Hg. Intermittent boluses of mannitol 0.25–1 g/kg as a 20% solution may be also be used. Mannitol, like sodium, lowers ICP by osmotically drawing water out of the brain into the vascular space. It also reduces blood viscosity, which elicits a vasoconstrictive response that decreases the cerebral blood volume. Normal saline may be needed to maintain cerebral perfusion pressure to counteract mannitol's diuretic effect. A bladder catheter must be in place to manage the resulting increased urine output, and central venous pressure monitoring should be considered. Serum osmolality should not exceed 320 mOsm/L to avoid precipitating acute renal failure in patients treated with mannitol, and 360 mOsm/L for those treated with hypertonic saline.

Mild hyperventilation may be used for brief periods, maintaining the $PaCO_2$ between 25 and 35 mm Hg. This leads to cerebral vasoconstriction and a reduction in cerebral blood flow and volume, decreasing ICP. This vasoconstrictor effect is transient, lasting less than 24 hr. More aggressive or prolonged hyperventilation may produce cerebral ischemia and should be avoided.

High dose barbiturate therapy should only be used when elevated ICP is resistant to these measures and only with ICP measurement. This is usually done with pentobarbital, loading with 10–15 mg/kg IV over 1 hr, titrating the dose to the point that a suppression-burst pattern is seen on EEG. Continuous EEG monitoring can be used as a guide to the infusion rate needed to maintain this state.

Metabolic Problems

Metabolic disturbances, such as hypoglycemia, electrolyte disturbances, or hyperammonemia should be corrected promptly. If the initial blood sugar is low, intravenous glucose should be given. If the serum sodium is below 120 mEq/L, slow correction with fluid restriction, loop diuretic, and isotonic/hypertonic saline should be instituted.

Ingestion

If ingestion is suspected, naloxone, 0.1 mg/kg intravenously or intratracheally should be given for children up to age 5. In adolescents, a minimum dose of 2 mg is recommended. This may be repeated every 2–3 min until at least 10 mg is given without a response. If there is a response, an infusion of two-thirds of the successful dose per hour may be necessary to avoid recurrent episodes of hypoventilation. This is necessary because the half-life of the opiate may be longer than the naloxone. If benzodiazepine ingestion cannot be excluded, there is no evidence of tricyclic antidepressant ingestion by history or EKG, and there is no history of seizures, flumazenil 0.02 mg/kg may be given over 30 sec up to a maximum of 0.2 mg. Use of these antagonist antidotes is safer in small children than in adults because it is unlikely they are on chronic opioid or benzodiazepine therapy. Gastric lavage, including nasogastric charcoal, may be used, if advised by poison control measures.

Nonconvulsive Status Epilepticus

Nonconvulsive status epilepticus should be suspected when a child is unresponsive, yet the eyes are open with nystagmus, gaze deviation, or lid flickering movements. An EEG may need to be performed urgently to confirm the diagnosis, followed by appropriate anticonvulsant therapy. Lorazepam 0.1 mg/kg is usually the first drug of choice, repeating the dose until there is a clinical or electrographic response. Alternatively, IV phenobarbital, phenytoin, or valproate may be used, depending on initial response and EEG findings.

Infection

If meningitis or encephalitis is suspected, then antibiotic therapy should be given. Where there is delay in performing a lumbar puncture, such as when increased intracranial pressure is suspected and a CT cannot be expedited, antibiotics may need to be initiated before cerebrospinal fluid can be obtained. For possible meningitis, empiric antibiotic therapy will depend on the child's age. Cefotaxime or ceftriaxone and vancomycin should be given to cover for *Streptococcus pneumoniae, Haemophilus influenzae*, and *Neisseria meningiditis*. If encephalitis is suspected because of a prodrome of altered mental status and seizures, IV acyclovir should be given. (See chapter on CNS infection.)

LONG-TERM MANAGEMENT AND PROGNOSIS

The prognosis for children with traumatic brain injuries may be better than for adults. Factors that have been associated with poor outcome after trauma include associated/total injuries, admission and 72 hr GCS scores, mass with increased intracranial pressure, diffuse axonal injury, and hyperglycemia. For near-drowning, there appears to be a bimodal distribution of outcomes. Children who survive tend either to return to normal or to remain in a vegetative state with few having intermediate impairment. For this and other cases of hypoxic–ischemic encephalopathy, initial cardiopulmonary resuscitation duration longer than 10 min, requirement of more than one bolus of epinephrine, and unreactive pupils in the emergency room or GCS less than 5 at 24 hr are predictive of poor outcome.

MR imaging, evoked potential studies, and EEG have been used to predict outcome. In coma due to hypoxia, ischemic lesions and edema seen early on MRI in arterial watershed regions and in the basal ganglia have been correlated with poor neurologic outcome. With the use of an MR imaging scoring system, these findings on early scans can be used to assess prognosis in children. Absence of cortical responses on somatosensory evoked potentials predicts an unfavorable outcome in most, but not all cases. Conversely, intact cortical potentials predict good outcome. The presence of organized sleep patterns on 24 hr polysomnographic EEG recordings, obtained 7–14 days after injury, has been shown to be highly predictive of better outcome in posttraumatic coma. With routine EEG, the most reliable indicator of a poor outcome is lack of variability and reactivity, including low-voltage undifferentiated tracings, burst-suppression, and electrocerebral inactivity. Clinically, the duration of coma remains an important indicator of long-term disability.

Long-term management of coma requires attention to nutrition and skin care, in addition to support of ventilation and perfusion. Once mechanical ventilation can be discontinued, circulatory function has stabilized, and intracranial pressure has normalized, early rehabilitation intervention should be considered, though the measurable impact on outcome remains unclear. Modalities used include various sensory stimulation techniques, along with standard physical, occupational, and speech therapies. This usually is best managed in a specialized rehabilitation care facility.

BRAIN DEATH

Determination of death using brain criteria is now equivalent to using cardiac criteria. Every state has adopted a version of the Uniform Determination of Death

Act, stating that "irreversible cessation of all functions of the brain including the brainstem is dead," just as with irreversible cessation of circulatory and respiratory function. Given the potential for organ donation, as well as the interest of humane care, timely identification of brain death is important in the child with coma. The determination of "irreversible cessation" of the brain is a clinical assessment. Before examining the patient, the cause of coma should be reasonably identified, the patient should be normothermic, and there should be no recent administration of interfering psychotropic or neuromuscular blocking pharmacologic agents. Complete unresponsiveness (GCS = 3) can be determined by the absence of anything more than spinal reflex activity to painful tactile stimulation. Brainstem pupillary, corneal, and vestibulo-ocular reflexes are absent. Determination of apnea is then made by removal of any external source of ventilation to allow a rise in pCO_2 to at least 60 torr or more than 20 torr above baseline with accompanying respiratory acidosis. Oxygenation is best maintained with a continuous flow of 100% oxygen. This may be done with a cannula placed down the endotracheal tube infusing at a low flow rate to avoid pneumothorax or with a source of continuous positive airway pressure. Observation is made for any evidence of respiratory effort. If none is seen, despite blood gas findings noted above, then complete apnea can be assumed and cessation of medullary function assumed. Current guidelines provide that, in infants age 7 days to 2 months, a repeat examination and EEG be performed in 48 hr; for age 2 months to 1 year, a repeat examination and ancillary testing in 24 hr; and for more than age 1 year, repeat exam in 12–24 hr. EEG may be used to provide ancillary confirmation at the discretion of the examining physician in children over 1 year. Use of ancillary imaging studies, such as radionuclide imaging, may be helpful where the child has been in drug-induced coma or when there is a medico-legal situation that warrants more extensive documentation. Once the examination has been performed, and brain death determined, then death should be pronounced and noted in the medical record. It is important to be clear with the family that death has occurred. If organ procurement is anticipated, mechanical ventilation is resumed, and circulatory support is maintained until donor organs are obtained. It may be difficult for the family, and for new intensive care staff, to understand or accept that the child has expired when color, perfusion, EKG tracing, and other signs of life persist. It is important that the clinician feels comfortable with the concept of brain death as equivalent to loss of life and that the apprehension and confusion of family members be dealt with sensitively and without ambiguity.

SUMMARY

Rapid assessment and skillful support are essential to the survival of any child presenting in coma. Once ventilation and perfusion have been assured, all possibly treatable etiologies need to be considered. If the severity of the brain insult prevents recovery, then serial estimates of prognosis can be made from clinical examination, MR imaging, and electrophysiologic measures. Early rehabilitation measures should begin in the intensive care unit. If treatment is unsuccessful and brain function is irreversibly lost, then this must be confirmed beyond doubt and communicated sensitively, but unequivocally, to the family.

APPENDIX

INITIAL EVALUATION OF UNEXPLAINED COMA

Support of airway, breathing, and circulation with cervical immobilization
Neurological examination

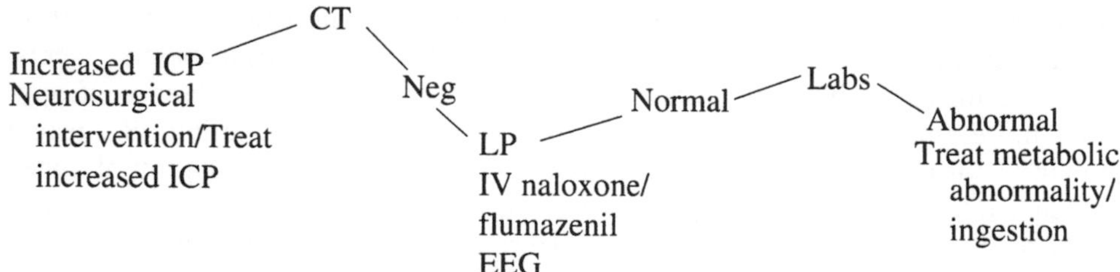

Glasgow Coma Scale

Sign	Behavior	Score
Eye opening	Spontaneous	4
	To command	3
	To pain	2
	None	1
Verbal response	Oriented	5
	Disoriented	4
	Inappropriate words	3
	Incomprehensible sounds	2
	None	1
Motor response	Obeys commands	6
	Localizes pain	5
	Withdraws	4
	Abnormal flexion to pain	3
	Abnormal extension	2
	None	1
Best total score		15

(From Ref. 1.)

Etiologies of Coma

Structural
- Trauma
- Hydrocephalus
- Neoplasm
- Hemorrhage
- Abscess
- Infarction

Hypoxia-ischemia
- Near-drowning

Continued

Etiologies of Coma *(Continued)*

- Near-miss SIDS
- Electrocution
- Strangulation

Metabolic-toxic
- Ingestion/inhalation
- Transient metabolic derangement
  - Electrolyte, glucose, calcium, magnesium
- Organ failure
  - Kidney, liver, adrenal, pituitary
- Hypothyroidism
- Inborn error of metabolism
- Drug reaction/anaphylaxis

Infection
- Sepsis
- Meningitis
- Encephalitis

Paroxysmal disorders
- Seizures
- Migraine

Guidelines for the Determination of Brain Death in Children

A. History:
1. Determine cause of coma to eliminate remediable or reversible conditions.

B. Physical examination criteria:
1. Coma and apnea must coexist.
2. Absence of brainstem function:
   (a) Midposition or fully dilated pupils unresponsive to light.
   (b) Absence of spontaneous oculocephalic (doll's eye) and caloric-induced eye movements.
   (c) Absence of movement of bulbar musculature, corneal, gag, cough, sucking, and rooting refleces.
   (d) Absence of respiratory effort with standardized testing for apnea.
3. Patient must not be hypothermic or hypotensive for age.
4. Flaccid tone and absence of spontaneous or induced movements excluding activity mediated at spinal cord level.
5. Examination should remain consistent for brain death throughout the predetermined period of observation.

C. Observation period according to age:
1. 7 days to 2 months: two examinations and EEGs 48 hr apart.
2. 2 months to 1 year: two examinations and EEGs 24 hr apart or one examination and an initial EEG demonstrating electrocerebral silence combined with a radionuclide angiogram demonstrating no cerebral blood flow, or both.
3. More than 1 year: two examinations 12–24 hr apart; EEG and isotope angiography are optional.

(From Ref. 1.)

REFERENCES

1. Teasdale G, Jennett B. Lancet 1974; 2:81.
2. Task Force for the Determination of Brain Death in Children. Guidelines for the determination of brain death in children. Pediatrics 1987; 80:298.

SUGGESTED READINGS

1. Bhardwaj A, Ulatowski J. Cerebral edema: hypertonic saline solutions. Curr Opin Neurol 1999; 1:179–187.
2. Carney N, et al. Guidelines for the acute medical management of severe traumatic brain injury in infants, children, and adolescents. Pediatr Crit Care Med 2003; 4(3): S1–S45.
3. Kirkham FJ. Non-traumatic coma in children. Arch Dis Child 2001; 85:303–312.
4. Luerssen TG. Intracranial pressure: current status in monitoring and management. Semin Pediatric Neurol 1997; 4(3):146–155.
5. Mandel R, et al. Prediction of outcome after hypoxic–ischemic encephalopathy: a prospective clinical and electrophysiologic study. J Pediatr 2002; 141:45.
6. Perry HE, Shannon MW. Diagnosis and management of opioid- and benzodiazepine-induced comatose overdose in children. Curr Opin Pediatr 1996; 8:243–247.
7. Plum F, Posner JB. The Diagnosis of Stupor and Coma 3d ed. Philadelphia: FA Davis, 1980.
8. Shewmon DA. Coma prognosis in children. Part I: definitional and methodological challenges and part II: clinical application. J Clin Neurophysiol 2000; 17(5):457–472.
9. Trubel HK, Novotny E, Lister G. Outcome of coma in children. Curr Opin Pediatr 2003; 15:283–287.

48
Postconcussion Syndrome

William R. Leahy
Neurological Medicine, Greenbelt, Maryland, U.S.A.

INTRODUCTION

During the past several decades, there has been a rapid proliferation of interest in both amateur and professional athletics. Head injury and the consequences of recurring head trauma have garnered interest among health professionals, from primary care pediatricians to neurologists, neurosurgeons, and psychiatrists. The result of this interest has led to research and long-term assessment of patients with head trauma and to the development of practice parameters such as the management of concussion in sports as established by the American Academy of Neurology (Table 1). This practice parameter is an essential guideline for all practitioners dealing with young athletes suffering concussions.

This chapter will address the postconcussion syndrome specifically. The postconcussion syndrome (PCS) can be a result of either minor or traumatic brain injury and is controversial. The debate arises due to conflicting findings regarding symptomatology, and the sparsity or absence of objective neurologic findings. Added to this dilemma are the inconsistencies in presentation, duration, and prognosis. The literature is also complex due to methodological problems.

DIAGNOSIS/CLINICAL FEATURES

Postconcussion syndrome is considered to be a relatively major public health issue, although it is rare in incidence. Most studies accept the definition of PCS to include the continuation of at least three of the following symptoms: headache, dizziness, fatigue, irritability, impaired concentration, insomnia, and photo or phonophobia. One therefore realizes the controversy as to the presence of true PCS as these symptoms are common with other etiologies such as migraine, depression, and systemic disorders. The duration of the symptoms can be weeks to months. Loss of consciousness does not have to occur to cause PCS.

Table 1 AAN Parameter on Concussion in Sports

Grade 1: Transient confusion, no LOC (loss of consciousness), resolves in 15 min
Remove from contest with neurologic examinations every 5 min
May return to game if symptoms clear within 15 min
If recurs, must stop competition and return no earlier than 1 week
Grade 2: Transient confusion, no LOC, lasts longer than 15 min
Remove from contest with no return that day
Can return in 1 week after physician examination
CT or MRI if symptoms last longer than 1 week
If recurs, must have at least 2 weeks symptom-free with rest
Grade 3: Any LOC
Transport to nearest emergency department for neurologic exam
May go home if findings normal upon initial hospital exam
If LOC is brief, can return after 1 week asymptomatic
If LOC is prolonged, can return after 2 weeks
CT or MRI if symptoms last longer than 1 week
If recurs, must have at least 1 month symptom-free

NATURAL HISTORY

The natural history (e.g., dates and times for resolution) for particular symptoms in individual patients is often variable. The severity of the injury, the effects of recurrent head trauma, and the predisposing neurologic state of the patient all influence the time to resolution.

In the first few days after the injury, the complaints are typically referable to the head (e.g., scalp, face, neck). Whiplash may occur in selected patients depending on the nature of the injury. Injury to the soft tissue of the cervical region may be associated with neck pain, musculoskeletal headaches, and dizziness.

The typical patient with PCS has a full recovery. Neural recovery often occurs immediately, with many patients back to baseline in 6–12 weeks. By one year, 85–90% of patients with PCS have fully recovered. These 10–15% of patients who have not returned to their baseline are often classified as having persistent postconcussion syndrome (PPCS).

In patients with PPCS, both cognitive and somatic complaints and/or emotional and vegetative symptoms may persist. Brain injury may manifest as forgetfulness, decreased concentration, and disturbances of the sleep–wake cycle. Impairment in attention may be long-lasting. Depression and anxiety appear to be highly correlated with the chronicity of this syndrome. Reviews in the literature have shown that the subset of PPCS often possesses premorbid psychiatric disorders and are typically under stress around the time of the head injury.

EVALUATION

Children with concussions and subsequent PCS often have CT scans and magnetic resonance imaging (MRI) at the time of injury. In the majority of cases, these studies are normal. However, the absence of loss of consciousness and neuroimaging does not rule out PCS. Findings, when present, can include petechial hemorrhage (often seen in the temporal lobes) or diffuse axonal injury.

Neuropsychological evaluation, often crucial to help treat these children, frequently demonstrates that cognitive symptomatology is not necessarily correlated with the degree of injury. Discrepancies between the signs of organic injury and symptoms may lead clinicians to question the diagnosis. Questions often arise in both PCS and PPCS as to the premorbid emotional and cognitive status of individuals with neuropsychologic difficulties.

TREATMENT

Treatment is directed to the symptom complex on an individual basis (Table 1). Simple reassurance is often the major treatment because most patients will improve within 3 months.

The management of muscle contraction type headaches on an acute basis is simple analgesics, NSAID, or muscle relaxants (methocarbamol). If headaches persist and become "chronic daily headaches" with effects on daily functioning, then prophylactic therapy is important.

Posttraumatic migraine is often responsive to abortive medications such as NSAIDs and the triptans (e.g., sumatriptan, zolmitriptan). More information about doses of all subsequently discussed medications are covered in both the abortive and preventative medications for migraine chapters in this textbook. Many of the newly approved triptans are not yet approved for the pediatric age group. If migraine begins to occur frequently, i.e., several times a week, and to interrupt daily function, then prophylaxis should begin. Prophylaxis of migraine includes beta blocking agents, calcium channel blockers, or antidepressants. Persistent vertigo or labyrinthine abnormalities with nausea and/or vomiting respond to antiemetics such as meclizine or metoclopramide. The prolonged postconcussive syndrome headaches and other nonspecific vegetative symptoms often require antidepressants, supportive psychotherapy, and cognitive rehabilitation (Table 2).

Table 2 Treatment for Postconcussion Syndrome

- Muscle contraction type of headaches
  - NSAIDs (ibuprofen, naproxen)
  - Antidepressants (amitryptline, sertraline)
  - Muscle relaxants (meclizine, metoclopramide)
- Migraine type headaches
  - Prophylactic drugs
    - Beta blockers (atenolol, propranolol)
    - Antidepressants
    - Calcium channel blockers (verapamil)
    - Anticonvulsants (valproate, topiramate)
  - Abortive drugs
    - Triptans
    - NSAIDs
- Psychological support
- Cognitive rehabilitation
- Psychotherapy
- Antidepressant medications

Antidepressants play a critical role in many levels of the postconcussive syndrome. Antidepressants, either the nightly administration of tricyclic antidepressants or the daily administration of SSRIs, may affect many of the myriad of complaints associated with postconcussive syndrome. Insomnia, anxiety, mood swings, and difficulty, in concentrating and remembering may all be positively influenced and diminished by the use of antidepressants. It is important to realize that patients may be extremely sensitive to the amount and the duration of these medications. The anticholinergic effects of tricyclic antidepressants, and the other potential side effects of SSRIs which might include emotional lability should be explained to the patient and the family prior to instituting these medications. Newer SSRIs are being approved and marketed while some of the older medications have been limited in their use because of side effects, especially depressive side effects. Consultation with psychiatrists who often use these mood-altering medications is very important for long-term use.

Management of PPCS is a mixture of medical treatment for somatic complaints, psychological and psychiatric management, and realistic occupational interventions. Cognitive therapy should be counseling, vocational supportive, adaptive therapy programs. Pharmacological treatment is for depression; SSRIs may be better than the tricyclic antidepressants. It is important to focus on the assistance in functional recovery for the persistent posttraumatic syndrome. The longer the posttraumatic symptom goes untreated, the more difficult the recovery and adjustment. Cognitive rehabilitation, biofeedback, and relaxation treatment can often be effective.

SUGGESTED READINGS

1. Evans RW. The post concussion syndrome and the sequelae of minor head injury. Neurol Clin 1992; 10:815–847.
2. McAllister TW, Archiniegas D. Evaluation and treatment of postconcussion symptoms. Neurorehabilitation 2002; 17:265–283.
3. Practice parameter: the management of concussion in sports (summary statement). Report of the Quality Standards Subcommittee. Neurology 1997; 48:581–585.

49
Neonatal Encephalopathy

Michael V. Johnston
Department of Neurology and Developmental Medicine, Kennedy Krieger Institute, Johns Hopkins University School of Medicine, Baltimore, Maryland, U.S.A.

INTRODUCTION

Neonatal encephalopathy manifested by seizures, lethargy or coma, hypotonia, poor feeding, and difficulty controlling respiration requires prompt evaluation because it often reflects a major neurological disorder. It occurs with an incidence of about 4/1000 term infants throughout the world. In 1976, Sarnat and Sarnat described encephalopathy from hypoxia–ischemia following fetal distress in full term infants and staged its severity by correlating clinical signs with electroencephalography. In 1998, Badawi and colleagues reported the first large prospective study of neonatal encephalopathy, the Western Australia study. In contrast to previous reports that focused on intrapartum asphyxia as the cause of newborn encephalopathy, the Western Australia study revealed a diverse group of antenatal etiologies unrelated to hypoxia in more than 70% of cases.

DIAGNOSIS AND CLINICAL FEATURES

Diagnosis of the presence of encephalopathy is made on the basis of observation by neonatal personnel and the neurologic exam, and its severity is graded into three numerical stages as described by the Sarnats or as mild, moderate or severe, in the Levene and Western Australia studies. In the Sarnat scale the EEG is normal in stage 1, slowed in stage 2 with a periodic or continuous delta pattern, and suppressed with infrequent discharges or isoelectric activity in stage 3. In the Levene study, the presence of seizures distinguished infants with moderate or severe encephalopathy from those with mild or no encephalopathy, but in the Western Australia study, infants were classified as having moderate encephalopathy without seizures if they had two of the following: abnormal consciousness, abnormal central breathing, poor feeding or abnormal tone and reflexes. There do not appear to be any specific clinical signs of encephalopathy that allow one to make a diagnosis of its cause. Although the EEG may suggest hypoxic-ischemic encephalopathy, it is often not specific.

Table 1 Differential Diagnosis of Neonatal Encephalopathy

Hypoglycemia
Infection
Primary: meningitis, encephalitis
Sepsis in infant
Congenital infections, TORCH
Maternal infection, sepsis syndrome
Electrolyte disturbances
Genetic/metabolic disorders
Brain malformations
Severe pre-eclampsia
Antenatal placental disorders
Stroke, in-utero or intrapartum
Asphyxia, in-utero or intrapartum
Trauma
Maternal thyroid disorders
Maternal medications/drugs/alcohol
Maternal nutritional/mineral disturbances
Venous sinus thrombosis
Intracranial hemorrhage
Kernicterus

DIFFERENTIAL DIAGNOSIS

The differential diagnosis of newborn encephalopathy is broad as shown in Table 1. Both primary central nervous system infections including meningitis and encephalitis as well as secondary effects of maternal infections are important to consider. Maternal infection can be associated with a sepsis-like syndrome that resembles the effects of direct infection. In the Western Australia study, maternal thyroid disease was associated with a ninefold increase in encephalopathy. Antenatal viral infections, placental disorders, and severe pre-eclampsia were also associated with an increase in encephalopathy. The likelihood that encephalopathy is associated with intrapartum asphyxia appears to be influenced strongly by country and level of medical care. In contrast to Western Australia, where more than 70% of cases were associated with non-hypoxic, antepartum events, a similar study in Nepal found that 60% were associated with an intrapartum event and factors including non-cephalic presentation, premature rupture of membranes and induction with oxytocin. Antenatal events such as multiple births, poor antenatal care, anemia, or maternal thyroid disease were also associated with neonatal encephalopathy in Nepal.

GENETIC AND METABOLIC DISORDERS CAUSING ENCEPHALOPATHY

A diverse group of genetic and metabolic disorders can also cause neonatal encephalopathy (Table 2). Hypoglycemia, non-ketotic hyperglycinemia, pyridoxine dependency, benign neonatal convulsions, ammonia cycle disorders, and peroxisomal disorders are fairly widely known, but it is less widely recognized that disorders such as Rett, Joubert, and Angelman syndrome can present with encephalopathy in the neonatal period, years before onset of other signs are recognized. In Rett syndrome,

Table 2 Genetic/Metabolic Causes of Neonatal Encephalopathy

Pyridoxine dependency
Benign neonatal seizures (K^+ channel genes)
Non-ketotic hyperglycinemia
Stroke/thrombophilic disorders (Leiden Factor V, etc.)
Zellweger syndrome
Neonatal adrenoleukodystrophy (peroxisomal disorders)
Ammonia cycle disorders
Congenital lactic acidosis
Mitochondrial disorders
Chromosomal disorders (e.g., trisomy 13, 18)
Smith–Lemli–Opitz
Methylmalonic academia
Angelman/Prader–Willi syndromes
Rett syndrome
Joubert syndrome
Cortical dysplasias (e.g., Miller–Dieker, 1p36 deletion)
Hemi-megalancephaly
Brain dysgenesis due to metabolic disorders
Neonatal epileptic encephalopathy (L-AADC deficiency)
Folinic responsive seizures
Ohtahara syndrome (EIEE)
Fumaric aciduria
Menkes' syndrome
Glutaric aciduria I and II
Other organic acid disorders
Sulfite oxidase deficiency (molybdenum cofactor)
Myotonic dystrophy, congenital muscular dystrophy

neonatal encephalopathy has been reported in both boys and girls. Infants with Joubert syndrome can present in the nursery with hypotonia, periodic breathing, and abnormal eye movements and have hypoplasia of the cerebellar vermis on brain imaging. Patients with Angelman syndrome can also present in the nursery with hypotonia, poor feeding, transient seizures and an abnormal EEG. It is noteworthy that in the Western Australia study, 28% of infants with encephalopathy had birth defects or other disorders (e.g., trisomy 13, 18, methylmalonic acidemia, Smith–Lemli–Opitz syndrome) compared with 4% of control infants, and in 37% of those cases the birth defect probably contributed to the encephalopathy.

DIAGNOSTIC EVALUATION

Information about the medical history of the mother and family, previous children and this pregnancy are valuable for suggesting possible causes for the encephalopathy. For example, the risk of encephalopathy is increased in families with a history of seizures or other neurologic disorders. A family history of thrombophilic disorders suggests the possibility of stroke or venous sinus thrombosis in the infant. Laboratory evaluation of the infant includes standard tests such as serum glucose, electrolytes, calcium, magnesium, and tests of renal and liver function, as well as umbilical cord arterial and venous blood gases if available. A cord pH of less than 7.0 with a severe metabolic acidosis with a base excess of 20 or greater suggests that the infant was asphyxiated, especially with a 5 min Apgar score of 3 or less at 5 min. Specialized metabolic tests may be useful for ruling out inherited metabolic diseases as listed in Table 2. Careful evaluation for sepsis, meningitis, and encephalitis is important, and a lumbar puncture should be considered. Results of fetal heart monitoring are sometimes useful, but they are often non-specific as many infants with prenatal brain disorders show abnormalities similar to those produced by intrapartum asphyxia.

EEG and brain imaging, especially magnetic resonance (MR) imaging, are valuable for determining the severity and cause of encephalopathy as well as for prognosis. Seizures are difficult to distinguish from other types of movements in sick neonates and EEG is useful for confirming their presence as well as for assessing the severity of background slowing. Cranial ultrasound is useful for detecting intracranial bleeding, hydrocephalus, and other malformations but is less sensitive for detecting early infarctions or hypoxic–ischemic injuries. Computerized tomographic (CT) scanning is rapid and readily available, but is far less sensitive than MR imaging for detecting ischemic or asphyxial injuries. Severe, "near-total" asphyxia in term infants produces a characteristic pattern of increased T1-weighted signal in the putamen, thalamus, and peri-Rolandic cerebral cortex that is often associated with extrapyramidal motor disability. In contrast, kernicterus produces increased signal in the globus pallidus. Magnetic resonance is also quite sensitive for detecting evolving infarctions, especially when diffusion and perfusion techniques are used.

THERAPY

Some causes of neonatal encephalopathy (e.g., hypoglycemia, pyridoxine dependency, infections) have specific therapies. Phenobarbital is the mainstay of treatment for seizures and is given intramuscularly or intravenously in boluses of 10 mg/kg. This is discussed in more detail in the chapter on neonatal seizures. Many clinicians consider a total dose of 40 mg/kg, producing a blood level of approximately 40 μg/mL, to be well tolerated and others use even higher doses. Respiration is monitored carefully, and patients are often placed on a ventilator to control breathing. Phenytoin (15–20 mg/kg) or fosphenytoin (equal dose in phenytoin equivalents) in a loading dose with monitoring for bradycardia is often used if a second drug is needed. However, in contrast to phenobarbital, which has a half-life of 2–3 days in neonates, the half-life of phenytoin is much shorter and less predictable. Lorazepam in boluses of 0.05–0.1 mg/kg are also useful for sustained seizures. These anticonvulsants appear to be less effective in neonates compared to adults. While it is prudent to treat seizures in the neonate, it has not been established if they damage the brain independently of the underlying pathology that causes them. For example in hypoxic–ischemic encephalopathy, seizures reflect the evolution of the cascade of excitotoxic events that cause damage, but it is not clear if they enhance the damage. A number of experimental therapies that might interrupt the neurotoxic cascade, such as hypothermia, are being evaluated for use in infants with hypoxic–ischemic encephalopathy, stroke or trauma, but none can be recommended at this time.

PROGNOSIS

Prognosis is linked to the cause of the encephalopathy as well as its severity. Levene and colleagues pointed out that the severity of encephalopathy from hypoxia–ischemia is more important than the Apgar score for determining neurological outcome in term infants with asphyxia. They reported that infants who had mild encephalopathy with minor disturbances of tone, hyper-alertness, and slight feeding difficulty with recovery in 48 hr were normal at follow-up, while 25% with moderate signs such as lethargy and seizures and 76% with more severe signs had adverse outcomes. Risk of death associated with encephalopathy in the Western Australia study was 9%, but in Nepal the death rate was 30%, probably reflecting the higher proportion of cases due to intrapartum asphyxial events in Nepal. EEG and brain MRI appear to be useful for estimating prognosis, and when both studies are normal within 72 hr, the outlook is generally favorable. However, the prognosis can be worse than the severity of encephalopathy if it is an early manifestation of a genetic disorder such as Rett syndrome or Angelman syndrome.

SUMMARY

Neonatal encephalopathy is caused by a diverse group of acquired and genetic disorders. Geographic location and level of medical care appear to affect the distribution of etiologies: less than 30% of cases are associated with intrapartum hypoxia in advanced countries such as Australia while more than half have been linked to intrapartum events in less advanced regions. A combination of EEG and brain imaging, especially MRI, is useful for establishing a diagnosis and prognosis. Specific therapies are available for some causes of encephalopathy, and anticonvulsants should be administered to treat seizures although their neuroprotective effects have not been established.

SUGGESTED READINGS

1. Cowan F, Rutherford M, Groenendaal F, et al. Origin and timing of brain lesions in term infants with neonatal encephalopathy. Lancet 2003; 361:736–742.
2. Johnston MV. MRI for neonatal encephalopathy in full-term infants. Lancet 2003; 361:713–714.
3. Johnston MV, Trescher WH, Ishida A, Nakajima W. Neurobiology of hypoxic–ischemic injury in the developing brain. Pediatr Res 2001; 49:735–741.
4. Levene MI, Sands C, Grindulis H, Moore JR. Comparison of two methods of predicting outcome in perinatal asphyxia. Lancet 1986; 1:67–69.
5. Sarnat HB, Sarnat MS. Neonatal encephalopathy following fetal distress. Arch Neurol 1976; 33:696–670.

50

Pantothenate Kinase-Associated Neurodegeneration (PKAN)

Susan J. Hayflick
Molecular and Medical Genetics, Pediatrics and Neurology, Oregon Health & Science University, Portland, Oregon, U.S.A.

INTRODUCTION

Pantothenate kinase-associated neurodegeneration (PKAN) is a genetic movement disorder that accounts for the majority of cases of what was formerly called Hallervorden–Spatz syndrome. In 1922, Hallervorden and Spatz reported an autosomal recessive neurodegenerative disorder with retinitis pigmentosa and high levels of iron in brain. Since then, the diagnosis has been expanded to encompass a heterogeneous group of disorders that share the feature of high brain iron. To discredit Hallervorden and Spatz for their objectionable actions during World War II, the eponym has been abandoned and replaced with the term "neurodegeneration with brain iron accumulation" (NBIA). NBIA includes neurological disorders in which basal ganglia iron levels are high. PKAN is one form of NBIA.

CLINICAL FEATURES AND DIAGNOSIS

The PKAN phenotype generally can be stratified into two groups: early onset, rapidly progressive disease, or later onset, more slowly progressive disease. The classic, more severe form of PKAN begins usually by age 5 years with gait abnormalities due to dystonia, rigidity, and spasticity. Though initially asymmetric and involving the limbs, the disease progresses to more generalized dystonia, including orofacial involvement. Pigmentary degeneration of the retina occurs in two-thirds of patients with classic PKAN. Patients with this form of disease experience periods of rapid clinical deterioration, with intercurrent plateauing. Skills, once lost, are only rarely regained. The HARP syndrome (hypoprebetalipoproteinemia, acanthocytosis, retinopathy, and pallidal degeneration) is in the PKAN disease spectrum and is caused by mutations in the same gene as PKAN.

In contrast to the homogeneous clinical profile of most patients with classic PKAN, atypical PKAN includes a broad spectrum of features including palilalia, parkinsonism, and neuropsychiatric disabilities. Eventually, these patients, too, develop dystonia with gait impairment that progresses to more generalized disease. Usually, the rate of progression is slower in atypical PKAN than that seen in classic disease, and the age at onset can be in the second or third decade of life. Careful history-taking often reveals that these patients were clumsy as children with frequent falls, impulsive behavior, and learning disabilities. Clinical retinal disease in atypical PKAN is rare. Seizures are not a common feature of either form of PKAN.

Suspicion of PKAN is raised in a patient with clinical features suggestive of this disease spectrum and in whom the brain MRI shows typical changes. These changes include a region of hypointensity in the globus pallidus surrounding a central area of hyperintensity on T2-weighted images (Fig. 1). The hypointense lesions indicate abundant iron, and the hyperintense signal suggests tissue edema. This pattern, called the eye-of-the-tiger sign, is virtually pathognomonic for PKAN occurring in both classic and atypical disease. In some patients, the MRI changes predate the onset of symptoms; in others, they become evident only following the initial period of clinical decline. The brain MRI changes in NBIA are distinct from those seen in PKAN and include only hypointense lesions in the globus pallidus on T2-weighted imaging.

The diagnosis of PKAN is strongly supported by the clinical and radiographic features. Since the discovery of the gene that is defective in PKAN, clinical molecular testing has become available (www.genetests.org). Demonstration of two deleterious mutations in the *PANK2* gene, which encodes pantothenate kinase 2, confirms the diagnosis. In some patients only one mutation can be found, most likely reflecting the limitations of current testing methods. As a general rule, patients with two null

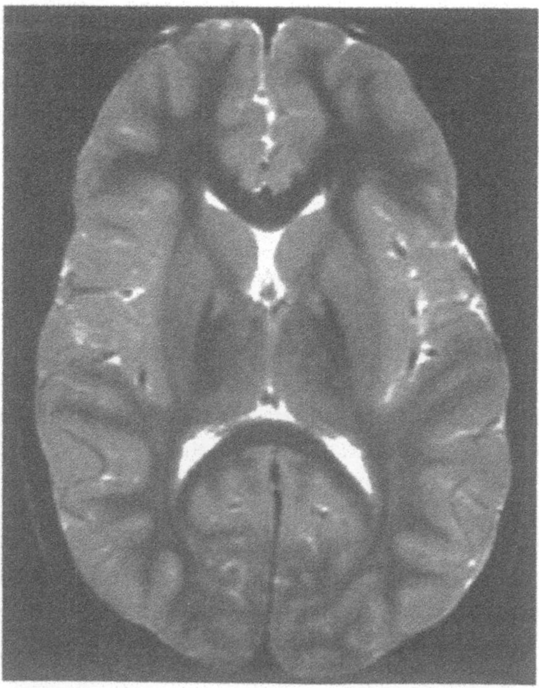

Figure 1 Pattern on T2-weighted brain magnetic resonance imaging. The image of a *PANK2*-mutation-positive patient shows hypointensity with a central region of hyperintensity in the medial globus pallidus (the eye-of-the-tiger sign).

mutations develop classic disease. To date, there is an absolute correlation between the presence of the eye-of-the-tiger sign and mutations in *PANK2*.

THERAPY

Until very recently, treatment of PKAN has been palliative. Drug regimens have been focused on managing the dystonia, rigidity, and pain associated with the disease. Following the discovery of the defect in the gene encoding pantothenate kinase 2, novel ideas for therapies that are based on predictions about the biochemistry of this disease have been proposed. Disease outcome measures are currently being studied in preparation for investigating rational treatments for PKAN.

PALLIATIVE THERAPIES

PKAN is primarily a disorder of the basal ganglia, with the most disabling features being dystonia, dysarthria, spasticity, and rigidity. Baclofen provides relief from the dystonia more consistently than any other medication. Both oral and intrathecal delivery have been used in PKAN with significant benefits. As their disease progresses, patients often require increasing doses in order to manage their worsening dystonia. Other drugs that have brought relief to some patients include trihexyphenydyl, clonazepam, and phenobarbital. As a rule, levo-DOPA offers no benefit to patients with PKAN.

Pain management is an important part of care in the later stages of PKAN. Foremost, it is essential to search for treatable causes of pain in these patients. The combination of severe dystonia with osteopenia in nonambulatory patients places them at high risk for fractures, even without obvious trauma. Orobuccal dystonia is common and can result in repeated trauma to the tongue. Bite blocks and other mechanical means to prevent this have generally proved unsuccessful. Full-mouth dental extraction has been used to allay this especially distressing problem. Involvement of a pain management team may eventually become necessary.

SUPPORTIVE CARE

Problems of feeding and breathing eventually complicate the course of most patients with classic PKAN. Early introduction of gastrostomy feeding helps to optimize nutrition and limit risks from aspiration. Laryngeal dystonia causes severe stridor, leading to distress for both the patient and their caregivers. This complication as well as the increasing risk of aspiration may compromise oxygen saturation sufficiently to warrant placement of a tracheostomy tube.

DEVELOPING ADDITIONAL RATIONAL THERAPIES

Ideas for rational therapies have followed the discovery of the genetic defect in PKAN. Pantothenate kinase catalyzes the phosphorylation of pantothenate (vitamin

B5) in a key regulatory step in the synthesis of coenzyme A, making PKAN the first recognized inborn error of coenzyme A metabolism (Fig. 2). Coenzyme A is important in numerous biochemical pathways, including energy and lipid metabolism, as well as neurotransmitter and glutathione synthesis. Since pantothenate kinase 2 is one of four human proteins predicted to carry out this enzymatic function and is now known to be uniquely targeted to mitochondria, limitation of the phenotype to brain and retina may reflect the high metabolic demands or susceptibility to oxidative damage that characterize these tissues.

The pathogenesis of PKAN is hypothesized to derive from a combination of product deficit and secondary substrate accumulation. Deficient pantothenate kinase is predicted to lead to low levels of coenzyme A in mitochondria causing a host of metabolic derangements. The cardinal feature of high basal ganglia iron levels in PKAN may be explained by tissue accumulation of two substrates of pantothenate kinase that contain cysteine, *N*-pantothenoylcysteine, and pantetheine. These compounds are predicted to chelate iron, though they also may cause direct toxicity. The globus pallidus may be especially susceptible to injury because of its high metabolic activity and normally iron-rich composition.

These hypotheses of pathogenesis have lead to novel ideas for therapeutic intervention in PKAN. Potential therapies aim to address the predicted deficiency of coenzyme A or the mechanisms leading to iron accumulation and the sequelae of oxidative damage. An obvious initial choice for therapy is the product of the enzyme that is deficient in PKAN, phosphopantothenate. This compound, however, is unlikely to traverse membranes and become bioavailable, and there is no ready source of phosphopantothenate. Ingested coenzyme A is metabolized to pantothenate, hence a direct attempt to supplement with CoA is probably no better than using pantothenate. For PKAN patients who are predicted to retain partial PANK2 enzyme function, substrate overload with high doses of pantothenate may be beneficial, and pantothenate has no significant toxicity.

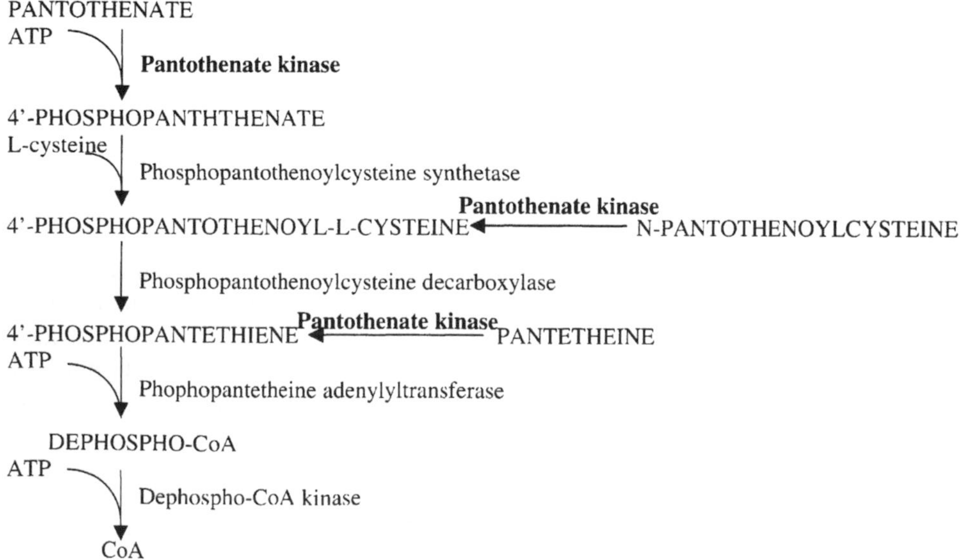

Figure 2 Pantothenate forms the chemical core of coenzyme A. Pantothenate kinase catalyzes the phosphorylation of pantothenate, *N*-pantothenoyl-cysteine, and pantetheine.

To address the pathologic sequelae of possible tissue accumulation of cysteine-containing compounds, cysteamine may be useful. Therapeutic iron-chelating agents have been tried in PKAN in order to decrease brain iron levels. Their use has lead to systemic iron deficiency with no apparent CNS benefits. Indirect approaches to limiting the toxic effects of high levels of iron in brain might include antioxidant therapy. However, there is a compelling argument against using antioxidants in PKAN since they may paradoxically fuel the redox cycle and worsen disease. Anecdotal reports of the use in PKAN of idebenone, a coenzyme Q analog, suggest that these compounds may indeed exacerbate disease and therefore may be contraindicated.

PROGNOSIS

The prognosis for patients with PKAN depends on the severity of their disease. Those with earlier onset consistently show a more rapid rate of disease progression than those who present later in life. In the classic form, most patients show relentless progression with loss of ambulation within 10–15 years of onset and death by the third decade of life. Causes of death are typically complications of a vegetative state, including pneumonia and sepsis, and are not directly from the disease. Adequate nutrition, prevention of aspiration, and attention to minor illnesses can extend the life of these patients. In atypical PKAN, patients often progress to loss of ambulation within 15–40 years of disease onset, though rarely a patient will show only minor neurologic impairment even into the eighth decade. Improvements in the prognosis for these patients have come mostly from better supportive care.

SUMMARY

Significant gains in our understanding of the biochemical defects in PKAN have shifted the therapeutic focus from palliative care to rational interventions. Novel therapies aimed at correcting specific perturbations in cellular metabolism hold great promise and are currently under investigation. Treatment of this rare neurodegenerative disorder is likely to change significantly over the next decade.

SUGGESTED READINGS

1. Coryell J, Hayflick S. Pantothenate kinase-associated neurodegeneration (updated March 8, 2003). In: GeneReviews: Medical Genetics Information Resource (database online). Copyright, University of Washington, Seattle, 1997–2003. Available at http://www.geneclinics.org. Accessed August 2003.
2. Hayflick SJ, Westaway SK, Levinson B, Zhou B, Johnson MA, Ching KHL, Gitschier J. Genetic, clinical, and radiographic delineation of Hallervorden–Spatz syndrome. N Engl J Med 2003; 348(1):33–40.
3. Zhou B, Westaway SK, Levinson B, Johnson MA, Gitschier J, Hayflick SJ. A novel pantothenate kinase gene (*PANK2*) is defective in Hallervorden–Spatz syndrome. Nature Genetics 2001; 28(4):345–349.

51
Copper (Menkes/Wilson)

Tyler Reimschisel
McKusick-Nathans Institute of Genetic Medicine, Johns Hopkins Hospital, Baltimore, Maryland, U.S.A.

INTRODUCTION

Copper is a heavy metal that is an essential cofactor for several important enzymes in humans. Known as *cuproenzymes*, these enzymes include cytochrome C oxidase (electron transport chain), dopamine β-hydroxylase (catecholamine synthesis), superoxide mutase (detoxification of free radicals), and lysyl oxidase (formation of collagen). The main source of copper is copper-containing foods, high quality sources being shellfish, nuts, chocolate, mushrooms, and liver. In the intestines, copper is transported into enterocytes and then transferred to the portal circulation by one of two mechanisms. Copper may bind to metallothioneins, proteins that bind metals, and then be transported to the liver. Alternatively, copper can be actively transported across the basolateral membrane of the enterocytes where it then binds to albumin and other proteins in blood. It is then transported to the liver through the portal circulation. Menkes disease is an X-linked disorder due to mutations in the gene *ATP7A* that encodes the ATPase-dependent copper transporter on the basolateral membrane of the enterocytes. In this disorder, there is a buildup of copper in enterocytes, leading to a secondary systemic copper deficiency. Without adequate copper, cuproenzyme function is impaired and the symptoms of Menkes disease develop.

Once copper reaches the liver, it is readily transported into the hepatocytes. A different membrane-associated ATPase transporter then incorporates copper into ceruloplasmin or excretes it into bile. Wilson disease is an autosomal recessive disorder due to mutations in *ATP7B*, the gene that encodes for this particular ATPase copper transporter. In Wilson disease, copper accumulates in hepatocytes, and this accumulation causes cell death. When the cells die, copper is released into the bloodstream. Copper then accumulates in the brain, eyes, kidneys, muscles, bones, and joints. Copper accumulation in the brain and liver leads to the clinical features of Wilson disease.

MENKES DISEASE

Clinical Features and Diagnosis

The characteristic features of Menkes disease include seizures, developmental regression, hypotonia, and failure to thrive. Seizures may present in the neonatal period, and infantile spasms may develop. Symptoms begin by 2–3 months of age in almost all boys with this disorder. Full rosy cheeks, coarse and sparse hair, and a highly arched palate are common. Microscopic evaluation of scalp hair reveals twisting of the hair shaft (*pili torti*). Individuals with Menkes syndrome may also have loose and redundant skin, episodic hypoglycemia, temperature instability, autonomic instability, hernias, retinal hypopigmentation, cataracts, and urinary bladder diverticula. Neuroimaging may show impaired myelination, diffuse atrophy, ventriculomegaly, and strokes due to fragile, tortuous cerebral vessels. Copper and ceruloplasmin levels are very low or undetectable. Dysfunction of dopamine β-hydroxylase, the cuproenzyme that converts dopamine to norepinephrine, leads to elevations of dopamine, dihydroxyphenylalanine (DOPA, a precursor of dopamine), and dihydroxyphenylacetic acid (a metabolite of dopamine). Norepinephrine and its metabolite, dihydroxyphenylglycol (DHPG), are low. The ratio of DOPA:DHPG is markedly elevated. Confirmatory DNA analysis is available. A fetus can be diagnosed with Menkes disease by measurement of copper concentration and direct genomic DNA analysis of amniocytes or chorionic villi cells.

Treatment

Due to the underlying defect in Menkes disease, oral administration of copper is ineffective. Parenteral administration of copper can be given in a variety of forms, including copper-acetate, copper-ethylenediamine tetraacetic acid, and copper-histidine. Copper-histidine is the form that is most efficiently taken up by the brain and is the best tolerated; therefore, it is the form that is used most commonly in Menkes patients. The dosage recommendation is 100–1000 μg per day given intramuscularly or subcutaneously. The efficacy of the medication can be monitored by following serum copper and ceruloplasmin levels and urinary copper excretion. On an adequate dose, the serum copper and ceruloplasmin levels should be within the normal limits.

Individuals with Menkes syndrome should also receive symptomatic management. The seizures can be very difficult to control, and the use of multiple anticonvulsants and the ketogenic diet may be necessary. If a bladder ultrasound reveals a structural abnormality that may predispose to urinary tract infections, then prophylactic antibiotics should be considered. Routine immunizations and the yearly influenza immunizations should be given to the child. Ongoing physical and occupational therapy should be provided. Genetic counseling should be offered to the parents. Since many children with Menkes disease have profound neurologic impairment, it may also be important to discuss end-of-life issues and palliative care options with the family.

Prognosis

There is a correlation between early, presymptomatic initiation of copper treatment and better neurologic outcome. If an infant with Menkes disease has neurologic deterioration before treatment is started, then full neurologic recovery is impossible. In some of these children, copper therapy may decrease the severity of the seizures, diminish irritability, and improve sleep hygiene. Nonetheless, these potential benefits must be weighed against the difficulty of providing daily to near-daily injections.

There are reports that normal development can be achieved in a subset of individuals with Menkes disease if the treatment is initiated before neurologic symptoms begin. Usually, a fetus or newborn is diagnosed with Menkes because he has a family history of death from the disease. In these cases, copper-histidine can be initiated in utero or in the newborn period. When treatment begins in the presymptomatic period, individuals may have no neurologic deficits. If they have impairment, it may be significantly less impairment than that seen in individuals who are treated after neurologic symptoms develop. However, presymptomatic copper therapy does not necessarily cure the nonneurologic characteristics of the disease, including the abnormal hair texture and connective tissue laxity.

WILSON DISEASE

Clinical Features and Diagnosis

Wilson disease can present with symptoms of hepatic, neurologic, or psychiatric dysfunction. Hepatic disease is most prevalent in those individuals who develop manifestations of the disease in adolescence. It causes nonspecific signs and symptoms of liver disease, including persistently elevated serum aminotransferase levels, jaundice, anorexia, vomiting, abdominal pain, ascites, weight loss, easy bruisability, bleeding, hepatomegaly, and splenomegaly. Individuals may also present with acute hepatitis or fulminant hepatic failure. Hemolytic anemia can be the presenting problem in children with Wilson disease and when noted is associated with mortality in up to 80%. In those with hepatic Wilson disease, there can be spontaneous remissions and exacerbations.

About 1/3 of individuals with Wilson disease present with neurologic problems, including dysarthria, dysphagia, and drooling. They also typically develop a movement disorder, including dystonia, rigidity, tremor, ataxia, ballism, or hypokinesia.

Wilson disease can also present with psychiatric symptoms, such as mood changes, frank depression, psychosis, and personality and behavior changes. Up to 60% of individuals with Wilson disease will have psychiatric manifestations of the disease at some point in the course of the illness. Other less common presentations include premature osteoporosis and arthritis, cardiomyopathy, pancreatitis, nephrolithiasis, generalized aminoaciduria, hypoparathyroidism, and infertility.

Multiple laboratory studies can be performed in the evaluation of Wilson disease. Ceruloplasmin is low in up to 95% of cases. However, ceruloplasmin is an acute phase reactant. Therefore, it can be within the normal range in affected individuals who have an intercurrent illness. Also, the ceruloplasmin level can be low in asymptomatic carriers. A 24-hr urine copper level is usually diagnostic. In affected individuals, the level is usually greater than 100 μg Cu/24 hr and a level less than 50 μg Cu/24 hr makes the disease highly unlikely. In half of individuals with only hepatic Wilson disease and in almost all individuals with neurologic or psychiatric symptoms from Wilson disease, slit-lamp examination reveals Kayser–Fleischer rings. They are benign copper accumulations in Decemet's membrane in the cornea. If the diagnosis is uncertain, then a liver biopsy can be performed to determine copper concentration. In affected individuals, the hepatic copper concentration is often significantly elevated (above 250–300 μg Cu/g dry weight), but the concentration can be elevated in any condition that causes impaired biliary excretion of copper. Neuroimaging is usually abnormal in individuals with neurologic or psychiatric problems, but may be normal in those with only hepatic dysfunction. The typical MRI abnormality is increased T_2-weighted signal in the caudate, putamen, subcortical white matter, and/or brainstem. DNA mutation analysis is not feasible since over 200 mutations have been identified in individuals with Wilson disease.

All first-degree relatives of affected individuals should have screening studies for the disease. This screen includes a complete history and physical examination; measurement of serum ceruloplasmin, liver aminotransferases, albumin, bilirubin, and 24-hr urine copper; and ophthalmology evaluation for Kayser–Fleischer rings. Enzyme linkage analysis of the family members of a proband can also be performed.

Serum copper analysis is not a reliable method for diagnosing Wilson disease.

Treatment

There are three phases in the treatment of Wilson disease: acute therapy, maintenance therapy, and prophylaxis of presymptomatic individuals. In affected individuals who present with acute liver failure, orthotopic liver transplantation may be necessary. In those who present with less severe liver dysfunction or neuropsychiatric symptoms, a chelating agent such as penicillamine, tetrathiomolybdate (TM), or trientine is indicated.

Penicillamine

Penicillamine, the first oral agent used to treat Wilson disease, promotes copper excretion in urine and induces metallothionein production. It is efficacious, but is associated with multiple side effects, including hypersensitivity reactions; production of autoantibodies that leads to Goodpasture disease, myasthenia gravis or systemic lupus erythematosis; pancytopenia; and nephrotic syndrome. Up to one quarter of the patients who begin penicillamine therapy discontinue it due to intolerable side effects.

The tolerability of penicillamine can be improved by starting it in adults at 250 to 500 mg per day and increasing by 250 mg every 4–7 days to a maximum of 1000 to 1500 mg per day in two to four divided doses. (All recommended doses are based on the excellent review by Roberts and Schilsky that is referenced in the Suggested Reading section.) In children, the recommended dose is 20 mg/kg per day (dose rounded to the nearest 250 mg) in two to three divided doses per day. The medication should be taken 1 hr prior to or 2 hr after meals. An effective dose of penicillamine will keep the 24-hr urinary copper excretion between 200 and 500 μg per day. Pyridoxine supplementation (25–50 mg daily) is also required.

The most troublesome and concerning side effect of penicillamine therapy is neurologic deterioration. Brewer has shown that up to 50% of individuals with neurologic symptoms have sudden neurologic deterioration after starting penicillamine therapy. Of those who develop neurologic deterioration, 50% have permanent disability that is worse than their pretreatment clinical status.

Tetrathiomolybdate

Tetrathiomolybdate (TM) is a newer, very effective chelating agent that has fewer side effects than penicillamine and rarely causes neurologic deterioration. Although a formal toxicity study of TM is currently in progress, investigators have shown that adverse effects from TM include mild bone marrow suppression that can cause anemia, leukopenia, and thrombocytopenia and minimal elevations in serum aminotransferase levels. Both adverse effects improve with a drug holiday or dose reduction. Only a small number of individuals on TM therapy have experienced worsening neurologic status while receiving TM. Thus, the risk of neurologic deterioration is much lower than the risk seen with penicillamine therapy.

The initial dose in adults is 120 mg per day. The dose may then be adjusted to a maximum of 200 mg per day to maintain the 24-hr urinary copper excretion at 250–500 μg per day. There is no recommended dose for TM in children. Tetrathiomolybdate is currently being used on an experimental basis in the United States.

Trientine

Trientine can also be used as a chelating agent for hepatic or neuropsychiatric symptoms. It chelates copper and promotes excretion by the kidneys. It is better tolerated than penicillamine, and in general individuals experiencing adverse effects from penicillamine get amelioration of their symptoms after switching to trientine. Possible side effects from trientine include pancytopenia, sideroblastic anemia (due to copper deficiency), aplastic anemia, gastritis, and lupus-like reactions. It is only rarely associated with neurologic deterioration.

In adults the typical initial dosage is 750–1500 mg per day in two to three divided doses. Maintenance dosage is 750–1000 mg per day. In children, the dose is not established, but investigators have recommended 250 mg/kg per day (dose rounded to nearest 250 mg) in two to three divided doses per day. Similar to penicillamine, the medication should be taken 1 hr before or 2 hr after meals. An effective dose of trientine will keep the 24-hr urinary copper excretion between 200 and 500 μg per day.

Zinc

Zinc is used in the maintenance phase of treatment or in individuals who are presymptomatic. It interferes with copper uptake in the intestines by inducing metallothionein synthesis. Metallothionein binds copper in the enterocyte and prohibits entry into the portal circulation. It has a relatively benign side effect profile, including gastric irritation and elevations in lipase and/or amylase without clinical evidence of pancreatitis. Neurologic deterioration occurs very rarely. The maintenance dose of elemental zinc is 150 mg per day in adults and 50–75 mg per day in children, divided into three daily doses. Desired 24-hr urinary copper excretion on treatment should be less than 75 μg per day.

Treatment of Presymptomatic Patients

Presymptomatic individuals over the age of three years, with biochemical, histological, or DNA evidence of Wilson disease should be started on prophylactic medication. Penicillamine or zinc can prevent the development and progression of symptoms. Treatment of children under the age of 3 is controversial.

All individuals on maintenance therapy with penicillamine, trientine, or zinc should regularly receive a complete blood count analysis with differential, liver aminotransferase levels, serum copper and ceruloplasmin levels, and urinalysis. If possible, one can also monitor the serum nonceruloplasmin-bound copper.

Foods that contain a high content of copper should be avoided by all individuals with Wilson disease or by presymptomatic individuals with biochemical evidence of the disease. Foods high in copper include shellfish, mushrooms, nuts, chocolate, and liver. Well water should be tested for copper content.

Symptomatic therapy may also be necessary. If affected individuals have problems with dysphagia, then a swallowing evaluation should be performed and appropriate diet modifications should be recommended. Psychiatric problems can develop even after acute treatment begins. Therefore, psychiatric evaluation and treatment may be necessary during acute and maintenance therapy.

Prognosis

In general, the prognosis for individuals with Wilson disease is reassuring, unless they have severe neurologic impairment or severe liver disease. In those with mild-to-moderate disease, recovery begins approximately 6 months after acute therapy begins. Recovery can continue for up to 2 years. It is likely that any neurologic disability or liver dysfunction that persists 2 years after the initiation of therapy will be permanent. Most patients who have mild-to-moderate disease when treatment is started will have complete or near-complete recovery.

SUGGESTED READINGS

1. Brewer GJ. Practical recommendations and new therapies for Wilson's disease. Drugs 1995; 50:240–249.
2. Brewer GJ, Hedera P, Kluin KJ, et al. Treatment of Wilson disease with ammonium tetrathiomolybdate. Archives Neurol 2003; 60:379–385.
3. Christodoulou J, Danks DM, Sarkar B, et al. Early treatment of Menkes disease with parenteral copper-histidine: long-term follow-up of four treated patients. Am J Med Genetics 1998; 76:154–164.
4. Gu Y, Kodama H, Sato E, et al. Prenatal diagnosis of Menkes disease by genetic analysis and copper measurement. Brain Devel 2002; 24:715–718.
5. Kaler SG. Menkes disease. Adv Pediatr 1994; 41:263–304.
6. Kodama H, Murata Y, Kobayashi M. Clinical manifestations and treatment of Menkes disease and its variants. Pediatr Int 1999; 41:423–429.
7. Roberts EA, Schilsky ML. A practice guideline on Wilson disease. Hepatology 2003; 37:1475–1492.

52
Metachromatic Leukodystrophy

Gerald V. Raymond
Kennedy Krieger Institute, Johns Hopkins University School of Medicine, Baltimore, Maryland, U.S.A.

INTRODUCTION

Metachromatic leukodystrophy (MLD) is a progressive genetic disorder affecting myelin of the central and peripheral nervous system. MLD results from an alteration in the gene for the lysosomal enzyme arylsulfatase A or its activator. Arylsulfatase A, in conjunction with its activator saposin, cleaves sulfatides from sphingoglycolipids. Defects in the process result in the accumulation of cerebroside sulfatides. This increase occurs predominantly in the nervous system resulting in dysfunction and progressive destruction of myelin. This demyelination results in the clinical syndrome of MLD.

There are three genetically and biochemically distinct disorders that can result in MLD—deficiency of arylsulfatase A; sulfatide activator deficiency due to a defect in sphingolipid activator protein (SAP1), required for the action of arylsulfatase A; or multiple sulfatase deficiency resulting from a defect in the gene sulfatase-modifying factor 1 (SUMF1). All three forms are autosomal recessive conditions. The gene that encodes arylsulfatase A is located on the terminal tip of chromosome 22. SAP1 is produced by the gene Prosaposin, which encodes several activators. The SUMF1 gene encodes the enzyme which converts a specific cysteine residue to formylglycine in the endoplasmic reticulum. Failure to carry out this transformation results in failure to activate a variety of sulfatases, including arylsulfatase A.

The presentation of MLD may occur in infancy, childhood, or rarely adulthood. The presentation varies to some extent depending on the age of the individual, but it is characterized by loss of previously acquired skills, progressive evidence of myelin destruction, and ultimately a vegetative state and death. The incidence of the condition is in the range of 1:40,000–100,000 and, as will be discussed below, is a rarer condition than the pseudodeficiency of arylsulfatase A, which complicates diagnosis.

DIAGNOSIS AND CLINICAL FEATURES

MLD is typically classified by age of presentation, but it is important to realize that there is great variability and may present at nearly any age. The infantile form of

MLD is usually noted around 18 months of age and is characterized by the slowed attainment of milestones followed by gradual loss of motor skills. The child who is just beginning to walk will stop, followed by the loss of the ability to feed himself and sit unsupported. Vision will become affected. Ataxia may also be present. The differential of such an individual will naturally be broad and will initially include both the static process of cerebral palsy as well as the progressive disorders including neoplasms, infections, inflammation, vascular disease, and other leukodystrophies (see Table 1 for leukodystrophies). Seizures may occur. A similar progression in the older child is characteristic of the juvenile form although the rate of progression may be slower. Peripheral neuropathy may be present and it is not unusual to have both loss of sensation and areflexia despite the presence of spasiticity. The adult presentation is characterized initially by psychiatric symptoms. Adult disease tends to be more slowly progressive and the diagnosis in affected individuals often is delayed.

MLD affects primarily the central and peripheral nervous system, but accumulation in the biliary tract and the kidneys has been reported. There are very rare reports of MLD producing symptomatic gall bladder disease.

The first clue to the diagnosis is usually neuroimaging with characteristic abnormalities noted on magnetic resonance imaging (MRI). There is hyperintensity of the myelin on T2-weighted or FLAIR images. Contrast enhancement is not typical. Magnetic resonance spectroscopy demonstrates a rise in choline and a decrease in *N*-acetyl aspartate (NAA) peaks.

The diagnosis of MLD rests on the demonstration of deficient arylsulfatase A activity in white cells or fibroblasts. In most affected individuals, levels will be markedly depressed. Caution must be exercised, however, because a significant percentage of the population carries a polymorphic alteration in the arylsulfatase A gene that results in a pseudodeficiency of arylsulfatase A. It is imperative that all abnormal values be confirmed with further testing for a defect in sulfatide metabolism either by measuring for an elevation in urine sulfatides or a defect in the ability of fibroblasts to metabolize sulfatides.

The pseudodeficiency allele interferes with the metabolism of the artificial substrate used in the assay, but does not result in disease. The frequency of the pseudodeficiency allele has been reported to be approximately 15% of the population and up to 2% of the population may be homozygous for this allele resulting in abnormal arylsulfatase levels on the standard assay.

Table 1 Leukodystrophies

Disorder	Enzyme/protein defect	Biochemical abnormality	Gene loci	Inheritance
Metachromatic leukodystrophy	Arylsulfatase A	Sulfatide accumulation	22q13	AR
Globoid leukodystrophy (Krabbe)	Galactocerebrosidase	Psychosine	14q25-31	AR
Adrenoleukodystrophy	ALD protein	Very long chain fatty acids	Xq28	XLR
Alexander	Glial fibrially acidic protein			Spontaneous rare—AD
Canavan	Aspartoacylase	*N*-acetylaspartate	17p13	AR
Pelizaeus Merzbacher	Proteolipid protein		Xq22	XLR

In families with documented arylsulfatase A deficiency, there is a 25% recurrence risk. It is very important for family counseling and therapeutic decisions that the disorder be diagnosed rapidly and accurately and younger siblings appropriately tested. Prenatal diagnosis is available using amniocytes for arylsulfatase A activity or DNA analysis.

In activator deficiency, presentation is usually in childhood, but enzymatic activity of arylsulfatase A will not be absent. Excreted amounts of urine sulfatides will be elevated. Children with multiple sulfatase deficiency have combined clinical features of the mucopolysaccharidosis and MLD.

TREATMENT

The observation that fibroblast cultures from patients with Hurler syndrome and Hunter syndrome could be corrected by cocultures with normal cell lines or lymphocyte extracts has led to hematopoietic cell transplantation for lysosomal disorders. Monocyte-macrophages are derived from bone marrow stem cells and provide the opportunity to transfer biochemically intact cells to an affected individual. However, for unclear reasons, not all lysosomal disorders have responded to this therapy.

Interpretation of the results of hematopoietic cell transplantation in MLD has been confounded by variations in disease, severity at the time of transplant, variation in regimen, post-transplant complications, and other confounders. At this time, it is accepted that MLD cannot be treated effectively by transplantation if neuropsychological or neurological signs are advanced in the late-infantile disease. Specific criteria for transplantation have not been established in childhood and adult disease forms. Transplantation with mesenchymal stem cells has been attempted in order to improve peripheral demyelination.

The best outcomes for hematopoietic cell transplantation have occurred in transplant centers experienced with performing transplantation in children who have metabolic storage diseases. This and similar storage disorders require a multidisciplinary team with the availability of a wide range of consultants both during the process and in follow-up.

It is expected that presymptomatic individuals would attain the greatest benefit from this therapy and it is important to evaluate younger at-risk siblings. This has prompted some to attempt to develop methods of newborn screening.

In those individuals who are not candidates for transplantation therapy, care should focus on symptoms including spasticity, feeding difficulties, mobility, communication, behavioral symptoms, and seizures.

A variety of agents have been used for spasticity and the resultant discomfort. Benzodiazepines including valium, lorazepam, or clonazepam have been the most used by our group, but often require elevated dosages with time. Dosages are outlined in the chapter on Spasticity. Baclofen, dantrolene, tizanidine, and other agents may also be used. Intrathecal baclofen pumps have an important role in selected patients.

Seizures may be treated by appropriate agent according to type. Sedative agents are sometimes required to assist with sleep. Psychiatric symptoms, especially in adults, require appropriate management with pharmacologic agents and support services. With loss of swallowing abilities, individuals may require gastrostomy placement.

PROGNOSIS

MLD is a progressive neurodegenerative disease and affected individuals will die of their disease. In most instances, the disorder results in a progressive bulbar and autonomic difficulties and individuals succumb to pulmonary complications.

Patients and their families require continuing care and support after the diagnosis is made. The depth of a discussion on the course of the disease will depend on where in the disease trajectory the patient is and given the nature of the news may need reiteration in future discussions. Hospice care and discussions on other end of life issues will need to be made in the course of the illness and adjusted depending on circumstances.

SUMMARY

MLD is a progressive, genetic demyelinating condition resulting from disruption of the action of arylsulfatase A with the accumulation of sulfated glycolipids in the nervous system of affected individuals. All the genetic leukodystrophies result in the loss of previously acquired skills, spasticity, cortical vision loss, and lead to spastic quadriparesis with bulbar dysfunction and the diagnosis rests on the accurate biochemical or genetic diagnosis. Curative therapy has been elusive, but the use of hematopoietic stem cell transplantation offers in selected individuals the ability to arrest the disease. Symptomatic care remains a mainstay for individuals and their families who are too advanced for transplantation.

SUGGESTED READINGS

1. Berger J, Moser HW, Forss-Petter S. Leukodystrophies: recent developments in genetics, molecular biology, pathogenesis and treatment. Curr Opin Neurol 2001; 14:305–312.
2. Gieselmann V. Metachromatic leukodystrophy: recent research developments. J Child Neurol 2003; 18:591–594.
3. Kim TS, Kim IO, Kim WS, Choi YS, Lee JY, Kim OW, Yeon KM, Kim KJ, Hwang YS. MR of childhood metachromatic leukodystrophy. AJNR Am J Neuroradiol 1997; 18:733–738.
4. Peters C, Steward CG, National Marrow Donor Program; International Bone Marrow Transplant Registry, Working Party on Inborn Errors, European Bone Marrow Transplant Group. Hematopoietic cell transplantation for inherited metabolic diseases: an overview of outcomes and practice guidelines. Bone Marrow Transplant 2003; 31:229–239.

53
Lesch–Nyhan Disease

H.A. Jinnah
Department of Neurology, Johns Hopkins University, Baltimore, Maryland, U.S.A.

INTRODUCTION

Lesch–Nyhan disease (LND) is an X-linked inherited disorder caused by deficiency of the purine salvage enzyme, hypoxanthine-guanine phosphoribosyltransferase (HPRT). Patients with severe enzyme deficiency exhibit a characteristic neurobehavioral syndrome along with evidence for systemic overproduction of uric acid. The neurobehavioral syndrome includes severely disabling generalized dystonia, mild-moderate cognitive impairment, impulsive and aggressive behaviors, and uncontrollable self-injury. The overproduction of uric acid leads to hyperuricemia, hyperuricosuria, uric acid kidney stones, early gouty arthritis, and rarely subcutaneous tophi. Patients with partial enzyme deficiency also overproduce uric acid but exhibit variable expression of the neurobehavioral syndrome. Some variants exhibit no detectable neurobehavioral defects or only mild subclinical clumsiness, while others have severe generalized dystonia and cognitive impairment but no behavioral manifestations.

DIAGNOSIS AND EVALUATION

A presumptive clinical diagnosis of LND is relatively straightforward when all of the major clinical features are manifest. Making the diagnosis is more challenging, however, early in the course of the disease when all of the features may not yet be evident and in those cases presenting with partial syndromes. Laboratory confirmation is essential, because of the implications for management and genetic counseling of family members. Hyperuricemia is characteristic but not sufficient for diagnosis because it lacks both sensitivity and specificity. Serum uric acid is sometimes elevated in disorders other than LND, and some LND patients have values that fall in the normal range. In most cases, definitive diagnosis is made with a combination of genetic and biochemical tests.

Genetic testing involves identifying a mutation in the HPRT gene by sequence analysis. Since the mutations are heterogeneous, the entire coding region must be sequenced. Genetic testing also allows for the screening of asymptomatic female carriers to determine their risk for having affected children. A major limitation of

Table 1 Therapy in Lesch–Nyhan Disease

Uric acid overproduction
Allopurinol
Hydration
Motor disability
Assistive devices
Benzodiazepines
Baclofen
Aberrant behaviors
Assitive devices
Behavior modification
Pharmacotherapy

genetic testing is that it does not provide reliable information on prognosis, information that is of particular interest because of the wide spectrum of disease severity.

Biochemical testing involves the measurement of HPRT enzyme activity, usually in erythrocytes or fibroblasts. Many different assays have been used, although those based on live cells (e.g., whole erythrocytes in suspension or cultured fibroblasts) are considered superior to lysate-based assays. In general, there is a good correlation between disease severity and residual HPRT enzyme activity in the live cell assays, allowing for some prediction of disease severity. However, the biochemical tests are technically demanding and more difficult to use for carrier detection.

TREATMENT

There are currently no therapies to directly correct or compensate for the deficiency of HPRT enzyme activity. As a result, the treatment strategy is largely symptomatic. The main clinical problems will be addressed separately, as the treatment of each is different (Table 1).

Uric Acid Overproduction

The overproduction of uric acid must be treated in all cases to prevent the occurrence of kidney stones and gouty arthritis. Proper treatment requires two main ingredients. The first is allopurinol, a drug that inhibits the production of uric acid by the enzyme xanthine oxidase. A dosage is selected to maintain serum uric acid values just below the upper limit of normal. Care must be taken to avoid using too much allopurinol, since it causes an increase in serum and urinary xanthine and hypoxanthine, which are also poorly soluble and can contribute to urinary stone formation. The second requirement in the treatment of uric acid overproduction is generous hydration at all times to maintain a high urinary flow rate. Some prefer to alkalinize the urine to promote the solubility of uric acid, but evidence for the efficacy of this approach is lacking.

Effective treatment brings serum uric acid to normal, reduces urinary excretion of uric acid, and lowers the risk of renal stone formation and gout. Despite optimal treatment, some patients continue to develop kidney stones. Because the risk of stones is reduced but not eliminated, a high index of suspicion must be maintained even among patients who are receiving allopurinol and hydration. In these cases, the stones may consist of combinations of uric acid, xanthine, hypoxanthine, or even oxypurinol (a metabolite of allopurinol). Renal ultrasound is the diagnostic modality of choice, because stones formed from purine compounds are radiolucent unless they are also calcified. Lithotripsy or surgical extraction is sometimes necessary, and chemical analysis of the stones may provide some guidance for future management.

Aberrant Behaviors

Aberrant behaviors, especially self-injurious behaviors, present the most challenging aspect of treatment. These behaviors wax and wane in severity and character and can be exacerbated by physical or psychological stressors. No single method can reliably control these problems. The best results are achieved with a combination of behavioral therapy, protective devices, and ancillary medications when required. Behavioral therapy that involves positive and negative reinforcement is generally not effective in LND. In contrast, favorable results are achieved by limiting stressors and using extinction methods which involve selectively ignoring unwanted behaviors along with positive reinforcement of acceptable behaviors. These methods are best employed by trained behaviorists, although some success can also be obtained through intensive training of family members.

Behavioral therapy is usually combined with various protective devices to assure that self-injury will not occur. Biting the fingers or hitting the face can be controlled with either strap-style restraints or elbow splints that prevent the hand moving to the face. Similar devices may be fashioned for the legs, if needed. Biting of the lips and tongue is more difficult to manage. Dental or lip guards can be useful if the problem is intermittent or mild, but extraction of thc offending teeth is very often required for severe and recurrent self-biting.

Some patients respond to medical therapy, although no single agent has proved consistently effective. Medications that are sometimes useful include benzodiazepines, neuroleptics, 5-hydroxytryptophan, gabapentin, and carbamazepine. Enthusiasm for the chronic use of these medications must be tempered by their known side effects such as sedation and other long-term side effects. However, periodic use may be very helpful during particularly difficult periods.

Motor Disorder

Although many early reports described the motor disorder of LND as a combination of choreoathetosis and spasticity, more recent studies have shown the predominant problem to be generalized action dystonia. Some patients also exhibit spasticity, but this is typically less prominent than dystonia. Medical treatments for the motor handicap are not satisfactory. Reductions in dystonia and/or spasticity can sometimes be achieved with oral benzodiazepines or baclofen (see elsewhere in this text for treatment of dystonia).

Despite optimal behavioral and medical treatment, most patients remain wheelchair-bound and need assistance for basic activities such as feeding and hygiene. A properly designed wheelchair, with all dangerous parts removed or covered with padding to prevent self-injury, is an important part of good supportive care.

Genetic Counseling

Genetic counseling plays a critical role in clinical management because there are currently no definitive methods for treatment. The disease is inherited in an X-linked recessive manner, so females are rarely clinically affected but they may be silent carriers. Genetic testing should be offered to the mother and any sisters to determine if they are carriers. Male offspring from a known carrier have a 50% risk of being clinically affected and a 50% risk of being normal. Female offspring have a 50% risk of being silent carriers and a 50% risk of being normal. Such information may affect reproductive decisions.

Experimental Treatments

A variety of experimental treatments have been considered. Gene therapy provides a theoretically attractive modality, but is not yet technically feasible in this condition. Bone marrow transplantation in an effort to replace cells with HPRT activity has not proven effective in several case studies. Deep-brain stimulation has been reported to attenuate both dystonia and self-injury in an isolated case. When considering any experimental therapy that may be offered, it is essential to ensure desperation does not unduly drive decision-making.

PROGNOSIS

Provided with good supportive care, patients with LND have lived until their 50s. Some succumb early to aspiration pneumonia, complications from recurrent nephrolithiasis, and a substantial proportion of patients expire suddenly and unexpectedly in their 20s through 40s. The cause of death in these cases remains unknown.

SUMMARY

Lesch–Nyhan disease is an inherited disorder associated with overproduction of uric acid and a characteristic neurobehavioral syndrome. The overproduction of uric acid and its associated consequences can usually be effectively treated with allopurinol and generous hydration. There are no definitive treatments for the neurobehavioral problems; but quality of life can be much improved with behavioral therapy, supportive care, and the judicious use of medications to target specific problems.

ADDITIONAL READINGS

1. Anderson LT, Ernst M. Self-injury in Lesch–Nyhan disease. J Autism Dev Disord 1994; 24:67–81.
2. Jinnah HA, Friedman T. Lesch–Nyhan disease and its variants. In: Scriver CR, Beaudet AL, Sly SW, Valle D, eds. The Metabolic and Molecular Bases of Inherited Disease. McGraw-Hill, NewYork, Chapter 107, 2001.
3. Olson L, Houlihan D. A review of behavioral treatments for Lesch–Nyhan syndrome. Behav Modif 2000; 24:202–222.

4. PUMPA, The Purine Metabolic Patients' Association. Caring for Children with Lesch–Nyhan Disease, East Sussex, U.K., 2002.
5. Visser JE, Bar PR, Jinnah HA. Lesch–Nyhan disease and the basal ganglia. Brain Res Rev 2000; 32:449–475.

54
X-Linked Adrenoleukodystrophy

Hugo W. Moser
Kennedy Krieger Institute, Johns Hopkins University, Baltimore, Maryland, U.S.A.

INTRODUCTION

X-linked adrenoleukodystrophy (X-ALD) is a genetically determined disorder that affects the nervous system, adrenal cortex, and testis. The defective gene, referred to as ABCD1, maps to Xq28, and codes for a peroxisomal membrane protein (ALDP) that is a member of the ATP binding cassette (ABC) transporter superfamily. X-ALD is associated with the abnormal accumulation of saturated very long chain fatty acids (VLCFA), such as hexacosanoic (C26:0) and tetracosanoic (C24:0) acids, in brain white matter, adrenal tissues, and plasma. The VLCFA excess is a diagnostic marker and may contribute to pathogenesis, but the pathogenetic mechanisms are complex and not yet understood. X-ALD affects approximately 1:21,000 males and 1:14,000 females are estimated to be heterozygous for X-ALD. It affects all ethnic groups with approximately the same frequency.

CLINICAL PRESENTATION

All affected males eventually develop some degree of nervous system involvement that can be subdivided into two major categories: (1) Cerebral forms (CCER) are the most common in childhood and progress rapidly. Pathology shows contiguous expanding lesions with a strong inflammatory component and breakdown of the blood–brain barrier near the advancing edge. The intense inflammatory reaction in white matter may be immune mediated. (2) Adrenomyeloneuropathy (AMN) a noninflammatory distal axonopathy that most severely affects the dorsal columns in the cervical segments and the corticospinal tract in the lower thoracic and lumbar segments. Most patients also have some degree of peripheral neuropathy with axonal changes. It manifests most commonly in young adults and progresses over decades leading to severe disability by the fifth decade. Some patients, however, remain relatively mildly involved until the seventh or even eighth decade. The two forms of X-ALD often coexist within the same family and do not correlate with the nature of the ABCD1 mutation.

X-ALD has a wide range of phenotypic expression and can easily be mistaken for other disorders (Table 1). Early manifestations of CCER often resemble

Table 1 Differential Diagnosis of X-ALD in Males

X-ALD phenotype	Differential	Recommended procedure
Asymptomatic		Plasma VLCFA in *all* at-riskrelatives of known X-ALD patients
Childhood cerebral	Attention deficit/hyperactivity disorder, anxiety disorder, personality disorder, learning disability, pervasive developmental disability, dementia, Asperger syndrome, autism, globoid leukodystrophy, metachromatic leukodystrophy, Batten disease, acute disseminated encephalomyelitis, childhood psychosis, drug use	Consider brain MRI and plasma VLCFA (see text)
Addison only	All types of Addison disease	Plasma VLCFA in all boys with Addison disease
Addison disease combined with neurological deficits	Glucocorticoid deficiency with achalasia and deficient tear production (Allgrove syndrome), X-linked glyceryl kinase deficiency, central pontine myelinolysis, hypoglycemic episodes in Addison disease due to other causes	Plasma VLCFA
Atypical presentations in childhood	Brain tumor, cerebellopontine degeneration, epilepsy, and coma	Plasma VLCFA
AMN in men and women	Multiple sclerosis, progressive spastic paraparesis, chronic nonprogressive spinal cord disease, amyotrophic lateral sclerosis, herniated disc in thoracic or lumbar region, cervical spondylosis, and spinal cord tumor	Plasma VLCFA

attention deficit hyperactivity disorders (ADHD) and from a therapeutic prospective, it would be highly desirable to diagnose cerebral X-ALD at this early stage. Clinically, the likelihood that ADHD is due to X-ALD is increased if symptoms develop de novo after age 3 or 4 years, are accompanied by cognitive, visual, or hearing deficits or by symptoms that suggest a psychosis. Most patients show biochemical or clinical evidence of primary adrenocortical insufficiency, but up to 30% of men with AMN have normal plasma levels of adrenal hormones and ACTH.

Approximately, 50% of women develop a neurological syndrome that resembles AMN clinically and pathologically, but is milder and progresses more slowly. Less than 1% of heterozygotes develop brain pathology or clinical evidence of adrenal insufficiency.

LABORATORY DIAGNOSIS

The definitive diagnosis of X-ALD requires the demonstration of the characteristic pattern of increased levels of VLCFA or the demonstration of a pathogenetic mutation in the ABCD1 gene (Table 2). The detection of MRI abnormalities often is the first clue to the diagnosis of CCER, but can be mimicked by other conditions. Eighty to 85% of CCER patients show parieto-occipital lesions; 15% have frontal lesions. In our experience, brain MRI is already abnormal at the time early behavioral manifestations of X-ALD develop.

The plasma VLCFA assay is the most frequently used diagnostic assay. Levels are increased in 99% of males with X-ALD irrespective of age (already increased on the day of birth) and in most circumstances can establish the diagnosis in males. Since plasma C26:0 levels may be elevated in normal persons after a high fat meal, in patients on the ketogenic diet or in individuals receiving intravenous lipids, the diagnosis of X-ALD should be confirmed by plasma assay in a second sample obtained after an overnight fast. Plasma VLCFA levels are increased in patients with other peroxisomal disorders, such as the Zellweger syndrome, neonatal adrenoleukodystrophy, and infantile Refsum syndrome, but these entities can be differentiated by their severe disability in early childhood, dysmorphic features, and involvement of multiple organs. We recommend an assay for VLCFA in all boys with ADHD in whom there is a family history of adrenal insufficiency or of progressive neurological diseases, and in all boys with idiopathic adrenocortical insufficiency. Plasma VLCFA are increased in approximately 80% of women who are heterozygous for X-ALD, but in 20% results are normal or equivocal. The occurrence of false negative results has led some women to conclude erroneously that they were not at risk of having affected children.

Mutation analysis can be performed in CLIA certified laboratories on lymphoblasts or cultured skin fibroblasts from affected males or obligate heterozygotes. Once the family mutation has been defined from among more than 500 pathogenic sites, targeted mutation analysis can be performed in at risk male and female members. Since this procedure has a false negative rate of 3% or less, it is the recommended approach, rather than the VLCFA assay, for the identification of women heterozygous for X-ALD. Affected male fetuses can be identified by demonstrating increased VLCFA levels in cultured amniocytes or chorion villus cells. Since false negatives have been reported with this assay, confirmation should be obtained by mutational analysis with comparisons to the documented family defect.

TREATMENT

Two forms of specific therapy are available: adrenal hormone replacement, which is mandatory for all X-ALD patients with adrenal insufficiency, and bone marrow transplantation (BMT), which is indicated only for selected groups of patients. Preliminary data also suggest that Lorenzo Oil may diminish the risk for latter neu-

Table 2 Laboratory Diagnosis of X-ALD

Procedure	Gender	Sensitivity	Specificity
Plasma VLCFA	Males	99%+	Differentiate from other peroxisomal disorders. False positive with ketogenic diet and occasionally postprandially.
	Females	80%	Differentiate from other peroxisomal disorders.False positive with ketogenic diet and occasionally postprandially.
VLCFA levels in cultured skin fibroblasts	Males	100%	Differentiate from other peroxisomal disorders.
	Females	85%	Differentiate from other peroxisomal disorders.
Mutation analysis	Males	99%	Differentiate from polymorphisms
	Females	95%	Differentiate from polymorphisms
ALDP immunocyto-chemistry	Males	70%	Differentiate from other peroxisomal disorders.
	Females	70%	Differentiate from other peroxisomal disorders.
Brain MRI	Male CCER	100%	High, but not 100%
	Asymptomatic boys with X-ALD	Approximately 30%	Uncertain
	AMN males	Approximately 30%	Uncertain
	Heterozygotes	1%	Low
Adrenal insufficiency	Males	70%	Low
	Females	1%	Low
LSH, FSH	Males	Increased in 30%	Low
Testosterone	Males	Low in 5%	Low

rological involvement in neurologically asymptomatic patients, and this therapy is being offered as part of an experimental study at the Kennedy Krieger Institute. Patients with CCER should be evaluated promptly in order to identify those who are candidates for BMT on the basis of current criteria, described below. The therapeutic approaches listed in Table 3 are described below. There is urgent need for additional therapies, several of which are under investigation.

Adrenal Hormone Replacement

More than 85% of boys and adolescents have or will develop primary adrenocortical insufficiency. Often this is evident clinically, but manifestations may be subtle, such as weakness and moderate hyponatremia associated with intestinal upsets or fever.

Table 3 Current Therapy for X-linked Adrenoleukodystrophy

Phenotype	Therapy	Comments
Adrenal insufficiency	Adrenal hormone replacement	Monitor adrenal function yearly in all males
Asymptomatic, normal MRI	Lorenzo's Oil[a]	Monitor brain MRI every 6 months at ages 3–7 years, yearly thereafter
CCER mild[b]	Bone marrow transplant	
CCER advanced[b]	Supportive care	
AMN	Supportive	Exercise, counseling, prevent complications

[a] Offered at Kennedy Krieger Institute under experimental protocol (see text).
[b] See text.

Adrenal function should be monitored at least yearly with measurements of plasma cortisol and ACTH levels. An increased ACTH level is often the first biochemical indication of adrenal insufficiency. Adrenal hormone replacement therapy should be provided for all X-ALD patients with adrenal insufficiency. Glucocorticoid dose requirements are generally similar to those used for other forms of primary adrenal insufficiency, such as hydrocortisone 10 mg/M^2/24 hr in divided doses, or equivalent doses (20–25% of hydrocortisone dosage) of prednisone or prednisolone. Patients should augment glucocorticoid coverage during physical or mental stress, be provided with a parenteral methylprednisolone dose for use if vomiting prevents oral dosing, and strongly encouraged to wear a Medic-Alert identification declaring their dependency on adrenal steroid therapy. Not all patients require mineralocorticoid replacement. When postural hypotension, hyponatremia, or hyperkalemia persist, in spite of adequate glucocorticoid therapy, fludrocortisone, 0.05–0.1 mg per day, is prescribed.

Bone Marrow Transplantation

Bone marrow transplantation can arrest further progression in boys and adolescents with X-ALD who have relatively mild inflammatory brain disease; stabilization maintained for an 8–10 year follow-up in several patients. The mechanism of this favorable effect is not yet fully understood, but includes the replacement of bone marrow-derived glia with normal cells and the effect of immunosuppression. In view of the high risk of the procedure, its indications must be considered with care. Present consensus is that BMT should be offered only to boys and adolescents with definitive, but still relatively mild, inflammatory cerebral involvement and not to those with advanced cerebral disease. Outcome in 126 X-ALD patients treated with BMT has been unsatisfactory, with respect to survival and quality of life, in individuals with a nonverbal IQ score of less than 80, a Loes MRI brain severity score greater than 9, and in those with multiple neurological deficits. On the basis of these studies, indications for transplantation have been expanded in the clinically asymptomatic or mild patient to include individuals with MRI abnormalities that progress over a 3–6 month period, particularly when the lesions enhance. The procedure is not recommended for patients who do not show clinical or MRI evidence of brain involvement, or for patients with AMN who do not have inflammatory cerebral disease. The technical aspects of the preparative regimens and the transplant procedure in X-ALD are being reviewed and revised in international collaborative studies. It is recommended that BMT be performed solely in centers experienced in transplant therapy for this disorder.

Additional Therapies Under Study

Several other therapeutic approaches, such as Lorenzo's Oil, lovastatin, 4-phenylbutyrate, coenzyme Q10, newer immunosuppressive agents, mesenchymal cell transplants, stem cell, and gene replacement, are under consideration, being studied in tissue culture or in the X-ALD animal model. None have been fully validated in clinical trials. Lorenzo's Oil, a 4:1 mixture of glyceryl trioleate and glyceryl trierucate, has the remarkable and so far unique capacity of normalizing plasma VLCFA levels within 4 weeks. Published clinical studies, however, have failed to demonstrate clinical efficacy in patients who were already symptomatic. Nevertheless, recent preliminary studies at the Kennedy Krieger Institute suggest that Lorenzo's Oil may lower the risk for later brain involvement in neurologically asymptomatic boys with X-ALD who have a normal brain MRI. Additional experimental studies are currently in progress.

SUPPORTIVE CARE

The progressive behavioral and neurologic disturbances associated with the childhood form of X-ALD provide an extreme challenge for the family. Treatment following confirmation of the diagnosis of X-ALD requires the establishment of a comprehensive management program and partnership between the family, physician, visiting nurses, dietitian, school authorities, and counselors. In addition, parental support groups such as the United Leukodystrophy Foundation (2304 Highland Drive, Sycamore, IL) have proven to be of great value. Under the provision of Public Law 94-142, Education for All Handicapped Children, an individual with leukodystrophy qualifies for special services under the "other health impaired" or "multihandicapped" designation. Depending on the rate of progression of the disease, special needs might range from relatively low-level resource services within a regular school program (to correct deficiencies in isolated academic subjects), to self-contained services (for children with ADHD and multiple academic deficiencies), to home-and hospital-based teaching programs (for children who are nonmobile). Management challenges vary with the stage of the illness. The early stages are characterized by subtle changes in affect, behavior, and attention span. Counseling and communication with school authorities are of prime importance during this period.

Painful muscle spasms often cause severe discomfort and can be treated with valium or baclofen. Valium is generally started at 1–2 mg every 4–6 hr, but since it has tachyphylaxis, it often needs to be increased rapidly. Some patients have required as much as 10 mg every 3–4 hr by mouth or gastrostomy tube. For baclofen, a starting dosage of 5 mg twice daily may be increased gradually to 25 mg four times daily. While respiratory depression is a concern, in our experience, this is always preceded by loss of alertness. If a patient who is awake continues to have painful spasms, it is our policy to increase the dosage of muscle relaxant. Other agents, such as dantrolene or tizanidine may also be tried, taking care to monitor for the occurrence of side effects and drug interactions.

PROGNOSIS

The prognosis of the cerebral forms of X-ALD is serious. In the past, most patients became totally disabled within 2–5 years, with death at varying intervals thereafter. Recent data, however, suggest that BMT performed in the early stages of this form considerably improves prognosis. Although AMN progresses more slowly, it often causes severe disability by the fourth and fifth decades.

PREVENTION OF X-ALD

It is estimated that only 5% of X-ALD patients have new mutations. Hence, extended family screening of at-risk relatives of known patients, with currently available, techniques offers the potential of identifying a substantial portion of all X-ALD patients. The identification of male patients before they are neurologically involved offers the possibility to provide therapies, such as bone marrow transplantation, at a time when they have the greatest chance of success. Early diagnosis also provides the opportunity to institute adrenal steroid replacement therapy before there is clinical evidence of adrenal insufficiency. Mutation analysis permits accurate identification of women heterozygous for X-ALD and provides a crucial opportunity for genetic counseling. Preimplantation diagnosis provides an additional new option for women who are known to be heterozygotes.

SUMMARY

X-linked adrenoleukodystrophy is due to a defect in a gene that has been mapped to X-q28 and codes for a peroxisomal membrane, the function of which has not yet been defined. Its frequency in males is estimated to be 1:21,000. Primary adrenocortical deficiency and progressive nervous system disability are the main clinical manifestations. Neurological manifestations vary widely and range from a rapidly progressive cerebral form that primarily affects boys to a slowly progressive adult form that involve the spinal cord. Analysis of very long chain fatty acids and mutation analysis permit accurate diagnosis of presymptomatic patients, prenatal diagnosis, and carrier identification. Adrenal steroid replacement therapy effectively corrects the adrenal insufficiency. Bone marrow transplantation stabilizes neurological deficits in the childhood cerebral and adolescent forms and offers the promise of long-term benefit, provided it is performed in the early phase of the disease.

SUGGESTED READINGS

1. Hershkovitz E, Narkis G, Shorer Z, Moser AB, Watkins PA, Moser HW, Manor E. Cerebral X-linked adrenoleukodystrophy in a girl with Xq27-Ter deletion. Ann Neurol 2002; 52(2):234–237.
2. Jorge P, Quelhas D, Oliveira P, Pinto R, Nogueira A. X-linked adrenoleukodystrophy in patients with idiopathic Addison disease. Eur J Pediatr 1994; 153(8):594–597.
3. Kemp S, Pujol A, Waterham HR, van Geel BM, Boehm CD, Raymond GV, Cutting GR, Wanders RJ, Moser HW. ABCD1 mutations and the X-linked adrenoleukodystrophy mutation database: role in diagnosis and clinical correlations. Hum Mutat 2001; 18:499–515.

4. Kumar AJ, Rosenbaum AE, Naidu S, Wenger L, Citrin CM, Lindenberg R, Kim WS, Zinreich SJ, Molliver ME, Mayberg HS, Moser HW. Adrenoleukodystrophy: correlating MR imaging with CT. Radiology 1987; 165(2):497–504.
5. Moser AB, Kreiter N, Bezman L, Lu S, Raymond GV, Naidu S, Moser HW. Plasma very long chain fatty acids in 3,000 peroxisome disease patients and 29,000 controls. Ann Neurol 1999; 45:100–110.
6. Moser HW, Smith KD, Watkins PA, Powers J, Moser AB. X-linked adrenoleukodystrophy. In: Scriver CR, Beaudet AL , Sly WS, Valle D, eds. The Metabolic and Molecular Bases of Inherited Disease. New York: McGraw Hill, 2000; 3257–3301.
7. Powers JM, DeCiero DP, Ito M, Moser AB, Moser HW. Adrenomyeloneuropathy: a neuropathologic review featuring its noninflammatory myelopathy. J Neuropathol Exp Neurol 2000; 59:89–102.
8. Shapiro E, Krivit W, Lockman L, Jambaque I, Peters C, Cowan M, Harris R, Blanche S, Bordigoni P, Loes D, Ziegler R, Crittenden M, Ris D, Berg B, Cox C, Moser H, Aubourg P. Long-term effect of bone-marrow transplantation for childhood-onset cerebral X-linked adrenoleukodystrophy. Lancet 2000; 356:713–718.

55
Mitochondrial Diseases

Adam L. Hartmanand and Anne M. Comi
Johns Hopkins Hospital, Baltimore, Maryland, U.S.A.

INTRODUCTION

Mitochondria serve a number of critical functions in the cell, including generation of energy, production of oxygen radicals, and regulation of apoptosis. In this chapter, a brief review of clinically relevant mitochondrial biology is followed by a description of the diagnosis and therapeutic approach to diseases that affect this critical organelle.

BACKGROUND

Although a detailed discussion of mitochondrial genetics is beyond the scope of this review (see Wallace in Suggested Reading section), a few comments are in order. The mitochondrial genome encodes proteins constituting the electron transport chain and ribosomal and transfer RNA. The nuclear genome also encodes many genes critical to mitochondrial function. For example, mitochondrial diseases such as Friedreich's ataxia and mitochondrial neurogastrointestinal encephalomyopathy (MNGIE) are caused by mutations in nuclear genes.

Certain properties of mitochondrial diseases distinguish them from other classes of disorders. Mutations are not carried in each copy of the mitochondrial genome. Normal copies can exist within the same mitochondrion with mutated copies, known as heteroplasmy. The phenotype of a cell is dictated in large part by the relative numbers of normal and abnormal genes (the "threshold effect"). The process of cell division can contribute to the seemingly nonrandom segregation of abnormal mitochondria and their respective mutations, so the same mutation can produce different phenotypes; conversely, similar phenotypes can be produced by different genotypes, making specific diagnosis and therapy a true challenge.

DIAGNOSIS

The laboratory work-up often includes the measurement of lactate, pyruvate, plasma amino acids, urine organic acids, and a carnitine analysis. Because of the phenotypic heterogeneity of these disorders, normal levels of lactate and pyruvate do not completely rule out mitochondrial disease as a cause of a patient's pathology. Analysis of the urine may demonstrate Fanconi's syndrome. Imaging may reveal stroke-like findings or basal ganglia calcifications. Tests can be done to look at the activities of various mitochondrial enzymes. Elevated lactate peaks may be seen on magnetic resonance spectroscopy of the brain. A muscle biopsy may demonstrate morphological abnormalities such as "ragged red fibers" or biochemical abnormalities based on various stains. Unfortunately, ragged red fibers (accumulations of morphologically abnormal mitochondria with dense cristae and inclusions) are not specific for mitochondrial disease and may occur in normal aging. Specific test panels for mitochondrial DNA mutations are available commercially or through various research laboratories.

Certain clinical findings have been clustered together into syndromes, some of which have been linked to various mutations. Examples include MELAS (mitochondrial encephalomyopathy, lactic acidosis, and stroke-like episodes), MERFF (myoclonic epilepsy, and ragged red fibers), and others. Diagnosis of these syndromes is discussed in greater detail in the Suggested Reading section.

THERAPY

General Management

Patients can be treated symptomatically for certain sequelae of their mitochondrial diseases. As an example, seizure management is fairly standard but some recommend levocarnitine supplementation for those taking valproic acid or avoidance of valproic acid altogether. Other examples include the use of pacemakers, cardiac transplants, and cochlear implants. Endocrinopathies, such as diabetes and hypoparathyroidism, can be treated as in patients without underlying mitochondrial disease. Renal complications can be treated with electrolytes.

Stresses such as exposure to temperature extremes should be avoided. Patients may benefit from a supervised aerobic exercise program undertaken in consultation with a physical therapist familiar with these disorders. Physical therapists can also provide input into assistive technology (including appropriate fitting of wheelchairs), should the need arise. Occupational and physical therapists can assist in assuring that activities of daily living consume a minimal amount of energy. Speech and language pathologists can assist with communication issues. Finally, support groups are available for patients and their families (see Patient Resources).

Genetic counseling should be made available to patients with mitochondrial disorders. Because of the nature of these diseases, including heteroplasmy, the threshold effect, and mitotic segregation, it may be difficult to make accurate predictions for prognosis and reproductive issues. Nonetheless, families need to understand the importance of these disorders in their own lives.

Diet

Prolonged fasting should be avoided. Frequent, small meals are recommended for some patients. Complex carbohydrates such as uncooked cornstarch or breads can be given before bedtime to patients who cannot tolerate an overnight fast, but these should be made palatable. The ketogenic diet has been reported to have variable clinical utility for patients with low pyruvate dehydrogenase (PDH) activity, in the belief that it bypasses the pyruvate dehydrogenase complex deficiency. However, it is thought that in most mitochondrial disorders, the ketogenic diet is relatively contraindicated. Conversely, a diet high in carbohydrates has been advocated for patients with long-chain fatty acid oxidation disorders; their best form of fat intake may be medium chain triglycerides (e.g., medium chain triglycerides, or MCT, oil). Nutritionists can assist with menu preparation for patients who need dietary interventions.

Medication and Supplementation

Numerous biochemical approaches have been attempted to augment or substitute for missing components in the respiratory chain, prevent the accumulation or formation of toxic metabolites, or "bypass" certain steps in metabolism. Their theoretical promise has not been fully realized in the clinic. One problem with assessing their efficacy arises from the varied definitions of these disorders (i.e., some patients have microscopic evidence of mitochondrial disease but negative genetic studies), and for most, our incomplete understanding of their molecular pathophysiology. The paucity of controlled studies, combined with the uncertain natural history of some disorders, makes outcomes challenging to assess. Some series suggest that there may be a subclass of therapy-responsive patients in many of these disorders. Table 1 summarizes the dose ranges noted in the literature for these medications. Doses in the following section have been recommended by the United Mitochondrial Disease Foundation and are what we use.

Table 1 Range of Doses and Various Regimens Used in the Treatment of Mitochondrial Disorders

Biotin	5–100 mg/day
l-Carnitine	Pediatric: 50 mg/kg/day po initially, then 50–100 mg/kg/day po; max: 1000 mg TID; adult: 1 g/day po initially, then max: 1000 mg TID; IV dosing and tablets available
Coenzyme Q10	5–15 mg/kg/day; 30–100 mg TID; up to 1000 mg/day in deficient patients
Creatine	0.08–0.35 g/kg/day or 5 g po BID × 14 days or 2 g po BID multi 14 days, then 2 g po BID × 7 days or 20 g/day div QID × 12 days, then 5 g/day div BID
DCA	25–100 mg/kg/day (regimens vary)
Idebenone	90–675 mg/day in mitochondrial encephalomyopathy; up to 5 mg/kg/day po in Friedreich's ataxia
Nicotinamide	50–100 mg/day (adult doses have been reported between 5–1000 mg po daily (larger doses divided QID)
Riboflavin	50–100 mg/day (doses of 10–400 mg/day have been reported)
Succinate	2–6 g/day
Thiamine	50–100 mg/day (doses of 10–3000 mg/day have been reported)
Vitamin C	100–500 mg TID (doses up to 4 g/day have been reported)
Vitamin E	400 IU QD-TID (doses of 200–400 IU/day or 300–500 mg po BID have been reported)
Vitamin K3	5–30 mg/day (doses up to 500 mg/day in divided doses have been reported)

First Line Therapy

Two compounds are frequently recommended for patients with mitochondrial disorders: coenzyme Q10 (CoQ10) and levocarnitine. Because they may play multiple roles in mitochondrial metabolism, facilitate the use of various fuel sources, and have limited toxicity, they are frequently included in therapeutic regimens for patients with a variety of mitochondrial disorders.

We typically dose CoQ10 at 5–15 mg/kg/day, up to 1000 mg/day. It is supplied in a variety of oral and intravenous forms. Side effects can include dizziness, fussiness, rashes, and gastrointestinal symptoms. CoQ10 is involved in an array of different processes involving transfer of electrons and protons and as an antioxidant. It is a ubiquitous component in various molecules involved in oxidative phosphorylation but its exact role is unclear. In case reports, it has been noted to improve muscle strength, ataxia, chorea, ptosis, ophthalmoplegia, and vital capacities. It has been associated with a decrease in stroke-like episodes, improved speech and auditory comprehension, and a decrease in delusions. There is conflict in the literature regarding recommendations of CoQ10 in the treatment of mitochondrial diabetes mellitus. The results of one blinded trial of CoQ10 are difficult to interpret, but suggest that there is a subpopulation of patients who respond to this therapy. Idebenone, a synthetic analog of CoQ10, has been used with mixed success, as well. Preliminary data suggest it might be particularly useful for the cardiomyopathy in Friedreich's ataxia.

We typically start levocarnitine with a dose of 50 mg/kg/day in children or 1000 mg/day in adults and titrate to a maximum of 100 mg/kg/day or 1000 mg po TID. It is supplied as an oral solution (1 g/10mL), injection (1 g/5 mL), and as a tablet (330 mg). Side effects can include worsening seizures, strange odors, and gastrointestinal symptoms. Carnitine plays a role in the transport of fatty acids and in acyltransferases. Levocarnitine has been given in states of primary deficiency (e.g., cardiomyopathies). Its efficacy has been variable in the treatment of secondary deficiencies, such as mitochondrial disorders. Reasons for this include its poor oral bioavailability and variable amounts of carnitine in certain formulations. Levocarnitine has been used in the treatment of medium- and short-chain fatty acid oxidation disorders; however, its utility in long-chain fatty acid oxidation disorders is debated.

Other Nutritional Supplements

If a patient does not have an adequate response to the interventions noted above, we move to one of a number of agents listed in this section. There is very little information available beyond case reports and series to guide the clinician. Some of these therapies may be particularly useful for certain classes of disorders, as noted below.

Thiamine (50–100 mg/day) is a cofactor for pyruvate dehydrogenase and has been a component of various cocktails used to treat mitochondrial disorders. Its effect as monotherapy has not been investigated.

Nicotinamide (50–100 mg/day) and riboflavin (50–100 mg/day) are precursors of NAD and flavin-containing compounds, respectively. They are critical to the function of complex I and II of the electron transport chain. Both have been used for patients with deficiencies in these compounds, including MELAS (mitochondrial encephalopathy, lactic acidosis, and stroke-like episodes), KSS (Kearns–Sayre syndrome), and others. Case reports have documented improvement in symptoms such as peripheral neuropathy, mental status changes, visual loss, and fatigability. Other PDH complex cofactors, such as pantothenic acid and lipoic acid, also have been used in various combination treatments.

Vitamin K3 (5–30 mg/day) and vitamin C (100–500 mg TID) have been used in an attempt to substitute electron acceptors in patients with cytochrome *b* dysfunction (i.e., to bypass complex III). Although surrogate markers have shown improvement, significant clinical benefits have been seen in only selected patients. Vitamin E was used with a similar rationale in one case report that demonstrated significantly improved physical activity levels (we use 400 units QD-TID).

Creatine (see Table 1 for dosing regimens) is believed to increase the availability of creatine phosphate, a storage form of high-energy phosphate bonds. There may also be a beneficial effect due to inhibition of platelet aggregation, which may be relevant for those prone to stroke-like events. A few case reports and randomized, blinded, controlled trials have shown symptomatic relief and improved exercise tolerance in patients with various mitochondrial disorders. Renal function should be monitored.

Biotin [5–10 mg/day], a key prosthetic group in mitochondrial and cytosolic carboxylases, is included in certain mitochondrial cocktails, but it has been mentioned only in case reports. Corticosteroids (varying doses) have been administered to some patients with mitochondrial diseases. Their mechanism of action and efficacy in this setting are uncertain. Various intermediates in the citric acid cycle (e.g., citrate and succinate) have been used, again with different degrees of success, as have other precursor molecules involved in other stages of cytoplasmic metabolism (e.g., aspartate).

Therapy for Specific Disorders

A patient may have a defined mutation or dysfunction of a particular component of the mitochondria. This section makes note of circumstances where certain agents may be helpful.

Pyruvate Dehydrogenase (PDH). Although not available commercially in the United States, dichloroacetate (DCA; 25–100 mg/kg/day) is used for its ability to maintain PDH in its active state by inhibiting its phosphorylation. This, in turn, prevents accumulation of lactate. It has been used in patients with PDH complex deficiencies, electron transport chain complex I deficiencies, cytochrome *C* oxidase deficiency, MELAS, KSS, NARP (neuropathy, ataxia, retinitis pigmentosa), Leigh syndrome, and undefined chronic congenital lactic acidemias. In pediatric case reports, DCA has been credited with modest decreases in abdominal pain, headaches, seizures, stroke-like episodes, improved cognitive function, reduced fatigability, and decreased visual and auditory hallucinations. Decreases in serum and CSF lactate and pyruvate have been noted, as have radiographic improvements. Dichloroacetate administration can cause a peripheral neuropathy as a result of decreased thiamine levels. Despite thiamine supplementation, nerve conduction velocity measurements suggest that a subclinical neuropathy still occurs.

Other PDH complex cofactors, such as thiamine, nicotinamide, riboflavin, pantothenic acid, and lipoic acid, also have been used in various combinations as treatments for patients with known PDH deficiencies. As noted previously, dietary interventions may be useful.

Complexes I and II. Nicotinamide and riboflavin have been supplemented in patients with known complex I and II deficiencies. Augmentation of the PDH complex and complex I is believed by some to facilitate energy production in the cell regardless of the primary molecular defect, so that many "general" mitochondrial therapeutic regimens include these compounds. These should be used cautiously, however, as an improved energy state of the cell may also lead to an increase in undesirable symptoms, such as seizures.

Complex III. Vitamin K3, vitamin C, and vitamin E have been used in attempts to substitute electron acceptors in patients with cytochrome *b* dysfunction (i.e., to bypass complex III).

Complex IV (Cytochrome c Oxidase). A variety of attempts have been made to treat patients with cytochrome *c* oxidase deficiencies, including treatment with carnitine, coenzyme Q10, thiamine, riboflavin, vitamin C, folate, biotin, and intravenous infusions of cytochrome *c*. Some clinical success has been reported up to 3 years after diagnosis.

Fatty Acid Oxidation Disorders. Carnitine, CoQ10, and flavoproteins are components of various molecules involved in fatty acid oxidation, and thus, there is a theoretical basis for their use. Dietary interventions may be useful.

Gene Therapy

Given the lack of consistent clinical improvement with the various therapies noted, there is new interest in treating mitochondrial disorders with gene therapy. One approach has used resistance exercise training (a signal for muscle growth and repair) to document the selective increase of wild-type mitochondrial DNA in muscle fibers of a patient. The theoretical basis for this approach is the heteroplasmy of mitochondrial DNA in various cells: in response to exercise, satellite cells (that serve as a source of wild-type DNA) fuse with existing muscle fibers and improve their mitochondrial function in the process. This approach has not resulted in large-scale clinical benefit yet.

CONCLUSION

Mitochondrial disorders are protean in their clinical manifestations. Their molecular pathology, mechanisms of disease, and natural history are not well understood, making specific therapy and large randomized, blinded trials difficult. Basic treatment of symptoms and dietary management is the first step in treatment. Support networks should be recommended for patients and their families. Certain compounds are used with the goal of augmenting cellular metabolism and protection from damage by radical oxygen species. The success in certain reports suggests that there may be a population of patients who respond favorably to administration of these compounds.

SUGGESTED READINGS

1. Dimauro S, Hirano M, Schon EA. Mitochondrial encephalomyopathies: therapeutic approaches. Neurol Sci 2000; 21:S109–S908.
2. DiMauro S, Schon EA. Mechanisms of disease: mitochondrial respiratory-chain diseases. New Engl J Med 2003; 348:2656–2668.
3. Gold DR, Cohen BH. Treatment of mitochondrial cytopathies. Sem Neurol 2001; 21: 309–325.
4. Przyrembel H. Therapy of mitochondrial disorders. J Inher Metab Dis 1987; 10:129–146.
5. Schapira AHV, DiMauro S, eds. Mitochondrial Disorders in Neurology. Vol.2. Blue Books of Practical Neurology Series. Boston: Butterworth, 2002.

6. Schmiedel J, Jackson S, Schafer J, Reichmann H. Mitochondrial cytopathies. J Neurol 2003; 250:267–277.
7. Wallace DC. Mitochondrial diseases in man and mouse. Science 1999; 283:1482–1488.

PATIENT RESOURCES

1. The Children's Mitochondrial Disease Network: www.emdn-mitonet.co.uk, EMDN, Mayfield House, 30 Heber Walk, Chester Way, Northwich, CW9 5JB, England, U.K.
2. The Mitochondria Research Society, www.mitoresearch.org, PO Box 306, Riderwood, MD 21139–0306, U.S.A.
3. United Mitochondrial Disease Foundation, www.umdf.org, 8085 Saltsburg Road, Suite 201, Pittsburgh, PA 15239, U.S.A.

56

Plumbism: Elevated Lead Levels in Children

Cecilia T. Davoli
Kennedy Krieger Institute, Baltimore, Maryland, U.S.A.

INTRODUCTION

Plumbism was first described as a pediatric environmental health concern during the latter part of the 19th century. To this day, children throughout the world continue to be identified with elevated blood lead levels because of environmental lead sources. Although any child in a leaded environment is at risk for lead exposure, children between 6 months and 6 years of age are at greatest risk for lead ingestion due to developmentally appropriate hand-to-mouth activity. An elevated lead level during early childhood places a child at potential risk for long-term developmental disabilities such as learning problems, hyperactivity, and attention deficit disorder.

DIAGNOSIS/CLINICAL FEATURES

In the United States, a blood lead level measured in micrograms/deciliter (mcg/dL) is used to determine diagnosis and direct treatment decisions. The Centers for Disease Control and Prevention (CDC) have defined 10 mcg/dL and above as an elevated lead level in the pediatric age group (Table 1). Since most children with an elevated lead level are asymptomatic, identification is heavily dependent on routine screening. Although a venous blood test is preferable, screening can be done with a capillary blood test if meticulous care is taken to clean the child's finger with alcohol.

Per current CDC guidelines, universal blood lead screening should be undertaken for all children who reside in an area with: (1) a high prevalence (≥12%) of children with elevated lead levels, or (2) a high concentration (≥27%) of housing built before 1950. These children should have a blood lead test at 1 and 2 years of age; children between the ages of 3 and 6 years who have never had a previous blood lead test should also receive one. In areas that do not meet universal screening criteria, a targeted screening approach can be taken, and a blood lead test is done only for children who meet specific local health department criteria. The CDC has

Table 1 CDC Classification of Elevated Lead Levels in Children

Class	Blood lead (mcg/dL)
I	≤9
IIA	10–14
IIB	15–19
III	20–44
IV	45–69
V	≥70

(Adapted from Centers for Disease Control and Preventive: Preventing lead poisoning in young children, Atlanta, 1991, CDC.)

recommended that these criteria include children in racial/ethnic minority groups, those who are poor, those who reside in geographic areas where there is known risk of lead exposure, and those whose lead screening questionnaire raises concern about possible risk of lead exposure/ingestion. Nonetheless, a child of any racial, ethnic, socioeconomic, or geographic background may be determined to be at risk for lead exposure/ingestion, and should be screened accordingly.

Because an elevated lead level is caused by environmental exposure to lead, the clinical and environmental history is of paramount importance in diagnosis and management. Routine well-child health surveillance visits should include questions about potential lead sources in the child's environment, especially between ages 6 months and 6 years. Positive or questionable responses merit a blood lead test, even if the child would not be at risk for lead exposure/ingestion based on other criteria. In addition, children who are newly arrived immigrants, international adoptees, and those with cognitive disabilities may require more stringent application of the CDC screening guidelines.

In general, almost all children with elevated blood lead levels are asymptomatic or their parents express concern about nonspecific symptoms that can only potentially be attributed to lead. Symptoms such as irritability, crankiness, behavioral changes, and high activity level may represent normal behavioral fluctuations of young children and are too vague to be of diagnostic value. Rarely, a child will present with more specific concerns such as colicky abdominal pain, developmental delay or loss of skills, appetite loss, constipation, or intermittent vomiting. Although these symptoms would not be considered "normal," they are also too nonspecific to be diagnostic for an elevated lead level. The inability to easily make a clinical diagnosis for the vast majority of children means that routine blood lead screening and the environmental history are the best diagnostic tools available to the clinician.

Although lead encephalopathy is extremely rare in the United States, it should remain in the differential diagnosis for an infant or child who presents with unexplained seizures, ataxia, or altered mental status. At or above a lead level of 100 mcg/dL, the potential for overt central nervous system decompensation increases rapidly and unpredictably due to an increased risk of breakdown of the blood–brain barrier. The resultant capillary "leakiness" increases the potential for cerebral edema, which may be manifested clinically by altered mental status (e.g., stupor, coma) and/or seizures. If this clinical progression occurs, the child is at high risk for permanent neurologic damage and death.

THERAPY

Decisions regarding chelation should be based on a *venous* lead level rather than a capillary level, except in the case of (1) a child with a blood lead level ≥70 mcg/dL, or (2) a child with overt neurologic signs, regardless of lead level. These two situations are considered medical emergencies, which require treatment without delay. A pre-chelation venous level should be drawn at the time that treatment is initiated, but treatment should not be withheld while awaiting the venous result. If necessary, treatment modifications can be made once the confirmatory blood test result is available.

Chelation is not currently recommended for children with blood lead levels between 10 and 44 mcg/dL. Hair, fingernail, tooth, bone, and urine lead levels are not currently used clinically for management, and chelation decisions are not based on these lead levels. If chelation is being considered, the clinician should ideally consult with a pediatric specialist who is experienced with use of chelating agents, and/or refer the child to the specialist for management. A pediatric environmental health specialist and a neonatologist should ideally manage neonates with elevated lead levels.

For all chelating agents, chelation is done in a documented lead-safe environment, such as an inpatient hospital unit, to protect the child from ongoing lead ingestion. The child should be well hydrated throughout chelation, to maintain steady renal excretion of lead. Prior to the initiation of any chelating agent, baseline bloodwork is done, including electrolytes, urea nitrogen, creatinine, complete blood count and differential, and liver function tests. Children who are identified to have iron deficiency should receive iron replacement therapy (3–6 mg/kg/day) concomitantly with chelation therapy, except when using British Anti-Lewisite (BAL), as described below. A pediatric enema is given twice before chelation to remove macroscopic lead particles from the lower gastrointestinal tract. During chelation, bloodwork is done on a weekly basis to monitor for potential medication side effects, such as depression of the absolute neutrophil count (ANC), elevation of the liver function tests, and thrombocytopenia. In most cases, it is not necessary to interrupt chelation if mild side effects occur, but the frequency of laboratory monitoring may need to be increased. Any drug-related laboratory abnormalities usually return to normal soon after chelation is complete, and sometimes even during the course of treatment. The weekly bloodwork during chelation should also include a venous lead level, which is done to monitor treatment efficacy. The response to chelation can be fairly dramatic, with the lead level falling by as much as 50% each week of treatment. Despite this decrease, chelation therapy should not be stopped until the full treatment course has been completed. Premature cessation of chelation usually results in rebound of the blood lead level due to incomplete treatment.

There are several chelating agents available for use in children, with the choice of agent being largely dependent upon the child's presenting lead level. For children with a venous lead level between 45 and 69 mcg/dL, the oral chelating agent, succimer, was approved for use in children by the Food and Drug Administration (FDA) in 1991. Succimer is frequently referred to as DMSA, which is an abbreviation of its chemical name, *meso*-2,3-dimercaptosuccinic acid. A course of chelation with succimer is 19 days, with the first 5 days dosed at 1050 mg/m^2/day in three divided doses per day, and the subsequent 14 days dosed at 700 mg/m^2/day in two divided doses per day. Succimer is only available as a 100 mg capsule, so the child's total daily dose usually needs to be rounded up (or down) slightly so that each dose is divisible by 100. Succimer is best absorbed on an empty stomach, so it is usually given 1 to 1-1/2 hr before or after a meal. It has a noxious sulfur smell and taste that can be masked by mixing the capsule beads in a small amount of ginger ale before administration.

If the child does not respond to succimer, or there is a drug reaction, intramuscular chelation should be carried out using edetate calcium disodium injection (Calcium Disodium Versenate or $CaNa_2EDTA$). This agent can also be used for lead levels between 70 and 90 mcg/dL to rapidly bring down a child's lead level, followed by a complete 19-day course of oral chelation with succimer. $CaNa_2EDTA$ is given via deep intramuscular (IM) injection for a 5-day course, and is dosed at 1000 mg/m^2/day in two divided doses per day. A topical anesthetic agent and/or dilution with procaine can be used to decrease the pain of the injections. Twelve hours after the 10th injection, a venous lead level and monitoring bloodwork should be done. If more than one course of chelation is required, the patient should have a 3-day "rest" between treatment courses. During treatment, a daily multivitamin should be provided to replace zinc and copper that is chelated along with the lead. Iron deficiency can be safely treated during administration of $CaNa_2EDTA$. Although this shorter treatment course may seem more desirable, $CaNa_2EDTA$ is less specific for lead, and will also chelate other trace metals. It may also result in less decrease in the child's pre-chelation lead level.

A lead level close to or above 100 mcg/dL requires admission to a monitored bed in a hospital that is capable of managing pediatric neurologic emergencies. Although many children with lead levels in this range will be asymptomatic, the potential risk of encephalopathy is greatly increased. A child may be stable until just before s/he decompensates precipitously, with a particular risk of clinical deterioration during the first 24–72 hr of chelation. If the child tolerates chelation well for the first 24–48 hr, then s/he can be transferred to a less acute setting for completion of treatment.

The CDC recommends combination therapy with British Anti-Lewisite (BAL or dimercaprol) and $CaNa_2EDTA$ for children with lead levels $\geq$70 mcg/dL, but is usually prescribed most frequently for those with lead levels close to or above 100 mcg/dL. BAL is the initial agent used, and is dosed at 75 mg/m^2 via deep IM injection. At least 4 hr later, a continuous intravenous (IV) infusion is started of $CaNa_2EDTA$ 1500 mg/m^2/day. BAL is then continued simultaneously at a dose of 75 mg/m^2 IM every 4 hr. If BAL is not given before IV $CaNa_2EDTA$ is started, clinical deterioration can occur, including the development of encephalopathy. Because of the increased renal excretion of lead, adequate hydration and good urine output must be maintained, except in the case of a child with cerebral edema. If there is concern that a child has developed or is developing cerebral edema, then fluid restriction can be maintained by administering the $CaNa_2EDTA$ via IM injection rather than the IV route. The venous lead level should be monitored every 48–72 hr, and combination therapy can be discontinued when the level falls below 70 mcg/dL. At that point, the child is given a 5-day course of IM $CaNa_2EDTA$ and then a 19-day course of DMSA. In general, there is no need for a rest period when transitioning from one chelating agent to the next, unless the child is exhibiting severe medication side effects. Bloodwork should be done every 5–7 days during the remainder of the chelation course to monitor treatment efficacy and medication side-effects as described earlier.

There are several precautions to keep in mind when using combination therapy for chelation. Because it is suspended in peanut oil, BAL can potentially precipitate anaphylaxis in children with peanut allergy. Children with glucose-6-phosphate dehydrogenase deficiency may experience severe hemolysis due to BAL. Iron cannot be administered simultaneously with BAL because of the risk of a severe toxic reaction, so treatment of iron deficiency must be delayed until several days after BAL is discontinued. Care should be taken that $CaNa_2EDTA$ is used instead of Na_2EDTA (disodium edetate), since the latter can induce hypocalcemia and tetany. In general, however, no special monitoring of calcium level is required when chelating with $CaNa_2EDTA$.

When the treatment course has been completed, chelation with succimer usually results in a decrease in blood lead level to 50–70% of the pre-chelation level. There is less decrease seen with the other chelating agents. A follow-up venous lead level is done about 2 weeks after chelation is complete, with subsequent monitoring occurring every 2–6 weeks for the first 3–4 months after chelation. Thereafter, monitoring frequency is dependent on the child's age, lead level, and environmental situation. After chelation therapy is stopped, the blood lead level will rebound due to tissue redistribution of lead within the child's body. This rebound usually occurs within 2–6 weeks after chelation is stopped, and the lead level may go above 44 mcg/dL if the pre-chelation level was high enough. In general, a child with a higher pre-chelation lead level will require a greater number of chelation courses. Chelation may be repeated for multiple treatment courses, with a two-week "rest" period between each course. In no case should the rebound lead level supersede the pre-chelation lead level; if this occurs, then new ingestion of lead has occurred due to ongoing or new environmental lead exposure.

Parents of all children with elevated blood lead levels should receive recommendations about optimizing the child's nutritional status, regardless of whether or not chelation is being administered. A diet that is reduced in fat assists in potentially reducing lead absorption and retention; the diet should be low in *excess* fat, such as fried foods, but not devoid of all fat. A daily multivitamin is given to ensure adequate trace elements. Iron deficiency, if present, should be corrected, except as described above when BAL is being administered. Since there is greater potential for efficient lead absorption when a child's stomach is empty, it is recommended that frequent nutritional snacks be given between meals.

ENVIRONMENTAL INTERVENTION

In addition to pharmacologic treatment, environmental remediation/intervention is essential in the management of a child with an elevated lead level. When blood lead screening is being considered or conducted, the clinical history should include questions about potential environmental sources of lead for the child(ren) in question. In the case of a child who has already been identified as having an elevated blood lead level, however, a *comprehensive* environmental history should be undertaken (Table 2). A child's elevated blood lead level usually results from multiple environmental lead sources, so identification of one potential source of lead exposure should not preclude completion of the environmental history in its entirety. The process of conducting the environmental history provides the opportunity for parental education about potential lead sources, while simultaneously identifying sources that need to be remediated or removed.

As soon as a child has been identified as having an elevated blood lead level, the local public health system should be notified so that information about available

Table 2 Chelating Agents and Recommended Lead Level for Use

Agent	Lead level
Succimer (DMSA)	45–69 mcg/dL
$CaNa_2EDTA$	70–90 mcg/dL (also alternative to succimer if allergic or lack of treatment response)
BAL and $CaNa_2EDTA$	≥70 mcg/dL (but usually used near or above 100 mcg/dL)

medical and environmental resources can be provided to the child and family. In many jurisdictions, a formal environmental assessment is provided free of charge. In some areas, the family will need to pay a private contractor or sanitarian to conduct the inspection. In addition to a visual assessment, environmental samples are usually taken, and may include paint chips, dust, water, and soil. The inspector often

Table 3 Potential Environmental Sources of Lead

Lead paint in an old house (pre-1978)
Recent or ongoing renovations in an old house
Secondary address (daycare or relative's house) containing lead hazards
Vinyl mini-blinds
Food canned outside the United States
Pottery, ceramics, or decorative tile (leaded glaze)
Leaded crystal
Prenatal exposure due to an elevated maternal lead level during pregnancy
Pica or eating dirt
Industry or factory involving lead emissions
Home remedies or medications (azarcon, greta, pay-loo-ah, bint al zahab)
Cosmetics used in some Indian or African cultures (kohl, surma)
Old plumbing or lead solder
Leaded gasoline (if living in this country less than 6 months, or after long visit to another country)
Ingestion of a leaded foreign body (fishing sinker, lead weight, lead bullet)
Colored newsprint or ink
Toys or clothing decorated with lead paint or dye (often seen in imported toys)
Parental occupational exposure:

- Construction
- Painting
- Auto body repair work
- Car radiator repair
- Lead smelting and brass foundaries
- Brass and copper manufacturing
- Battery and aircraft manufacturing
- Bridge building or repair
- Sandblasting
- Firing ranges
- Valve and pipe fittings
- Plumbing fixtures
- Shipbuilding or ship repair

uses an x-ray fluorescence (XRF) instrument, which is a hand-held spectrum analyzer that requires training and expertise for use. It provides on-site, immediate analysis of painted surfaces and other objects to determine their lead content.

The information gleaned by a formal environmental inspection can be used to remediate the child's environment to decrease exposure to potential lead hazards. In many cases, mobile leaded objects can be easily removed from the dwelling. Parents can be taught housekeeping methods that can significantly reduce the child's lead exposure/ingestion. Interventions such as paint stabilization or minor repairs can also decrease potential lead hazards. In some cases, the parents may choose to remove the child to a safer environment. Families often use an interim lead-safe environment such as the home of a relative or neighbor temporarily. Prior to relocation of a child or family, the "new" home should be determined to be lead-safe. Environmental intervention that includes renovation or repainting should only be undertaken by individuals who have been trained and certified in safe lead abatement practices. When a home is undergoing active abatement, all children, adults, and pets should vacate the property. Home renovations that are improperly conducted are a leading cause of elevated lead levels in both children and adults.

Resources that are available to all families of children with elevated lead levels include the local health department, the state public health system, and local citizen advocacy groups. These organizations usually have the most up-to-date information about certified lead abatement contractors, abatement loan and grant information, and other services/programs related to lead remediation. The public health nurse or health outreach worker usually makes home visits to do on-site family education about nutrition, handwashing, wet-cleaning, and other prevention/intervention measures. Case management services by a nurse or clinical social worker are often available through the child's insurance carrier, managed care organization, or local health department.

PROGNOSIS

In children with elevated lead levels, the potential target organ of greatest concern is the central nervous system. Because a child's brain is undergoing rapid change and development, it is potentially more vulnerable to damage. Research has demonstrated an association between an elevated childhood lead level and developmental disabilities such as language delay, hyperactivity, behavior problems, attention deficit disorder, and learning disabilities. Some research has suggested an association between early childhood lead exposure and delinquent or criminal behavior. It is not possible to predict the potential impact of an elevated lead level on an individual child, and there is no direct linear relationship between a specific lead level and a child's developmental outcome. As a broad generality, a higher lead level and/or more chronic exposure is theoretically more potentially harmful. Although chelation is recommended at a lead level $\geq$45 mcg/dL, it is used to rapidly decrease the child's lead level, and has not been proven to ameliorate developmental outcome. Environmental remediation/intervention to decrease lead hazards is usually the most effective "treatment" for a child with an elevated lead level. In a lead-safe environment, a child's blood lead level will eventually fall as urinary lead excretion supersedes lead ingestion. Whether or not a child has been chelated, the eventual fall in lead level is more dependent on a child's individual physiology than on other factors. There is no predictable linear relationship between the interruption of lead ingestion and the rate of fall in lead level.

SUMMARY

Over a century after the first reported cases in the pediatric literature, children with elevated lead levels continue to present an environmental health challenge. An elevated lead level during early childhood places a child at potential risk for long-term developmental disabilities. Management of children with elevated lead levels is most effective when there is a team approach among medical, environmental, and public health personnel. Although there are resources and chelating agents available to assist children with elevated lead levels, the best intervention is primary prevention.

SUGGESTED READINGS

1. Centers for Disease Control and Prevention. Screening Young Children for Lead Poisoning: Guidance for State and Local Public Health Officials. Atlanta: CDC, 1997.
2. Chisolm JJ. Safety and efficacy of meso-2,3-dimercaptosuccinic acid (DMSA) in children with elevated blood lead concentrations. Clin Toxicol 2000; 38:365–375.
3. Consumer Product Safety Commission. http://www.cpsc.gov.
4. Davoli CT, Serwint JR, Chisolm JJ. Children with blood lead levels $>100\,\mu g/dL$. Pediatrics 1996; 98(5):965–968.
5. Environmental Protection Agency. http://www.epa.gov.lead.
6. Johnston MV, Goldstein GW. Selective vulnerability of the developing brain to lead. Curr Opin Neurol 1998; 11:689–693.
7. Pueschel SM, Linakis JG, Anderson AC. Lead Poisoning in Childhood. Baltimore: Brookes Publishing, 1996.
8. Treatment of Lead-Exposed Children (TLC) Trial Group. The effect of chelation therapy with succimer on neuropsychological development in children exposed to lead. NEJM 2001; 344(19):1421–1426.

57
Stroke in Childhood

Rebecca N. Ichord
Department of Neurology, Children's Hospital of Philadelphia, Philadelphia, Pennsylvania, U.S.A.

INTRODUCTION

Stroke encompasses several distinct cerebrovascular disorders traditionally defined by clinical criteria, in which the sudden onset of an acute focal neurological deficit is a cardinal clinical sign. Stroke includes ischemic infarction from arterial occlusion or hypoperfusion (arterial ischemic stroke, AIS), venous infarction related to cerebral sinovenous thrombosis (SVT), and primary intracranial hemorrhage (ICH). Events resembling TIAs in children should be evaluated and managed with the same level of urgency and completeness as for completed stroke.

The design and rationale for diagnostic and treatment guidelines in childhood stroke rest on the results of epidemiological cohort studies, as there are no prospective randomized clinical trials for treatment of childhood stroke outside of transfusion for sickle cell anemia. Incidence estimates vary depending on definitions and inclusion criteria, ranging from 3.3 to 6/100,000/year, with 1/3 of all strokes occurring in neonates. Risk factors for stroke in children are very different than in adults, where atherosclerosis, hypertension, and diabetes predominate. A recent 22-year consecutive cohort study of children with AIS found that 46% of cases had a pre-existing condition known to be associated with stroke (symptomatic), and 54% did not (cryptogenic). After full investigation for risk factors after the index event, risk factors can usually be identified in >95% of cases, including cervical or intracranial arteriopathies in up to 80%, and prothrombotic risk factors in 10–40%, more often in neonatal stroke and in SVT.

EVALUATION AND TREATMENT: PARALLEL PROCESSES IN STROKE

Stroke syndromes represent one of the few true emergencies in pediatric neurology. Diagnosis and management should occur in parallel, and are presented as such here. Evidence-based diagnostic and treatment guidelines are not presently available. The guidelines provided here represent a consensus based on data from cohort studies, and the experience and results of trials in adult stroke. In all matters of treatment, it is reasonable to assume that the principle of "time is brain" applies equally to children as it does to adults.

Acute Management—Initial Supportive Care

A stroke management protocol begins with defining inclusion criteria: (1) acute onset focal neurological deficit of any duration, (2) unexplained altered consciousness, particularly with headache, (3) seizures in a near-term newborn, and (4) seizures in an infant recovering from cardiac surgery. Upon identification of a child with suspected stroke, a series of treatment and diagnostic procedures should be simultaneously activated. Treatment prior to definitive diagnosis is by necessity supportive, and can be critical to the evolution of the deficit, as described in Table 1. While initial supportive care begins, diagnostic studies should be performed promptly, which will then guide further management decisions.

Acute Management—Initial Diagnostic Studies

Admitting laboratory studies should include comprehensive chemistry and hematologic profiles, PT, PTT, and INR. Other admission diagnostic studies commonly obtained in the setting of acute stroke include urinalysis and EKG, and more specific testing as indicated by patient history and exam findings, for example in case of fever or in a patient with sickle cell anemia, or in suspected metabolic disease, rheumatologic disease, or HIV. All patients with arterial or venous thrombotic or thromboembolic syndromes should be evaluated for prothrombotic risk factors. The specific studies to be obtained may be worked out in consultation with pediatric thrombosis experts, as these tests and their results are subject to change as research progresses in this area. An example of a list of studies to evaluate for thrombophilia is shown below in Table 2. Cardiac evaluation is commonly recommended in children with AIS

Table 1 Acute Supportive Care of Acute Ischemic Stroke in Children

1. Assure airway, oxygenation, and air exchange, providing supplemental oxygen to maintain $SaO_2 \geq 95\%$.
2. Monitor cardiopulmonary status continuously, with intermittent frequent checks of blood pressure, temperature, neurologic status (GCS), and bedside blood glucose levels.
3. Restrict activity to bed rest until the clinical deficit is stable or improving (24–72 hr), to avoid potential posturally triggered fluctuations in perfusion.
4. Establish IV access and provide maintenance volume with nondextrose-containing isotonic fluids, aiming for normovolemia, and blood glucoses levels of 60–120 mg/dl.
5. Maintain blood pressure around the 50 percentile for the child's age- or height-related norms. Treatment of hypertension in the setting of acute stroke is controversial. Unless BP is extremely elevated, or suspected to be a cause of acute heart failure, elevated blood pressure should not be treated with acute blood pressure-lowering agents.
6. Prevent and treat hyperthermia aggressively, aiming for core temperatures $< 37.0°C$.
7. Treat seizures with anticonvulsants, taking care to avoid transient blood pressure depression from rapid dosing.
8. Institute DVT prophylaxis for children and adolescents who are seriously immobilized by their deficit.
9. Hold oral intake pending 24 hr of hemodynamic and respiratory stability, and evaluation of adequate swallowing function by a speech therapist.

Table 2 Laboratory Evaluation for Prothrombotic Risk Factors

Laboratory test	Comments
CBC, PT/PTT	Must be sent prior to giving heparin
Protein C-functional activity	Not helpful if pt. is on coumadin
Protein C–immunologic if <6 months	Normal levels in neonates are based on immunologic test
Protein S-functional and free	Not helpful if pt. is on coumadin
Antithrombin III	Must be sent prior to giving heparin
Factor V Leiden mutation	This is not a factor V level
Prothrombin mutation 20210A	
Lupus inhibitor screen	Includes anticardiolipin Ab, anti-2GPI, dRVVT, and TTI
MTHFR gene mutation	Methylenetetrahydrofolate reductase
Plasma homocysteine level	Fasting specimen
Lipoprotein(a)	

stroke, and usually involves minimally a transthoracic echocardiogram. Transesophageal echocardiogram may be considered for patients in whom no other major vascular cause is identified, and in whom the transthoracic echo was normal or equivocal

The key to diagnosis lies in neuroimaging. While MRI is superior to CT in confirming and characterizing acute stroke syndromes, there is a significant time delay involved in obtaining MR imaging in most facilities. An urgent head CT is usually obtained in all children with a clinical suspicion of a stroke syndrome, and may narrow the differential diagnosis quickly to a limited number of possibilities which have immediate treatment implications. For example, venous thrombosis may be apparent on head CT in severe cases, and if so should prompt immediate therapy with heparin and IV fluids, and lead to urgent venography. All children with suspected stroke should go onto have brain MRI as soon as possible, with careful attention to sedation and monitoring during radiologic procedures so as to prevent secondary hypoxemia, hypercarbia, or aspiration. A reasonable MRI protocol for acute stroke will include axial T2, gradient echo, FLAIR, and diffusion weighted sequences as a minimum. Vascular imaging should be included with the initial MRI. Clinical assessment, and sometimes the admission CT, may provide an indication as to whether MR angiography or venography should be obtained. Vascular imaging should include cervical vessels in all patients with a posterior circulation stroke syndrome, and in any patient with an anterior circulation stroke syndrome who complains of significant headache or neck ache, or has a history of possible triggering factors for dissection, such as weight-lifting, chiropractic manipulation, head or neck trauma, amusement park rides, or prolonged or forceful vomiting. Repeat imaging will be needed in selected patients who develop new or progressive deficits during the first week. Standard angiography should be considered in cases with equivocal or negative findings on MR vascular imaging, or where no other risk factor is identified. Results of diagnostic studies are critical in guiding both acute management and secondary prevention.

Acute Management—Specific Stroke Therapy

The only proven effective therapy for children with acute stroke is exchange transfusion for children with sickle cell anemia. Most centers that care for patients with sickle cell anemia have in place procedures for transfusion therapy for acute stroke, which is beyond the scope of this chapter. In all other patients with acute stroke syndromes confirmed by MRI, treatment at present is essentially based on consensus and the judicious and selective application of treatments used in adults. Therapeutic options for children with stroke commonly in use include anticoagulation and antiplatelet agents. Systemic anticoagulation acutely may have a role, provided the initial infarct is nonhemorrhagic, in selected groups of patients considered to have a high risk of clot propagation or of recurrent embolization: sinovenous thrombosis, arterial dissection, cardiogenic embolus, or high-grade intracranial focal segmental stenosis. Low molecular weight heparin has the advantages of ease of administration and predictable effect on coagulation parameters, and a good safety record in children treated for a wide variety of thrombotic conditions. Standard unfractionated heparin has the advantage of being able to be reversed quickly in patients at high risk of hemorrhage or who might need emergency surgery for other problems. Dosage recommendations and monitoring are best worked out in advance as part of an institutional stroke protocol in consultation with local thrombosis specialists, with examples of dosage guidelines shown in Table 3.

By the end of the first week, most diagnostic studies have been complete, and the patient's clinical deficits have stabilized. Decisions can then be made concerning secondary preventive treatments, which may include systemic anticoagulation with LMWH or coumadin, or antiplatelet agents, or a definitive procedure such as closure of a patent foramen ovale. The decision to maintain long-term anticoagulation vs. treat with antiplatelet agents is individualized depending on the risk factors. Patients with an estimated high risk of stroke recurrence from thromboembolic events should be considered for long-term anticoagulation (e.g., recurrent cardiogenic stroke from fixed structural heart defect, or a patient with a severe permanent thrombophilia), short-term anticoagulation for 3–6 months, (arterial dissection, SVT related to head/neck infection). Other patients with known risk factors such as intracranial arteriopathy other than dissection, or with no identifiable risk factors, may be considered for antiplatelet agents. Aspirin is started at 3–5 mg/kg/day. Reyes syndrome is a traditional concern in children treated with aspirin, but is extremely rare. Most experts feel that aspirin is a reasonable and safe choice, although vaccination for influenza and varicella should be considered.

Rehabilitation should be started in the acute hospital unit as soon as the patient is hemodynamically stable. Discharge planning needs to start early, leading to a transfer to in-patient rehabilitation or home with outpatient rehabilitation. Appropriate family and patient psychosocial supportive services will usually be necessary at all stages of the illness and its treatment. A list of parent-oriented resources is shown at the end of this chapter.

In rare cases, there may be a role for two additional interventions for extreme or rare circumstances. Timely decompressive craniectomy may be both life-saving and function-sparing in children with large middle cerebral artery stroke syndromes who display rapid deterioration in level of consciousness or progress to signs and symptoms of impending herniation. The second controversial intervention is thrombolysis. Current standard of care for adult stroke involves using IV tPA only for patients 18 years and older meeting strict inclusion criteria, which are described in detail in the American Heart Association (AHA) website. The role of thrombolysis for children under age 18 years is much more controversial. The major limiting factor is that IV thrombolysis must be started within 3 hr

Table 3 Treatment Guidelines for Systemic Anticoagulation

Anticoagulant	Dose	Monitoring	Comment
Low molecular weight heparin LMWH (enoxaparin)	For age < 2 months: 1.5 mg/kg/dose SQ q 12 hr For age > 2 months: 1.0 mg/kg/dose SQ q 12 hrs	Four hours after second or third dose obtain an antifactor Xa level	Therapeutic anti-Xa level for treatment dose therapy is 0.5–1.0 units/ml
Unfractionated heparin	Loading dose: 75 units/kg IV over 10 min Initial maintenance: For age < 1 yr 28 units/kg/hr For age > 1 yr 20 units/kg/hr	Check PTT 4 hr after administration of the heparin loading dose and 4 hr after every change in the infusion rate	Adjust heparin to maintain PTT 60–85 sec. When PTT values are therapeutic, check daily CBC and PTT

Heparin dose titration

PTT (sec)	Bolus (units/kg)	Hold (min)	Rate change	Repeat PTT
< 50	50	0	+10%	4 hr
50–59	0	0	+10%	4 hr
60–85	0	0	0	Next day
86–95	0	0	−10%	4 hr
96–120	0	30	−10%	4 hr
> 120	0	60	−15%	4 hr

of symptom onset, which is defined as the time the patient was last seen well. Children with stroke rarely meet this time limit. Evidence as to the safety and efficacy of thrombolysis for children with stroke are extremely limited, and that existing for thrombolysis for systemic clots suggests a high risk of hemorrhagic complications. Until more evidence is available, decisions about using thrombolysis for children less than 18 years are best handled with extreme caution, and in consultation with an affiliated adult stroke program experienced in the use of thrombolysis in adults.

PROGNOSIS

Stroke in childhood is associated with significant morbidity and mortality even in the current era of high quality and availability of tertiary care. Case fatality rates in children range from 5 to 18% for AIS, 22 to 36% for hemorrhagic stroke and 8 to 10% for sinovenous thrombosis. Morbidity among survivors is reported in the range of 20–40% with mild and 15–40% with severe impairments 3–7 years after stroke onset, and epilepsy in 10–15%. There is very limited data concerning predictors of the poor outcome, with age < 1 year, depressed consciousness at presentation, and large hemisphere infarcts associated with poorer outcomes. Estimates for 2–5-year recurrence rates range from 5% to 39% in children with AIS, with higher recurrence rates seen in children with vasculopathies and with multiple risk factors, and with up to one-third of recurrences being clinically "silent".

SUMMARY

Stroke is one of the few neurologic emergencies in pediatric medicine, for which there are no proven therapies outside of transfusion for sickle cell anemia. The incidence is highest among neonates, and overall is similar to that of childhood brain tumors. Morbidity is high, and mortality remains signficant. Evaluation and treatment should proceed in parallel, and with the understanding that "time is brain". This begins with clinical suspicion of a stroke syndrome in any child with a new focal neurologic deficit or unexplained acute encephalopathy, relies heavily on timely and comprehensive brain and vascular imaging, and finishes with evaluation in all patients for underlying cardiac, prothrombotic, and cerebrovascular risk factors. Treatment is initially supportive, aiming to minimize stroke progression by optimizing perfusion and preventing hyperthermia. Judicious and selective use of platelet inhibitors and systemic anticoagulation may limit progression or recurrence. Early and aggressive rehabilitation are necessary to optimize recovery. There is very little data concerning safety or efficacy of thrombolysis at present. Long-term follow-up with clinical and neuroimaging assessment are necessary to fully ascertain recurrence rates and support recovery.

SUGGESTED READINGS

1. Chabrier S, Husson B, Lasjaunias P et al. Stroke in childhood: outcome and recurrence risk by mechanism in 59 patients. J Child Neurol 2000; 15:290–294.
2. Chan AK, deVeber G. Prothrombotic disorders and ischemic stroke in children. Semin Pediatr Neurol 2000; 7:301–308.
3. De Schryver EL, Kappelle LJ, Jennekens-Schinkel A, et al. Prognosis of ischemic stroke in childhood: a long-term follow-up study. Dev Med Child Neurol 2000; 42:313–318.
4. deVeber G. Stroke and the child's brain: an overview of epidemiology, syndromes and risk factors. Curr Opin Neurol 2002; 15:133–138.
5. deVeber GA, MacGregor D, Curtis R, et al. Neurologic outcome in survivors of childhood arterial ischemic stroke and sinovenous thrombosis. J Child Neurol 2000; 15: 316–324.
6. deVeber G, Andrew M. Cerebral sinovenous thrombosis in children. N Engl J Med 2001; 345:417–423.
7. Ganesan V, Prengler M, McShane MA, et al. Investigation of risk factors in children with arterial ischemic stroke. Ann Neurol 2003; 53:167–173.
8. Strater R, Vielhaber H, Kassenbohmer R, et al. Genetic risk factors of thrombophilia in ischaemic childhood stroke of cardiac origin. A prospective ESPED survey. Eur J Pediatr 1999; 158(suppl 3):S122–S125.

RESOURCES

American Heart Association Stroke site: http://www.strokeassociation.org

Parent Support Resources: http://www.hemikids.org, http://www.pediatricstroke network.com

NIH Stroke Information Page: http://accessible.ninds.nih.gov/health_and_medical/disorders/stroke.htm

58
Vascular Malformations

Judy Huang and Rafael J. Tamargo
Department of Neurosurgery, Johns Hopkins University School of Medicine, Baltimore, Maryland, U.S.A.

Philippe H. Gailloud
Division of Interventional Neuroradiology, Johns Hopkins University School of Medicine, Baltimore, Maryland, U.S.A.

INTRODUCTION

Cerebral vascular malformations occurring in the pediatric population that may require specialized neurosurgical and neurointerventional care include arteriovenous malformations (AVMs), cerebral aneurysms, cavernous malformations, vein of Galen aneurysmal malformations (VGAMS), and dural arteriovenous fistulas (DAVFs). Venous angiomas and capillary telangiectasias are typically incidental findings that require no specific treatment. These cerebral vascular lesions are varied in their pathophysiology, treatment options, and prognosis. Although some of these malformations exist more commonly in adults, the principles of treatment may be extended to pediatric patients.

ARTERIOVENOUS MALFORMATIONS

Background

Arteriovenous malformations are high-flow vascular malformations comprised of arteries shunting blood into an abnormal tangle of vessels known as the "nidus" and draining directly into veins without an intervening capillary bed. These congenital lesions occurring within the brain parenchyma are likely the result of incomplete differentiation of the embryonic arteriovenous network of vessels into separate arterial and venous systems between 3 and 12 weeks of gestation. Arteriovenous malformations may occur superficially in the cortex, buried deep in the basal ganglia, or less commonly in the posterior fossa. The estimated incidence of cerebral AVMs in childhood is 1 per 100,000, with only 12–18% becoming symptomatic during the childhood years.

Clinical Presentation

Not only are AVMs the most common cause of intracranial hemorrhage occurring in children, but hemorrhage is also the most common initial presentation of these lesions (50–80%). Presentation with seizures occurs in 12–25% of cases. A child with an acute hemorrhage may complain of sudden headache and develop nausea, vomiting, progressive neurological deficits, and seizures. In adults, the annual risk of hemorrhage is estimated at 2–4%. Children with AVMs are thought to have a higher cumulative risk of bleeding and rebleeding than adults since their risk period is longer. In pediatric AVM patients who present with an intracerebral hemorrhage, the mortality rate is approximately twice that of adults, which is estimated at 10%.

Diagnosis

Children who present acutely will initially undergo computed tomography (CT) or magnetic resonance imaging (MRI). CT will readily identify the presence of a hemorrhage. MRA may be used to detect the presence of an AVM. MRI is invaluable in delineating the anatomic localization of the AVM with respect to normal surrounding structures as well as cortical and ventricular surfaces, providing information that subsequently directs treatment strategies. The areas of the AVM nidus as well as abnormal feeding and draining vessels manifest as flow-voids. Cerebral angiography is necessary to define the vascular anatomy of the AVM, namely the vascular territories contributing to its arterial supply, the size and architecture of the nidus, and the number and location of the draining veins.

Treatment

The management of a child presenting with an acute hemorrhage is aimed at management of elevated intracranial pressure and may require craniotomy for hematoma evacuation or external ventricular drainage for intraventricular hemorrhage in selected cases. Following neurological stabilization, definitive treatment with the objective of complete AVM obliteration is then considered.

The size, location, and venous drainage are crucial in the decision to pursue either surgical resection or radiosurgery, with or without preoperative embolization. Endovascular embolization is an adjunctive rather than a stand-alone treatment for most AVMs with the exception of small AVMs with a limited number of feeders. The clear advantage of microsurgical removal is that it provides immediate cure and eliminates the risk of rebleeding. However, small, deep-seated lesions in inoperable locations may be safely and effectively treated by Gamma Knife radiosurgery. There is a latency period of approximately 2 years, during which the annual risk of hemorrhage remains the same as that of an untreated lesion. Treatment outcomes have improved in recent decades due to the multidisciplinary team approach to these lesions that is commonly employed at highly specialized centers.

CEREBRAL ANEURYSMS

Background

Pediatric cerebral aneurysms are extremely rare, with a reported incidence ranging from 0.5% to 4.6%. Patients less than 18 years old account for less than 2% of all patients with cerebral aneurysms. They are even less common in the youngest age groups, with only a small number of patients less than 5 years of age.

Several features of aneurysms found in the pediatric age group distinguish them from their adult counterparts. A male-to-female preponderance of 1.75:1

exists. The terminal bifurcation of the internal carotid artery is the location of one quarter of pediatric aneurysms. One-fifth are "giant" (larger than 2.5 cm) in size and one-fifth occur in the posterior circulation. In addition, an infectious etiology is more commonly associated with aneurysms occurring in this young population.

Clinical Presentation

Aneurysms in the pediatric population are most likely to present with subarachnoid hemorrhage. This can be manifested as headache, irritability, nausea, vomiting, nuchal rigidity, seizure, lethargy, cranial nerve palsy, weakness, or coma. Giant aneurysms in particular may present with headaches or cranial nerve palsies from local mass effect, prompting radiographic evaluation and leading to early detection prior to rupture and subarachnoid hemorrhage.

Diagnosis

Subarachnoid hemorrhage and the presence of hydrocephalus requiring ventriculostomy placement may be easily detected on CT. Although techniques such as magnetic resonance angiography and CT angiography are continuing to undergo refinement, the mainstay of diagnosis for cerebral aneurysms in the pediatric population remains conventional digital subtraction cerebral angiography.

Treatment

The treatment of cerebral aneurysms in the pediatric age group has undergone dramatic advances in the recent decade with significant improvements in patient outcomes. Multimodality treatment strategies at specialized neurovascular centers are widely adopted as a standard approach in the care of these rare patients. Lesion characteristics such as clinical condition at presentation, size, and location in the cerebral vasculature determine the suitability of surgical, endovascular, or combined approaches in the treatment of individual patients. Fortunately, in contradistinction to adults, cerebral vasospasm causing delayed cerebral ischemia is not a characteristic problem associated with subarachnoid hemorrhage in young patients. Taken together, good outcomes may be expected in greater than 90% of this patient population.

CAVERNOUS MALFORMATIONS

Background

Cavernous malformations are vascular malformations comprised histologically of sinusoidal vascular channels lacking the structures of normal blood vessel walls. The lesion is typically filled with blood and hemosiderin in varying stages of degradation, leading to their characteristic radiographic appearance on MRI. Approximately one-fifth of these vascular malformations are found in the pediatric population. The anatomical distribution of cavernous malformations is directly related to the volume of tissue in each region, with the vast majority occurring in the frontal and temporal lobes, with proportionally fewer located in the brainstem, cerebellum, and spinal cord. Familial cases of cavernous malformations account for about 20–50% of all cases and are more likely than sporadic cases to have multiple lesions. An association with chromosome 7 has been implicated and these familial cases appear to be inherited in an autosomal-dominant fashion.

Clinical Presentation

Insufficient information exists to allow distinction between the features of presentation of cavernous malformations in pediatric compared to adult patients. The most common clinical presentations are headaches, seizures, and hemorrhage. With the advent of CT and MRI in recent decades, a large number of these lesions are now incidentally discovered in the course of radiographic evaluation for other clinical indications. Therefore, the current understanding of the natural history of these lesions is evolving.

Diagnosis

The preferred diagnostic study for the detection of cavernous malformations is MRI, and in particular, gradient echo sequences. CT scanning is suboptimal in sensitivity and specificity for identification of cavernous malformations. These vascular malformations are angiographically occult, rendering angiography, MRA, or CT angiography extraneous in the diagnostic evaluation.

Treatment

Although the inherent biological behavior of cavernous malformations is believed to be relatively more benign than AVMs and cerebral aneurysms, cavernous malformations that hemorrhage may cause significant neurologic sequelae depending on their specific location. Therefore, symptomatic lesions in surgically accessible locations should be considered for removal as a definitive cure. The rate of seizure control with lesion resection is excellent. However, cavernous malformations in highly eloquent locations such as the brainstem or spinal cord present a particularly challenging problem in which the risk of surgical excision must be individually balanced with nonsurgical management.

VEIN OF GALEN ANEURYSMAL MALFORMATIONS

Background

Vein of Galen aneurysmal malformations (VGAMs) are rare intracranial vascular anomalies typically found in the pediatric population. The anatomic landmark of a VGAM is the presence of multiple arteriovenous shunts draining into a dilated median cerebral venous collector. This median vein corresponds to an embryonic channel, the median prosencephalic vein, which normally only partially persists at the adult stage as the vein of Galen. VGAMs represent approximately 30% of the pediatric vascular malformations.

Clinical Presentation

Neonatal Period

Newborns typically present with severe cardiorespiratory alterations at or shortly after birth. The volume overload imposed by a high-flow VGAM rapidly induces cardiovascular and respiratory distress syndromes. In the past, the mortality rate for this group was close to 100%. Recent advances made in the acute management of these neonates, in particular the use of endovascular techniques in a dedicated neonatal intensive care environment, have significantly improved this dark prognosis.

Infancy

Infants characteristically present with increased head circumference, hydrocephalus, psychomotor delay, and/or seizures. Noncommunicating hydrocephalus results from direct compression of the aqueduct or posterior third ventricle by the venous aneurysm itself. Communicating hydrocephalus is related either to impaired cerebrospinal fluid reabsorption caused by subarachnoid blood, or to VGAM-induced intracranial venous hypertension. Among less constant signs and symptoms are a cranial bruit, dilated scalp veins (in particular in the periorbital region and the glabella), proptosis, and recurrent epistaxis.

Older Child and Adult

Older children tend to present with headache that may or may not be associated with subarachnoid hemorrhage. Diagnosis of a VGAM at the adult age is rare. A small cerebral arteriovenous malformation draining into an enlarged but otherwise normal vein of Galen has to be considered in the differential diagnosis.

Treatment

The advent of endovascular therapy and the development of neonatal intensive care units have radically changed the treatment and prognosis of VGAM patients. Surgical options are reserved for particular situations that include the evacuation of intracranial hematomas and the placement of ventricular shunts. The optimal management of patients with a VGAM can be achieved only through the comprehensive, multidisciplinary approach offered by specialized tertiary care centers.

The endovascular treatment of VGAM includes transarterial and transvenous percutaneous embolization. In our institution, a transarterial approach through the umbilical artery or via a femoral puncture is favored whenever possible. Superselective catheterization and embolization of the arterial feeders with a cyanoacrylate embolic agent is the technique of choice. The transvenous approach, performed via a femoral or jugular access followed by retrograde catheterization of the venous aneurysm, or via direct puncture of the torcula, offers an alternate route that should be reserved to VGAMs that cannot be accessed transarterially. The endovascular treatment of a VGAM often requires staged embolization procedures, initially aimed at controlling cardiac failure. This helps avoid the occurrence of parenchymal bleedings secondary to a "perfusion breakthrough phenomenon" or to massive venous thrombosis potentially endangering the normal venous drainage. Ideally, when the hemodynamic conditions allow it, embolization should be deferred until 5–6 months of life.

SUGGESTED READINGS

1. Burrows PF, Robertson RL, Barnes PD. Angiography and the evaluation of cerebrovascular disease in childhood. Neuroimaging Clin N Am 1996; 6(3):561–588.

2. Smith ER, Butler WE, Ogilvy CS. Surgical approaches to vascular anomalies of the child's brain. Curr Opin Neurol 2002; 15(2):165–171.
3. TerBrugge KG. Neurointerventional procedures in the pediatric age group. Childs Nerv Syst 1999; 15(11–12):751–754.

59
Ataxia

Donald L. Gilbert
Cincinnati Children's Hospital Medical Center, Movement Disorders Clinics, Cincinnati, Ohio, U.S.A.

INTRODUCTION

Ataxia refers to impaired ability to coordinate muscle activity in the execution of voluntary movement. Clinically, important findings include broad based gait, errors in range and force of limb movement (dysmetria), errors in rate and regularity of repetitive and alternating movements (dysdiadochokinesia), and tremor that is usually most marked at the end of movement. Anatomically, this involves most prominently pathology of the cerebellum and/or its afferent or efferent connections. A clinician's efforts primarily involve diagnosis and supportive care, as few useful specific medical therapies are available. Challenges to proper diagnosis of genetic causes include: (1) variable phenotypes and ages of onset within individual genotypes, and (2) overlapping phenotypes among different genotypes.

APPROACH/CLINICAL FEATURES

The Uncoordinated Child

Parents may seek evaluation for a young child with subnormal fine or gross motor skills, often as the child enters preschool or kindergarten. Typically, such children have a nonspecific constellation of motor difficulties, which may include tremor, incoordination, and learning and behavioral difficulties. A follow-up examination in 6–12 months to ensure there is no regression may be all that is required diagnostically. Referral for occupational/physical/speech therapy or special education evaluation may be important.

The Child with Acute Ataxia

Acute ataxia in a previously well child often presents with gait impairment. A large number of acute processes (partial list in Table 1) can affect the cerebellum. A careful thorough history and examination is essential to identify serious causes. *Intoxications* may cause ataxia, sometimes in conjunction with an acute confusional state. Anticonvulsant medications, alcohol, stimulants, and other causes can often be

Table 1 Differential Diagnosis of Acute Ataxia in Childhood

Category	Examples	Clinical features
Toxic	Acute ingestion: EtOH, anticonvulsants, antihistamines, benzodiazepines	Toddlers—accidental ingestion; adolescents—substance abuse. Mental status changes common, urine/serum toxicology screen in ER may detect unsuspected ingestions
Inflammatory	Acute cerebellar ataxia	Symmetric cerebellar findings, gait impairment, truncal ataxia (titubation), may include nystagmus. Mental status normal. Usually postinfectious
	Acute disseminated encephalomyelitis (ADEM)	Mental status changes and multifocal neurologic deficits
	Miller Fisher variant of Guillain–Barre syndrome	Oculomotor paresis, bulbar weakness, hyporeflexia, pain. Admit, monitor for respiratory/autonomic failure. Treat pain. Nerve conduction studies to assess demyelinating vs. axonal forms. Treat with IVIG or plasmapheresis if moderate or severe to shorten course
	Opsoclonus myoclonus	Paraneoplastic or postinfectious
Mass lesions	Posterior fossa neoplasms	Usually more chronic. Headaches, vomiting, papilledema, cranial nerve palsies
Vascular	Stroke, vertebrobasilar dissection	Consider after neck trauma or if hypercoagulable
Metabolic	Many inborn errors of metabolism	Can be triggered by intercurrent illness. Consider if child has preexisting developmental impairment, positive family history, consanguinity; or if current encephalopathy, vomiting
Migrainous	Basilar migraine, benign paroxysmal vertigo	Initial episode suggests focal pathology
Functional	Abnormal illness behavior, "psychogenic" gait disturbance	Dramatic or variable symptoms which do not conform to neuroanatomic distributions

A vast number of acute processes can affect cerebellar function. This partial list contains relatively more common causes.

identified by history, and urine/serum drug screening. *Acute cerebellar ataxia* may occur after a clinical or subclinical infection or vaccination. Gait ataxia occurs in 100%, truncal ataxia in 60–80%, and nystagmus in 10–20% of affected children. CSF abnormalities, if present, are nonspecific: elevated WBC in 30–50%, elevated protein in 6–27%. Recovery is complete in approximately 90%, with mean time to normal gait of 2–3 months. Treatment is not recommended.

A preceding history of headaches with vomiting, double vision, high fevers, or mental status changes prior to the onset of ataxia suggests more severe pathology. Similarly, findings on examination of mental status changes, cranial nerve palsies, and hypo- or hyper-reflexia raise concerns for serious etiologies including acute disseminated encephalomyelitis, basilar migraine, Miller Fisher variant of acute inflammatory demyelinating polyneuropathy, vascular events, hydrocephalus, and subacute onset neoplasms. Children with the Miller Fisher syndrome are at risk for respiratory failure or autonomic decompensation and should be admitted and monitored aggressively.

The Child with Subacute or Chronic Progressive Ataxia

Because a large variety of diseases can produce similar ataxic syndromes, the diagnostic evaluation should be thoughtful, to avoid needless testing where possible, yet thorough. Key questions are similar to those involved in most neurologic assessments: (1) localization of the lesion? Unilateral or predominantly midline cerebellar signs may indicate focal cerebellar pathology. Depending on the time course, accompanying symptoms, and MRI findings, possible causes of focal cerebellar disease include congenital malformation, neoplasm, demyelination, abscess, or vascular event. Treatment of focal processes may be surgical and depends on the cause identified or suspected; (2) what is the time course? Subacute, intermittent, or chronic progressive patterns narrow the diagnostic considerations; (3) is there a pattern of inheritance? A large proportion of intermittent and chronic progressive ataxias are heritable, and many causative genes have been identified. Careful pedigrees and examination of relatives aid in diagnostic decision making; (4) is there a highly characteristic phenotype? The presence of certain findings can limit the differential diagnosis quickly and allow for more focused diagnostic testing. Diagnosis depends on the presence and pattern of neurologic and nonneurologic symptoms and confirmatory laboratory testing.

DIAGNOSTIC GENETIC TESTING FOR PROGRESSIVE AND FAMILIAL ATAXIAS

After synthesis of the patient's history, family history, and detailed general, ophthalmologic, and neurological examinations, the use of updated web-based databases is recommended. For example, the National Center for Biotechnology Information's Online Mendelian Inheritance in Man (OMIM) at http://www.ncbi.nlm.nih.gov/Omim/ allows searches based on signs and symptoms, and each entry contains useful text and a clinical synopsis in outline form. The NIH/DOE-funded GeneTests website at http://www.geneclinics.org/ provides helpful disease descriptions and contact information for laboratories where testing may be obtained.

Dominant ataxias, mostly referred to as Spinocerebellar ataxias (SCAs), can be subcategorized as: (1) CAG repeat expansion disorders within gene reading frames (SCA 1, 2, 3, 7, 17); (2) disorders with noncoding repeats (SCA 8, 10, 12); (3) disorders with chromosomal linkage only (SCA 4, 5, 11, 13, 14, 15, 16, 19, 21); and (4) episodic ataxias (EA) due to channelopathies/ion channel defects (EA1, EA2/SCA6). Results from genetic testing often broaden our understanding of the phenotype. Dominant, recessive, and episodic ataxias known to have possible childhood onset are listed in Table 2.

Table 2 Heritable Ataxias that May Present with Chronic Progressive or Intermittent Ataxia in Childhood

Disease	Classic features	Earliest onset	Inheritance	Diagnostic tests	Medical treatment
Friedreich's ataxia	Gait ataxia, axonal neuropathy, extensor plantar, cardiomyopathy, diabetes	>2 years, mean 15 years	AR	>90 GAA expansion in frataxin	idebenone or anti-oxidants for cardiomyopathy
Ataxia telangiectasia	Progressive ataxia, oculomotor signs, telangiectasias (later) recurrent sinopulmonary infections (60%)	Ataxia at 2–4 years	AR	Elevated AFP; ATM mutation screening difficult	IVIG for immune deficiency
SCA1	Ataxia, dysarthria, pyramidal tract signs, brain stem symptoms, peripheral neuropathy	15 years (mean 35 years)	AD	>40 CAG repeats in ataxin-1	None
SCA2	Ataxia, dysarthria, tremor, slow saccades, hyporeflexia	6 months (mean 30 years)	AD	>33 CAG repeats in ataxin-2	None
SCA3/MJD type 1	Ataxia, dystonia, spasticity, rapid progression	10 years	AD	>74 CAG repeats in MJD1	None
SCA7	Ataxia, macular degeneration	1 year (mean 29 years)	AD	>36 CAG repeats (>> in childhood cases) in SCA7 gene	None
EA-1	Episodic bouts of ataxia lasting minutes, with Myokymia between spells	2 years	AD	Mutation in KCNA1 gene	Acetazolamide 250–750 mg per day
EA-2	Episodic bouts of ataxia lasting hours to days with abnormal eye movements between spells	2 years	AD	Mutation in CACNA1A	acetazolamide 250–750 mg per day

AD, autosomal dominant; AFP alpha feto protein; AR autosomal recessive; ATM ataxia telangiectasia mutation; CAG/GAA, trinucleotide sequences; CACNA/KCNA calcium and potassium channel subunit genes; EA, episodic ataxia; MJD, Machado–Joseph disease; SCA, spinocerebellar ataxias; IVIG; Intravenous Immunoglobolin.

SELECTED CATEGORIES OF ATAXIA AND THEIR THERAPY

Ataxia Associated with Congenital Malformations

A large number of congenital malformation syndromes may be associated with ataxia. Unilateral cerebellar malformations are generally acquired due to pre-, peri-, or postnatal insults.

Multiple syndromes are associated with dysgenesis of the midline cerebellar structures. *Dandy-Walker malformations*, characterized by large posterior fossa cystic dilation, upward displacement of the tentorium, midline communication with the fourth ventricle, and complete or partial agenesis of the vermis, can present with early hydrocephalus and later cranial nerve palsies, nystagmus, truncal ataxia, seizures, or mental impairments. Dandy-Walker malformations have been associated with over 100 chromosomal disorders, gene mutations, inborn errors of metabolism, and teratogens. There is no specific medical therapy for these patients, but neurosurgical consultation for shunting or fenestration of the ventricles or posterior fossa cysts may be needed. *Joubert's syndrome* is an autosomal recessive syndrome characterized by agenesis of the vermis, dysplasia and heterotopias of cerebellar nuclei, and other brainstem anomalies. Clinically, patients have episodic hyperpnea and apnea, abnormal eye movements, mental retardation, and ataxia. *Cerebellar hypoplasia* and *pontocerebellar hypoplasia* may be part of multiple syndromes that clinically include ataxia as well as other neurologic or organ system dysfunction. Examples include several familial autosomal recessive or X-linked syndromes, multiple chromosomal trisomies, Smith–Lemli–Opitz syndrome, bilateral periventricular nodular heterotopia/mental retardation syndrome, pontocerebellar hypoplasias types I and II, congenital disorders of glycosylation syndromes types I and II. No specific medical therapies are available for the ataxia symptoms.

Metabolic Ataxias

A number of metabolic disorders can be associated with *acute intermittent ataxia.* Specific examples include Maple Syrup Urine Disease (branched chain aminoaciduria), Hartnup Disease, hyperammonemia, biotinidase deficiency, mitochondrial disorders, and pyruvate dehydrogenase complex deficiency.

Pyruvate dehydrogenase (PDH) deficiency, resulting from mutations in components of the PDH enzyme complex, can present with intermittent bouts of ataxia which last for days. Supportive laboratory findings include elevated serum pyruvate and alanine, and a CSF lactate levels exceeding that in the serum. Administration of 100–200 mg per day of thiamine (B1) and reducing carbohydrate intake may diminish the duration of symptoms and frequency of episodes. Cost/benefit ratio of the ketogenic diet for treatment of patients with the intermittent phenotype is unclear.

Examples of *chronic progressive ataxia* include storage disorders, cerebrotendinous xanthomatosis, Neimann Pick type C, gangliosidoses, adrenoleukodystrophy, Refsum disease, abetalipoproteinemia, and vitamin E deficiency.

Ataxia with isolated vitamin E deficiency, due to malabsorption or to mutation of the gene for alpha-tocopherol transfer protein, is associated pathologically with degeneration of posterior column axons and mild loss of cerebellar Purkinje cells. Early treatment with large doses, e.g., 300 iu/kg/day of vitamin E, can reverse symptoms in some cases.

Refsum disease (heredopathia atactica polyneuritiformis) is a rare, autosomal recessive disorder associated with mutations in the phytanic acid hydrolase (PAHX) gene, resulting in elevated plasma phytanic acid and deposition in brain, spinal cord, and nerves. Onset can occur between ages 10 and 20, with impaired night and peripheral vision due to retinitis pigmentosa initially, and ataxia, polyneuropathy, nystagmus, anosmia, and ichthyosis occurring later. Reducing dietary intake of phytanic acid containing foods (meats, dairy products) can be helpful.

Cerebrotendinous xanthomatosis is an autosomal recessive disorder due to the absence of chenodeoxycholic acid, used in bile acid synthesis. It is characterized neurologically by progressive ataxia, spasticity, neuropathy, and dementia. Tendon xanthomas and cataracts, associated with elevated serum cholestanol levels, are present. Treatment with chenodeoxycholic acid (750 mg/day or 15 mg/kg/day orally divided TID) expands the deficient bile acid pool and reduces elevated plasma cholestanol, partially reversing neurologic symptoms. HMG CoA reductase inhibitors, e.g., simvastatin 10–40 mg daily or pravastatin 10 mg daily, are also helpful.

Hereditary Degenerative Ataxias

Ataxia telangiectasia is a rare, autosomal recessive neurodegenerative disorder associated with mutations in the ATM (ataxia telangiectasia mutated) gene. Affected individuals have gait and ocular control impairments, immunologic and endocrine disturbances, neoplasms, and skin manifestations. There is no curative or preventative treatment for the ataxia and neurologic degeneration. Aggressive treatment of infections, IVIG for patients with recurring infections, and treatment for malignancies may be required.

Friedreich ataxia (FA) is the most common autosomal recessive degenerative ataxia and one of the most prevalent inherited ataxias. Clinical features include progressive, mixed sensory and cerebellar ataxia, dysarthria, areflexia, pyramidal leg weakness, sensorineural hearing loss, hypertrophic cardiomyopathy, and diabetes. It most commonly occurs due to expanded GAA triplet repeats within the first intron of the frataxin (FRDA) gene, causing impaired exon splicing and reduced expression. Frataxin may function as an iron storage or transport protein in mitochondria. Due to the relatively high prevalence of this etiology, FA patients have been included with various SCA patients in a large number of trials of nonspecific therapy for ataxia, with similar negative results. However, evidence of mitochondrial functional abnormalities in FA has led to several open and controlled clinical trials of antioxidants. A 12 month, randomized, blinded, placebo-controlled trial of idebenone, a free radical scavenger, showed moderate improvement in echocardiographic measures of hypertrophy. Unfortunately, no improvement was identified in neurologic symptoms.

Spinocerebellar ataxia type 3 (SCA3; Machado–Joseph disease), a CAG repeat disease, has a highly variable presentation. Clinical subphenotype 1 has an onset between 10 and 30 years of age, can progress rapidly and involve extrapyramidal, pyramidal, and cerebellar systems. Clinical studies of trimethoprim-sulfamethoxazole (TMP/SMZ) have been performed, based on data suggesting it could correct abnormally low CSF biopterin and homovanillic acid levels, thereby increasing levels of dopamine, norepinephrine, and serotonin. A recent randomized, placebo-controlled trial failed to confirm benefit suggested by open label studies.

Episodic Ataxias Due to Channelopathies

Episodic ataxia type 1 is characterized by childhood onset, brief attacks of dysarthria, and incoordination. Sudden movement, anxiety, excitement, fevers, and other factors can be triggers. Between attacks, myokymia—semirhythmic twitching in hand, tongue, or in skin around the eyes and mouth—is usually present, although this may be subtle in children. Inheritance is autosomal dominant, penetrance is believed to be complete, and the responsible gene codes for the potassium channel KCNA1. Treatment, if desired, is with carbonic anhydrase inhibitors (acetazolamide), up to 375 mg per day. This is not always effective chronically, and some patients take small doses intermittently, e.g., prior to playing sports.

Episodic ataxia type 2 is characterized by episodes of ataxia lasting hours to days, with gaze-evoked nystagmus between episodes. Triggers for the ataxia episodes include emotional upset, exercise, alcohol, phenytoin, and caffeine. Some patients ultimately have chronic, slowly progressive ataxia. Inheritance is autosomal dominant, and this disorder is allelic with another episodic disorder, familial hemiplegic migraine; both involve point mutations in the calcium channel subunit gene CACNA1A. An expanded CAG repeat in an open reading frame of this gene causes SCA type 6, a degenerative ataxia. Treatment of EA2 with doses of acetazolamide of 250–750 mg per day can be dramatically effective.

Nonspecific Medical Treatments for Ataxia

A number of studies in the past 20 years have been performed in patients with degenerative ataxias, prior to knowledge of, or without consideration of, the specific genetic basis of these diseases. Apparent benefit seen in open label studies often failed to be confirmed with randomized controlled trials. Trials of cholinergic medications, including L-acetylcarnitine, a cholinomimetic compound, phosphatidylcholine, choline, and physostigmine, and of amantadine, lecithin, and vigabatrin have been essentially negative. Studies of buspirone, a serotonin receptor 1A agonist, and 5 hydroxy-tryptophan have shown minimal effects. At present, there are no symptom-suppressing medications that can be recommended for childhood onset ataxias. The use of these largely benign medications in hopes of limited benefit depends on the clinician's pharmacologic activism or nihilism.

Nonmedical Management

Physical and occupational therapy are important for ameliorating complications, such as contractures, that occur in some progressive neurologic disorders, and in assisting with mechanisms to enhance mobility and performance of activities of daily living. Specific diagnoses may be helpful in linking families through the internet to appropriate support groups and to research studies. Clinicians should be mindful of the effects of progressive disorders on nonneurologic organ systems, as these may be more amenable to therapy.

SUMMARY

A large number of congenital, degenerative, and acquired processes affect cerebellar function, producing ataxia. Diagnosis of chronic progressive cases is complex, but advancing rapidly. There is hope that rational therapeutic advances may follow.

SUGGESTED READINGS

1. Albin RL. Dominant ataxias and Friedreich ataxia: an update. Curr Opin Neurol 2003; 16:507–514.
2. Connolly AM, Dodson WE, Prensky AL, Rust RS. Course and outcome of acute cerebellar ataxia. Ann Neurol 1994; 35:673–679.
3. Klockgether T. Handbook of Ataxia Disorders. New York: Marcel Dekker, 2000.
4. Ryan MM, Engle EC. Acute ataxia in childhood. J Child Neurol 2003; 18:309–316.

60
Dysautonomias

Natan Gadoth
Department of Neurology, Meir General Hospital, Kfar Saba, Israel

INTRODUCTION

Autonomic dysfunction or "dysautonomia" accompanies a variety of metabolic, toxic, autoimmune, and genetic peripheral neuropathies. In general, those disorders affect mainly adults; only rarely will children present with acute or chronic dysautonomia. The pediatrician and the pediatric neurologist will often have difficulties in interpreting published treatment guidelines that are based on anecdotal data.

Dysfunction of the autonomic nervous system in children might be acute, as in Guillain–Barré syndrome (GBS) or chronic, as in some forms of hereditary autonomic and sensory neuropathies (HSAN). Familial dysautonomia (FD), also known as HSAN III, is an autosomal recessive disorder affecting exclusively infants and children of Jewish Ashkenazi origin (MIM 223900). Although rare worldwide, it is relatively common in certain parts of the United States and Israel, where a considerable number of Ashkenazi Jews are living. Thus, patients with FD may serve as a "human model" for the understanding and management of systemic autonomic dysfunction manifested throughout a life span. During the last 30 years, we have taken care of a relatively large number of infants, children, and adults with FD and this chapter summarizes the experience others and we have had in treating the acute and chronic manifestations of autonomic dysfunction. Although the clinical features of FD are unique to this rare disease, the experience gained from treating those children and summarized here may serve as treatment guidelines for other forms of childhood dysautonomia.

DIAGNOSIS AND EVALUATION

The main target of autonomic dysfunction is the cardiovascular system, manifested as orthostatic hypotension and intolerance, bouts of hypertension, and poor peripheral circulation. Disordered pulse regulation in the form of arrhythmias may be life threatening. Gastrointestinal tract motility impairment can manifest as cyclic vomiting with recurrent aspirations, diarrhea and or constipation, and impaired sphincter control. As autonomic dysfunction is frequently associated with axonal small fiber neuropathy, patients may suffer from pain, discomfort, allodynia, and painless mutilation. The evaluation of autonomic dysfunction can be difficult, especially in a young child in whom it is almost impossible to perform the battery of tests recommended for adults with autonomic failure.

As the treatment outlined in this chapter is based on experience gained with FD patients, a short note regarding the diagnosis seems appropriate. Familial dysautonomia should be considered in a Jewish Ashkenazi child who has a combination of characteristic somatic abnormalities associated with marked autonomic dysfunction. Children typically have absence of tongue fungiform papillae, short stature, peculiar facies, decreased to absent pain sensation, markedly diminished or completely absent deep tendon reflexes, absent corneal reflexes, lack of tearing, and progressive scoliosis. The diagnosis can be confirmed by genetic testing for IKBKAP (IkB kinase complex-associated protein) mutations.

TREATMENT

The main targets for treatment are labile blood pressure, the so-called "dysautonomic crisis," recurrent aspiration, disordered sleep, hypersalivation, lack of tearing, and oral self-mutilation.

Labile Blood Pressure

The most common clinical manifestation of impaired blood pressure control in FD is postural hypotension without compensatory tachycardia. This differs from chronic orthostatic intolerance associated with postural tachycardia known as postural tachycardia syndrome (POTS), a leading cause of postural intolerance in adults, which has been increasingly recognized in children. Less common is episodic hypertension.

The clinical spectrum caused by postural hypotension includes spells of dizziness, headaches, attacks of sudden pallor and nausea, and occasional loss of consciousness. Occasionally, these episodes are instinctively ameliorated by squatting. Sometimes, a prolonged bout of cough or laughter leads to sudden loss of consciousness, which may be misdiagnosed as epilepsy. Fainting occurs mainly during early morning hours, on hot and humid days, when the bladder is distended, while straining before a bowel movement, and following an emotional upset. Episodic hypertension is frequently induced by excitement, emotional upset, and not infrequently, visceral pain.

Treatment should be initiated only when postural hypotension becomes symptomatic. One should always start with physical measures. Hypovolemia is frequent in FD due to excessive sweating and inadequate feeding, mainly secondary to anorexia. Hydration (monitored by blood urea nitrogen), promotion of venous return by leg exercise, and a diet rich in sodium may be sufficient. Other measures known to be helpful in children with orthostatic intolerance are not very helpful in FD. Tilt training was not beneficial in our experience. Inducing lower body negative pressure and wearing elastic stockings is not recommended for children with FD. Tight dressings may be painful, unpleasant, or ticklish; they may also induce skin sores due to the decreased pain sensation, poor skin circulation, and excessive sweating. When indicated, oral fludrocortisone acetate 0.1 mg should be given in the morning. The putative mechanism of action is water retention at the expense of some urinary potassium loss. The drug may also aid in sensitizing alpha-receptors and block peripheral vasodilatation. Addition of the alpha-blocker midodrine 0.05–0.1 mg/kg in the morning and in repeated doses every 4 hr (not within 4 hr of bedtime) may be required.

As hypertension is usually episodic, long-term antihypertensive drug therapy is not recommended. For refractory hypertension accompanied by headache, nausea, and agitation, diazepam and clonidine may be tried before the administration of ACE inhibitors or beta agonists. One should be aware of the possibility of paradoxical responses to those drugs as a consequence of denervation supersensitivity causing an exaggerated peripheral response to endogenous and exogenous catecholamines.

Similar cardiovascular problems may accompany the acute phase of GBS. Autonomic neuropathy affects most patients with GBS. Mild manifestations such as tachycardia and postural hypertension are quite common, but life-threatening arrhythmias leading to sinus arrest may occur. Rarely, paroxysms of severe autonomic dysfunction may cause sudden death. In patients with GBS, limb blood flow fails to increase in response to rise in blood pressure (indicating the presence of elevated vascular resistance due to excessive sympathetic activity); thus, hypertension should be treated cautiously. Vasodilatating agents should be avoided because of their potential to induce reflex tachycardia. The potential risk for an excessive response to antihypertensives and vasopressors calls for the use of agents with a short half-life, preferably by the intravenous route, with careful monitoring and titration of dose-to-response. Esmolol, a short acting beta-blocker, has been successfully used in GBS. Although the safety of this drug in children has not been established, its use in pediatric hypertensive emergencies has been beneficial. Initially, 600 μg/kg is infused for 2 min and followed by an infusion of 200 μm/kg/min. The dose is increased by 50–100 μg/kg/min every 5–10 min until a reduction greater than 10% in mean blood pressure is reached. The mean dose required to reach beta blockade in children aged 2–16 years was 550 μg/kg/min (range 3300–1000).

Recurrent Aspiration

Upper gastrointestinal tract motor dysfunction is the main cause for this serious complication. Bouts of protracted vomiting, gastroesophageal reflux due to irregular esophageal peristalsis, and impaired oropharyngeal motor coordination can all cause recurrent aspiration, frequently resulting in recurrent aspiration pneumonia. Avoiding liquid foods with thickening of feeds, increasing and regulating peristalsis by antacids and H_2-antagonists, and sleeping in a semisupine posture may be tried but are often insufficient. Progressive scoliosis with restriction of lung volume is another burden on the pulmonary system.

Children with FD have an outstanding ability to withstand prolonged breath holding. These children repeatedly challenge normal peers with diving competitions (which they always win), but may die underwater of CO_2 narcosis because their brainstems are unable to respond adequately to hypoxia and hypopnea due to decreased sensitivity of the chemoreceptors.

A relatively large number of patients with FD have had fundoplication with gastrostomies. Fifty-five patients aged 5 weeks to 40 years received this treatment and were available for follow-up a year later. Cyclic vomiting initially reported by 42 patients was experienced in 20 on follow-up. Twenty of the 52 patients still had recurrent pneumonias. The nutritional status improved in 27 patients. However, there were 30 patients with recurrent aspiration pneumonia, recurrent GI reflux, and exacerbation of previously documented lung disease in those who were followed-up beyond the first postoperative year.

More recently, laparoscopic fundoplication was found to be safer while retaining the beneficial effect observed with the previous technique. Unfortunately, precise guidelines, indications, and timing of this operation are still not established. The institution of this mode of oral feeding bypass at a very young age, which is aimed at preventing the development of chronic lung disease may cause a permanent loss of swallowing reflexes.

The "Dysautonomic" Crisis

Dysautonomic crisis consists of an acute onset of recurrent retching and vomiting every 15–20 min, which typically lasts up to 72 hr and is frequently associated with aspiration, hypertension, profuse sweating, and widespread skin blotching. The child is irritable, frightened, dehydrated, and in a state of profound agitation leading to total exhaustion. The precise mechanism responsible for the crisis is yet unknown. It was postulated that a sudden rise of plasma dopamine and to a lesser extent, norepinephrine, might be responsible. During the crisis, most patients need hospitalization in an intensive care setting.

Intramuscular injection of chlorpromazine 25 mg is the classical treatment. In addition to its antiemetic action, it also lowers the high blood pressure and acts as a tranquilizer. Intravenous diazepam, together with chlorpromazine, is sometimes required. Recently, intranasal midazolam at a dose of 0.2 mg/kg to a maximum of 10 mg per dose every 6 hr was found safe and beneficial.

Disordered Sleep

Disordered sleep is reported quite frequently. This takes the form of sleep apnea with difficulty in getting up in the morning, excessive daytime sleepiness and prolonged sleep latency. Treatment with imipramine 25 mg and modafinil 100 mg at bedtime can be beneficial. Tricyclic antidepressants may improve sleep by increasing the shortened REM latency present in FD, while modafinil may be beneficial due to its ability to increase the low blood norepinephrine in those patients.

Hypersalivation

Hypersalivation and drooling have been attributed for many years to swallowing difficulties and impaired oral-motor coordination. We have recently shown that there is an increased production of saliva in FD, probably secondary to denervation supersensitivity of the major salivary glands that contribute to drooling. Interestingly, excessive production of saliva may be one of the mechanisms that protects children with FD from dental caries. The constant drooling is unpleasant and can be cosmetically disturbing.

Until recently, atropine and trihexyphenidyl were commonly used despite lack of proven efficacy. Children with severe cerebral palsy have received ultrasound-guided injections of small amounts of botulinum toxin A (50–65 units) into parotid and submandibular glands led to a considerable reduction of salivary flow rate and subjective improvement. The procedure seems to be safe and with no adverse clinical effects or structural changes at the injection sites.

Alacrima

Alacrima, or lack of tearing, may be seen in FD or the rare autoimmune autonomic neuropathy associated with sicca complex. The simplest method to avoid dry eyes is to keep the cornea moist with artificial tears. We used tarsorrhaphy for many years; however, disuse atrophy of the levator palpebrae superior muscle after a long period of forced immobilization can occur. This procedure can be used temporarily, especially during periods of acute corneal ulcerations and infection. Thermal lacrimal punctum occlusion, which increases eye moisture, is another option. In somewhat older patients, goggles with rubber edges fitted to the face contour were helpful. Along with these measures, there is a need for frequent slit lamp examinations to prevent the development of corneal ulcerations and subsequent scarring.

Oral Self-Mutilation

Patients with FD and congenital insensitivity to pain with anhidrosis (CIPA) suffer from the consequences of severe self-mutilation (SM), which is prominent in the oral cavity but affects also other body parts. The reason why SM occurs in FD and CIPA but not in other forms of HSAN is unknown. However, it might be the result of loss of small myelinated fibers in the peripheral nerves, which is common to both conditions. Another explanation might be the fact that patients with FD have skin dysesthesias rather than anesthesia. When the hair is gently combed, they often perceive severe pain and when the skin is vigorously pinched, they report being extremely ticklish. The same aberrant perception is also manifested in their tasting ability. While they have a high threshold for sweet tastes, they show hypersensitivity to sour tastes. It is possible that the self-injurious behavior in FD is due to skin dysesthesia (i.e., gaining pleasure from the injury instead of perceiving pain).

We have applied some protective measures in a number of young children who were in the habit of tongue-sucking and -thrusting against the sharp edges of the erupting primary teeth (in the form of grinding the irritating sharp edges of the offending teeth). Covering the sharp edges with small protective appliances may be dangerous, as those tend to become loose and may be aspirated. A more radical approach is tooth extraction, which might be needed to avoid chronic tongue and cheek injury, resulting in a traumatic eosinophilic ulcer known as Riga-Fede's disease. Self-mutilation of fingers, nails, and skin of limbs is of concern as this can lead to traumatic amputations and sometimes, severe local infection and in extreme cases, osteomyelitis. Bandaging or casting the target of injury and administration of various tranquilizers was not helpful in our experience.

PROGNOSIS

As "dysautnomia" occurs in a variety of conditions, it is difficult to establish precise prognostic criteria, especially for children. Published data are available on adults and even those are based on small numbers of patients. Autonomic failure in GBS is an important cause of death. In one series of 16 children with GBS treated in an intensive care unit, two died of arrhythmia. In chronic autonomic dysfunction such as

FD, life expectancy is relatively shortened by the disease. In a recently published survey on 551 patients, 4 died of cardiac reasons, 72 of "sudden death," and 5 of "vasovagal" causes.

With better understanding of the disease and earlier intervention, life expectancy as well as life quality has significantly improved. The mortality during infancy is quite significant; however, 40% of those who survive are over 20 years of age. Milder forms may have a somewhat shortened life expectancy. Our oldest patient was 63 when first diagnosed by us although he was mildly symptomatic most of his life. He died 2 years later during a cold winter night probably from CO_2 narcosis due to heating with insufficient ventilation.

SUMMARY

Childhood dysautonomia is fortunately quite rare. It is difficult to diagnose, often resistant even to vigorous treatments and carries a significant risk of mortality. Long-term observations on specific disease entities such as the HSAN will result in better treatment modes and improved quality of life.

SUGGESTED READINGS

1. Axelrod FB. Genetic disorders as models to understand autonomic dysfunction. Clin Auton Res 2002; 12(suppl 1):1/2–1/14.
2. Bos AP, van der Meche FG, Witsenburg M, van der Voort E. Experience with Guillain-Barré syndrome in pediatric patients. Intensive Care Med 1987; 13:328–331.
3. Ellies M, Rohrbach-Volland S, Arglebe C, Wilkins B, Lakawi R, Hanfeld F. Successful management of drooling with botulinum toxin A in neurologically disabled children. Neuropediatrics 2002; 33:327–330.
4. Gadoth N. Familial dysautonomia. Handbook of autonomic nervous system dysfunction. New York: Marcel Dekker Inc., 1995:95–115.
5. Lahat E, Goldaman M, Barr J, Bistrizer T, Berkovitch M. Intranasal midazolam as a treatment of autonomic crises in patients with familial dysautonomia. Pediatr Neurol 2000; 22:19–22.
6. NIH conference. Dysautonomias: clinical disorders of the autonomic nervous system. Ann Intern Med 2002; 137:753–763.
7. Shatzky S, Moses S, Levy J, Pinsk V, Hershkovitz E, Herzog L, Shorer Z, Luder A, Parvari R. Congenital insensitivity to pain with anhidrosis (CIPA) in Israeli-Bedouins: genetic heterogeneity, novel mutations in the TRKA/NGF receptor gene, clinical findings and results of nerve conduction studies. Am J Med Genet 2000; 92:353–360.
8. Stewart JM. Orthostatic intolerance in pediatrics. J Pediatr 2002; 40:404–411.

61
Syncope

Xue Ming and Sina Zaim
UMDNJ-New Jersey Medical School, Newark, New Jersey, U.S.A.

INTRODUCTION

Syncope or fainting refers to a sudden and transient loss of consciousness resulting from temporarily inadequate cerebral blood flow. A population-based study found an incidence of 126/100,000 during childhood and adolescence with a peak in the 15- to 19-year old group for both sexes. Up to 15% of children may experience one syncopal episode before the age of 18. The prognosis is dependent on the etiology of syncope. In most cases, there is full recovery without sequelae and recurrence is rare.

PATHOPHYSIOLOGY

The most common cause of syncope in children is vasovagal, also referred to as neurally mediated, or neuro-cardiogenic syncope. Studies suggest that a sudden excessive venous pooling, occurring during upright posturing, results in an abrupt decrease in venous return to the heart. The "empty heart" contracts forcefully to compensate the volume loss. This in turn activates the ventricular mechanoreceptors and vagal efferent pathways with resultant enhanced parasympathetic activity and reduced sympathethic tone. Consequently, bradycardia and vasodilatation ensue which leads to syncope, the so-called Bezold–Jarisch reflex.

A less common etiology, associated with the heart itself, is classified under the heading of structural or functional abnormalities. Some of the structural abnormalities that can lead to syncope include aortic stenosis, hypertrophic cardiomyopathy, atrial myxoma, etc. Ventricular tachycardia/fibrillation secondary to long-QT syndrome, Brugada syndrome, hypertrophic cardiomyopathy, right ventricular dysplasia, accessory pathways with concurrent atrial fibrillation, and bradyarrhythmia associated with congenital heart block and Kearns–Sayre syndrome have been associated with syncope. Brugada syndrome is a relatively new described condition linked to mutations in SCN5A. Patients with this syndrome have normal cardiac structures but display ST-segment elevations and right bundle branch block pattern in leads V1–V3 and are prone to recurrent syncope and sudden cardiac death.

DIAGNOSTIC EVALUATION

The initial effort should be directed towards establishing a diagnosis of syncope with exclusion of other clinical diagnosis that may resemble it (Fig. 1). A thorough personal and family history, physical examination, and a 12-lead ECG are usually the most fruitful for establishing the diagnosis. A dramatic reaction to an emotionally disturbing event such as the sight of blood, sudden stressful or painful experience, surgical instrumentation, or trauma suggests vasovagal syncope.

Fainting while standing in a hot, crowded public gathering is also frequently reported, especially if the patient has not eaten or slept well the night before. Premonitory signs and symptoms of syncope often include dizziness, lightheadedness, nausea, blurred vision, pallor, and clammy extremities. Recovery of consciousness is complete and rapid although the patient may feel fatigued for a prolonged time afterwards.

Physical examination at time of referral in otherwise healthy children is generally unrevealing, and a baseline 12-lead ECG or 24-hour Holter recording system is usually normal. Further diagnostic tests are not necessary although a tilt table test can be helpful in recurrent syncope.

A child with history of syncope during exertion or while supine or immobile requires detailed investigation. Similarly, a patient with syncope and a heart murmur should be evaluated thoroughly and an echocardiographic study is warranted to look for structural abnormalities. Prolonged monitoring using an implantable loop

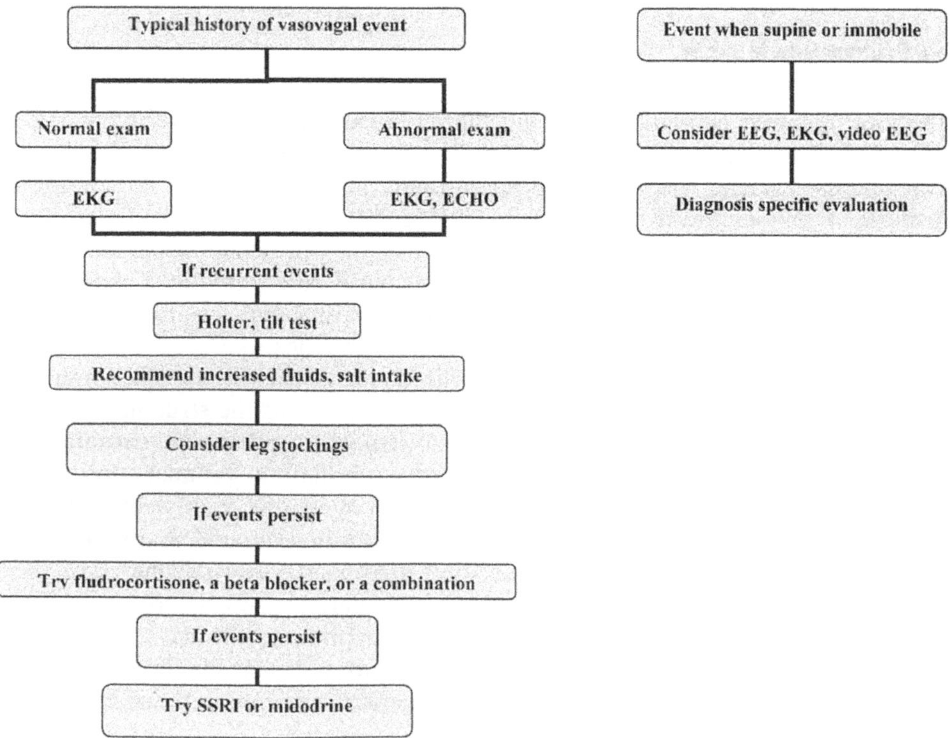

Figure 1 Algorithm for the diagnosis and management of syncope.

recorder can be helpful. A patient should be referred to a pediatric cardiologist when there is evidence of a primary cardiac structural or functional disorder.

Patients who demonstrate prolonged convulsion, significant postictal phase, or urinary incontinence should undergo an electroencephalogram (EEG) and possibly a prolonged video EEG monitoring to rule out epilepsy. Sometimes, syncope and seizure may coexist in patients with temporal lobe epilepsy, because of a secondary sinus arrest or, less often, atrioventricular block, triggered by the seizure. A history of hyperventilation in children with anxiety, panic disorders, or hysteria suggests psychogenic syncope due to hypocapnia. Medication history can be revealing in patients with orthostatic hypotension.

THERAPEUTIC APPROACH

The therapeutic approach to a child with vasovagal syncope must be individualized. The first step is to educate the child and the family as to the nature of the condition and to caution the patient to avoid known predisposing factors. These may include extreme heat, dehydration, abrupt postural changes after prolonged kneeling or squatting, and abrupt immobilization after prolonged exercise. Furthermore, the patient should be advised to lie down when premonitory symptoms become apparent. This conservative approach of reassurance, avoidance of known triggers, and assuming a supine position during prodromal symptoms, will reduce or eliminate the problem in the majority of patients. Increase of fluid and salt intake with resultant increase in intravascular volume may be required in some patients. Supportive long leg stockings can be helpful.

A pharmacological treatment approach, usually empiric, is often necessary for those patients who experience frequent recurrent vasovagal syncope despite following conservative therapies. Several agents are used for treatment of recurrent syncope. Patients who have associated medical problems such as hypertension will need an individualized approach to the selection and use of these medications. Similarly, patients whose syncopal episodes are due to abnormal cardiac structure or an arrhythmia will require diagnosis-specific therapy.

First-Line Medication Therapy

Fludrocortisone is used to expand volume and diminish the central hypovolemia that can initiate the syncope cascade. When the history suggests hypovolemia is contributing to syncope, fludrocortisone may be chosen in addition to increasing fluid and salt intake. Although fludrocortisone is well tolerated and inexpensive, its efficacy has not been established in a prospective controlled trial. The dose for fludrocortisone acetate is 0.05–0.2 mg qd. The side effects of fludrocortisone include hypokalemia, hyperglycemia, hypertension, acne, rash, headaches, gastric discomfort or even ulcer, cataracts, muscle weakness, and growth suppression.

Beta blockers (e.g., propranolol and atenolol) are used as a first-line agent in treating syncope as well. The proposed mechanism of action includes a decreased stimulation of mechanoreceptors in the afferent limb of the pathway through blunting the excitatory effect of released catecholamines and via the inherent negative inotropy of the drug. A difference in efficacy among the different beta blockers used has not been found. However, its efficacy, as with fludrocortisone, has also not yet been established. Sometimes a combination of a beta blocker and fludrocortisone can be effective. The dose for atenolol in children is 1.0 mg/kg qd. Side effects of atenolol include bradycardia, fatigue, lethargy, and headache. The dose for propranolol is 0.6–1.5 mg/kg which can be divided as b.i.d. The side effects of propranolol are insomnia, lethargy, vivid dreams, depression, bradycardia, hypotension, worsening of A–V conduction block.

Second-Line Agents

Vasoconstrictors such as midodrine, an alpha-1 agonist, can be considered when fludrocortisone, a beta blocker, or their combination fail. This agent increases venous vasomotor tone, thereby reducing venous pooling and causing arterial vasoconstriction. This acts to diminish the vasodilatation induced by the efferent response. The efficacy of midodrine is also not well established.

Selective serotonin reuptake inhibitors (SSRI) have also recently been used in treating vasovagal syncope. Serotonin is reported to play a role in the development of hypotension and bradycardia during vasovagal syncope. Paroxetine was found to be helpful in patients with refractory vasovagal syncope in a single placebo-controlled study. The use of paroxetine in the pediatric population has recently been discouraged, however, secondary to increased risk of suicide. Studies have demonstrated that sertraline is effective in children with vasovagal syncope. The dosage of either paroxetine or sertraline for syncope in pediatric population has not been well established.

SUGGESTED READINGS

1. Benditt DG, Fahy GJ, Lurie KG, Sakagushi S, Fabian W, Samniah N. Pharmacotherapy of neurally mediated syncope. Circulation 1999; 100:1242–1248.
2. Calkins H. Pharmacologic approaches to therapy for vasovagal syncope. Am J Cardiol 1999; 84:20Q–25Q.
3. Di Gerolamo E, Di Iorio C, Sabatini O, Leonzio L, Barbone C, Barsotti A. Effects of paroxetine hydrochloride, a selective serotonin reuptake inhibitor, on refractory vasovagal syncope: a randomized, double-blind, placebo-conrolled study. J Am Coll Cardiol 1999; 33:1227–1230.
4. Driscoll DJ, Jacobsen SJ, Porter CJ, Wollan PC. Syncope in children and adolescents. J Am Coll Cardiol 1997; 29:1039–1045.
5. Task Force on Syncope, European Society of Cardiology. Guidelines on management (diagnosis and treatment) of syncope. Eur Heart J 2001; 22:1256–1306.
6. Hainsworth R, Syncope and fainting: classification and pathophysiological basis. In: Mathias C, Bannister R, eds. Autonomic Failure: A Textbook of Clinical Disorders of the Autonomic Nervous System. 4th ed. 1999:428–436.
7. Lewis DA, Dhala A. Syncope in the pediatric patient. The cardiologist's perspective. Pediatric Clin North Am 1999; 49:205–219.

62
Acute Disseminated Encephalomyelitis

Anita L. Belman
Department of Neurology, School of Medicine, State University of New York (SUNY) at Stony Brook, Stony Brook, New York, U.S.A.

INTRODUCTION

Acute disseminated encephalomyelitis (ADEM) is an acute inflammatory demyelinating disorder of the CNS characterized by new onset focal or multifocal neurological signs and symptoms coupled with neuroimaging evidence of multifocal demyelinating lesions. ADEM (also referred to as post- or para-infectious encephalomyelitis) frequently follows a recognized prodromal infectious illness (most often viral) or antecedent event such as vaccination or immunization, administration of serum, or as an adverse reaction to drugs. ADEM typically follows a monophasic course.

In the past, ADEM was most often associated with exanthemata infectious illnesses and certain vaccines. Morbidity and mortality rates were high (up to 20–30% after measles), and for those who recovered, neurological sequelae was common. The virtual eradication of natural smallpox disease, successful immunization programs for prevention of measles, mumps and rubella, and development of vaccines devoid of neural elements have lead to a marked decrease in the frequency in ADEM from these causes. Currently nonspecific (less easily identifiable) viral illnesses, most often during the winter months, appear to be the most common antecedent, with a predominance of those viruses causing upper respiratory infections.

DIAGNOSIS AND EVALUATION

The diagnosis of ADEM is based on clinical presentation, signs, and symptoms of CNS dysfunction, coupled with typical MRI findings (other possible causes excluded). The differential diagnosis includes Lyme disease, vasculitis, multiple infarctions (possibly embolic), encephalitis, neurocysticercosis, and multiple sclerosis.

Clinical Features

Onset is acute, even at times explosive, or subacute. Neurological signs and symptoms (aphasia, seizures, bilateral optic neuritis, visual field defects, motor and sensory deficits, ataxia, dysmetria, and movement disorders) occur as isolated features or in various combinations. Systemic symptoms (fever, malaise, myalgias, headache, decreased appetite, nausea, and vomiting) usually occur prior to the onset of neurological problems, beginning 4–42 days following the antecedent event. Behavioral and mental status changes (irritability, emotional lability and even frank psychosis; lethargy, depressed level of consciousness, ranging from lethargy to coma) are common. Meningismus with or without signs of an acute meningoencephalitis may occur, as may focal or generalized seizures. The differential diagnosis is broad including infections, leukodystrophies, neoplasms, sarcoidosis, and vasculitis. MRI findings need to be correlated with the clinical picture.

Laboratory Findings

Cerebrospinal fluid (CSF) findings are variable. CSF may or may not show a mild to moderate lymphocytic pleocytosis, elevation in protein content, detectable levels of myelin basic protein, intrathecal production of oligoclonal bands or immunoglobulin G. CSF studies are most valuable for excluding other illnesses (especially direct viral or bacterial infection) rather than establishing the diagnosis of ADEM.

MRI is the neuroimaging study of choice. Hyperintense lesions imaged on T2-weighted/proton density/FLAIR are often diffuse and highly variable in size and number (Fig. 1). These include few to multiple predominantly white matter (WM) lesions throughout the brain (subcortical WM, grey–white junction, periventricular regions, corpus callosum, basal ganglia, thalamus, midbrain, brain stem, cerebellar WM, cerebellar peduncles) and spinal cord (segmental or contiguous). Lesions are often bilateral and asymmetric ranging from small punctate (<1 cm) to moderate size (4–5 cm) lesions, with or without a "cotton ball" appearance, to large and confluent, or "tumor-like" lesions. Enhancement with gadolinium is variable. MRI abnormalities may lag behind clinical signs and symptoms.

Clinical features and MRI findings can also be discordant. For example, some children present with relatively mild focal deficits yet have extensive bihemispheric MRI abnormalities. Conversely, other children with widespread multifocal clinical

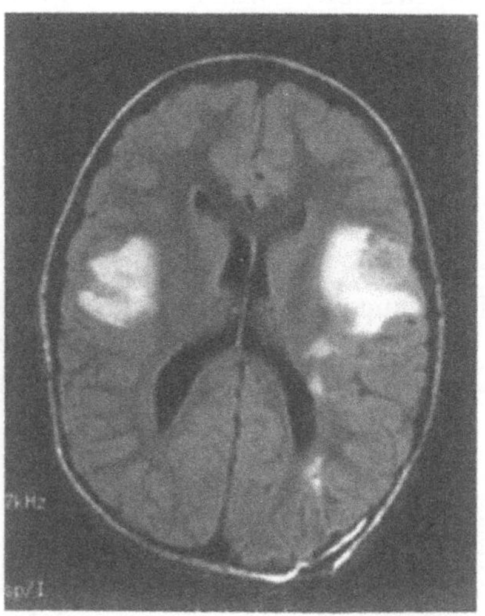

Figure 1 MRI of a case of ADEM.

signs and symptoms may have only a few small lesions imaged on MRI. MRI abnormalities can clear completely, show partial resolution, or persist for months.

Clinical Course

ADEM is considered a monophasic illness. Evolution of signs and symptoms usually appear over time with maximal deficits often reached within one to two weeks. Resolution may occur rapidly (with or without treatment), or may take weeks to months and may not be complete.

Although ADEM is classically considered a monophasic illness, most clinicians acknowledge the course may be biphasic, and thought by some to represent a protracted single episode rather than a new event. "Relapses" or recurrence within the first several months of the initial illness, or relapse as steroids are tapered, may also represent part of the same acute monophasic immune process, in some cases. Some authors report RDEM (recurrent) after events recur several times. When this condition becomes multiple sclerosis is unclear.

THERAPY

Supportive care, symptomatic treatment (including physical and occupational therapy), and therapy targeted to the immune-mediated processes are the mainstays of treatment. There have been no controlled treatment trials for ADEM and most references in the literature are collections of case series. As such, the best therapy has not been determined and there is no established treatment protocol. A suggested algorithm is presented in Fig. 2.

Corticosteroids (methylprednisolone or dexamethasone) are commonly used based on (1) their anti-inflammatory and immunosuppressive properties, and (2) anecdotal reports (case reports and case series). Many children recover spontaneously showing signs of rapid improvement by the time other etiologies (e.g., direct viral or bacterial infections) have been ruled out. In these cases, some clinicians do not elect to treat with steroids.

Review of the literature shows the most common treatment regimens are a 3–5 day course of intravenous (IV) methylprednisolone (10–30 mg/kg/day for children under 30 kg; 1 g/day for children > 30 kg) or dexamthasone (0.5–1 mg/kg/day). Regimens of orally administered steroids [dexamethasone (0.5–1 mg/kg/day), prednisolone (2 mg/kg/day)] for 5–10 days have also been used.

Some clinicians advocate a slow 2–6 week orally administered prednisolone taper (especially for children who presented with changes of mental status, impairment of consciousness, brain stem or spinal cord involvement, and those with MRI findings of large lesions with mass effect). Regimens include PO prenisolone 1–2 mg/kg/day for 10–14 days followed by a 4 week taper.

Recently four case series with larger numbers of children (three retrospective, one prospective study) have been published suggesting high dose IV methylprednisolone (20–30 mg/kg/day) followed by a slow prednisolone taper over 4–6 weeks, shortens the course of the illness, may prevent recurrence and is associated with a better outcome.

For patients who fail to respond to methylprednisolone (persisting, severe neurologic deficits) or who have a fulminant course, or who progressively deteriorate during methylprednisolone therapy, administration of intravenous IVIG

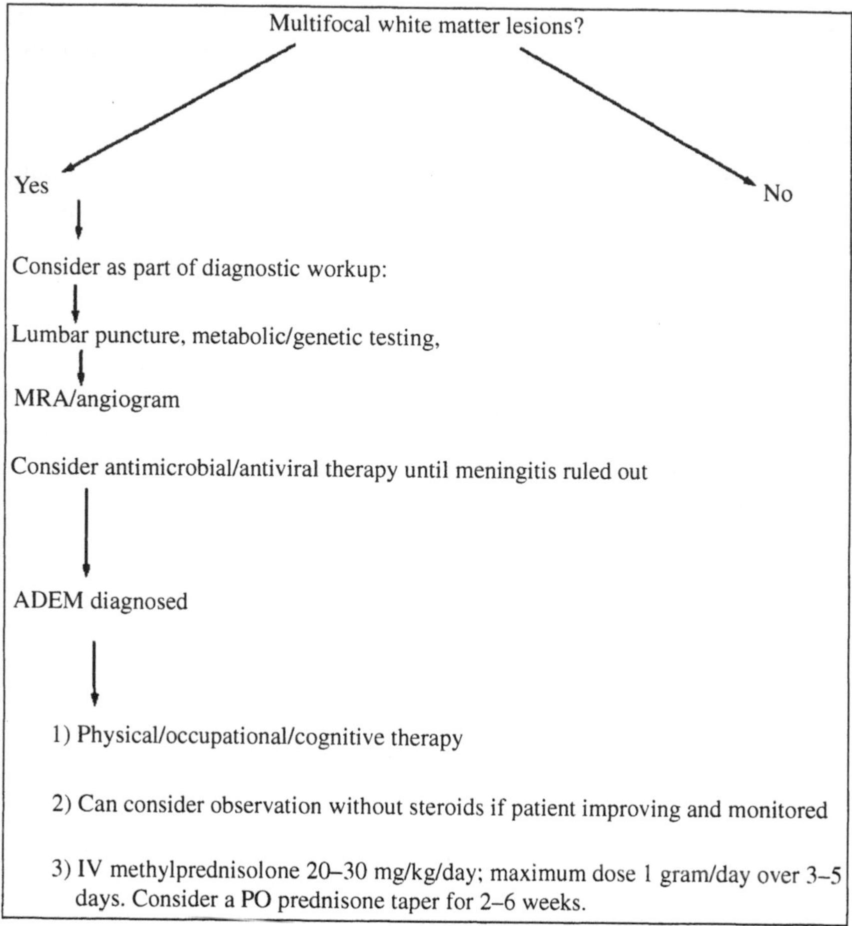
Multifocal white matter lesions?
Yes
No
Consider as part of diagnostic workup:
Lumbar puncture, metabolic/genetic testing,
MRA/angiogram
Consider antimicrobial/antiviral therapy until meningitis ruled out
ADEM diagnosed
1) Physical/occupational/cognitive therapy
2) Can consider observation without steroids if patient improving and monitored
3) IV methylprednisolone 20–30 mg/kg/day; maximum dose 1 gram/day over 3–5 days. Consider a PO prednisone taper for 2–6 weeks.

Figure 2 Suggested treatment and evaluation algorithm for ADEM.

(400 mg/kg/day for 5 days) is reported to be an effective mode of therapy. Plasma exchange is also reported to be beneficial in some fulminant cases that have failed methylprednisolone therapy.

PROGNOSIS

Childhood ADEM has a favorable outcome. Review of the most recent published case series shows a survival rate of 100% with complete functional recovery noted in 57–89% of children at follow-up. The biphasic course carries a similarly good prognosis. For those children with incomplete recovery, neurological sequelae can include behavioral, cognitive, visual, or motor deficits.

SUMMARY

ADEM is an acute inflammatory demyelinating disorder of the CNS characterized by the new onset of focal or multifocal neurological signs and symptoms coupled with neuroimaging evidence of multifocal demyelinating lesions. ADEM frequently follows a recognized prodromal infectious illness or event. Maximal deficits are usually reached within one to two weeks. Treatment consists of supportive and symptomatic care and therapy targeted to the immune-mediated process. No controlled clinical trials have been conducted to define the most effective therapy. It is suggested that high dose IV methylprednisolone shortens the course of the illness and is associated with a better outcome. Resolution of signs and symptoms typically occurs rapidly, but in some cases may take weeks to months to resolve and may not be complete.

SUGGESTED READINGS

1. Dale RC, de Sousa C, Chong WK, Cox TCS, Harding B, Neville BGR. Acute disseminated encephalomyelitis, multiphasic disseminated encephalomyelitis and multiple sclerosis in children. Brain 2000; 123:2407–2422.
2. Hyson JL, Kornberg AJ, Coleman LT, Shield L, Harvey AS, Kean MJ. Clinical and neuroradiologic features of acute disseminated encephalomyelitis in children. Neurology 2001; 56:1308–1312.
3. Johnson RT, Griffin DE, Gendelman HE. Postinfectious encephalomyelitis. Semin Neurol 1985; 5:180–190.
4. Murthy SNK, Faden HS, Cohen ME, Bakshi R. Acute disseminated encephalomyelitis in children. Pediatrics 2002; 110:e21.
5. Sahlas DJ, Miller SP, Guerin M, Veilleux M, Francis G. Treatment of acute disseminated encephalomyelitis with intravenous immunoglobulin. Neurology 2000; 54:1370–1372.
6. Sharar E, Andraus J, Savitzki D, Pilar G, Zelnik N. Outcome of severe encephalomyelitis in children: effect of high-doase methylprednisolone and immunoglobulins. J Child Neurol 2002; 17:810–814.
7. Tenembaum S, Chamoles N, Fejerman N. Acute disseminated encephalomyelitis. A long term follow-up study of 84 pediatric patients. Neurology 2002; 59:1224–1231.

63
Childhood Multiple Sclerosis

Annapurna Poduri and Gihan Tennekoon
Division of Pediatric Neurology, Children's Hospital of Philadelphia, University of Pennsylvania, Philadelphia, Pennsylvania, U.S.A.

INTRODUCTION

Although Charcot is accredited with some of the earliest descriptions of multiple sclerosis (MS) in 1868, Jean Cruveilhier was the first to publish an account of the disease in 1842. Since then, most of the medical literature concerning MS focuses on the diagnosis and management of the disease in adults. To date, there are no compelling data suggesting a fundamental difference between the disease in children compared to adults. One difference that has been observed between the two populations is a higher female:male ratio among patients in adolescents and adults compared to more even ratios in preadolescent children. While some groups suggest that children with MS have a less progressive disorder than adults, others describe a more severe condition in children with very early age of onset.

EPIDEMIOLOGY

Multiple sclerosis is defined as a demyelinating disease of the central nervous system white matter, which over time affects multiple noncontiguous areas of the neuraxis. The typical age of onset is the third or fourth decade. It is not surprising, however, that a disease that is presumed to involve autoimmune pathophysiology would present in childhood. In children, cases have been reported as young as 10 months of age. Pediatric cases are estimated to comprise 1.8–5% of all cases. While young children, particularly under age 6 years, have a roughly equal female : male ratio, in patients presenting over the age of 12 years, the female : male ratio is as high as 3:1.

ETIOLOGY

The etiology of MS is likely multifactorial. An attractive hypothesis is that in genetically susceptible individuals, a viral trigger produces a T-cell-mediated inflammatory response via molecular mimicry. A number of viruses, including EBV, measles, human herpes virus 6, or human papilloma virus, have been suggested as inciting the process that targets myelin antigens such as myelin specific–myelin oligodendrocyte glycoprotein, myelin basic protein, or proteolipid protein. Once the activated T-cells penetrate the blood–brain barrier, it is thought that they are responsible for the recruitment of macrophages and activation of microglia that, in turn, destroy the myelin sheath, oligodendrocytes, and axons. Although there is good evidence that the T helper 1 cells (Th1) are the major effectors of the autoimmune response, there is evidence to support a role for Th2 and B cells contribute to the disease process.

CLINICAL PRESENTATION

Over time, there are multiple clinical attacks, or episodes of demyelination, but each individual episode is likely to present discretely. Thus, any monophasic demyelinating event may be part of a larger picture of MS. Presentations include optic neuritis—typically unilateral painful loss of vision, transverse myelitis or another spinal cord syndrome, or any focal neurological presentation associated with demyelination. In children with MS, brainstem symptoms are seen frequently at the onset of disease. Other common presenting symptoms are sensory or motor dysfunction, ataxia, and bladder dysfunction. Seizures occur in 10–22% of children with MS, with higher frequencies associated with younger ages of onset. A history of L'Hermitte's phenomenon, an electrical sensation down the arms following neck flexion, presumably perturbing a cervical spinal cord lesion, can sometimes be elicited. Uthoff's phenomenon refers to a history of symptoms worsening or even brought on by heat.

Each episode may last from days to weeks. Attacks may occur without apparent provocation, or may be precipitated by acute infection or metabolic derangement. About two-thirds of children with MS have full recovery to baseline neurological status between each attack, thus fitting the description of relapsing-remitting MS. The time between attacks may range from less than 1 year, in more than half of the patients of some series of children, to several years.

Other presenting patterns of MS include primary progressive, secondary progressive, and progressive relapsing MS. The progression refers to the evolution of baseline neurological dysfunction over time. In general, half of the adults with relapsing-remitting MS become progressive within 10 years of presentation.

The differential diagnosis includes recurrent ADEM; symptoms from prior ADEM exacerbated in the setting of physiologic stress; autoimmune disease such as systemic lupus erythematosus, Sjögren's syndrome, antiphospholipid antibody syndrome, neurosarcoidosis, Behçet's disease, and primary CNS vasculitis; CNS infection, including syphilis, HIV, and Lyme disease; myelopathy from B12 deficiency; Alexander's disease; and CADASIL. Table 1 provides a list of recommended laboratory tests to be considered in the initial evaluation of a patient with suspected MS.

A careful history and physical examination in a patient with multiple episodes of neurological symptoms over time should raise suspicion for MS. The possibility of MS may not be so apparent, however, when a patient presents with his or her first episode. There are no unique diagnostic criteria for MS in children, so the adult criteria have been adopted in practice.

The currently accepted criteria stratify patients into four groups, reflecting the level of certainty of the diagnosis: clinically definite MS, laboratory supported definite MS, clinically probable MS, and laboratory supported probable MS. Table 2 summarizes the key criteria required to satisfy each diagnostic category. Clinical

Table 1 Diagnostic Evaluation for the Child with Suspected Multiple Sclerosis: Laboratory Studies

Antinuclear antibodies (ANA)
Anti-neutrophil cytoplasmic antibody (ANCA)
Anti-ssA, anti-ssB
Angiotensin converting enzyme (ACE)
Anti-scl70
Anticardiolipin Ab
Sedimentation rate (ESR)
C-reactive protein (CRP)
With history of oral and genital ulcers, skin pathergy test for Behçet's
Rapid plasma reagent (RPR)
Human immunodeficiency virus (HIV)
Lyme IgM and IgG
B12 level

attacks must last at least 24 hr, and the time between separate attacks must be at least 1 month. Clinical evidence refers to evidence of a lesion on neurological examination, preferably performed by a neurologist. Paraclinical data are considered to be extensions of the neurological examination and include abnormal MRI with gadolinium of the brain and spine, abnormal visual evoked responses (e.g., prolonged P100 latency), abnormal brainstem auditory evoked responses (e.g., increased I–III to I–IV interval), and demonstration of urological dysfunction. Laboratory support includes cerebrospinal fluid evidence of oligoclonal bands or elevated IgG index.

Table 2 Poser Criteria for the Diagnosis of Multiple Sclerosis

Clinically definite multiple sclerosis
Two clinical attacks AND clinical evidence of two lesions
OR
Clinical evidence of one lesion and paraclinical evidence of a second lesion
Laboratory supported definite multiple sclerosis
Two clinical attacks AND clinical or paraclinical evidence of one lesion
AND CSF oligoclonal bands or elevated IgG index
Clinically probable multiple sclerosis
Two clinical attacks AND clinical evidence of one lesion
OR
One clinical attack AND clinical evidence of two lesions
OR
One clinical attack AND clinical evidence of one lesion
AND paraclinical evidence of a second lesion
Laboratory supported probable multiple sclerosis
Two clinical attacks AND CSF oligoclonal bands or elevated IgG index

Note that clinical attacks refer to episodes lasting at least 24 hr and separated by a minimum of 1 month. Clinical evidence refers to abnormality on neurological examination. Paraclinical evidence refers to abnormalities on extensions of the neurological examination, including MRI, VER, BAER, and evidence of urological dysfunction.

MRI with gadolinium has been shown to be a useful tool in establishing the diagnosis of MS in children and in monitoring disease progression. When the diagnosis is not certain at the onset of symptoms, MRI can aid in predicting whether a patient with an isolated demyelinating syndrome, such as optic neuritis or myelitis, will progress to clinically definite MS. A detailed model of MRI criteria presented by Barkhof et al. suggests that lesions that are juxtacortical, infratentorial, periventricular, and enhancing with gadolinium are the most predictive of disease progression.

MANAGEMENT

Once the diagnosis of MS is made with reasonable certainty, patients and their families should be counseled about the variety of symptoms that may represent clinical episodes or exacerbations. Clinicians should stress the importance of seeking medical attention when these symptoms arise, particularly when there is loss of vision or substantial weakness.

The two major aspects of the management of relapsing-remitting MS are the acute management of an attack and prevention of disease progression, or disease modification. While there is no cure for the disease itself, appropriate management of acute exacerbations may limit morbidity and may, in fact, play a role in long-term disease modification. In progressive forms of the disease, chronic symptoms such as spasticity, fatigue, and urinary incontinence may require pharmacological management. Patients with progressive disease will also likely benefit from long-term physical and occupational therapy, and eventually may require assistance with activities of daily living. Since these latter issues tend to arise in the later stages of the disease, they will not be the focus of this discussion of management of children with MS. A summary of treatment strategies is presented in Table 3, and a more detailed discussion of these treatments follows below.

Management of Acute Exacerbations

Acute neurological symptoms in a child with MS may represent the evolution and presentation of new inflammatory white matter lesions or exacerbations of previous

Table 3 Summary of Treatments for Multiple Sclerosis

Acute treatment for exacerbations
Methylprednisolone
For younger children: 30 mg/kg/dose (maximum 1 g) IV daily for three to five days
For older children: 1 g IV daily for three to five days
Consider short oral taper, depending on evolution of symptoms

Chronic immunomodulatory regimens
Avonex, 30 μm intramuscularly each week
Betaseron, 8 million IU subcutaneously every alternate day
Copaxone, 20 mg subcutaneously every day

Treatment of chronic symptoms
Spasticity: baclofen, tizanidine
Neuropathic pain: carbamazepine, amitryptiline, gabapentin
Fatigue: amantadine

lesions. As with any neurological condition, any perturbation of the child's systemic milieu—such as fever, infection, dehydration, electrolyte imbalance, or other metabolic disturbance—can precipitate an exacerbation. This must be considered if a patient is presenting with the reappearance of prior symptoms or even with new complaints, since a previously asymptomatic lesion may produce symptoms for the first time in the setting of systemic illness. Thus, an age-appropriate infectious evaluation, including urinalysis and possibly chest radiography, should be performed. This is of utmost importance, since steroids may exacerbate an untreated infection rather than alleviate symptoms.

The use of intravenous steroids should be considered when symptoms of an acute MS exacerbation are severe and progressive. A typical steroid regimen for an acute MS exacerbation in an adolescent or adult is methylprednisolone 1 g intravenously each day for three to five days. In young children, the highest appropriate weight-based dose, typically 30 mg/kg/dose (maximum 1 g), should be administered intravenously each day for three to five days. The decision of whether or not an oral taper is required must bc decided on an individual patient basis.

Chronic Therapy

Though acute exacerbations cause neurological deficit and can be distressing to patients, in a patient with relapsing-remitting MS, the natural history of an acute exacerbation is to gradually wane with rcturn to neurological baseline. Nevertheless, the natural history of the disorder is to progress. Thus, pharmacological research has focused on developing agents that can prevent or delay the evolution from relapsing-remitting MS to a more progressive form of the disease. Several immunomodulatory and immunosuppressive strategies have been employed in adults with MS.

To date, the interferon beta medications have shown the most promise in reducing the rate of exacerbations by nearly one-third. Interferon beta 1a (Avonex, Rebif) has also been shown to delay the development of neurological disability in patients with clinically definite MS, to delay the progression to clinically definite multiple in monosymptomatic patients with MRI findings highly suspicious for MS, and to decrease the number of gadolinium-enhancing lesions on MRI. The standard adult dose in the United States for Avonex is 30 µm intramuscularly each week. Side effects include flu-like symptoms for one to two days after each injection. These symptoms typically last only a few months from initiation of the medication. Patients and families must also monitor for injection site complications.

Interferon beta 1b (Betaseron) also reduces relapse frequency and disease activity on the basis of MRI, but it has not yet been shown to affect a decrease in progression of neurological disability. The standard dose is Betaseron 250 µm subcutaneously every alternate day. In addition to the side effects encountered with Avonex, Betaseron has been associated with the onset or worsening of depression, anemia, and leukopenia. Some patients may reach a major limitation of both forms of interferon beta if neutralizing antibodies develop, usually after two to three years of treatment.

Glatiramer acetate (Copaxone) is a synthetic copolymer that has been shown in adults to decrease relapse rates by nearly one-third in patients with relapsing-remitting MS. The rate is comparable to that seen with the interferons. There is evidence that glatiramer acetate decreases the chance of progressing to worsening disability, but in a major two-year study performed to show efficacy, there was no improvement in the status of patients' MRIs when they were on this agent. The typical dose is Copaxone 20 mg subcutaneously each day. Injection site reactions are common but mild, and other potential side effects include shortness of breath, chest tightness, and anxiety. The development of antibodies to Copaxone does not interfere with the efficacy of the medication.

While the aforementioned agents now comprise the standard armamentarium for neurologists treating adults with relapsing-remitting MS, very little investigation into the use of these agents in children has been undertaken, and there is a paucity of studies in the literature to guide a purely evidence-based approach. Almost all recommendations for treatment are therefore based on extrapolations from the data in adults. In a study of 16 patients under 16 years of age with MS, Mikaeloff demonstrated the safety of interferon beta treatment. Fifteen of the patients received interferon beta 1a, 12 Avonex at adult doses, one Avonex at half-adult dose, and one Rebif; the other two patients received Interferon beta 1b (Betaseron). Efficacy was not established in this small trial.

Overall, we believe that Avonex has the most potential benefits and fewest serious side effects, and is our first choice for immunomodulatory therapy in children with MS. If problems are encountered with tolerability or neutralizing antibodies, a good second choice is Copaxone, since it also offers the possibility of delaying the development of disability.

Other Treatment Strategies

Other medications that have been studied in adults include intravenous immunoglobulin (IVIg) and azathioprine for relapsing-remitting disease and methotrexate, cyclophosphamide, cyclosporine, and novantrone for progressive MS. Monthly IVIg has produced a small decrease in disability in adults, but there has been no evaluation of this modality in children with MS. Azathioprine has been well studied in adults and shown to be effective in decreasing the rate of exacerbations, but it has not been shown to alter progression to disability. If the interferons and glatiramer acetate are not tolerated, azathioprine may be considered in the treatment of children with MS, but should be reserved for only the most severely affected cases, since there are no data to date to support its use and the potential side effect profile includes an increased risk of non-Hodgkin's lymphoma. The other agents, such as mitoxantrone, have not been studied in children and have side effect profiles sufficiently worrisome that at this time their use cannot be recommended.

SUGGESTED READINGS

1. Goodin DS, Frohman EM, Garmany GP et al. Disease modifying therapy in multiple sclerosis. Report of the Therapeutics and Technology Assessment Subcommittee of the American Academy of Neurology and the MS Council for Clinical Practice Guidelines. Neurology 2002; 58:169–178.
2. Rudick RA, Cohen JA, Weinstock-Guttman B, et al. Drug therapy: management of multiple sclerosis. N Engl J Med 1997; 337(22):1604–1611.

64
Acute Transverse Myelitis

Douglas Kerr and Chitra Krishnan
Department of Neurology, Johns Hopkins University School of Medicine, Baltimore, Maryland, U.S.A.

Frank S. Pidcock
Department of Pediatric Physical Medicine and Rehabilitation, Johns Hopkins University School of Medicine, Kennedy Krieger Institute, Baltimore, Maryland, U.S.A.

INTRODUCTION

Acute transverse myelitis (ATM) is a focal inflammatory disorder of the spinal cord resulting in motor, sensory, and autonomic dysfunction. It is a rare disorder with an estimated 1400 new cases diagnosed in the United States per year (between 1 and 8 per million per year). This leads to a total prevalence of approximately 34,000 people chronic sequlae of ATM; approximately 20% of these individuals had the acute illness before the age of 18 years. Idiopathic ATM must be distinguished from acute myelopathy secondary to a definable cause and from compressive myelopathies to insure appropriate management. Between 6% and 43% of patients with ATM will be diagnosed with multiple sclerosis (most with the benefit of longitudinal follow up), 8–16.5% may have an associated systemic mixed connective tissue disorder, and up to 5% may have features suggesting that the acute myelopathy is caused by direct infection of the spinal cord (i.e., mycoplasma or herpes virus family). Up to 14% of patients who present with an acute noncompressive myelopathy appear to have had a vascular cause (i.e., infarct or vascular malformation) (JHTMC case series). Ten to 45% patients with an acute myelopathy who have no clearly established etiology are classified as having idiopathic ATM.

DIAGNOSIS AND CLINICAL FEATURES

Acute transverse myelitis is usually a monophasic and monofocal disorder. Most often, it presents with sudden onset of rapidly progressive weakness of the lower extremities, loss of sensation, loss of sphincter control, and pain with no signs of spinal cord compression or other systemic neurologic disease.

The weakness of ATM develops generally as a progressive flaccid paraparesis that occasionally progresses to involve the arms as well. Pyramidal signs generally appear by the second week of the illness. More than 80% patients reach their clinical nadir within 10 days of the onset of symptoms. Although the temporal course may vary, neurologic function usually deteriorates progressively during the acute phase between 4 and 21 days.

A sensory level can be documented in most cases and is usually reported as located between T5 and T10; in about 20% of cases, there is a cervical sensory level and in 10% the level is in the lumbar region. In the case series followed at our institution, cervical myelopathy with a cervical sensory level is more frequent than a thoracic level. Pain may occur in the back, extremities, or abdomen. Neck stiffness has been reported to occur in about a third of the cases. Adults with ATM often note parethesias at the outset of the disorder; this is an unusual complaint in children.

A preceding illness within 3 weeks of the onset of ATM, including nonspecific symptoms such as fever, nausea, and muscle pain, has been reported in about 40% of children. Although a history of an immunization preceding the onset of ATM has been reported to be common, the relationship of ATM to immunization is unclear because of limited unbiased data. Thirty percent of all cases of pediatric ATM referred to Johns Hopkins Transverse Myelitis Center reported retrospectively an immunization within one month of the onset of symptoms.

DIAGNOSTIC EVALUATION

The first priority in the diagnostic approach of acute myelopathy is to rule out a compressive lesion. In cases with a consistent history and physical examination, a gadolinium-enhanced MRI of the spinal cord should be obtained as soon as possible. If there is no structural lesion such as epidural blood or a spinal mass, then the presence or absence of spinal cord inflammation should be documented by evaluation of the cerebrospinal fluid. The absence of pleocytosis would lead to consideration of noninflammatory causes of myelopathy such as arteriovenous malformations, epidural lipomatosis, fibrocartilaginous embolism or possibly early inflammatory myelopathy (i.e., a false negative CSF). In the presence of an inflammatory process (defined by gadolinium enhancement and CSF WBC pleocytosis), one should determine whether there is an infectious cause. Viral polymerase chain reaction assays should be performed to determine whether there is the presence of viral gene expression within the CNS (herpes simplex 1 and 2, varicella zoster, cytomegalovirus, Epstein–Barr virus, and enterovirus). Detection of lyme infection of the CNS typically is based on antibody detection methods (ELISA with confirmatory western blot) and the CSF/serum index is often helpful in determining whether there is true neuroborreliosis. Evidence of *M. pneumoniae* infection may be determined by seroconversion, which is defined by a four-fold increase in titer or a single titer of $\geq$1:128.

The next priority is to define the extent of demyelination within the CNS, since several disorders (i.e., multiple sclerosis or acute disseminated encephalomyelitis) may present with ATM in the setting of multifocal disease. A gadolinium-enhanced brain MRI and visual evoked potential should be ordered to look for these entities. The absence of multifocal areas of demyelination would suggest the diagnosis of idiopathic ATM and lead to appropriate treatment measures.

Acute transfer myelitis is often misdiagnosed as acute inflammatory demyelinating polyradiculoneuropathy (AIDP) because both conditions may present with rapidly progressive sensory and motor loss involving principally the lower extremities. A pure paraplegia or paraparesis with a corresponding distribution of sensory loss may favor ATM, while AIDP may present with a gradient of motor and sensory loss involving the lower extremities greater than the upper extremities. When weakness and sensory loss involve both the upper and lower extremities equally with a distinct spinal cord level, ATM is highly likely. Enhanced deep tendon reflexes generally support the diagnosis of ATM, however, patients with fulminant cases of ATM with inflammation in the central spinal cord gray matter may present with hypotonia with decreased or absent deep tendon reflexes, while some cases of AIDP may have retained tendon reflexes early in the course. Urinary urgency or retention is a common early finding in ATM and is less common in AIDP. Dysesthetic pain, involvement of the upper extremity and cranial nerve 7, and absent deep tendon reflexes involving the upper extremities are more common features of AIDP. An MRI of the spinal cord may show an area of inflammation in ATM but not in AIDP. Although cerebral spinal fluid findings in ATM are not consistent and an elevated cell count may be absent, there is usually a moderate lymphocytic pleocytosis and elevated protein level. This is in contrast to the albumino-cytologic dissociation of the CSF most often seen in AIDP.

THERAPY (FIG. 1)

Intravenous steroid therapy for three days followed by an oral taper is often instituted. A study of five children with severe ATM who received Solumedrol (1 g/1.73 m squared per day) for 3 or 5 consecutive days followed by oral prednisone for 14 days reported beneficial effects compared to 10 historic controls. In the steroid treated group, the median time to walking was 23 days vs. 97 days, full recovery occurred in 80% vs. 10%, and full motor recovery at 1 year was present in 100% vs. 20%. No serious adverse effects from the steroid treatments occurred. However, this was a small group and the study was not controlled or prospective.

Dunne compared a steroid treated group of 14 children with ATM with a group that did not receive steroids. He concluded that there was no evidence that steroids improved outcomes, but does not present any specific details to support his beliefs. In 1998, Knebusch was unable to determine whether a pulse of intravenous steroids led to improved outcome.

Plasma exchange (PE) can be initiated if a patient who has moderate to severe ATM (i.e., inability to walk, markedly impaired autonomic function and at least some sensory loss in the lower extremities) with little clinical improvement within 5–7 days of intravenous steroids. Although its efficacy is unproven in children, and the potential for vascular and hemodynamic complications with PE increases with small body size, PE has been shown to be effective in adults with ATM and other inflammatory disorders of the CNS. Predictors of good response to PE include early treatment (less than 20 days from symptom onset), male sex, and a clinically incomplete lesion (i.e., some motor function in the lower extremities, intact, or brisk reflexes).

Chronic immunomodulatory therapy should be considered for the small subgroup of children affected by recurrent disease. These patients are usually adolescents and typically have a multifocal demyelinating process. The differential diagnosis includes multiple sclerosis, CNS neuroborreliosis, neuromyelitis optica, or a systemic inflammatory disorder (e.g., neurosarcoidosis, Sjogren's syndrome, systemic or lupus erythematosus) and an appropriate workup should be conducted.

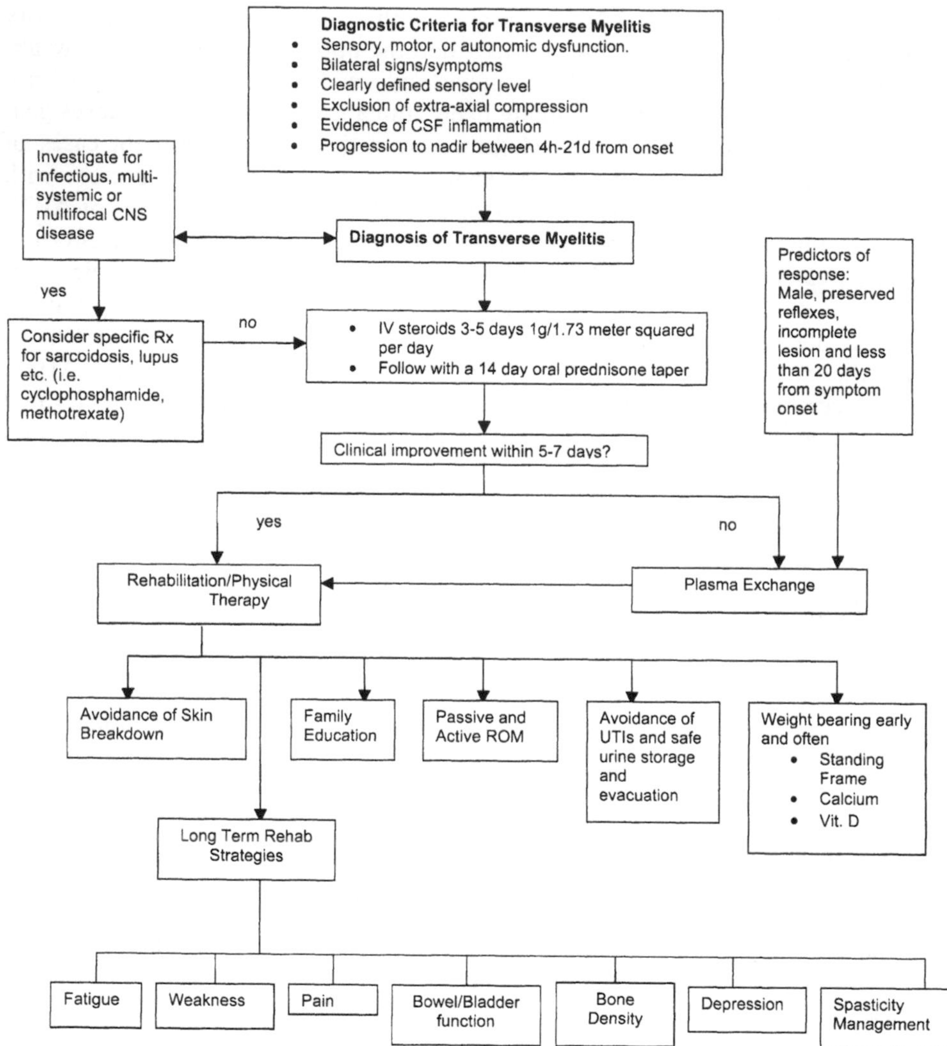

Figure 1 Evaluation and treatment of patients with acute transverse myelitis.

Adolescents diagnosed with MS may be treated with interferon-β or Copaxone. If a systemic inflammatory disease is diagnosed, treatment specific for the particular disorder should be started. Unfortunately, the effectiveness of these treatment regimens has not been studied in children, and consultation with the appropriate subspecialist is recommended. Since many of these treatments (i.e., azathioprine, methotrexate, cyclophosphamide) have a risk of long-term toxicity including myelodysplastic disorders or leukemias, they should be reserved for the most aggressive inflammatory disorders.

Many children with ATM will require rehabilitative care to prevent secondary complications of immobility and to improve their functional skills. It is important to begin occupational and physical therapies early during the course of recovery to prevent the inactivity-related problems of skin breakdown and soft-tissue contracture with associated loss of joint range of motion. This should include daily weight bearing as soon as possible after the loss of the ability to ambulate. During the early recovery period, family education is essential to develop a strategic plan for dealing with the challenges to independence following return to the community. Assessment and fitting for splints designed to passively maintain an optimal position for limbs that cannot be actively moved is an important part of the management at this stage.

The long-term management of ATM requires attention to a number of issues. These are the residual effects of any spinal cord injury including ATM. Table 1 describes therapeutic options that may be considered for treating these complications. In addition to chronic medical problems, there are the ongoing issues of ordering the appropriate equipment, re-entry into the school and community, and coping with the psychological effects of this condition by the patients and their families.

Spasticity is often a very difficult problem. The key goal is to maintain flexibilitywith both passive and, where possible, active stretching exercises accompanied by bracing where necessary to retard the development of contractures where joints are inclined to a single position by flaccid or spastic weakness. Splints are commonly used at the ankles, wrists, and elbows. A strengthening program for the weaker of the spastic muscle, acting on a joint and aerobic conditioning regimens, can also be recommended. These interventions are supported by adjunctive measures that include antispasticity drugs (e.g., valium, baclofen, dantrolene), therapeutic botulinum toxin injections, and serial casting. The therapeutic goal is to improve the function of the patient in performing specific activities of daily living (i.e., feeding, dressing, bathing, hygiene, mobility) through improving the available joint range of motion, teaching effective compensatory strategies, and relieving pain.

Another major area of concern is effective management of bowel and bladder function. A high fiber diet, adequate and timely fluid intake, medications to regulate bowel evacuations, and a clean intermittent urinary catheterization are the basic components to success. Regular evaluations by medical specialists for urodynamic studies and adjustment of the bowel program are recommended to prevent potentially serious complications.

PROGNOSIS

Longitudinal case series of ATM reveal that approximately 1/3 of patients recover with little to no sequelae, 1/3 are left with moderate degree of permanent disability, and 1/3 have severe disabilities. From a series of nine children with ATM, Knebusch found that 44% evolved to a good outcome defined by an essentially normal gait, mild urinary symptoms, minimal sensory and upper motor neuron signs, or a combination of these features. A fair outcome with mild spasticity but independent ambulation, urgency, constipation, and some sensory signs developed in 33%, and a poor outcome with severe gait disturbance or complete inability to walk, absence of sphincter control, and substantial sensory deficit was the long-term outcome of 23%.

Symptoms associated with poor outcome include back pain as an initial complaint, rapid progression to maximal symptoms within hours of onset, spinal shock, and sensory disturbance up to the cervical level. The presence of 14–3-3 protein, a marker of neuronal injury, in the CSF during the acute phase may also predict a poor outcome.

Table 1 Long-Term Management of Patients with Transverse Myelitis

Fatigue	Bladder dysfunction	Bowel dysfunction	Weakness	Pain or dysesthesias	Spasticity	Fragile bones
Amantidine	Urodynamics	High fiber diet	Strengthening program for weaker muscles	ROM exercises	ROM exercises	Bone densitometry
Methylphenidate	Clean intermittent catheterization if possible	Increased fluid intake	Aquatherapy	Medications (gabapentin, carbamazepine, nortriptyline, tramadol)	Orthotics	Vitamin D
Modafinil	Anticholinergic drug if detrusor hyperactive	Digital disimpaction	Orthoses, ambulation devices when appropriate	TENS unit	Aquatherapy	Calcium
CoQ10	Adrenergic blocker if sphincter dysfunction	Bowel med program colace, senokot/ dulcolax, docusate PR, bisacodyl in a water base, miralax, enemas PRN	Biofeedback	Intrathecal opioids	Hippotherapy	Standing frame if nonambulatory
Consider depression	Cranberry juice for urine acidification		Fampridine		Medications (Baclofen, tizanidine, dantrolene)	
	Sacral nerve stimulation				Therapeutic botulinum toxin	
	Biofeedback				Intrathecal baclofen	

SUMMARY

Acute transverse myelitis is a rare disorder of children and adults. It presents with rapidly progressive weakness of the legs accompanied by sensory loss and sphincter control. The first priority is to rule out a compressive lesion of the spinal cord and a gadolinium-enhanced MRI of the spinal cord should be obtained as soon as possible after presentation. The role of steroids is unclear in the treatment of this condition, however can be used. Rehabilitation interventions are an essential component to managing the chronic aspects of this disorder.

SUGGESTED READINGS

1. De Seze J, Stojkovic T, Breteau G, Lucas C, Michon-Pasturel U, Gauvrit JY, Hachulla E, Mounier-Vehier F, Pruvo JP, Leys D, Destee A, Hatron PY, Vermersch P. Acute myelopathies: clinical, laboratory and outcome profiles in 79 cases. Brain 2001; 124:1509–1521.
2. Kerr DA, Ayetey H. Immunopathogenesis of acute transverse myelitis. Curr Opin Neurol 2002; 15:339–347.
3. Knebusch M, Strassburg HM, Reiners K. Acute transverse myelitis in childhood: nine cases and review of the literature. Dev Med Child Neurol 1998; 40:631–639.
4. Paine RS, Byers RK. Transverse myelopathy in childhood. AMA Am J Diseases of Children 1968; 85:151–163.
5. Sebire G, Hollenberg H, Meyer L, Huault G, Landrieu P, Tardieu M. High dose methylprednisolone in severe acute transverse myelopathy. Arch Dis Child 1997; 76:167–168.
6. Transverse Myelitis Consortium Working Group. Proposed diagnostic criteria and nosology of acute transverse myelitis. Neurology 2002; 59:499–505.
7. Weinshenker BG, O'Brien PC, Petterson TM, Noseworthy JH, Lucchinetti CF, Dodick DW, Pineda AA, Stevens LN, Rodriguez M. A randomized trial of plasma exchange in acute central nervous system inflammatory demyelinating disease. Ann Neurol 1999; 46:878–886.

65
Optic Neuritis

Linda M. Famiglio
Geisinger Health System, Danville, Pennsylvania, U.S.A.

INTRODUCTION

The diagnosis and treatment of optic neuritis require a team approach. Although the child usually presents to the pediatrician or family doctor, consultation is rapidly sought with the neurologist or ophthalmologist for diagnostic help. Parental, patient, and primary care physician anxiety over the acute presentation of significant eye pain and the loss of vision often leads to urgent consultation in the emergency room or office setting. Ophthalmologists provide an analysis of visual function and fundoscopic detail. Neurologists usually direct the care by providing an overall context that guides treatment and prognosis. Prognosis is the key issue in optic neuritis, not as much for visual recovery as for the development of symptoms and signs that support the diagnosis of multiple sclerosis (MS). After vision recovers, anxiety may continue to build over the possibility of later development of MS.

DIAGNOSIS/CLINICAL FEATURES

Unilateral or bilateral ocular pain with evolution of visual loss over hours to days is typical and diagnostic of childhood onset optic neuritis (Table 1). Parents first seek advice from the pediatrician or family physician for the pain that may be described as a headache in up to one-third of children. Older children can describe localized orbital or retro orbital pain. The pain arises from inflammation of the optic nerve sheath itself. Orbital pressure and eye movements increase the pain by causing traction on the sheath at the extraocular muscle insertion points.

Visual dysfunction is bilateral in about 60% of children, slightly higher than reported in adults. Patients may present with bilateral involvement, develop involvement of the second eye within weeks or may have a recurrence months later in the previously unaffected eye. Young children may not complain of visual loss but may describe room darkening or blurring. Older, more verbal children can describe loss of central vision and decreased visual acuity. With direct questioning and observation of the child while attempting to read or name pictures, the accompanying visual loss is almost always apparent. Loss of color vision and contrast sensitivity can be reported as things looking dark, drab, or blurry.

Table 1 Clinical Features of Optic Neuritis

Clinical features
Decreased visual acuity
Central visual field defect
Color desaturation
Decreased contrast sensitivity
Afferent pupillary defect
Orbital or retroorbital pain
Headache
Disc edema
Disc pallor

Disc edema is present acutely in most children with optic neuritis, but can be absent also. Ophthalmologic consultation is necessary for confirming the visual function and documenting disc edema, hemorrhage, macular exudates, and any cells in the vitreous. As the clinical symptoms resolve, the disc becomes pale especially along the temporal aspect due to loss of axons. Rarely epiretinal membrane formation can complicate recovery from optic neuritis and lead to further visual loss. Ophthalmologists also may contribute retinal photographs, documentation of visual fields, and measurement of visual acuity. Hand-held color plates may document loss of color vision. The remainder of the neurologic examination is usually normal.

Although optic neuritis is described most often as primary idiopathic inflammation of the optic nerve, the same picture can be seen in disseminated or systemic conditions. The extended history and review of systems may uncover chronic systemic illnesses, prior demyelinating events, transient neurologic symptoms, or acute exposure to infectious diseases. Many children have a history of a viral illness during the 2 weeks prior to the episode. Optic neuritis can occur in combination with other demyelinating lesions especially transverse myelitis. In this condition, Devic's disease, flaccid weakness with decreased or absent reflexes, decreased sensation, and bowel and bladder dysfunction are found on examination (Table 2).

Other diagnosis must be considered in the proper setting. For example, in the context of blood pressure instability as seen in trauma, renal disease or dialysis, children can develop anterior ischemic optic neuropathy. Also, papilledema and visual field loss can be due to increased intracranial pressure; the pattern of headache and disc swelling with central sparing of vision distinguishes the presentation of elevated intracranial pressure from that of optic neuritis (Table 3).

Magnetic resonance imaging (MRI) may be normal or demonstrate white matter high-intensity lesions suggestive of subclinical plaques of MS. Rarely, optic

Table 2 Conditions Reported in Association with Optic Neuritis

Acute disseminated encephalomyelitis	Viral encephalitis
Devic's disease/optic neuritis with transverse myelitis	Measles
Bone marrow transplant	Mumps
Postvaccination	Varicella
Postinfection	EBV
Allergic reaction to bee sting	HSV
Paranasal sinus inflammation	Parvo
Multiple sclerosis	Lyme's

Table 3 Distinguishing Features of Optic Neuritis, Elevated ICP, and Anterior Ischemic Optic Neuropathy

	Optic neuritis	Elevated ICP	Anterior ischemic optic neuropathy
Pain	Orbital or retro orbital	Headache	None
Visual field loss	Central vision loss	Occasional obscuration or no loss	Altitudinal Loss with sparing of central vision
Unilateral/bilateral	Can be unilateral	Bilateral	Bilateral
Pupil response	Afferent pupillary defect	Normal early	Absent
PREP	Delayed P100	Variable	Decreased amplitudes
MRI abnormality	Normal or white matter lesions	Hydrocephalus or mass occupying lesion predominates	Rarely abnormal
Treatment	Steroids	ICP measures	Maintain volume and BP; decrease intraocular pressure; correct anemia
Prognosis for visual recovery	Good	Variable	Poor

nerves may be enlarged. Spinal tap is not essential, but cerebrospinal fluid (CSF) may show pleocytosis and a mild protein elevation. Investigations to elucidate associated conditions should be considered in context.

TREATMENT

Visual recovery usually takes place spontaneously within a few weeks. The Optic Neuritis Study Group found no difference in long-term visual outcome between adults assigned to intravenous methylprednisolone, oral prednisone, or placebo treated groups at 1 year and 10 year follow up. However, the intravenous methylprednisolone treatment group experienced more rapid resolution of visual field, contrast sensitivity, and color vision defects. Thus, many physicians treat optic neuritis with intravenous methylprednisolone for more rapid relief of visual symptoms, especially when bilateral visual loss is present.

Methylprednisolone sodium acetate (Solumedrol) can be administered intravenously in a high dose, anti-inflammatory regimen of 10–30 mg per kilogram per day for 3 days followed by oral prednisone 1 mg per kilogram per day tapered over 11 – 21 days. Prophylaxis against steroid-induced ulcers with an H2 blocker such as ranitidine is recommended.

Oral acetaminophen, ibuprofen, or aspirin may improve the child's acute pain. Extended analgesics are rarely necessary, as the pain associated with optic neuritis usually resolves within days. School adaptations for visual loss are sometimes warranted.

PROGNOSIS

In children, vision recovery is complete in about one-third, improved but abnormal in an additional one-half and minimally improved in the remaining 15% of patients. A trend towards better visual outcome is noted in children with normal MRI and also in children younger than six years old. No difference in visual outcome has been identified between unilateral and bilateral cases.

The effect of treatment on risk of recurrence and of development of MS is extrapolated from pediatric case series and reports of adult patients in the Optic Neuritis Study Group. Early results of the Optic Neuritis Study Group suggested increased risk of recurrence in adults treated with oral prednisone when compared to intravenous methylprednisolone and placebo. The largest published series of children by Lucchinetti with optic neuritis identified 79 children by record review over 38 years. Although this analysis did not focus on treatment effect, univariate analysis found no statistical association between steroid treatment and further development of MS.

The Optic Neuritis Study Group has identified groups of adults at high and low risk of developing MS. At 10 year follow up, 56% of adults with one or more white matter lesions on baseline MRI developed MS compared to 22% of those with a normal baseline MRI scan. Thus, a baseline MRI is recommended in order to contribute to the discussion of prognosis. Adults with optic neuritis who are at high risk for developing MS may receive a theoretical benefit from beginning immunomodulatory therapy early, before the second clinical attack.

Children have a lower risk of developing MS than adults and, especially in the context of preceding viral illness, may have a different underlying disease process. In childhood chart review series of optic neuritis, the estimated probability of developing MS within 10 years is 0.13 (95% CI 0.05 – 0.20). The percent cumulative probability for developing MS was highest in children with recurrent or sequential episodes. Those patients with a preceding infection appeared to be at decreased risk of developing MS. Elevated CSF protein was weakly associated with developing MS.

Based on the current studies, children cannot be recommended to receive early immunomodulatory treatment even if they have white matter lesions on baseline MRI. However, continued follow up with a neurologist for early recognition of demyelinating events, reassessment of risk and initiation of early treatment if MS develops is recommended.

SUMMARY

Optic neuritis can occur spontaneously or following infection. The prognosis for visual recovery is good. Intravenous methylprednisolone can shorten the time for visual recovery. The risk of developing MS following optic neuritis appears to be lower than in adults.

SUGGESTED READINGS

1. Brady KM, Brar AS, Lee AG, Coats DK, Paysse EA, Steinkuller PG. Optic neuritis in children: clinical features and visual outcome. J AAPOS 1999; 3:98–103.
2. Lucchinetti CF, Kiers L, O'Duffy A, Gomez MR, Cross S, Leavitt JA, O'Brien P, Rodriguez M. Risk factors for developing multiple sclerosis after childhood optic neuritis. Neurology 1997; 49:1413–1418.
3. Optic Neuritis Study Group. High- and low-risk profiles for the development of multiple sclerosis within 10 years after optic neuritis. Arch Ophthamol 2003; 121:944–949.

66
Rett Syndrome

Genila M. Bibat and SakkuBai Naidu
Neurogenetics Unit, Kennedy Krieger Institute, Johns Hopkins Medical Institutions, Baltimore, Maryland, U.S.A.

INTRODUCTION

Rett syndrome (RS) is one of the many mental retardation syndromes for which the genetic basis was recently identified. It is a neurodevelopmental disorder predominantly affecting females, associated with devastating loss of function between infancy and the fifth year of life. Thereafter, its course is relatively static, distinguishing it from most neurodegenerative disorders of childhood. Rett syndrome is pan-ethnic, affecting patients worldwide. The prevalence of the RS phenotype among females is estimated at 1:10,000–1:22,000, with 99.5% of all cases occurring in a sporadic manner. There are reports of males with molecular defects in the MeCP2 gene that present with a widely variable phenotype.

Identified as a distinct entity initially by Andreas Rett in the 1960s, the disorder was mapped to chromosome Xq28 in 1998 and identified a year later, as being secondary to mutations in the methyl CpG binding protein-2 (MeCP2) gene located in this region. MeCP2 is a transcription repressor that silences an as yet unknown number of genes. Seventy to eighty percent of patients with the RS phenotype demonstrate mutations in MeCP2.

DIAGNOSIS AND EVALUATION

RS is characterized by a period of apparent normal development followed by arrest of developmental skills. The symptomatology and pattern of evolution in classic RS patients have been remarkably consistent. RS patients are reported to have normal prenatal and perinatal history; however, close inspection reveals hypotonia, tremulousness, and reduced social interaction in early infancy. Characteristic features of RS include deceleration in velocity of head growth between 3 months and 4 years of age resulting in microcephaly, stereotyped hand movements, psychomotor retardation, impaired language development, gait dysfunction, and loss of purposeful hand use. A distinctive phase in the disease between 1 and 5 years of age may resemble autism and also manifests the above-mentioned pathognomonic clinical features of RS. The majority of patients have EEG abnormalities (central sharp waves), but only half have recognizable clinical seizures. Magnetic resonance imaging is within normal limits. Respiratory irregularities in RS occur only during wakefulness and include periodic apnea and intermittent hyperventilation. Sleep is fragmented and problematic in infancy and early childhood. Autonomic nervous system dysfunction can cause peripheral vasomotor instability and disturbances in the gastrointestinal system resulting in oropharyngeal dysphagia, severe constipation, gastroesophageal reflux, and failure to thrive.

Since the identification of a genetic marker, diagnosis of classical and atypical RS has become possible much earlier than when the stereotyped behaviors become evident in the second year of life. Mutations in the MeCP2 gene cause partial or complete loss of function of the MeCP2 protein leading to a failure of repression of a variety of genes. The resulting alterations in expression of genes responsible for early postnatal development of the nervous system coincide with the reduction in velocity of brain growth noted in infancy. Neuropathological studies point to anatomical abnormalities such as simplified inferior olivary nucleus in the brain stem. These changes must occur during the late second or third trimester when MeCP2 is normally expressed in this region. However, postnatal brain development, when MeCP2 is expressed in cortical neurons, is markedly affected with poor neuronal maturation, dendritic arborization, and synapse formation. Reported alterations in dopaminergic, cholinergic, and glutaminergic neurotransmitters play a vital role in activity-dependent synaptic plasticity and morphogenesis of the developing nervous system.

With the increase in clinical recognition and recent advances in the understanding of the neurobiology and molecular genetics of RS, a wide clinical spectrum has been recognized. A subgroup of mutation positive patients with very mild symptomatology, normal head growth, or preserved speech have been identified, while another group presents with severe and early onset of motor disability, scoliosis, and seizures. The site of mutation in MeCP2, X-inactivation status, and possibly as yet unidentified factors can modify the severity of the disease.

TREATMENT

Presently, specific therapies are not available for RS. However, the realization that the disorder advances slowly or not at all in later stages highlights the importance of early intervention with symptomatic and palliative care.

Seizures

Epileptic seizures of myoclonic, partial or generalized variety, respond to most standard anticonvulsants, such as carbamazepine, valproic acid, lamotrigine, and benzodiazepine. The ketogenic diet and vagal nerve stimulation have been reported as effective in some RS patients. Seizures are often overdiagnosed because of breath-holding, cyanotic spells, inattention, and eye rolling movements, which are presumed to be ictal events. Appropriate use of antiepileptic drugs may be guided by such EEG correlations. Topiramate, an anticonvulsant that antagonizes the α-amino-3-hydroxy-5-methylisoxazole-4-propionic acid (AMPA) subtype of glutamate receptor, has been shown to exert some influence in regulating respiratory irregularities, and is a good adjunct for the management of seizures in RS.

Gastrointestinal Dysfunction and Failure to Thrive

Pervasive growth failure is a chronic issue in the majority of RS children despite a caloric intake of up to 125% of the recommended daily allowance for age in some cases. Dietary supplementation may still be required under the guidance of a nutritionist; in some gastrostomy feeding becomes a necessity to optimize for growth failure due to oropharyngeal dysfunction. Swallow studies as well as endoscopy and esophagogastric motility studies aid in the identification of feeding impairment and rectify nutritional status and prevent pneumonia due to aspiration. The RS individuals with mild chewing and swallowing problems may benefit initially from a variety of palliative interventions such as optimal posture and seating, manipulation of food texture, use of adaptive utensils, and altering the pace of feeding. Gastroesophageal reflux (GER), manifesting as irritability, poor feeding, and regurgitation, is best managed by thickening feeds and antacids (e.g., ranitidine). Prokinetic agents (e.g., metoclopramide) to increase lower esophageal sphincter tone and enhance gastric emptying are used in severe and persistent cases of GER.

A serious day-to-day care issue is functional constipation that results from the generalized autonomic dysfunction. High fiber diet, stool softeners, and lactulose can ameliorate it. It is not unusual to have RS patients requiring daily Miralax therapy. Occasionally, the constipation can be severe enough to necessitate the use of Fleets enemas for initial relief of stool compaction. Rarely, intestinal perforation may result from severe, chronic constipation. Increased fluid intake to 1.5 times maintenance is suggested to prevent aggravation of constipation and compensate for excessive drooling and hyperventilation.

Gallstones reported in some RS patients might be the cause of unexplained irritability, and needs evaluation if all other etiologies for irritability are excluded.

Behavior

Severe sleep disturbance, mainly fragmented sleep pattern, benefits from melatonin (1–3 mg) or chloral hydrate use (50 mg/kg, with maximum of 500 mg in children and 1 g in adults) at bedtime. Adequate seizure control may also improve sleep disturbance as seizure activity maximizes during non-REM sleep in RS patients. Daytime behavior problems such as irritability, screaming spells, and self-abuse occur more intensely during the autistic phase of the disease. These behaviors may be due to pain, discomfort from gastrointestinal dysfunction such as severe constipation or reflux, and increased muscle tone and contractures in later years. It is thus, important to exclude medical causes before considering pharmacotherapy for behavior modification. Medications to improve behavioral abnormalities such as screaming or self-injury include carbamazepine, valproic acid, or low-dose risperidone. Music has a particularly calming effect and has been used effectively by parents.

Bone Density

Individuals with RS are at risk for developing osteoporosis. DEXAscan is a valuable study to determine bone density. Pamidronate has been used for therapeutic intervention; however, its efficacy is uncertain.

Scoliosis

Scoliosis occurs in RS individuals, especially those with truncal hypotonia, and its frequency rises dramatically to about 60–80% with increasing age. Spine films are obtained as needed to monitor the progression of scoliosis as it may be mild (with a 25° curvature), slowly progressive, and amenable to body brace. In contrast, scoliosis may progress rapidly and when the curvature exceeds 40° can cause respiratory compromise warranting spinal fusion and rod placement. Rett syndrome patients tolerate general anesthesia and postoperative complications of surgical procedures well, such as scoliosis repair, indicating their ability to handle physiologic stress.

Habilitation

Intensive habilitation and close developmental surveillance are warranted to prevent progressive disability and functional impairment. Active physical and occupational therapy are advocated to prevent contractures. Individuals with weak ankles and excessive valgus may benefit from ankle/foot orthoses (AFOs) to help improve gait. Ambulation needs to be encouraged. Weight bearing and upright positioning by the use of prone standers or standing frames should be encouraged in those who are not walking independently. Increased muscle tone may interfere with therapy sessions and ambulation, and in nonambulatory patients may affect transfers, seating, and hygiene. Botulinum toxin injections may be necessary to treat complex abnormalities. Baclofen should be given with caution as it may lower seizure threshold. Orthopedic surgical intervention may be necessary to treat complex abnormalities resulting from rigidity and contractures.

Communication skills can be improved through the use of sign language and picture cards. Those with preserved hand use can benefit extensively with augmentative communication devices. These modes of intervention can be remarkably effective in improving the quality of life of the patients and their family.

Previous Drug Trials

Drug trials in RS included dietary supplementation with L-carnitine, and naltrexone, an opiate antagonist. These were placebo-controlled double-blind studies with improvement in motor and behavioral skills as outcome variables. Both showed no evidence of improvement in the clinical features of RS, although social interaction and general well being were said to be better with carnitine therapy.

PROGNOSIS

Life expectancy varies widely. Some RS patients, frequently children under the age of 15 years, die unexpectedly in sleep with no identifiable cause. A direct relationship of such deaths to seizure or medications has not been established. The possibility of cardiac dysfunction with prolonged QT interval has been suggested as a cause of sudden death. The identification of a 77-year-old female with preserved speech that tested positive for the mutation indicates a potential normal life span. In a few others, death resulted from respiratory infections in the second and third decades of life. The survival rate by age 35 years is reduced to 70%, compared to 98% in the general U.S. female population, and 27% for profoundly mentally retarded individuals.

Social interaction and hand use show considerable improvement in the later phases of the disease. Older children acquire minimal skills such as playing with interactive toys with reduction in stereotyped hand movements. Many adult RS women have been identified in whom seizures and respiratory irregularities have improved or abated; however, rigidity, dystonia, scoliosis, contractures, and muscle wasting gradually increase. Prominent vasomotor instability with wasting of the distal portions of the extremities and curled toes are noted despite lack of evidence for a myopathy or peripheral neuropathy.

SUMMARY

Rett syndrome is a neurological disorder with severe mental retardation seen among all ethnic groups. It primarily affects females and a small number of males particularly among familial cases. Rett syndrome causes early developmental stagnation, and later striking cognitive and motor delays, followed by partial recovery and cognitive stability. Mutations in the MeCP2 gene causing RS are identified in a majority of the patients. In 99.5% of cases, the disease arises from sporadic de novo mutations. Mutational analysis identifies a subgroup of patients both males and females with milder symptomatology. Currently, specific therapies are unavailable for RS. In view of the nonprogressive nature of this disease in later stages, symptomatic care and intensive habilitation are extremely important and needs to be maintained.

SUGGESTED READINGS

1. Amir RE, Van den Veyver IB, Wan M, et al. Rett syndrome is caused by mutations in X-linked MeCP2, encoding methyl CpG-binding protein 2. Nat Genet 1999; 23:185–188.
2. Hoffbuhr K, Devaney J, LaFleur B, Sirianni M, Scacheri S, Giron J, Schuette J, Innis J, Marino M, Philippart M, Narayanan V, Umansky R, Hoffman E, Naidu S. MeCP2 mutations in children with and without the phenotype of Rett syndrome. Neurology 2001; 56:1486–1495.
3. Naidu S. Rett syndrome: a disorder affecting early brain growth. Ann Neurol 1997; 42: 3–10.
4. Percy A. Clinical trials and treatment prospects. Mental Retard Dev Disabilities 2002; 8:106–111.

67

Treatment of Obsessive-Compulsive Disorder

Marco A. Grados
The Johns Hopkins Hospital, Department of Psychiatry, Division of Child and Adolescent Psychiatry, Baltimore, Maryland, U.S.A.

INTRODUCTION

Obsessive-compulsive disorder (OCD) is characterized by disabling obsessions and/or compulsions. Originally thought to be a rare condition, epidemiologic studies have shown that OCD is the fourth most common psychiatric disorder, more common than schizophrenia or bipolar disorder. Onset of symptoms at an early age is common, with up to 80% of adults with OCD reporting symptoms before age 18. A childhood prepubertal variant of OCD can be observed, most often in males, associated with "sensory" compulsions and tics. After puberty, rates of OCD in males and females are similar.

DIAGNOSIS AND EVALUATION

Obsessions are intrusive thoughts, images or urges that are senseless, unpleasant, frightening, or distressing. Clinically, it is critical to differentiate obsessions from ruminations, general worrying, restrictive ego-syntonic interests, and organically based perseverative thoughts. Ruminations on themes of low-self-worth and hopelessness are common in depression; generalized worrying about daily life activities occurs in generalized anxiety disorder; overly restrictive interests are present in pervasive developmental disorders (autism and Asperger disorder); and organically based perseverative thoughts can appear in children with cerebral palsy or other brain insults.

Compulsions are rigid, repetitive behaviors that a child is compelled to complete, often in response to an obsession. Compulsions include hand washing or bathing, hoarding, perfectionist tendencies, ordering and checking, and mental rituals such as counting and praying. Children with a tic history can have sensory-based compulsions such as touching rituals, evening up compulsions, difficulty with certain types of clothing, sensitivity to loud sounds, strong food preferences based on texture and sometimes a need to smell objects.

The measure of the severity of the obsessions and compulsions can differentiate clinical OCD from OC behaviors. The time spent, the degree of interference with daily activities, and the extent of distress caused by obsessions or compulsions are the main parameters. The OCD is diagnosed when obsessions and/or compulsions occupy more than 1 hr of the day and cause at least moderate interference or distress (Table 1). The Children's Yale-Brown Obsessive-Compulsive Scale (CY-BOCS) is a valuable tool for quantifying symptoms and following treatment effects; the CY-BOCS measures the severity of OCD symptoms using time, interference, distress, resistance, and control for both obsessions and compulsions. The OCD shows frequent comorbidity with depression, anxiety disorders (separation anxiety, generalized anxiety disorder), impulse control disorders, (trichotillomania, skin picking), body dysmorphic disorder, and eating disorders.

There are no laboratory studies that confirm the diagnosis of OCD, but when considering the use of psychotropic medications a baseline electrocardiogram, hematological profile, and hepatic and renal function tests may be indicated. Pediatric

Table 1 DSM-IV Criteria for Diagnosis of Obsessive-Compulsive Disorder

A. The person exhibits either obsessions or compulsions

Obsessions are indicated by the following:

- The person has recurrent and persistent thoughts, impulses, or images that are experienced, at some time during the disturbance, as intrusive and inappropriate and that cause marked anxiety or distress
- The thoughts, impulses, or images are not simply excessive worries about real-life problems
- The person attempts to ignore or suppress such thoughts, impulses, or images or to neutralize them with some other thought or action
- The person recognizes that the obsessional thoughts, impulses, or images are a product of his or her own mind (not imposed from without as in thought insertion)

Compulsions are indicated by the following:

- The person has repetitive behaviors (e.g., hand washing, ordering, checking) or mental acts (e.g., praying, counting, repeating words silently) that the person feels driven to perform in response to an obsession or according to rules that must be applied rigidly
- The behaviors or mental acts are aimed at preventing some dreaded event or situation; however, these behaviors or mental acts either are not connected in a realistic way with what they are designed to neutralize or prevent or are clearly excessive

B. At some point during the course of the disorder, the person has recognized that the obsessions or compulsions are excessive or unreasonable. (note: this does not apply to children)

C. The obsessions or compulsions cause marked distress, are time consuming (take more than 1 hr a day), or significantly interfere with the person's normal routine, occupational/academic functioning, or usual social activities or relationships

D. If another axis I disorder is present, the content of the obsessions or compulsions is not restricted to it (e.g., preoccupation with drugs in the presence of a substance abuse disorder)

E. The disturbance is not due to the direct physiologic effects of a substance (e.g., drug abuse, a medication) or a general medical condition

(Diagnostic and Statistical Manual-IV. Washington DC: American Psychiatric Association Press, 1994.)

autoimmune neuropsychiatric disorder associated with streptococcal infection (PANDAS) should be considered in a child with prepubertal OCD and the acute fulminant onset/exacerbation of symptoms in association with a streptococcal infection. Other laboratory tests should be considered, if there is reason to suspect a developmental diathesis.

TREATMENT

The treatment of OCD includes three separate lines of intervention: (a) illness education; (b) cognitive-behavioral and other psychological therapies; and (c) psychopharmacological strategies.

Illness Education. Guiding the family to understand the nature of the illness, to structure the environment for the child, to enhance therapeutic interventions, and to provide information on course and prognosis are essential interventions in treating OCD. Since OCD tends to develop gradually and parents often have subclinical symptoms, treatment is often delayed. It is therefore often necessary to correct patterns of family accommodation which have been implemented to cope with the child's repetitive behaviors. Similarly, it must be recognized that aggressive behaviors or emotional outbursts may result from the inability to complete rituals in the home.

Cognitive-Behavioral Therapy (CBT). In recent years, CBT with an exposure-response prevention paradigm has been used successfully in children with OCD. A hierarchy of avoidance and ritualistic behaviors is formulated, and the child is guided to self-regulate anxiety and overcome fears while engaging in behaviors that counter the OCD symptoms. A map of behaviors is created with "territory" being conquered from OCD by the child. As the child overcomes his/her first OCD symptoms, renewed self-confidence and decreased anxiety ensue, and major symptoms can be then confronted in a planned fashion. Prognostic factors for the success of CBT in children with OCD include greater insight, older age, fewer comorbid conditions, and the absence of strong oppositional traits. Psychodynamic and family therapy approaches may provide further support to address internal conflicts and developmental issues in the child and highly emotional family environments.

Pharmacological Interventions. Pharmacological trials have shown that drugs that increase serotonin in the synaptic clefts of cortico-subcortical-thalamic-cortical pathways, such as serotonin re-uptake inhibitors, improve OCD symptoms. In contrast, those that only affect norepinephrine do not improve OCD symptoms. Dopamine antagonists, including newer atypical neuroleptics, are useful in augmenting pharmacologic response when trials of serotonin augmenting agent have not been sufficient.

SSRIs. The original drug used to treat OCD was a non-selective reuptake inhibitor of serotonin, clomipramine (CMI; Anafranil). Given its nonselective properties, and concomitant side effects, it is currently a second-line agent, but is at least as effective as the newer SSRIs. CMI has FDA approval for use in children with OCD. There are several SSRIs currently available for use in OCD; these include fluoxetine (Prozac), fluvoxamine (Luvox), paroxetine (Paxil), sertraline (Zoloft), and citalopram (Celexa) (Table 2). Fluoxetine, fluvoxamine, and sertraline have undergone double-blind clinical trials in children and have FDA approval for use

Table 2 Psychotropics in Obsessive-Compulsive Disorder in Children and Adolescents

Medication	Final dose range	Indication	Most frequent side effects	Comments
SSRIs				
Fluoxetine (Prozac)	10–40 mg	First-line agent	Nausea, diarrhea, dry mouth, anorexia, insomnia, headaches (all); hyperkinesia/agitation, urinary frequency (children)	FDA-approved in children
Fluvoxamine (Luvox)	25–150 mg	First-line agent	Insomnia, asthenia, diarrhea, hyperkinesia	FDA-approved in children
Sertraline (Zoloft)	25–200 mg	First-line agent	Nausea, diarrhea, insomnia, somnolence, fatigue, tremor, headaches	FDA-approved in children
Citalopram (Celexa)	10–40 mg	Alternative agent	Dry mouth, nausea, somnolence or insomnia, tachycardia, weight changes, polyuria	May have less frequentcy of side effects
Neuroleptics				
Haloperidol (Haldol)	0.25–2 mg	2 SSRIs not effective or severity warrants	Extrapyramidal syndrome (EPS), tardive dyskinesia, dystonia, dry mouth, akathisia	Add to first agent, used in tic-related OCD Monitor EPS
Risperidone (Risperdal)	0.25–2 mg	2 SSRIs not effective or severity warrants	Weight gain, EPS, drooling	Add to first agent Monitor weight
Pimozide (Orap)	0.5–2 mg	2 SSRIs not effective or severity warrants	EPS, tardive dyskinesia, dystonia, QTc prolongation	Add to first agent Monitor EKG
Tricyclics				
Clomipramine (Anafranil)	25–150 mg (3 mg/kg)	Single agent or SSRI augmentation	Dry mouth, constipation, blurry vision, somnolence, QTc prolongation	As effective or more than SSRIs; more side effects Monitor EKG

in children with OCD. Multiple clinical trials, both open label and double blind, have generally confirmed the utility of the other SSRIs to treat OCD in children. Few head-to-head comparisons among SSRIs in the treatment of OCD are available; one such study in adults showed that sertraline may produce a slightly faster and better response compared to fluoxetine. Recently, reports have surfaced of paroxetine causing suicidal ideation in pediatric depression, and this drug is not currently advised for new use in children. There is less clinical experience with citalopram in OCD compared to other agents. The main side effects of SSRIs in children, as in adults, include nausea, tiredness, nervousness, dizziness, and difficulty concentrating. Younger children may be more prone to behavioral activation and slow titration, as tolerated, is recommended. Activation and easy bruising for fluoxetine, tiredness for fluvoxamine, and tremor for sertraline may be more specific side effects to each drug.

Drug interactions with SSRIs are important to monitor. Fluoxetine uses the P-450 cytochrome system for its metabolism, with preference for the 2D6 variant; it has a long half-life and an active metabolite, nor-fluoxetine. Up to 5–10% of Caucasians and 1–2% of Asians may have slow metabolism of 2D6. Other drugs that use the 2D6 system are tricyclics, haloperidol, risperidone, amphetamines, venlafaxine, trazodone, codeine, and dextrometorphan. Fluvoxamine uses the 1A2 P-450 enzyme for its metabolism. Grapefruit juice, brussel sprouts, broccoli, and cabbage inhibit the 1A2 system and drugs that use this system include clomipramine, imipramine, clozapine, haloperidol, naprosen, acetaminophen, theophylline, and warfarin. Sertraline has a milder effect on the 2D6 system, but its effect on the 3A4 system requires monitoring with use of tricyclics, nefazodone, alprazolam, carbamazepine, erythromycin, lidocaine, and others.

Neuroleptic Augmentation. If a trial of two consecutive SSRIs does not produce significant clinical benefit, and symptoms continue to impair daily functioning, a neuroleptic (e.g., haloperidol), augmentation strategy may be indicated. Originally found to be helpful in tic-related subtypes of OCD, newer atypical neuroleptics (e.g., risperidone) have been found useful in neuroleptic augmentation both for tic- and non-tic-related OCD (Table 2).

Clomipramine Augmentation. Published case reports in adolescents show that CMI may be useful as a single agent or as an adjunct to the SSRI in select cases with poor response to traditional regiments. Care must be taken to monitor levels of CMI given metabolism interaction with most SSRIs.

Other Drugs Used in Augmentation. Drugs that have been found to be equal to placebo in OCD when used for augmentation include lithium (Lithobid) and buspirone (Buspar). Case reports point to possible usefulness of clonazepam (Klonopin).

Combination Treatment. A combination of CBT and psychopharmacology approaches is indicated in moderate–severe OCD. An assessment of family resources, coping mechanisms in the child, psychiatric comorbidity, and susceptibility risk factors should guide the decision to use combined modalities of treatment.

PROGNOSIS

There are few long-term outcome studies in childhood OCD. A waxing and waning course with metamorphosis of symptoms over time is not uncommon. In small clinic-based studies, up to one-third of children initially treated are symptom free on follow-up years later. Results appear to be similar for medication- and psychotherapy-treated patients.

SUMMARY

Obsessive-compulsive disorder is a condition with frequent onset in childhood. Neurobiological research shows that OCD is a brain-based condition with neuropsychiatric correlates. Interventions include illness education of the family, cognitive-behavioral therapy, and use of pharmacologic strategies. Prognosis can be favorable with early, directed intervention.

SUGGESTED READINGS

1. Bergeron R, Ravindran AV, Chaput Y, Goldner E, Swinson R, van Ameringen MA, Austin C, Hadrava VJ. Sertraline and fluoxetine treatment of obsessive-compulsive disorder: results of a double-blind, 6-month treatment study. Clin Psychopharmacol 2002; 22:148–154.
2. Cook EH, Wagner KD, March JS, Biederman J, Landau P, Wolkow R, Messig M. Long-term sertraline treatment of children and adolescents with obsessive-compulsive disorder. J Am Acad Child Adolesc Psychiatry 2001; 40(10):1175–1181.
3. Grados MA, Riddle MA. Pharmacological treatment of childhood obsessive-compulsive disorder: from theory to practice. J Clin Child Psychol 2001; 30:67–79.
4. Leonard HL, Swedo Se, Rapoport JL, Koby EV, Lenane MC, Cheslow DL, Hamburger SD. Treatment of obsessive-compulsive disorder with clomipramine and desipramine in children and adolescents. A double-blind cross-over comparison study. Arch Gen Psychiatry 1989; 46:1088–1092.
5. March JS, Franklin M, Nelson A, Foa E. Cognitive-behavioral psychotherapy for pediatric obsessive-compulsive disorder. J Clin Child Psychol 2001; 30(1):8–18.
6. McDougle CJ, Epperson CN, Pelton GH, Wasylink S, Price LH. A double-blind, placebo-controlled study of risperidone addition in serotonin reuptake inhibitor-refractory obsessive-compulsive disorder. Arch Gen Psychiatry 2000; 57:794–801.
7. Miguel EC, do Rosario-Campos MC, Prado HS, do Valle R, Rauch SL, Coffey BJ, Baer L, Savage CR, O'Sullivan RL, Jenike MA, Leckman JF. Sensory phenomena in obsessive-compulsive disorder and Tourette's disorder. J Clin Psychiatry 2000; 61(2):150–156.
8. Riddle MA, Reeve EA, Yaryura-Tobias JA, Yang HM, Claghorn JL, Gaffney G, Greist JH, Holland D, McConville BJ, Pigott T, Walkup JT. Fluvoxamine for children and adolescents with obsessive-compulsive disorder: a randomized, controlled, multicenter trial. J Am Acad Child Adolesc Psychiatry 2001; 40:222–229.

68
Learning Disabilities

Martha Bridge Denckla
Johns Hopkins University School of Medicine, Kennedy Krieger Institute, Baltimore, Maryland, U.S.A.

INTRODUCTION

Consultation for the possible diagnosis of a learning disability (LD) is far less common than one for attention deficit hyperactivity disorder (ADHD) and/or developmental motor coordination disorder (DMCD). Nevertheless, because of a substantial overlap (about a third either way) between LD and ADHD, and because superficially diagnosed ADHD may actually be secondary to LD, the clinician must know how to evaluate for LD in all "school problem" referrals. Unfortunately, the "official" manner in which educational and legal systems define LD differs from state to state depending on variations in statistical comparisons of aptitude and achievement scores. In general, however, the term implies a significant deficit in learning relative to expectations based on intellectual ability, not explained by environment or psychological symptoms. While mention is sometimes made of "underlying psychological processes," even after aptitude-achievement discrepancies are judged statistically significant, these descriptors of the student are remote from concepts in cognitive neuroscience/neuropsychology. Additionally, the roles of subcategories of DMCD in various aspects of child development (e.g., handwriting, neatness of appearance, ability to participate in sports or music or art) should be of special concern to the pediatric neurologist, whose training equips him or her to appreciate the motor status of the student in ways that other specialities do not.

DIAGNOSIS

Establishment of the diagnosis of DMCD and/or ADHD does not rule out comorbid LD. Absence of motor inadequacies/anomalies and/or unconvincing history of any type of ADHD, however, should heighten and sharpen the suspicion that LD are more likely the central issue(s). Most LD are language based, running the gamut from the subtle phonological "tin ear" of the "pure dyslexic" to the more common, moderately linguistically impaired "expressive word-finding" type. Rarely, one will also identify a receptively impaired student who has managed to elude diagnosis. Any suspicion (whether from history or during visit) concerning possible

Table 1 Some Tests to Identify Children at Risk for Dyslexia (Reading Disability)[a]

1. Comprehensive Test of Phonological Processing (C-TOPP) (For five years of age through adult)
2. Lindamood Auditory Conceptualization (LAC) (For kindergarten through sixth grade)
3. Test of Phonological Awareness (TOPA) (For kindergarten through second grade)
4. The Phonological Awareness Test (PAT)[a] (For five, six, and seven years of age)

[a] Available from LinguiSystems; others (1, 2, 3) available from PRO-ED, Inc.

articulation, word pronunciation (even malapropisms), word-finding hesitations, circumlocutions, or incomprehension of instructions/directions should lead to a referral for speech/language evaluation, preferably outside of the school system. Parental concerns about underachievement in reading, mathematics, or written composition, even if already dismissed by school personnel as insignificant, should trigger referral to an evaluator or evaluation team experienced in finding the evidence of specific neurocognitive weaknesses.

Subtypes

With the exception of basic reading disability and the manual aspects of handwriting, diagnosis of LD is predominantly psychoeducational. The diagnosis of mathematics disability is made superficially on the basis of achievement unexpectedly discrepant from aptitude and/or other school achievement. Reading disability, to which many (but not all) equate the term developmental dyslexia, is currently diagnosed primarily on the basis of tests of phonological (speech sound) processing and secondarily by rapid naming tests (Table 1). Conventionally, intelligence/aptitude must be within normal limits, but the trend is away from discrepancy formulae and towards documentation of the underlying phonolinguistic deficit(s). Visual processing remains a research issue, but which has been dislodged from any central position is diagnosis; certainly, letter and word reversals are currently considered trivial epiphenomena. Criteria for the diagnosis of reading comprehension disability or written expression disability remain unclear. Spelling, while entering into written expression, currently functions as a side-issue or an output-side manifestation of the phonological processing deficit underlying reading disability; for decades, the term dyslexia has implied both reading and spelling impairment. Although, not strictly defined as LD, spoken developmental language disorder (DLD) should be considered whenever the diagnosis of dyslexia is at issue. Either the medical practitioner needs to screen for aural comprehension (of sentences with syntax not just single words) or be sure to refer for psychoeducational testing by a neuropsychologist.

ACCOMMODATIONS AND THERAPY

General

Guiding choices among therapeutic interventions and recommending accommodations that substantially alter the academic atmosphere are the major contributions to intervention of the medical clinician. For example, when selecting an evidence-based reading–remediation program, it is crucial to be guided by the individual child's "assets" in graphomotor (handwriting) and/or speech–articulatory skills.

Simply put, advice is needed in order to avoid the frustration engendered by attempting to compensate for phonological weakness by putting emphasis on another weakness! Accommodations, especially those providing extended time (and reduced load, its logical reciprocal) and technological detours around handwriting "pain and suffering," are all important because they provide opportunities to make academic progress, experience success, and keep alive both hope and courage for the bright LD student.

Motor Issues

With pressure for earlier handwriting (even as young as age three years) and with much of the recently increased homework load consisting of written exercises, it has become important for medical practitioners to become diagnosticians not only of motor anomalies but often of the neurodevelopmental motor status of young children. Physicians need to know (and to inform educators) that pencil grasp is the observable result of the neurodevelopmental "readiness" of the child, no matter how often corrected or given physically modified writing implements.

Slow-for-age, qualitatively dysrhythmic or mis-sequenced fingers-to-thumb performance is robustly correlated with poor handwriting; so also are the subtle postural instabilities seen on examination as choreiform movements, elicited on sustained posture tasks and seen in the wavering line quality of simple from copies (Table 2). These "minor" neurodevelopmental signs justify graphomotor accommodations; often the use of word processing but avoiding a requirement for "proper keyboarding" or finger sequencing.

Dyslexia

Specific educational interventions addressing phonological processing and the sound-symbol (phoneme–grapheme) code, such as "sounding out" programs, have resulted in dramatic gains in basic reading skills in children with dyslexia. All such successful interventions are systematic, explicit, and build upon phoneme awareness to establish phoneme–grapheme correspondences. Programs differ in terms of what sensorimotor linkages are used to reinforce the grapheme–phoneme connection (Table 3). Much less is established about the effects of other cognitive processes, which tutors of the dyslexic population bring to bear on reading comprehension, e.g., fluency, oral vocabulary and syntax, verbal working memory, and visual

Table 2 Neuromotor Signs of Diagnostic and Prognostic Utility in an LD Examination

- Overflow excess for age indicates inhibitory insufficiency, confirmatory of ADHD neurobiology
- Choreiform movements (unsteady hand) directly impair handwriting as an academic skill and as reading–remedial "multisensory" component
- Dysrhythmic/disorganized/mis-sequenced foot, hand, and finger patterned movement coordinations indicate likelihood of ADHD neurobiology (slow[a] feet discriminate ADHD best)
- Slow[a]/mis-sequenced fingers-successively-to-thumb performance highly predicts and correlates with impaired handwriting

[a] "Slow" requires PANESS timed motor administration with stopwatch and reference to PANESS age-specific norms.

Table 3 Principles of Intervention for Children With Dyslexia (Reading Disability)

- Start intense help early and keep help at some level of maintenance/monitoring
- Intensity means frequent sessions (e.g., four per week), tiny groups or individual (even better), and at least 1.5 school years in duration
- Quality control the instructors' credentials and the evidence-based nature of the reading program, e.g., Orton-Gillingham exemplified by Wilson Reading System, Lindamood Phoneme Sequencing Program, among others

imagery. Treating "dyslexia" alone when it occurs within a broader/deeper language disorder is a major diagnostic failure and results in poor outcomes.

PROGNOSIS

Published literature on outcomes is limited in scope, both of sampling populations and the endpoints of quality-of-life outcome. There is no definite knowledge about mental health morbidity or mortality, although one respected research center has reported unexpectedly gloomy data on depression (and suicide) in a well-educated and high-income-earning adult follow-up group. It is probable that until diagnosis becomes more biologically grounded, we will have difficulty interpreting prognostic associations with what we now call "comorbidities." Factors frequently associated with positive outcomes appear to be the predictable interdependent ones including robust aptitude or measured intelligence and socioeconomic advantage. These overarching "covariates" are also highly correlated with the availability of optimal interventions, currently rarely available within the majority of public schools, despite the about-to-be reauthorized (but still unfunded) federal mandate for appropriate special education.

SUMMARY

Over the past two decades, research relevant to understanding learning disabilities, particularly reading disability or "dyslexia," has made much progress aided by improved cognitive neuroscience and neuroimaging. Translation into intervention is in its infancy, except for the basic steps involved in reading, and even that restricted (early educational) range has only recently been informed by evidence. Even greater than the gap between brain research and knowledge about intervention is the gap between what is known and what is implemented in schools. A frustration for clinicians advocating for patients with LDs is that the most important interventions must be implemented outside the sphere of influence of medicine, in the zone where health and education overlap. Pressures to over-emphasize the diagnosis of ADHD (even when it is legitimate comorbidity of LD) and to exaggerate the benefits of stimulant medication (even when this is a legitimate part of a multifaceted intervention program) converge upon the medical clinician not only from schools but also from desperate parents. Clinicians and educators must join together in the use of biomedical research methods to establish the nature of LD as well as provide evidence for effective interventions.

SUGGESTED READINGS

1. Denckla MB. In: Feinberg TE, Farah MJ, eds. The Neurobehavioral Examination in Children. 2d ed. Chapter 61, Part 9. New York: McGraw-Hill 2003:765–771.
2. Fisher SE, DeFries JC. Developmental dyslexia: genetic dissection of a complex cognitive trait. Nat Rev Neurosci 2002; 30:767–780.
3. Shavelson R, Towne L, eds. Scientific Research in Education. Washington, DC: National Academies Press (www.nap.edu), 2002.
4. The Report of the National Reading Panel. Teaching Children to Read: An Evidence-Based Assessment of the Scientific Research Literature and Its Implications for Reading Instruction. Washington, DC: U.S. Department of Health and Human Services, Public Health Service, National Institutes of Health, National Institute of Child Health and Human Development, 2000.

69
Behavioral Interventions

Dana D. Cummings
Kennedy Krieger Institute, Baltimore, Maryland, U.S.A.

INTRODUCTION

Behavioral interventions can be broadly divided into two categories: the management of disruptive behaviors and pain management. Approaches should be planned and implemented in consultation with a psychologist experienced in behavioral treatment. Parent/patient education, longitudinal follow up, and a consistent approach are keys to the success of these techniques. Behavioral treatments can be used in isolation or as a means to maximize the effectiveness of pharmacotherapy. Interventions based on the principles of applied behavioral analysis, including operant conditioning, can be effective in ameliorating oppositional and disruptive behaviors, aggression, inattention, academic difficulties, impulsivity, deficiencies in communication skills, self-injurious behavior, and sleep problems. Relaxation training in conjunction with biofeedback techniques can be successful in treating chronic pain syndromes such as migraine.

Benefits of a behavior intervention program are far more likely to occur when a therapeutic alliance exists among physician, behavioral psychologist, educational specialists, school teachers, and family. Families face multiple challenges and to persist with a behavioral intervention program requires frequent encouragement and a consistent approach. Caregivers must also have realistic expectations for the child's behavioral progress. The behavioral psychologist has a critical role and should provide the treatment program, frequent follow up, and feedback regarding progress. The physician should support interventions of the behavioral psychologist by repeatedly emphasizing the importance of behavior interventions. For example, in children with attention-deficit hyperactivity disorder (ADHD), parents are often eager to start pharmacotherapy, but less willing to pursue concurrent behavior interventions and regular follow up with a psychologist. In some situations, it may be necessary for the physician to "contract" with the family and not provide pharmacotherapy unless behavior interventions are also pursued. Occasionally, a family's lack of enthusiasm for a behavioral intervention program may result from financial concerns due to the failure of health insurance companies to reimburse services provided by behavioral psychologists. The specific goals of the behavioral intervention program and its finite duration should be emphasized to both the family and health insurance providers.

In this author's opinion the Multimodal Treatment Study of Children with ADHD (MTA) serves as a model for effective behavior interventions. The MTA behavior modification program began with parent training and a child-focused intensive summer program that included group-based interventions, social skills training, and reinforcement of appropriate classroom behavior. The school year program included biweekly teacher consultation focused on classroom behavior management and regular contact with a behavioral therapist aide who reinforced skills learned in the summer program. This approach provided additional benefits compared to medication treatment alone for oppositional/aggressive behaviors, internalizing symptoms, teacher-rated social skills, parent–child relations, and reading achievement. Improvements in parental attitudes and disciplinary practices were major components of the success attributed to this behavior modification treatment protocol.

In situations where the services of a behavioral psychologist are not available to the family, it may be necessary for the physician to provide a plan as well as to make suggestions for how the family can conduct behavioral interventions. Because education of the family cannot be overemphasized, a list of parent resources are provided and basic concepts of a behavior modification programs are reviewed.

BEHAVIOR MODIFICATION

Basic Principles

Behavior modification includes interventions that increase the frequency of desirable behaviors and/or decrease the frequency of undesirable behaviors. Selection of an appropriate behavior modification protocol requires identification of desirable and undesirable behaviors and the identification of the situations in which behaviors occur (antecedents). The selection of an appropriate behavioral modification protocol, often referred to as applied behavior analysis, necessitates data collection through direct observation of behavior, self-report and caregiver questionnaires, and structured interviews and checklists. It is also strongly recommended that a child's functional ability be evaluated prior to initiating behavioral intervention in order to ensure appropriate programming. The behavioral intervention program should be periodically assessed to determine its effectiveness.

Positive reinforcement occurs when the behavior is encouraged to repeat itself. *Positive reinforcers* are the specific factors that encourage the individual to increase the frequency of the desired behavior. Positive reinforcers may include personal praise, activities involving joint participation (playing games or reading together), or the receipt of tangible rewards such as toys and food. Since positive reinforcers can only be defined based on the child's behavior, caregiver's knowledge of the child's preferences can be valuable in their selection. The effectiveness of each positive reinforcer depends on a consistent delivery. The shorter the time span between the targeted behavior and the delivery of the reinforcer, the more effective the positive reinforcement. Positive reinforcers should also be varied to enhance their novelty and effectiveness, e.g., trading points for different reinforcers. As caregivers become more skilled in positive reinforcement techniques, it should be possible to recognize situations in which they unintentionally provide positive reinforcement for maladaptive behaviors such as "whining."

Negative reinforcement is a process in which a desired behavior leads to avoidance, removal, or cessation of an adversive stimulus or *negative reinforcer.* Hence, in order to decrease the frequency or stop the presentation of the negative reinforcer, the child increases the targeted behavior. *Punishment* is a process in which either an imposed penalty or withdrawal of a positive reinforcer results in the decreased frequency of a behavior. Punishment can be used to immediately suppress an inappropriate behavior, but it should only be used in conjunction with other methods including positive and negative reinforcement. While punishment helps the child learn what inappropriate behavior is, positive and negative reinforcement emphasize appropriate behavior. In general, without a caring, affectionate, and supportive relationship, punishment interventions may actually provide positive reinforcement of inappropriate behavior. The physician/therapist must carefully monitor the caregivers' punishment procedures to assure they do not constitute child abuse. *Extinction* is defined as the consistent withholding of positive reinforcement during inappropriate behaviors or the planned ignoring of inappropriate behaviors such as "whining." As many parents can attest, extinction typically results in an initial increase in the inappropriate behavior. Nevertheless, parents and other caregivers should be encouraged to persevere through this initial escalation of inappropriate behavior and subsequent "testing."

Interventions in Language and Communication Disorders

Behavior modification can also be applied to enhance communication skills in children with mental retardation, autistic spectrum, and developmental language disorders. Skinner's analysis of language in *Verbal Behavior* (1957) serves as a framework for behavioral interventions in language and communication skills. In children with neurologic disorders accompanied by deficits in language and communication, improvement in communication skills often results in improvement of neurobehavioral problems including aggression, self-injury, and other disruptive behaviors. Therefore, whenever possible, a behavioral intervention program in this group of children should combine positive reinforcement, to enhance language skills, with interventions to improve neurobehavioral disorders. For example, in children with severe mental retardation accompanied by communication deficits and severe destructive behavior, a combination of positive reinforcement of communicative responses and extinction and/or punishment for inappropriate behavior is often more effective than individual behavioral interventions.

RELAXATION TRAINING AND BIOFEEDBACK

Stress can often exacerbate neurologic disorders including headache, chronic pain, and sleep disturbances. There are few studies in pediatric populations to guide physicians, but recent work supports the application of *relaxation training* in children with disorders including tension and migraine headache. Relaxation training techniques are varied and include autogenic training, meditation, progressive muscle relaxation, and paced or deep breathing. In *autogenic training*, the subject imagines a peaceful setting while focusing on a comforting body sensation such as coolness in the forehead or warmth in the limbs. In *progressive muscle relaxation*, the individual systematically tenses and relaxes muscle groups, while focusing on contrasting sensations accompanying muscle tension and relaxation. To aid training, younger children are instructed to use mental imagery along with muscle tension and relaxation.

Although younger children with average cognitive ability may be able to comply with directives, the utility of these types of interventions may not generalize beyond the training environment. Because relaxation training is a treatment technique based on the assumption of at least average cognitive ability, young and/or cognitively impaired individuals may have extreme difficulty learning the technique, understanding why they are doing it, and carry it out beyond the training environment. Furthermore, cognitive techniques are very dependent on the ability of the individual to think about their difficulties and process ways to ameliorate them.

Relaxation training is often used in conjunction with biofeedback to either enhance relaxation training or to alter autonomic nervous system function. Biofeedback involves the use of monitoring equipment to show internal physiological events in the form of visual or auditory signals. These displayed signals, in turn, enable modification of otherwise involuntary or unfelt events. Examples of monitoring equipment include thermometry, electromyography, anorectal manometry, and heart rate or blood pressure monitors. Biofeedback has been used to treat pediatric neurologic disorders ranging from fecal incontinence accompanying myelomeningocele to migraine headaches. For migraine headaches, the child completes four to six one hour training sessions over a six week period, each consisting of progressive muscle relaxation, deep breathing techniques, age-appropriate stress management skills, and thermal biofeedback training. It is important that the child understand the rationale for intervening in the headaches because nonspecific treatment benefits maybe affected by patient-rated "credibility" of the treatment. During training, the child is encouraged to practice biofeedback-assisted relaxation at least 15 min daily at home as well as at the time of headache onset. Thermal biofeedback consists of warming the hands to increase skin temperature, measured by a biofeedback thermometer reading to a designated point. Biofeedback-assisted hand warming has been correlated with an increase in hemispheric cerebral blood flow and improvement in headache symptoms. However, since improvements in headache severity and frequency have also occurred with "hand-cooling" biofeedback, the therapeutic benefit of thermal biofeedback-assisted relaxation training maybe nonspecific. Improvement has also been speculated to be related to development of a sense of control or empowerment accompanying success in regulating hand temperature.

Relaxation training and biofeedback techniques are best implemented in collaboration with a psychologist experienced in these techniques. Initial training sessions include learning relaxation techniques and the use of biofeedback instrumentation. Ongoing educational aids, such as instructional audio recordings and periodic retraining are beneficial.

ADDITIONAL READINGS

1. Hughes JN. Cognitive Behavior Therapy with Children in Schools. New York: Pergamon Press, 1988.
2. Kazdin AE. Behavior Modification in Applied Settings. 5th ed. Pacific Grove, CA: Brooks/Cole Publishing Company, 1994.
3. Kerr MM, Nelson CM. Strategies for Managing Behavior Problems in the Classroom. 3d ed. Upper Saddle River, NJ: Merrill, 1998.
4. Mercugliano M, Power TJ, Blum NJ. The Clinician's Practical Guide to Attention-Deficit/Hyperactivity Disorder. PH Brookes Publishing, 1999.
5. Parrish JM. Child behavior. In: Levine MD, Carey WB, Crocker AC, eds. Developmental-Behavioral Pediatrics. 3d ed. Saunders, 1999:767–780.

6. Scharff L, Marcus DA, Masek BJ. A controlled study of minimal-contact thermal biofeedback treatment in children with migraine. J Pediatr Psychol 2002; 27(2):109–119.
7. Schwartz M. Biofeedback. 2d ed. A Practitioner's Guide. Guilford Press, 1998.
8. The MTA Cooperative Group. A 14-month randomized clinical trial of treatment strategies for attention-deficit/hyperactivity disorder. Arch Gen Psychiatry 1999; 56:1073–1086.

FAMILY RESOURCES

1. Barkley R. Taking Charge of ADHD, Revised Edition: The Complete, Authoritative Guide for Parents. Guilford Press, 2000.
2. Ozonoff S, Dawson G, McPartland. A Parent's Guide to Asperger Syndrome and High-Functioning Autism. Guilford Press, 2002.

70
Interpretation of Neuropsychological Testing

E. Mark Mahone
Department of Neuropsychology, Kennedy Krieger Institute, Baltimore, Maryland, U.S.A.

INTRODUCTION

The primary aim of this chapter is to provide an understanding of the indications, components, and expectations of neuropsychological testing. The neuropsychological examination provides the clinician with an additional method for diagnosing neurodevelopmental, neurodegenerative, and acquired disorders of brain function. It should be considered a valuable addition to the overall neurodiagnostic assessment that includes other techniques such as the neurological examination and appropriate laboratory tests. The goal of the neuropsychological examination is to assess the clinical relationship between the central nervous system and a behavioral dysfunction. The Social Security Administration defines neuropsychological testing as the administration of standardized tests that are reliable and valid with respect to assessing impairment in brain functioning. Procedurally, neuropsychological services are designated as *medicine, diagnostic* by the federal Health Care and Financing Administration (HCFA), and are subsumed under *Central Nervous System Assessments* in the CPT 2002 Code Book, with corresponding ICD diagnoses. The American Academy of Neurology has rated neuropsychological assessment as *Established* with Class II evidence, and a Type A recommendation. In contrast to a clinical psychological evaluation, the neuropsychological assessment is not a primary mental health/psychiatric service and does not use corresponding DSM IV diagnostic codes.

Neuropsychological examinations are performed by qualified specialists who have undergone intensive training in the clinical neurosciences, including inter-relationship among behavioral functions and neuroanatomy, neurology, and neurophysiology. Pediatric neuropsychologists have additional training and experience in the application of developmental and neuropsychological principles to children with neurological disorders. They typically work closely with consulting pediatric physicians and surgeons in the assessment of a child's neurological development and cerebral status. Neuropsychological examinations are clinically indicated and medically necessary for children with known congenital or acquired neurological disorders and for those suspected of these conditions. Referral should be made for children who display signs or symptoms of cognitive and/or neurobehavioral dysfunction that involve attention or memory deficits, language disorders, learning disabilities, neuromotor impairment, developmental disabilities, pervasive developmental disorders, impairment of organization and planning, and perceptual abnormalities.

OVERVIEW OF PEDIATRIC NEUROPSYCHOLOGICAL ASSESSMENT

The goal of the neuropsychological assessment is to understand a child's current functioning, predict future needs, and provide appropriate recommendations. The examination of the child involves the dynamic integration of information from a thorough history, observation in multiple settings, and the use of standardized psychometric tests. The child's performance on formal tests and standardized observations of behavior is then compared to available normative data for age and sex. Often, the actual tests used in neuropsychological examinations are identical to those used by clinical or school psychologists, including measures of intellectual functioning, academic achievement, language competence, attention, memory, or perceptual/motor skills (Table 1). There is little about the tests themselves that make an examination "neuropsychological." Rather, it is the way tests are interpreted, including the process by which children obtain their scores, which is different in a neuropsychological examination. The pediatric neuropsychologist seeks to gain a fuller understanding of how and why a child is having cognitive and behavioral problems, and, using history, observations and testing, makes inferences about brain development.

The neuropsychological examination in many ways parallels that of a physical examination, and involves a review of neurobehavioral systems or domains, Pediatric neuropsychologists typically assess the following domains in a comprehensive assessment: (1) intelligence; (2) adaptive/self-help skills; (3) academic achievement; (4) emotional status and personality; (5) language and language-related processes (especially those skills crucial for the development of reading and writing); (6) attention and executive functions; (7) memory and learning; (8) visuospatial, visuoperceptual, and visuoconstructional skills; (9) sensory and perceptual skills; and (10) neuromotor skills and praxis. In addition to performance-based assessment, neuropsychologists also use structured interviews as well as caregiver and teacher rating scales to augment the office assessment, and add to the ecological validity of the conclusions that can be drawn. The age and functional level of the child and the availability of standardized instruments often determine how extensively these domains can be assessed. Some domains (particularly the sensory perceptual examination) are difficult and often unreliable in children under age 9, and are often omitted in this age group. Application of neuropsychological principles to children requires more than "downsizing" adult models, theories and tests to children. While the majority of our early knowledge about brain–behavior relationships was based on observations of adults with acquired lesions, direct application of these models to children is inappropriate because they have developing brains. Early neurological insults can change the course of learning and the availability of systems to learn new skills.

The essential question in the adult neuropsychological assessment is location of the lesion, and secondarily, the type of lesion or disorder. In children, there is often no focal lesion, but rather a disruption of overall brain development, typically affecting multiple neurobehavioral systems. Thus, the critical concepts for understanding neurobehavioral processes in children are: *what* processes are disrupted (e.g., cell migration, myelination), *when* were these processes were disrupted, *when* is the child assessed, and lastly, *where* is the lesion. The impact of atypical brain development in children is affected by timing, chronicity, prior development, and development not yet completed at time of insult. In children, development is not a linear process. Rather there are critical periods that involve rapid development of skills and simultaneously great periods of vulnerability.

CHALLENGES FOR THE CONCEPTUALIZATION AND DESCRIPTION OF VARIOUS CONDITIONS

The term *delay* signifies slower than expected development in one or more domains of behavior. While it does not imply cause, it carries the assumption (often incorrectly to parents) that the child will eventually catch up. Thus, use of the term "developmental delay" interchangeably with mental retardation in young children can be problematic and misleading. The term *deficit* refers to an absence of, or a significantly impaired performance, and should only be applied to children when referenced in comparison to clearly defined expectations for age. It usually implies that the child will remain significantly impaired in relation to peers in the identified area; in some cases, however, improvement in skill can be observed, especially in individuals in which the assessment was completed shortly postinsult (e.g., infection, trauma). *Deviant* behavior does not typically occur in the repertoire of normal children (e.g., self-injury, stereotypies), and is considered abnormal across settings and times. While some deviant behavior may improve (e.g., post-trauma), in other cases improvement is not expected. Parents and physicians often have concerns with regression or decline in functioning. In these instances, a neuropsychologist can provide objective information to differentiate a decline in relative standing to peers vs. a true *loss of skill*; done by comparing a child's raw score performance on one or more standardized tests to his/her score raw performance on the same tests at a later point in time. *Failure to keep pace* in skill acquisition in relation to peers is commonly observed in children with neurological disorders and is generally associated with increased environmental demands.

STEPS IN THE ASSESSMENT PROCESS

Step 1: Review of History. The medical history is essential to determine whether the lesion is static or unstable. Conditions such as cerebral palsy or Fragile X syndrome imply *static* neurological conditions, such that the underlying biologic problem causing the cognitive deficit is presumed to be stable, even if the functional outcome (based on interaction with the demands of the child's life) changes. Disorders considered to be potentially *unstable* (e.g., epilepsy, hydrocephalus) require closer or more frequent follow up and neuropsychological management. Conditions such as congenital HIV or neurodegenerative disorders can show true decline and loss of skill over time, while others such as traumatic brain injury are expected to show initial improvement in functioning. Multiple psychological assessments (especially IQ testing) can raise concerns about practice effects. Similarly, the presence of sensory and/or motor impairments can negatively impact test administration and results.

Table 1 A Selected List of Commonly Used Neuropsychological Tests for Children

Indication	Name	Ages	Interpretation/scales
Broad developmental assessment	NEPSY: A Developmental Neuropsychological Assessment	3–12	5 core domains: language, visuospatial, memory/learning, attention/executive, sensorimotor; supplementary scales; qualitative observations
	Woodcock–Johnson Tests of Cognitive Abilities and Achievement, Third Edition	2–90+ years	Broad cognitive abilities, broad range of academic achievement scales; English and Spanish versions
General intelligence	Wechsler Intelligence Scale for Children, Fourth Edition (WISC-IV)	6–16	Verbal comprehension, perceptual reasoning, working memory, processing speed indices; full scale IQ
	Stanford Binet, Fifth Edition (SB-V)	2–85+	5 factors (all with verbal and nonverbal domains): fluid reasoning, knowledge, quantitative reasoning, visual-spatial processing, working memory; IQ
Nonverbal intelligence	Leiter International Performance Scales-Revised (Leiter-R)	2–20	When English is not first language; language or hearing impaired; cultural deprivation
	Universal Nonverbal Intelligence Test (UNIT)	5–17	For individuals with speech/language impairment, different cultural backgrounds, or those who are verbally uncommunicative
Preschool intelligence	Wechsler Preschool and Primary Scale of Intelligence, Third Edition (WPPSI-III)	2.5–7.25	Verbal IQ, performance IQ, processing speed index, general language index, full scale IQ
Infant development	Bayley Scales of Infant Development-II	1–42 months	Mental, motor and behavior scales
	Mullen Scales of Early Learning	Birth to 68 months	Measures five areas of development: gross motor, fine motor, visual reception, receptive language, and expressive language.
Memory	Children's Memory Scale (CMS)	5–16	Visual and verbal memory and learning; attention, short and long delay memory
	Wide Range Assessment of Memory and Learning-2 (WRAML-2)	5–90	Verbal memory, visual memory, and attention/concentration indices
Executive functions	Delis–Kaplan Executive Function Scales (DKEFS)	8–89	Planning, organization, reasoning, set-shifting, inhibitory control, fluency
	Behavior Rating Inventory of Executive Functions (BRIEF)	5–18	Parent and teacher rating scales; eight scales: inhibit, shift, emotional control, working memory, initiate,plan/organize

			monitor, organization of materials; behavior regulation, metacognition, and global executive composite indices
Language	Clinical Evaluation of Language Functions, Fourth Edition (CELF-4)	5–21	Broad range of receptive and expressive language
	Preschool Language Scale, Fourth Edition (PLS-4)	Birth–6 years	Auditory comprehension, expressive communication, total language composite
Attention	Test of Everyday Attention for Children (TEA-Ch)	6–16	Selective, sustained, divided attention; attentional control/switching
	Conners' Continuous Performance Test-II (CPT-II)	6–adult	Sustained attention, inhibitory control
Visuospatial, visuoperceptual, visuoconstruction	Beery Developmental Tests of Visuomotor Integration	3–18	Three forms: motor control, visual perception, visuomotor integration (copying)
	Wide Range Assessment of Visual Motor Ability (WRAMVA)	3–17	Fine motor, visual–spatial, and visual motor abilities scales
Sensorimotor	Grooved Pegboard	5–adult	Motor coordination and speed
	Purdue Pegboard	3–70+	Finger and hand dexterity and speed
Adaptive skills	Vineland Adaptive Behavior Scales	Birth–adult	Communication, daily living skills, socialization, motor skills; adaptive skills composite
	Scales of Independent Behavior Revised (SIB-R)	Birth–adult	Motor skills, personal living skills, communication, community living skills; behavior problems scales
Academic skills	Wechsler Individual Achievement Test-II (WIAT-II)	5–85	Reading, math, written expression cores
	Wide Range Achievement Tests, Third Edition (WRAT-3)	5–75	Three scales: reading, arithmetic and spelling; alternate forms
Behavior rating scales	Child Behavior Checklist (Parent, Teacher and Self-Report Forms)	6–18	Aggressive behavior, anxious/depressed, social problems, somatic complaints, attention problems, thought problems, withdrawn/depressed; internalizing/externalizing/total problems scales
	Conners' Rating Scales-Revised (Parent and Teacher Scales; CPRS-R, CTRS-R) Self report	3–17	Broad range of problem behavior in children and adolescents; assesses behaviors present in attention-deficit hyperactivity disorder (ADHD)

Step 2: Development of a Flexible Assessment Plan. Observation of *how* tasks are completed is essential in order to uncover the source of the problem and to consider implications for brain development and treatment. Early insults often lead to alternative neural pathways that can assume the affected function. The formulation of alternative pathways affects not only the target function, but also those for which the compensating structures were originally intended. The neuropsychologist can provide observations both on the adequacy of the product and how the child goes about accomplishing the task. Depending on the purpose and type of assessment, the consulting neuropsychologist can devise a flexible assessment battery that efficiently reviews each relevant neurobehavioral domain (Table 2).

Step 3: Interpretation. The neuropsychologist interprets findings in a way that has maximal impact for the treatment team, keeping in mind the specific referral question, and the framework of long-term behavioral support. Patterns of observations and test scores in children are interpreted with regard to what is known about

Table 2 Types of Pediatric Neuropsychological Assessment

Type	Format	When used	Purpose
Baseline	Broad-based, comprehensive	Early in life, infancy/preschool; immediately after identification of neurological condition	Establish general approach and context for intervention; document initial functioning for planned future follow up
Planned follow up	Broad-based, comprehensive	Annually in preschool years; every 1–2 years during elementary school; prior to known academic or life stress points	Document changing needs associated with early neurological disorder; proactively assess needs prior to known times of increased academic and life skill demand
Screening	Brief, but covering major neurobehavioral domains; 15–20 min	With at risk populations; in schools with all students; inmedical clinic appointments	Briefly and efficiently document need for more comprehensive cognitive assessment; provide brief, frequent documentation of progress following comprehensive assessments
Problem focused	Focused on neurobehavioral domain of interest	Pre- and postmedical surgical or behavioral intervention	Document response to intervention; document askills/deficits present prior to intervention

the individual's brain development to date and the presence of potentially interfering behaviors (e.g., motor overflow, stimulus bound behavior) that impact test performance. Observed test scores should be considered only estimates of constructs (e.g., memory), and a variety of factors can reduce their accuracy. Attention problems can be observed secondary to a neurological disease or in the context of fatigue related to motor dysfunction. Atypical behaviors (e.g., stereotypies, self-injury, or compulsive behaviors observed in autism) can also interfere with the child's production of responses, and can lower test scores (relative to presumed ability). If the child's condition is considered static, statements can be provided about the child's trajectory relative to peers and discussion of prognosis. If the child's condition is unstable, statements can be made about cognitive stability and the need for additional intervention. Longitudinal data are often required.

Step 4: Recommendations. After providing recommendations for the child's current situation, the neuropsychologist should be able to make recommendations on what is expected over the next several years using his/her understanding of the child's current brain functioning. Additionally, information on long-term prognosis can be provided based on knowledge of upcoming environmental challenges. Specific recommendations for the home environment can include those regarding the need for supervision and independence. Recommendations for school made at the start of elementary classes often need to be amended around fourth grade (to take into account the increased reading and writing demands of the daily school schedule), and again around sixth grade as the emphasis on organization and self-study skills increases. Results of neuropsychological testing can be used to determine the intensity of special education services (especially the need for extended school year), and to define the need for pharmacotherapy, family respite, and appropriate leisure activities. Often, children with neurological disorders and associated cognitive problems are eligible for special education services under the "Other Health Impaired" category.

SUMMARY

Children with neurological disorders have dynamic cognitive and behavioral profiles, calling for flexible management. Frequently, these children have longstanding disabilities, requiring interdisciplinary and multidisciplinary approaches for assessment and intervention. While many of these children have considerable impairments, a thorough neuropsychological assessment can be helpful in pinpointing strengths and weaknesses and planning appropriate interventions. While many individuals have static "lesions," the impact of the CNS impairment can change throughout the child's life. A developmental framework to neuropsychological assessment is essential, and the pediatric neuropsychologist should be considered an important part of the child's interdisciplinary treatment team.

WEBSITES

http://www.nanonline.org/downloads/paio/NANPedNeuroPhy.pdf
http://www.nanonline.org/downloads/paio/NANPedNeuroPar.pdf
http://www.ssa.gov/disability/professionals/bluebook/ChildhoodListings.htm
http://www.nanonline.org/content/pages/prof/houston.shtm

SUGGESTED READINGS

1. American Medical Association. CPT: Current Procedural Terminology. Chicago: AMA Press, 2002:368.
2. Baron IS. The Neuropsychological Evaluation of the Child. New York: Oxford University Press, 2004.
3. Bernstein JH, Waber D. Developmental neuropsychological assessment: the systemic approach. In: Boulton A, Baker G, Hiscock M, eds. Neuromethods: Neuropsychology. New Jercy:Humana Press, 1990:311–371.
4. Denckla MB. The neurobehavioral examination in children. In: Feinberg TE, Farah ME, eds. Behavioral Neurology and Neuropsychology. New York: McGraw-Hill Professional, 1996.
5. Simeonssen RJ, Rosenthal SL. Psychological and Developmental Assessment: Children With Disabilities and Chronic Conditions. New York: Guilford Press, 2001.
6. Spreen O, Strauss E. A Compendium of Neuropsychological Tests. New York: Oxford University Press, 1998.
7. Yeates KO, Ris MD, Taylor HG. Pediatric Neuropsychology: Research, Theory, and Practice. New York: Guilford Press, 2000.

71
Autism Spectrum Disorders

Andrew W. Zimmerman
Kennedy Krieger Institute, Baltimore, Maryland, U.S.A.

INTRODUCTION

Autism spectrum disorders (ASDs) are common heterogeneous neurobehavioral syndromes that result from abnormal neural development and present before 3 years of age. Known etiologies are detectable in up to 10% of patients, although the causes in most children are still unknown. Children typically present with the triad of delayed or disordered language development, abnormal social relatedness, and repetitive odd behaviors. Autistic symptoms and cognitive deficits vary widely among patients in their age of onset, severity, and clinical course. Regression in previously acquired language and social skills occurs in approximately 30%, usually between 18 and 24 months. "Classic" or Kanner-type autism is grouped with other ASDs (or pervasive developmental disorders, PDDs, in DSM-IV), including Asperger syndrome and PDD/NOS (not otherwise specified). Childhood disintegrative disorder and Rett syndrome are related disorders that also have autistic symptoms.

Idiopathic autism is genetic; concordance for the broad autism spectrum in monozygotic twins is 90% and in dizygotic twins is 10%. The recurrence risk for a family with one child with autism is up to 9%. The disorders typically affect boys more than girls (4:1) and occur in all cultural and racial groups. The estimated incidence of ASDs is 1:250–1:500, and their prevalence appears to be increasing. However, this may result in part from broader definition and improved recognition of symptoms in recent years.

Neuropathological findings in autism postmortem brain tissue include altered neuronal populations in the limbic system, decreased Purkinje cells, altered cortical minicolumns, increased white matter and neuroglial activation. Most of the findings are consistent with abnormal developmental programs of prenatal onset. These altered programs could result in observations of altered neuropeptides at birth, accelerated brain growth during infancy and increased platelet serotonin. In addition to genetic influences, epigenetic and environmental factors may affect selectively vulnerable networks through multiple mechanisms. Several neurobiological processes have been implicated in the pathogenesis of autism, including abnormal neurotransmitters, experience-dependent synaptic plasticity, glutamate excitotoxicity, and neuroimmune mechanisms.

DIAGNOSIS AND EVALUATION (FIG. 1)

Initial detection and screening for ASDs take place through primary care practitioners, referral from infant and early childhood development programs, and therapists. Early detection is important because early intensive intervention improves outcomes for most children. An effective screening tool for autism is the Modified Checklist for Autism in Toddlers (M-CHAT). Clinical indictors for a more structured evaluation include: failure to point at objects with the intent to get another's attention (normally present at 12 months of age); impaired receptive and expressive language [e.g., failure to use single words by 18 months; 2-word phrases by 2 years; answer "what," "where," and "who" questions by 3 years; and the use of sustained high-pitched sounds ("eeeee") or echolalia]. An exception is Asperger syndrome, in which semantics are usually spared. Early signs of abnormal social relatedness may include difficulty engaging in "peek-a-boo" games, making and maintaining eye contact, and showing reciprocal emotion. The child may be affectionate on his or her own terms, or relate to older children and adults rather than peers. Children and adults with ASDs lack "theory of mind": they are unable to perceive the thoughts and feeling states of others. Repetitive and stereotyped behaviors may include an insistence on "sameness" without apparent meaning, such as waving the hands in the lateral visual fields, flapping the hands and ordering objects. Certain autistic behaviors, such as covering the ears, scratching the skin and repeating visual patterns, may result from abnormal neurophysiological processing of sensory inputs.

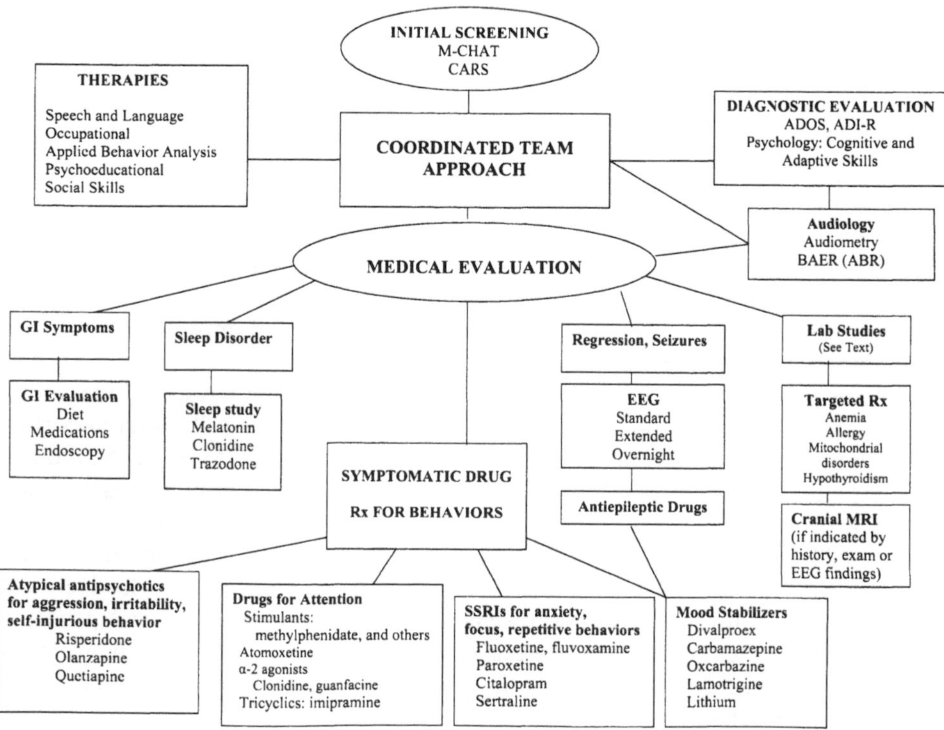

Figure 1 Evaluation and treatment of autism (see text for abbreviations).

Table 1 Conditions That May Be Concurrent with Autism Spectrum Disorders

1. Congenital hearing loss
2. Developmental language disorder
3. Genetic disorders: Down, Rett, fragile X, Williams syndromes
4. Phakomatoses: tuberous sclerosis, neurofibromatosis
5. Metabolic disorders: glutaric aciduria, phenylketonuria, mitochondrial disorders
6. Congenital infections: rubella, toxoplasmosis, cytomegalovirus
7. Seizures; generalized tonic clonic; Landau–Kleffner variant
8. Autoimmune disorders
9. Macrocephaly: familial megalencephaly, hydrocephalus
10. Movement disorders: Tourette syndrome, Sydenham chorea
11. Obsessive compulsive disorder
12. Bipolar disorder
13. ADHD

A preliminary impression of ASD in preschool children, based on observation and screening tests (e.g., M-CHAT or Childhood Autism Rating Scale, CARS), should be followed by a coordinated team evaluation (physician, speech and language pathologist and psychologist). The diagnosis is confirmed and further defined using the Autism Diagnostic Observation Schedule (ADOS) or Autism Diagnostic Interview-Revised (ADI-R), both of which are well standardized and are administered by specially trained testers. Evaluations should also include assessments of cognitive functions and adaptive skills. All children should have audiological, speech and language (SLT) and occupational therapy (OT) evaluations. It is important to rule out hearing loss using age-appropriate audiometric techniques or auditory evoked responses (BAER) if necessary. Structured behavioral therapies (e.g., applied behavioral analysis or ABA) should be considered for young children, with assisted programming based on psychological and educational testing in school aged children. Additional help with play or social skills groups may be needed.

The differential diagnosis of ASD includes over 100 known conditions (see partial list in Table 1). Many of these include "double syndromes," in which the phenotype of autism is associated with another disorder of known cause, such as tuberous sclerosis, Down's, and fragile X syndromes. It is important to note that "autism" by itself, in most cases, will not have an identifiable cause. Identification of a specific etiology can have important implications for prognosis and treatment, e.g., seizures and mitochondrial dysfunction.

The medical and neurological evaluations of ASD should include histories of the pre- and perinatal periods, early development, infections, gastrointestinal and immune functions, and seizures. The family history may reveal conditions concurrent with autism (Table 1) or elements of ASDs (such as difficulties with social or pragmatic language skills). The physical examination, often a challenge to perform, should be comprehensive as well as include direct observation of the child's communication and play behaviors, evaluation of receptive, expressive and social aspects of language, measurements of growth, notation of dysmorphic features and Wood's lamp exam.

LABORATORY TESTING

The extent of required laboratory testing in children with autism is uncertain, ranging from no studies to a comprehensive evaluation. In the author's opinion basic laboratory studies for children with ASDs should include complete blood count, serum chemistries (including AST/ALT and CK), red blood cell lead and thyroid function. Marginal or low hemoglobin levels occur frequently, especially in children with restricted food preferences. Genetic testing should include a karyotype, subtelomere screening by fluorescence in situ hybridization (FISH), and fragile X by DNA (in girls as well as boys).

If there has been regression of language and/or other skills, further testing of mitochondrial function is indicated, including fasting lactic acid, plasma amino and urinary organic acids. The ratio of alanine:lysine should normally be less than 3:1. An overnight or extended EEG study including deep natural sleep is also suggested to evaluate for seizure activity (atypical Landau–Kleffner syndrome). Other tests may be indicated for specific syndromes, such as 7-dehydrocholesterol for Smith–Lemli–Opitz syndrome, FISH for velocardiofacial syndrome and Angelman syndrome, transferrin electrophoresis for congenital disorders of glycosylation, 24 hr urinary uric acid for "purine autism," and serum ammonia levels. Cranial CT, SPECT, and MRI scans are generally not performed routinely, and should be reserved for those with special indications based on the history and neurological examination. Other imaging methods, such as PET, functional MRI and MR spectroscopy, are strictly research tools.

TREATMENT (FIG. 1)

Established therapies for autism should include individualized special school programs, speech and language and behavioral therapies in a setting that is coordinated, structured and predictable, as well as containing visual supports and high degrees of reinforcement. Beginning therapies early takes advantage of potential synaptic plasticity. Although most children improve, an individual child's trajectory for improvement varies over time. Outcomes for independent functioning correlate with attainment of functional language and adaptive skills by school age. Periodic, regular assessments should include cognitive, social skills and educational testing, in additional to SLT, OT, and occasionally physical therapy (PT).

Drug therapies for ASDs are symptomatic and chosen to improve short-term functions and behaviors, e.g., improved attention or reduced aggression to enable the child to remain in the classroom. There is no evidence to suggest that pharmacotherapy affects long-term outcomes. In individual cases, therapy targeted to the treatment of concurrent medical disorders, such as mitochondrial dysfunction, allergy, or hypothyroidism, can be beneficial. Children with gastrointestinal (GI) symptoms (recurrent loose stools or constipation in 50%) may benefit from GI evaluation and elimination diets (e.g., gluten and casein free). Sleep is disordered in 60% of ASD patients (more in young children), and abnormal REM arousals can be observed in sleep studies. Treatment with melatonin (up to 3 mg/day) or clonidine at bedtime (0.025–0.1 mg) may help to initiate—but not maintain—sleep, whereas trazodone (25–75 mg) may benefit both.

Anticonvulsants: EEGs following language regression or seizures may reinforce a decision to treat with anticonvulsant medications, such as divalproex or carbamazepine. Although guidelines for the evaluation, treatment, and prognosis of children with abnormal EEGs (but without clinical seizures) have not been determined, experience suggests that approximately one-half of these patients will improve in their behavior and language when treated with anticonvulsants. Such improvements, however, likely result from the effect of these medications as mood stabilizers and suggest that epileptiform activity on EEGs reflects, rather than causes, underlying CNS dysfunction.

Drugs for Attention: Although symptoms of attention deficit hyperactivity disorder (ADHD) occur frequently, children with ASDs are less likely than typical children with ADHD to respond favorably to stimulant medications. Children with ASDs *overfocus* and have selective attention. Brief medication trials with stimulants (such as methylphenidate) are indicated, but may lead to irritability and increased hyperactivity. Clonidine, guanfacine, imipramine, or atomoxetine are often good alternatives.

Selective Serotonin Reuptake Inhibitors (SSRIs): The SSRIs improve function in the majority of children with ASDs. Multiple clinical and experimental studies over 30 years have shown that altered serotonin (increased in platelets; decreased transport in CNS) is a critical component of ASDs in many patients and suggest that treatment may improve outcome. Unfortunately, currently available clinical assays of circulating serotonin are not useful to guide treatment. The SSRIs decrease anxiety and repetitive behaviors, and improve attention and mood. Experience shows that most children with ASDs have *increased sensitivity* to SSRIs and respond to small doses: a small minority of children show *decreased sensitivity* and require high doses. The author prefers to begin therapy with very small doses of citalopram (using liquid preparations of 0.5–1 mg daily, usually in the morning) and to increase weekly by a similar amount, being cautious to avoid *overstimulation* as the dose increases. This may occur when the dose exceeds the individual's "therapeutic window," usually in doses from 1 to 5 mg in young children. Individual responses vary among different SSRIs, so repeated trials of different medications may be needed, each over 2–3 months. Full therapeutic benefits may not become apparent for 6–8 weeks, and may be superseded by side effects if the dose is increased too rapidly. Treatment should continue for 6–12 months, then be tapered slowly over 6–8 weeks. Most young children maintain their gains after the SSRI is discontinued, although loss of function may dictate restoration of drug therapy.

Atypical Antipsychotics: Atypical antipsychotic medications are helpful for aggression and adverse behaviors in ASDs. Despite their demonstrated efficacy in short-term trials, risperidone and related drugs deserve cautious follow up for side effects, including extrapyramidal movements, weight gain, and hyperprolactinemia. Olanzapine and other atypical antipsychotics may induce diabetic changes that require glucose monitoring.

SUMMARY

Methods and medications for the evaluation and treatment of ASDs are improving rapidly, along with increased emphasis on basic science and clinical research. Although optimal treatments await discoveries of the ultimate pathophysiologies involved, thoughtful physicians, psychologists, and therapists can all contribute to improving the lives of children with ASDs and their families.

SUGGESTED READINGS

1. Anderson GW, Zimmerman AW, Akshoomoff N, Chugani DC. Autism clinical trials: biological and medical issues in patient selection and treatment response. CNS Spectr 2004; 9:57–64.

2. Bauman ML, Kemper TL, eds. The Neurobiology of Autism. 2d ed. Baltimore, MD: The Johns Hopkins University Press, 2004.
3. Filipek PA, Accardo PJ, Ashwal S, Baranek GT, Cook EH Jr, Dawson G, Gordon B, Gravel JS, Johnson CP, Kallen RJ, Levy SE, Minshew NJ, Ozonoff S, Prizant BM, Rapin I, Rogers SJ, Stone WL, Teplin SW, Tuchman RF, Volkmar FR. Practice parameter: screening and diagnosis of autism: report of the Quality Standards Subcommittee of the American Academy of Neurology and the Child Neurology Society. Neurology 2000; 55:468–479.
4. Gillberg C, Coleman M. Biology of the Autistic Syndromes. 3d ed. London: MacKeith Press, 2000.
5. Robins DL, Fein D, Barton ML, Green JA. The modified checklist for autism in toddlers: an initial study investigating the early detection of autism and pervasive developmental disorders. J Autism Dev Disord 2001; 31:131–44.
6. Zimmerman AW, Gordon B. Neural mechanisms in autism. In: Pasquale Accardo, Christy Magdnusen, Arnold J. Capute, eds. Autism: Clinical and Research Issues. Baltimore, MD: York Press, 2000.
7. Zimmerman AW, Bonfardin B, Myers SM. Neuropharmacological therapy in autism. In: Pasquale Accardo, Christy Magdnusen, Arnold J. Capute, eds. Autism: Clinical and Research Issues. Baltimore, MD: York Press, 2000.

72
ADHD

Stewart Mostofsky
Kennedy Krieger Institute, Baltimore, Maryland, U.S.A.

INTRODUCTION

Attention deficit hyperactivity disorder (ADHD) is the most common developmental disorder of childhood. It affects approximately 3–9% of schoolchildren and is one of the more common reasons for pediatric neurology referral. Among the clinical specialists involved in the assessment and treatment of ADHD, the pediatric neurologist is best trained to approach the evaluation based on his/her knowledge of the neurological basis of the disorder. The focus of this chapter will be to provide a review of ADHD in which the diagnosis and treatment will be discussed in light of the current understanding of the neuropathophysiology of ADHD.

CLINICAL FEATURES

ADHD is characterized by symptoms of hyperactivity, impulsivity, and a decreased ability to maintain on-task behavior, particularly during nonpreferred tasks. Currently, the DSM IV includes three subtypes: "predominantly inattentive," "predominantly hyperactive/impulsive," and a combined type. By definition, signs must be observed prior to age seven years. The forms can change over the lifespan; an individual can have the hyperactive/impulsive type as a preschooler, the full syndrome until middle school, and the inattentive type thereafter. Studies have found a higher incidence of ADHD in males than females, with a ratio of approximately 3:1. Gender-biased diagnostic criteria may, however, account for the size, if not the direction, of the ratio, since girls more commonly present with the inattentive symptoms, which are less likely to be identified as a problem in school, home, and social settings.

While ADHD was originally conceived of as a developmental disorder occurring in childhood, it has become increasingly apparent that symptoms often persist into adulthood. Thirty to seventy-five percent of individuals diagnosed with ADHD in childhood continue to have symptoms into adult life. Furthermore, it is not uncommon for patients to present during adulthood, despite a lifelong history of symptoms. ADHD is often associated with comorbid conditions such as oppositional defiant disorder, conduct disorder, anxiety disorders, mood disorders, dyslexia, and other language-based learning disabilities.

PATHOBIOLOGY

The etiology of ADHD appears to be heterogeneous. Various adverse environmental factors including infection, toxins such as lead and prenatal exposure to cigarettes or alcohol have been associated with symptoms of ADHD. Genetic factors have also been identified. Several genetic disorders have ADHD as part of the phenotype and twin studies report a heredibility of approximately 0.75 for ADHD. Linkage studies have implicated two dopaminergic system genes; the dopamine transporter locus (DAT1) and the seven-repeat allele in the locus for the D4 dopamine receptor gene (*DRD4*7*).

Current nomenclature stresses abnormalities of "attention" as being central to ADHD. Neurologic models of attention emphasize posterior parietal "sensory" attentional systems important for stimulus detection, vigilance, disengagement and shifting, and frontal-subcortical "motor" intentional systems important for initiating and sustaining a response to a stimulus and inhibiting inappropriate responses. Most researchers suggest that ADHD is fundamentally the result of a dysfunction within frontal-subcortical intentional networks. In this model, the core symptoms of ADHD are thought to be secondary to the abnormal selection of motor response to stimuli (i.e., difficulty in preparing the response to, rather than attending to, stimuli). The result is unresponsiveness to stimuli that should lead to action and defective inhibition of responses to those that should not, with the latter contributing to impulsive and hyperactive behavior. Neuropsychological findings of impairment on response inhibition tasks, both skeletomotor and oculomotor, lend support to this hypothesis.

Findings from functional imaging, lesion, and electrophysiology studies implicate frontal-subcortical circuits in response inhibition. At its most basic level, premotor circuits, including those originating in the supplementary motor area, are likely critical for selection of motor responses, including inhibition, with prefrontal circuits important for processing of cognitive and socioemotional information necessary to guide response selection. Abnormalities within frontal regions and interconnected subcortical regions—the basal ganglia and cerebellum—are consistent findings in anatomic magnetic resonance imaging (MRI) studies of ADHD, and decreased volume has been observed within both premotor and prefrontal regions, suggesting that the clinical picture of ADHD encompasses dysfunctions that are attributable to anomalous development of both premotor and prefrontal circuits. Findings from neurologic and neuropsychologic studies also implicate abnormalities within both premotor and prefrontal systems. Subtle motor abnormalities (e.g., slow speed and excessive overflow movements) suggest dysfunction of motor/premotor circuits; evidence of impaired prefrontal function includes difficulties with working memory and planning, organizing, and generating strategies for future actions, often collectively referred to as "executive functions."

Evidence from linkage analysis, metabolic imaging studies, and medication effects strongly suggests that catecholamine dysregulation within frontal-subcortical systems contributes to the pathophysiology of ADHD. PET studies have shown increased dopamine transporter (DAT) density in adults with ADHD, but results showing changes in [^{18}F] F-DOPA studies have been inconsistent. The high response rate of ADHD symptoms to stimulant medications, which blocks catecholamine reuptake and facilitates release of dopamine and norepinephrine, further supports this hypothesis.

DIAGNOSIS AND EVALUATION

ADHD is diagnosed by the individual having a history that typically reveals problems with maintaining on-task behavior and impulsivity, associated inhibitory insufficiencies, and difficulties with executive functions (planning, organizing, strategizing). Multiple techniques should be used to obtain an accurate diagnosis and to assess for the presence of comorbid diagnoses including clinical interviews and rating scales/questionnaires. Diagnosis requires that difficulties be present in at least two settings, so it is important that historical information be obtained from multiple sources that should, at the very least, include parents and teachers. Available school records and teacher observations should be reviewed, since they are an important source of information. In children with the hyperactive/impulsive or combined forms of the disorder, signs are typically recognizable at an early age and often include behavioral as well as academic difficulties. In the inattentive form, signs may not be evident until the child enters school and begins engaging in nonpreferred activities that require a much greater ability to inhibit off-task behavior. With persistent, focused questioning, however, the clinician can often find a history of off-task behavior during the preschool years.

Past medical history should focus on developmental history, including history of neurologic signs and conditions that can be associated with difficulty staying on-task, such as seizures and tics. Birth history should be reviewed; low birth weight has been found to be a risk factor for ADHD, although most children with ADHD do not have a history of perinatal complications. Family history is often positive for impulsivity and off-task behavior. Nevertheless, because the formal diagnosis of ADHD has existed only since 1980, a history of diagnosed ADHD in family members born before 1970 is somewhat uncommon. Inattentiveness and off-task behavior can be presenting signs of neurodegenerative disorders (adrenal leukodystrophy, neuronal ceroid-lipofuscinosis) or be seen in other medical conditions including neurocutaneous disorders (neurofibromatosis type 1), endocrine disorders (hypo- or hyperthyroidism) and toxic exposures (lead toxicity). Comorbid disorders (oppositional defiant disorder, conduct disorder, anxiety disorders, mood disorders, and language-based learning disabilities) must also be considered as part of the differential diagnoses, since each can result in inattentiveness or cause a lack of task completion.

Particularly relevant signs on neurological examination are abnormalities on motor examination including the presence of subtle motor signs and increased overflow movements. The latter includes feet-to-hand overflow observed during stressed gait maneuvers such as heel and toe walking and mirror and proximal overflow movements observed during rapid sequential movements of the hands and feet (e.g., toe tapping, hand pronation/supination, finger sequencing). Children with ADHD also show excessive motor impersistence, motor slowing, and impaired performance on tasks of motor response inhibition. Abnormal findings on neuropsychological evaluation include changes on computerized continuous performance tests, tests of "cognitive" inhibition (e.g., Stroop interference test), and measures of more complex aspects of executive function including organization/

planning and working memory are important for assessing subtle but long-lasting aspects of the disorder.

THERAPEUTIC INTERVENTIONS

The approach to the treatment of children presenting with ADHD is multimodal, involving the use of behavior modification techniques to improve on-task performance maintenance, the use of academic accommodations to help create an academic environment in which the child is better able to learn, and the use of medications.

Behavior modification utilizes techniques of operant conditioning, stressing positive reinforcement to alter behavior. It is optimal to have a behavioral psychologist involved who would work not only with the child, but also with the parents, teachers, and other supervisory adults. Consistency is extremely important, and the psychologist can help in establishing a coordinated program in which caregivers provide defined responses to both positive and negative behavior. For children with ADHD, it is important that consequences be immediate and consistent and that praise and reward for good behavior and performance be emphasized. These approaches are particularly critical when ADHD is comorbid with oppositional defiant disorder and/or conduct disorder.

Academic accommodations are important for providing a child with ADHD a school setting in which maximum learning can take place. Teachers should attempt to provide as much structure and routine as possible. Classrooms should be small in size and the child should be given preferential seating towards the front of the class. Frequent changes of teachers during the day should be avoided. Given the known difficulties with motor speed and response preparation, untimed tests are an essential accommodation as is limiting the length of homework assignments. Attempts should also be made at helping to provide organization by using a combination of techniques including keeping an extra set of textbooks at home and using a daily assignment notebook (or school website) that allows the teacher to communicate directly with parents regarding homework assignments.

The use of medications is the most well known and most controversial aspect of treatment in ADHD (Table 1). Stimulant medications, including methylphenidate (Ritalin, Concerta, Metadate) and amphetamine preparations (Dexadrine and Adderall), are highly effective with response rates estimated at 70%. The stimulants are thought to affect dopaminergic or noradrenergic systems within frontal-subcortical circuits, enhancing inhibitory control systems and potentiating delays between stimuli and responses, reducing impulsive and off-task behavior. Controversy emerges from the fact that although a multimodal approach to ADHD is recommended, it is the highly publicized stimulant therapy that is frequently the first and sole treatment. Further, since typically-developing children administered stimulant medications may show improved performance on continuous performance tasks, there are concerns that stimulants are being prescribed to make perfectly acceptable students into even better ones ("cosmetic" use). Side effects may include insomnia, appetite suppression, and possibly transient tics (see chapter on Tourette syndrome). If stimulants are not effective or cause unmanageable side effects, several alternative medications can be considered, although none are nearly as efficacious as the stimulants. Tricyclic antidepressants, which are nonselective monoamine reuptake inhibitors, can be helpful, particularly in individuals with comorbid anxi-

Table 1 Medications Used for the Treatment of ADHD

Medication	Dose (mg/kg/day)[a]	Daily schedule	Common side effects
Stimulants			
Amphetamine	0.3–1.5		Common to all stimulants:
Short acting (Dexedrine tablets)		Two or three times	Insomnia Appetite suppression
Intermediate acting (Adderall, Dexedrine spansules)		Once or twice	Tic exacerbation Depression, anxiety
Long acting (Adderall-XR)		Once	Preparation-specific: Reboundphenomena (more common with short-acting preparations) Hepatitis (pemoline only)
Methylphenidate	0.5–2.0		
Short acting (Ritalin, metadate)		Two to four times	
Long acting (Concerta, Ritalin SR,Ritalin LA, Metadate CD, Metadate ER)		Once	
Pemoline (Cylert)	1.0–3.0	Once	
Selective Norepinephrine Reuptake Inhibitors			
Atomoxetine (Strattera)	0.5–1.4	Once or twice	Abdominal pain nausea/vomiting constipation dry mouth appetite suppression fatigue
Antidepressants			
Tricyclic Antipressants (TCAs)[b] (e.g., imipramine, nortryptiline)	2.0–5.0 for imipramine 1.0–3.0 for nortryptiline	Once or twice	Dry mouth Constipation Weight change EKG changes
Bupropion	1.0–6.0		Irritability, insomnia
Short acting (Wellbutrin)		Three times	Lower seizure threshold
Long acting (Wellbutrin SR)		Once	Contraindicated in bulimia
Antihypertensives			
Clonidine (Catapress)	3–10	Two to four times	Sedation (less with guanfacine) Dry mouth Depression
Guanfacine (Tenex)	30–100	Two	Hypotension (including orthostatic) and associated symptoms of lightheadedness, dizziness

[a] Recommended doses by weight (mg/kg/day) serve only as a guide. Optimal dose varies across patients and several medications have maximum doses recommended by the manufacturer. For all medications, slow titration is recommended to achieve a dose that provides maximal benefit with minimal side effects.
[b] Monitoring of blood levels can be useful in guiding TCA dosing.

ety; however, these have fallen somewhat out of favor due to the known, but uncommon, side effect of cardiac toxicity. More recently, atomoxetine, a specific norepinephrine reuptake inhibitor, has been found to be effective. Antihypertensive medications (alpha-2 antagonists), clonidine and guanfacine, may help in reducing impulsive and hyperactive behavior, but can be sedating. Bupropion has also recently been reported to be effective in decreasing symptoms/signs of impulsivity and off-task behavior, particularly in individuals with comorbid depression. Therapy for comorbid conditions including anxiety, depression, and conduct disorder are discussed in separate chapters.

SUMMARY

ADHD is a highly prevalent developmental disorder that is one of the more common reasons for pediatric neurology referral. Evidence from neuroimaging and neuropsychological studies suggests that the excessive impulsivity, hyperactivity, and offtask behaviors that characterize ADHD are secondary to impaired response inhibition associated with anomalous development within frontal-subcortical circuits. Comprehensive history is necessary for diagnosis as well as to assess for comorbid and differential diagnoses, many of which are one and the same. While not diagnostic, neurologic and neuropsychologic examinations are important for assessing often observed motor and cognitive signs reflecting dysfunction within motor, premotor, and prefrontal circuits. Treatment is multimodal and targeted at addressing the primary behavioral symptoms of ADHD as well as motor and executive deficits that can affect school performance.

SUGGESTED READINGS

1. Barkley RA. Behavioral inhibition, sustained attention, and executive functions: constructing a unifying theory of ADHD. Psychol Bull 1997; 121:65.
2. Denckla MB. ADHD: topic update. Brain Dev 2003; 25:383–389.
3. Durston S. A review of the biological bases of ADHD: what have we learned from imaging studies? Mental Retardation Dev Disabilities Res Rev 2003; 9:184–195
4. Jensen PS, Hinshaw SP, Swanson JM, Greenhill LL, Conners CK, Eugene AL et al. Findings from the NIMH Multimodal Treatment Study of ADHD (MTA): implications and applications for primary care providers. J Dev Behav Pediatr 2001; 22:60–73.
5. Rowland AS, Lesesne CA, Abramowitz AJ. The Epidemiology of attention-deficit/hyperactivity disorder (ADHD): a public health view. Mental Retardation Dev Disabilities Res Rev 2002; 8:162–170.
6. Solanto MV. Dopamine dysfunction in AD/HD: integrating clinical and basic neuroscience research. Behav Brain Res 2002; 130:65–71.
7. Wilens TE, Biederman J, Spencer TJ. Attention deficit/hyperactivity disorder across the lifespan. Ann Rev Med 2002; 53:113–131.
8. Mostutsky SH, Newsehaffer CJ, Derekla MB. Oveflow movements predict impaired response inhibition in children with ADHD. Perceptual and Motor skills 2003; 97: 1315–1331.

73
Anxiety Disorders in Children

Julie Newman Kingery and John T. Walkup
Division of Child and Adolescent Psychiatry, Johns Hopkins University School of Medicine, Baltimore, Maryland, U.S.A.

INTRODUCTION

It is common for children to experience fears and worries. There is cause for concern, however, when anxiety leads to excessive distress, avoidance behavior, or the need for constant reassurance. Early detection and intervention are crucial, as anxiety can be very responsive to both psychological and pharmacological treatment. Anxiety disorders in children have a prevalence rate of 5–18% and can present with physical complaints suggesting underlying medical or neurological disorders. Anxiety disorders can also complicate the presentation of neurological problems and if unrecognized, can negatively impact treatment outcome.

ETIOLOGY

Both genetic and environmental factors are implicated in the etiology of anxiety disorders. An increased concordance for anxiety in monozygotic as compared to dizygotic twins suggests a direct genetic contribution. Additionally, genetic effects on temperament and cognitive style may put children at risk for an anxiety disorder. Environmental factors, such as stressful life events and the family environment (e.g., overprotective parenting style), have also been implicated. Neuroanatomically, the amygdala appears to be the central location for the fear and anxiety circuitry. Based on the beneficial effects of antidepressants and benzodiazepines, various neurotransmitters, including serotonin, norepinephrine and gamma-amino butyric acid, have been suggested to have a role in the pathophysiology of anxiety disorders.

DIAGNOSIS AND CLINICAL FEATURES

Children with anxiety disorders experience *distress* associated with anxiety, fear, or worry, *avoid* situations that provoke anxiety, *seek reassurance* in their interactions with adults. There are currently nine different anxiety disorders that are diagnosed in childhood: separation anxiety disorder (SAD); specific phobia (SP); social phobia

(SoP); agoraphobia; obsessive-compulsive disorder (OCD); generalized anxiety disorder (GAD); panic disorder; post-traumatic stress disorder (PTSD); and acute stress disorder. Since differentiating each of these disorders is essential for diagnosis and treatment, the various types will be discussed in more detail.

Specific Phobia

Simple and short-lived fears are developmentally normal in children. Children and adolescents who have a marked, persistent (>6 months) and impairing fear of a particular object or situation (e.g., flying, heights, darkness, loud noises including thunder, insects, dogs and other small animals, blood or injections) are diagnosed with SP. Specific phobias can lead to *avoidance* behavior out of proportion to the potential for encountering the feared situation (e.g., not going outside in the winter because of a fear of bees) and can lead children to excessive *reassurance seeking* from their parents. Upwards of 70% of children with a specific phobia will have another anxiety disorder. The average age of onset of SP is between 7 and 8 years, with a peak between the ages of 10 and 13. If untreated, some SPs will persist into adulthood.

Separation Anxiety Disorder

Children with SAD experience a pattern of inter-related symptoms—*distress* when separation from home or attachment figures is anticipated or occurs, *avoidance* of situations that may result in separation from a major attachment figure, and *reassurance seeking* by maintaining physical or psychological proximity. Children with SAD experience an overwhelming fear of losing or becoming separated from major attachment figures through catastrophic means (e.g., fears of being kidnapped from bed or that a parent will die in an accident). These concerns are particularly intense when leaving home for school, going to a friend's house, attending after school activities, and going to summer camp or sleepovers. This intense fear of separation may lead children to avoid out of home activities altogether. Desperate means to *seek reassurance* are often pursued (e.g., begging not to be separated, arguing, temper tantrums, sleeping in the caretaker's bedroom, following the parent around the house). Children with SAD often voice a variety of physical complaints (e.g., stomachaches, headaches, nausea, fear of vomiting) when separation from a caregiver occurs or is anticipated. These children may be inattentive and restless in the classroom, frequently being misdiagnosed with the inattentive subtype of attention deficit hyperactivity disorder (ADHD). The peak age of onset is between 7 and 9 years. Girls are more likely than boys to experience SAD.

Social Phobia

Children with SoP are excessively shy and fearful of embarrassment in one or more social or performance situations. Children with SoP either *avoid or endure social situations with extreme distress,* including speaking or reading aloud in class, asking or answering questions, and joining group activities. At home and when comfortable, children with SoP are capable of normal interpersonal interactions, but may avoid answering the door or the phone, having peers visit, or ordering their own food when out with the family at a restaurant. Children and adolescents with SoP may voice complaints about attending school or they may completely refuse to attend school related to fear that they will be do something to embarrass themselves (e.g., fears of being teased by peers or called on by a teacher in class, concerns about appearance). Physical complaints (e.g., headaches, stomachaches) are common when facing embarrassing situations. Similar to SP, children and adolescents with SoP often express their anxiety through crying, tantrums, freezing, or shirking away from social situations. The average age of onset is between 11 and 12 years.

Generalized Anxiety Disorder

Children with GAD experience *excessive distress* about a number of events and activities, including academic challenges, extracurricular activities, and peer relationships. This worry or apprehension usually occurs despite the fact that there is no reasonable cause for concern. For example, they are earning good grades, but worry about failure at school. These children also have unrealistic and extreme worries about future events (e.g., an upcoming vacation, the start of school, changes in family routines) and adult-like concerns about issues such as family finances or the birth of a new baby. They frequently request, but are not relieved by *reassurance*. In contrast to children with SP who have fears of specific stimuli or situations, the fears of children and adolescents with GAD are both more general and global. The frequency of worries held by children with GAD ranges from several times per week to nearly constant worrying. Although it is developmentally normal for children to occasionally worry about low-frequency events, children with GAD do not seem to recognize that these events are unlikely to actually occur. The GAD symptoms are more common in older children (ages 12–19) than in younger children (ages 5–11).

Panic Disorder

Panic attacks are characterized by an abrupt onset of intense anxiety that peaks and then subsides over approximately 15–20 minutes. Symptoms during an attack include shortness of breath (dyspnea), chest tightness, fears of dying or losing control, shaking, palpitations, and dizziness. Children describe their symptoms in more concrete terms (e.g., a fear of suddenly becoming sick, vomiting, or chest pain). Panic attacks may be spontaneous or situationally cued (e.g., seeing a dog triggers a panic attack). Spontaneous panic attacks are rare in childhood and more common in late adolescence. Situationally cued attacks are more common in children than spontaneous attacks. Panic disorder is characterized by the occurrence of at least one spontaneous panic attack followed by a minimum of 1 month of a persistent fear of experiencing future attacks or significant avoidance behavior. Although panic attacks are physically uncomfortable, they are usually not disabling in and of themselves. Persistent fear of having a subsequent panic attack may actually be more disabling than the attack itself. Following a panic attack, an individual may falsely assume that an environmental factor caused the attack leading to *avoidance* of certain settings (e.g., malls, movie theaters). Although this disorder can be diagnosed in children, the typical onset occurs in late adolescence.

Post-traumatic Stress Disorder

Acute stress disorder (ASD) occurs when a child or adolescent is directly exposed to a significant traumatic event (e.g., physical injury, natural disaster, witness of a car accident), and for a limited time subsequent to the event has problems with re-experiencing the event and increased autonomic arousal as described below. Children with PTSD continue to be symptomatic longer than expected (>than 1 month). They re-experience the traumatic event in at least one of the following ways: intrusive thoughts, nightmares, and distress or physiological reactivity when exposed to cues related to the event. Stimuli associated with the trauma are *avoided,* and persistent symptoms of arousal occur (e.g., difficulty falling asleep, tension, exaggerated startle response). Generally, the more extensive the exposure to the traumatic event, the more PTSD symptoms a child is likely to experience.

Other Anxiety Disorders

Other anxiety disorders seen in childhood include agoraphobia (the fear of being in situations from which escape may be difficult or embarrassing, or in which help is not readily available in the event of a panic attack), and OCD.

Common Clinical Features

Children are more likely than adults to express their anxiety in the form of physical complaints. The somatic complaints that are common across all of the anxiety disorders fall into the following categories: *head related* (e.g., headaches, feeling dizzy or lightheaded), *chest and cardiac functioning* (e.g., accelerated heart rate, difficulty breathing, feeling of choking, chest pain or discomfort), *abdomen* (e.g., fear of choking/gagging, nausea, stomachaches, vomiting, frequent urge to urinate or defecate), *sleep* (e.g., difficulty falling asleep, restless sleep, nightmares), *appetite* (e.g., decreased appetite, picky eating or refusal to eat in front of others because of fear of embarrassment), *other body complaints* (e.g., feeling easily fatigued, muscle tension, sweating, trembling or shaking, dry mouth, exaggerated startle response), and *mood or mental state* (irritability, difficulty concentrating, feeling restless or on edge, fear of losing control or getting sick/passing out, fear of dying). It is essential for neurologists to inquire about *behavioral manifestations* of anxiety in children and adolescents (e.g., clinging to parent, refusal to attend school, refusal to sleep alone or away from home, crying or having a tantrum when exposed to feared situation or stimulus, general avoidance of certain feared objects or situations). Additionally, the physician should discuss with the youngster and his/her parents the extent to which the above symptoms are interfering with the child or adolescent's functioning (e.g., social, academic) or the normal family routine (e.g., attending social events, parents leaving the home while children stay with a babysitter).

TREATMENT FOR ANXIETY DISORDERS

Psychotherapy

Cognitive-behavioral therapy (CBT) has received empirical support for the treatment of anxiety disorders in children and adolescents. CBT is based on the assumption that anxiety symptoms develop through behavioral and learning processes. To reduce the symptoms of anxiety, children and adolescents are taught to recognize the physiological responses of anxiety, implement specific relaxation skills, identify maladaptive thought patterns and use more adaptive self-talk, and gradually face anxiety-provoking situations by applying the skills learned in treatment.

Involving parents in treatment is extremely important (e.g., to provide a weekly update for the therapist and to assist the child with practicing new skills learned in treatment).

Medication

The Food and Drug Administration (FDA) has approved the use of several different psychotropic medications for treatment of anxiety disorders in adults (e.g., antidepressant and anxiolytic groups). Many of these medications have been used clinically in children and adolescents, but only a few have FDA indications, including the selective serotonin reuptake inhibitors (SSRIs)—fluvoxamine (≥age 8 years for OCD), sertraline (≥age 6 for OCD); and the tricyclic antidepressants (TCAs)—clomipraime (≥age 10 for OCD). The SSRIs are currently the treatment of choice for anxiety in children and adolescents based on superior efficacy and low side effect profile. See Tablc 1 for a listing of medications that may be useful in treating anxiety.

Treatment duration necessary for remission of symptoms is likely greater than one year. Some children are able to come off of medication and not require long-term treatment.

Combination of Medication and Therapy

Research has not yet answered the question of which approach is the most effective for the treatment of anxiety in children and adolescents. A multisite study sponsored

Table 1 Medications That May Be Useful for Anxiety Disorders in Children and Adolescents

Generic name	Trade name	FDA indication for < 18 years	Starting dose[a] (mg/day)	Smallest effective dose[b] (mg/day)	Highest safe dose[c] (mg/day)
Sertraline	Zoloft®	OCD to age 6	25	25–50	150–200
Fluoxetine	Prozac®	OCD to age 7; depression to age 7	5–10	10–20	20–40
Fluvoxamine	Luvox®	OCD to age 8	25	25–50	150–200
Paroxetine	Paxil®	None	10	10–30	40–60
Citalopram	Celexa®	None	10	10–30	40–60
Venlafaxine	Effexor® and Effexor XR®	None	25–37.5	50–100	150–225
Nefazadone	Serzone®	None	50	100–200	300–600
Escitalopram	Lexapro®	None	5–10	10	20
Mirtazapine	Remeron®	None	15	30	30–45

[a] Starting dose refers to a reasonable dose for initiating treatment. Smaller or larger doses are possible.
[b] Smallest effective dose is the smallest dose that might be beneficial. Some will require higher doses, but it is unlikely that lower doses will be effective.
[c] Highest safe dose is the highest dose that is commonly tolerated. Higher doses may not be more effective and may be likely to be associated with more side effects.
This chart is not intended to be used as a guide for treatment of anxious youth. Effective treatment requires a comprehensive evaluation and a treatment plan tailored to a patient's individual needs.

by the National Institutes of Mental Health is currently examining the efficacy of CBT, medication, and the combination of these two treatments in comparison to pill placebo over a 12-week treatment trial. Long-term benefits of the active treatment conditions are also being assessed. Results of this clinical trial will help to answer the question of which treatment is the most effective for stopping the progress of anxiety in children and adolescents.

SUMMARY

Anxiety disorders are arguably the most common psychiatric disorder in childhood. Although the anxiety disorders have many different symptom patterns, all anxiety disorders include an anxious target symptom (e.g., separation, humiliation, etc.), avoidance behavior and reassurance seeking that can be significantly distressing and impairing. Despite the prevalence of these disorders, they are often not diagnosed and more often not treated effectively. Treatment can be extremely helpful in reducing symptoms and improving function. If left untreated, anxiety disorders can complicate the presentation of neurological disorders and have a negative impact on treatment outcome.

SUGGESTED READINGS

1. Albano AM, Chorpita BF, Barlow DH. Childhood anxiety disorders. In: Mash EJ, Barkley RA, eds. Child Psychopathology. New York: The Guilford Press, 2002.
2. Albano AM, Kendall PC. Cognitive behavioral therapy for children and adolescents with anxiety disorders: clinical research advances. Int Rev Psychiatry 2002; 14:129–134.
3. Charney DS. Neuroanatomical circuits modulating fear and anxiety behaviors. Acta Psychiatr Scand Suppl 2003; 417:38–50.
4. Silverman WK, Ginsburg GS. Anxiety disorders. In: Ollendick TH, Hersen M, eds. Anxiety Disorders. Handbook of Child Psychopathology. 3rd ed. New York: Plenum Press, 1998.
5. Walkup JT, Labellarte MJ, Ginsburg GS. The pharmacological treatment of childhood anxiety disorders. Int Rev Psychiatry 2002; 14:135–142.

74
Mood Disorders in Children

Helen E. Courvoisie
Division of Child and Adolescent Psychiatry, Department of Psychiatry and Behavioral Sciences, The Johns Hopkins Medical Institutions, Baltimore, Maryland, U.S.A.

INTRODUCTION

Major depression disorder (MDD), a common psychiatric disorder, is characterized by a depressed mood, anhedonia, hopelessness, sleep and weight problems, suicidal thoughts and actions, a depressed appearance, and somatic complaints. Depression is both an inability to regulate emotion and a persistence of negative affect. The MDD is traditionally considered to be an episodic disorder, but in youth it often manifests as a disease with protracted periods of illness and with a chronic pattern.

Depression, a treatable illness, occurs in 1–5% of children and 15% of adolescents. Children with depression are vulnerable to the development of other psychiatric disorders including bipolar disorder, anxiety, behavioral problems, and substance abuse. Youth with major depression are at increased risk for suicide, early pregnancy, poor academic performance, and impaired psychosocial functioning. There is evidence that this social impairment can continue beyond the episode of depression. Depression has been shown to complicate the treatment and outcome of neurologic illnesses.

ETIOLOGY

Genetic and Psychosocial Factors

Twin studies have shown that there is a markedly higher rate of mood disorders found in the general population, with a significantly higher monozygotic than dizygotic psychiatric concordance. A family history of mood disorders in parents is associated with a high incidence of mood disorder in their children. Children of parents with MDD exhibit a lifetime risk of developing a mood disorder ranging from 15% to 45%. A high incidence of depression in family members predicts earlier onset of MDD and recurrence in prepubertal-onset MDD.

There are numerous factors associated with the onset, duration, and recurrence of MDD. These factors include demographic factors such as age and gender; familial determinates such as parental psychopathology; history of early onset mood disorders; psychopathologic factors, such as pre-existing diagnoses and subsyndromal depressive symptoms; and psychosocial causes, such as stressful life events. Preliminary evidence suggests that MDD may be increasing in the pediatric population in a cohort fashion with psychosocial factors associated with this increase. There is a small body of literature that indicates that juvenile affective disorders are associated with neurodevelopmental delays.

DIAGNOSTIC AND CLINICAL FEATURES

Depression

Childhood depression is thought to be continuous with adult depression, exhibiting the same symptom profile. Children exhibit their symptoms at their developmental stage (e.g., lack of interest in studies or play vs. decreased ability to work in adults). Children have shown higher rates of hallucinations than any other age group. The development of delusions is more commonly seen in adolescents. Physical complaints such as headaches and abdominal pain are a part of symptom presentation in 100% of depressed preschool children.

The onset of depression is often gradual, with changes in personality such as depressed mood, irritability, and anhedonia, being noted months to years later. Frequent episodes are seen in children associated with increasing severity that lead to fewer recoveries, longer episodes, and an increased rate of recurrence. Chronic waxing and waning of depressive symptoms are common and, when remission of MDD occurs, relapse rates are relatively high (40–50%). Rates of remission are low in untreated samples (35%). When depressive episodes last at least 2 years, children and adolescents have significantly higher rates of suicidal ideation, attempts, and lethality than those with depressions of shorter duration.

Rates of comorbidity of MDD in children and adolescents are similar to rates in adults. The most common comorbid diagnoses are separation anxiety disorder in children and generalized anxiety disorder in adolescents. Dysthymic disorder coexists with MDD in approximately 30% of youngsters.

There is a pronounced gender effect with a prevalence of depression being roughly equal in boys and girls in early adolescence, but by age 14, the incidence of MDD in girls rapidly begins to exceed that for boys. Many, if not most, depressed adolescents suffer from more than one disorder, more commonly externalizing in boys and internalizing in girls.

The MDD can present with psychotic features, with auditory hallucinations more prominent in children and delusions being more common in adolescents. Of those youth who suffer psychotic features, one-third of child patients will go on to develop bipolar disorder.

Dysthymia

Dysthymia is defined as chronic low-level depression that does not meet all the criteria for MDD. While the severity of dysthymia is not as great as with MDD, dysthymic disorder is characterized by a persistent and long-term depressed or irritable mood with a mean episode duration of 3–4 years and a worse outcome than major depression. These long-lasting depressive symptoms seem to be responsible for long-term disabling consequences of social skill learning and psychosocial functioning. There is a higher risk of relapse or development of major depression. Double depression (DD) refers to dysthymia plus a MDD episode. The first episode of major depression occurs 2–3 years after the onset of dysthymic disorder. Anxiety disorders arecommonly comorbid with DD.

The goals of treatment for dysthymic disorder are resolution of the depressive symptoms in order to reduce the risk of developing recurrent mood disorders, and psychotherapy and psychoeducation to prevent the progression of the serious sequelae.

Depression in Bipolar Disorder

A smaller number of children who present with depression, perhaps 1 in 200, go on to develop bipolar affective disorder (BPAD), especially bipolar II (i.e., no manic or mixed episodes) and cyclothymia (i.e., swings of mood to a lesser degree than bipolar disorder). This switch to mania is often preceded by several episodes of depression. The rate of bipolar outcome is threefold higher in childhood-onset depression than in later onset and the presence of psychotic symptoms during a depressive episode predicts bipolar outcome in 60% of child patients. Patients who switch polarity usually do so approximately 4 years after onset of depression. The switch is most likely to occur after two to four episodes of MDD. Children often exhibit a mixed state of depression and mania (i.e., coexistence of depression with mania) or rapid cycling of mood states (i.e., rapid switching from depression to mania). Children appear to cycle faster than adolescents and adults, with some cycling several times a day.

There is comorbidity present with BPD, with attention deficit-hyperactivity disorder (ADHD) seen in 89% of affected individuals. Other comorbidities include anxiety, oppositional defiant disorder, conduct disorder, and substance abuse.

There is increasing evidence that treatment with antidepressants and stimulants may increase cycling or contribute to mixed states. Those children and adolescents with BPD who have received prior antidepressants or stimulants were shown to have an earlier diagnosis (10.7 ± 3.1 years) than those who were never exposed to these medications (12.7 ± 4.3 years). Treatment with antidepressants for the depressed component of the bipolar picture should be judicious with stabilization using mood stabilizers before treatment with antidepressants.

Depression and Neurological Diseases

Depression is one of the most frequent psychiatric disorders found to be comorbid in patients with neurologic diseases such as epilepsy, stroke, head trauma, and other disorders. It is under-recognized and under-treated in neurology patients.

Depression is more common and more severe in patients with epilepsy than in patients with other chronic medical or neurologic illnesses. The causes of depression in epileptic patients include clinical factors, such as seizure type and frequency and epilepsy duration, and psychosocial factors such as quality of life and life stressors. There is some evidence that depression precedes the onset of epilepsy up to 6 times more often than depression in normal controls. The phenomenology, clinical course, or response to treatment do not appear to be different in youth with epilepsy compared with depression in youths without epilepsy.

Genetic factors account for at least 50% of the variance in the transmission of mood disorders in children with neurologic disorders. Family history of depression is reported in about 50% of patients with epilepsy and depression. Twenty percent of children and adolescents with depression and epilepsy develop mania or hypomania within 5 years after the onset of depression.

TREATMENT

Psychotherapy

The empirical literature on treating pediatric major depression is more supportive for problem-specific psychotherapies than for medication management. Several controlled trials have now shown that individual or group-administered cognitive-behavioral psychotherapy (CBT) is an effective treatment for depressed children and adolescents. A recent meta-analysis of 6 controlled CBT studies in depressed adolescents yielded a reasonably robust overall post-treatment effect size.

The CBT is a time-limited, goal directed therapeutic technique, based on social learning. It uses a blend of other psychotherapeutic techniques, many of which are based on classical operant conditioning models. Social learning theory is based on the assumption that a person's environment, personal dispositional characteristics, and situational behavior reciprocally determine each other and that behavior is an evolving dynamic phenomenon. The negative cognitive triad characterizes depressive behavior: self-criticism, negative view of experiences/other people, and a pessimistic view of the future. The therapeutic experience is focused on problem solving, self-monitoring, pleasant activity scheduling, self-instructional approaches, and rational analysis techniques.

Other forms of psychotherapy, including interpersonal therapy and social skills training, are also beneficial in the treatment of depression. Interpersonal psychotherapy (ITP) is based on the theory that interpersonal conflicts or changes maintain depression. Treatment is short term and focused on one or more problem areas in the current functioning of interpersonal relationships. Studies comparing CBT to the more traditional therapies showed a better initial response to treatment than those given more traditional therapies; however, 6 months after treatment, all groups showed about equal improvement in relief of symptoms.

Psychopharmacology

The literature on psychopharmacological interventions in pediatric MDD is sparse. There are now three published controlled trials in which selective serotonin-reuptake inhibitors (SSRI) proved more effective than pill placebo in depressed children and adolescents. The SSRIs studied were fluoxetine, citalopram, and sertraline. A recent multisite placebo-controlled study also showed benefit for paroxetine (SSRI), but not for the active comparator (imipramine). Fluvoxamine, which has antianxiety qualities as well as antidepressant effects, has been shown in a double-blind study to be well tolerated by children. Because a substantial proportion of the fluoxetine sample relapsed during the first year of follow up of the off-medication extension of this study, this may indicate that longer-term drug treatment is essential.

Despite a dearth of data, the SSRIs are widely used as first-line treatments for depressed youth because these medications are well tolerated with few side effects. Fluoxetine and citalopram should be started at 10 mg and raised to 20 mg; if after 4 weeks there is only a partial response, the dosage can be raised up to 40 or 60 mg. Sertraline dosages range from 50 to 100 mg, with raising the dose to 150–200 mg if there is a partial response. Treatment should last at least 9 months, with tapering of dosage recommended to ascertain if there has been remission of the depressive episode. If the patient becomes symptomatic during the taper, then increasing the dosage to its former level is indicated.

Common side effects include behavioral activation such as restlessness, anxiety and agitation, as well as nausea, drowsiness, and constipation. Sexual side effects can occur in youth that may lead to noncompliance in teenagers. Antidepressants can cause a switch to a manic episode in those youth predisposed to BPD.

Recently, paroxetine has been reported to increase suicidal ideation in children and adolescents who are treated with these medications. Until this issue is clarified, this medication should not be initiated in children and adolescents. Those patients who are being treated with these medications and have not reported increased suicidal ideation may be continued on this treatment.

Other antidepressants reported in open label studies to be of some benefits in youth include venlafaxine, bupropion, nefazadone, and mirtazapine. Venlafaxine should be dosed to 75–150 mg: if there is partial response, the dosage can be raised to 225 mg. Venlafaxine can cause hypertension so blood pressure should be monitored; otherwise, the side effect profile is similar to the SSRIs.

There is some evidence that bupropion does not introduce switching to mania as often as other antidepressants. However, bupropion has a rate of association of 0.4–0.8% with seizures when taken at high total daily doses. Therefore, alternatives should be considered in patients with epilepsy. Dosing is usually 75–300 mg bid.

Mirtazapine, dosed at 15–39 mg, has sedative properties that are useful in patients with insomnia; however, weight gain can be problematic. Nefazodone received a black box warning about the occurrence of hepatic failure in adults, and is not currently recommended for use in the pediatric population.

The antiepileptic drugs (AEDs) or mood stabilizers such as valproate and carbamazepine are reported to elevate mood. Treatment of children with bipolar disorder using AEDs may be efficacious in relieving depressive symptoms. Also, these drugs may be useful in depressed patients with epilepsy. Interactions between antidepressants and AEDs include hepatic enzyme induction, resulting in toxic levels of the anticonvulsants. When antidepressant therapy is initiated while patient is on an AED, anticonvulsant levels should be monitored.

More than a dozen negative random-controlled trials using various tricyclic antidepressants (TCAs) have now been conducted, essentially ruling out this group as effective for treating MDD as the TCAs were found to be no better than placebo.

Light Therapy

Seasonal affective disorder (SAD) is a recurrent affective disorder with mood changes and vegetative symptoms regularly occurring during the winter months and that disappear completely during the spring and summer. One open label study with a seven-year follow up and 2 double-blind studies of children with SAD demonstrate significant improvement from baseline in affected patients with light therapy. Both bright light therapy as well as dawn simulation contributed to improvement.

Electroconvulsive Therapy

Recently, there has been a resurgence of interest in the use of electroconvulsive therapy (ECT) in children and adolescents with two recent reviews of the child literature as to the use, safety and efficacy of ECT. There are also a number of case reports that have documented robust treatment response and efficacy. This therapy has been used in those adolescents and children who are treatment resistant. Follow up of adolescents treated with ECT indicate that the response can have long-lasting benefits, and that the adolescents who responded to ECT and their parents felt positive about the experience.

SUMMARY

Approximately 1% of children and adolescents in the United States receive outpatient treatment for depression each year. This rate of treatment falls substantially short of the epidemiological estimates of the prevalence of major depression in childhood. There are no data from controlled studies to help treating physicians develop an optimal treatment algorithm in order to decide rationally between starting treatment with an antidepressant or with psychotherapy in an individual. However, it is important to treat adequately and for a sufficient period of time in order to ameliorate the psychosocial and developmental sequelae of these illnesses.

SUGGESTED READINGS

1. Birmaher B, Ryan ND, Williamson DE, Brent DA, et al. Childhood and adolescent depression. A review of the past ten years. Part I. J Am Acad Child Adolesc Psychiatry 1996; 35:1427–1439.
2. Birmaher B, Ryan ND, Williamson DE, Brent DA, Kaufman J. Childhood and adolescent depression. A review of the past ten years. Part II. J Am Acad Child Adolesc Psychiatry 1996; 35:1575–1583.
3. Davidson RJ, Pizagalli D, Nitschke JB, Putman K. Depression: perspectives from affective neuroscience. Ann Rev Psychol 2002; 53:545–574.
4. Harden CL. The co-morbidity of depression of depression and epilepsy. Epidemiology, etiology, and treatment. Neurology 2002; 59:S48–S55.
5. Kanner AM, Barry JJ. The impact of mood disorders in neurological diseases: should neurologists be concerned? Epilepsy Behav 2003; 4(S3):3–13.
6. Plioplys S. Depression in children and adolescents with epilepsy. Epilepsy Behav 2003; 4(S3):35–39.

75
Conduct Disorder

Shannon Barnett and Mark Riddle
Department of Psychiatry, The Johns Hopkins Hospital, Baltimore, Maryland, U.S.A.

INTRODUCTION

Conduct disorder (CD) differs from mood, anxiety, and psychotic disorders because the diagnosis is defined solely by the behavior of an individual as directed at others, their property, or the presence of other rule violations (see Table 1 for list of symptoms). The youth does not need to endorse any physiologic or mental distress to meet criteria for CD, although these youth often have poor self-esteem, are often irritable, and have rates of suicidal ideation, suicide attempts, and completed suicides that are higher than the general population. Conduct disorder differs from personality disorders, in that for most individuals, the pattern of defiant behaviors remits prior to adulthood, although for a subgroup of these youth, CD is a precursor to antisocial personality disorder and/or substance-related disorders. A second diagnosis that is defined by behavior, oppositional defiant disorder (ODD), occasionally develops into CD. Conduct disorder is distinguished from ODD because the behaviors in CD are more confrontational and destructive, and because CD has a poorer prognosis.

The severity of CD ranges from a mild form, in which the negative behaviors consist mainly of rule violations such as staying out at night without permission, a moderate form, with behaviors such as stealing without confrontation, to a severe form, which includes criminal behavior such as using a weapon or forced sexual acts. Individuals with the child-onset form (symptoms beginning before age 10), when compared to youth with an adolescent-onset (absence of meeting any criteria prior to age 10), have a higher high risk for developing chronic aggression and antisocial personality disorder in adulthood. The diagnosis is occasionally made as young as age 5–7 years of age or between the ages of 16 and 18 years of age, but is most frequently diagnosed in late childhood or early adolescence.

A diagnosis of CD is not made if the disorder can be fully explained by the presence of another axis one disorder, such as bipolar disorder, or if the behaviors can be fully explained as an expected response to a social situation (stealing food for survival). When the axis I diagnosis follows a lapsing and remitting course or when psychosocial stressors are intermittent, the clinician can determine whether or not the deviant behaviors occur only in the context of other co-morbid disorders or only in the context of a particular stressor. However, when a youth has chronic

Table 1 Symptoms of Conduct Disorder

Symptoms
Harassment or threatening towards others
Instigating physical fights
Use of a weapon against others
Physically malicious towards others
Physically cruel to animals
Stealing by confrontation
Forced sexual activity
Deliberate fire setting with the intent of causing serious damage
Vandalism
Breaking into buildings or cars
Lying to obtain stuff or avoid obligations
Stealing without confrontation
Staying out all night without permission prior to age 13
Running away from home overnight at least two times
Frequent truancy from school

(Modified from DSM-IV-TR.)

psychiatric symptoms that are refractory to treatment and/or is chronically exposed to psychosocial stressors that cannot be removed, it may be impossible to know whether a diagnosis of CD is appropriate. The downside of diagnosing CD in these youth includes the negative stigma associated with a diagnosis of CD and the poor prognosis of CD, which in combination can lead mental health providers, educators, parents, and workers in other involved agencies to blame all negative behaviors on the CD, and to not provide adequate interventions for other contributing factors. However, missing a diagnosis of CD may lead the clinician away from treatments that specifically target CD.

Risk factors for the development of CD include a family history of CD, diagnosis of attention-deficit hyperactivity disorder (ADHD), low social economic status (SES), reading disorders, harsh and inconsistent parenting style, and history of being a victim of abuse or neglect. The pathway between risk factors and the disorder is unknown.

Children and adolescents with CD create a significant burden on society by having frequent contact with the juvenile justice system, creating disruptions in the school system, and burdening their families. Individuals with CD are more likely than peers to engage in risky behaviors such as fast driving, drug use, and parenting children during adolescence. Educational and occupational achievement is frequently lower than expected. While effective treatment programs are labor intensive and expensive, it has been estimated that the successful treatment of one individual with conduct disorder may save society close to $2 million.

CO-MORBIDITIES AND DIFFERENTIAL DIAGNOSIS

A thorough evaluation should be performed to determine the presence of criteria for conduct disorder, co-morbid disorders, or outside factors that reinforce the deviant activities. Several disorders may mimic or occur in association with CD including ADHD, bipolar disorder, depression, anxiety, and developmental disorders.

ADHD: ADHD is the most common disorder found in youth with disruptive behavior including those with CD. Severe ADHD symptoms can lead to frequent truancy, defiant behaviors, rule braking, and physical aggression.

Bipolar Disorder: Individuals with this diagnosis typically have obvious changes in mood with grandiose delusions, marked decrease in need for sleep, and impaired judgment. A challenging population includes youths who present with chronic irritability, sleep disturbance, and frequent mood swings, but who do not meet strict criteria for bipolar disorder. Common symptoms in this group include episodes of inappropriately acting silly, severe psychomotor agitation, and sudden mood change to severe anger with minimal provocation.

Depressive Disorders: The combination of irritability with psychomotor agitation, changes in school performance, and withdrawal from previously pleasurable activities, should lead to the consideration of a depressive disorder (see chapter on depression). Parents may not suspect depression, especially when the primary affect is anger, not sadness, and because youths with depressive disorders may briefly cheer up when engaging in pleasurable activities.

Anxiety Disorders: Children with undetected anxiety disorders are often seen as oppositional and disruptive (see chapter on anxiety). Some may be oppositional in order to avoid anxiety-producing situations. Post-traumatic stress disorder (PTSD) may be co-morbid with CD, since youth exposed to chronic violence may develop aggressive behavior.

Learning Disorders, Mental Retardation, Speech and Language Disorders: Children with speech and language problems are more likely to develop behavior problems, in part because they become frustrated when trying to communicate. Similarly, children with severe learning disorders, especially those with poor executive function, may also become aggressive during school secondary to frustration.

PREVENTION

Children at high risk for developing CD, including those with low SES or those who live in areas with high rates of crime, may benefit from preventative interventions. Successful interventions combine community participation, parent training, and classroom interventions that include teaching skills in self-control, emotional awareness, peer relations, and problem solving.

TREATMENT

Treatment begins by using interventions that stop dangerous and disruptive behaviors. Behavioral interventions include parent training, providing high structure both at school and in the community, and, when appropriate, working with the juvenile justice system to enforce compliance with the treatment plan. If required, brief inpatient hospitalizations or partial hospitalization can be used to control acute aggressive behavior. If a particular youth cannot be maintained in the community, then residential treatment, therapeutic group home, or placement in a juvenile justice facility must be considered.

Additional treatments should be directed to address co-morbid psychiatric problems and substance abuse disorders. Individuals with psychiatric disorders should

Table 2 Treatment of Co-morbid Psychiatric Disorders

Disorder	Effective treatments
ADHD	Stimulants (methylphenidate, dextro-amphetamine, amphetamine), atomoxitine, school interventions
Bipolar disorder	Lithium, divalproate, carbamazepine, neuroleptics
Depressive disorders	SSRIs, cognitive behavioral therapy, venlafaxine, mirtazepine, buproprion
Anxiety disorders	SSRIs, cognitive behavioral therapy, (benzodiazepines should be used only rarely in this population because of the risks of dependency, concurrent substance use, and the possibility that the youth might sell the medication)
Substance use disorders	Frequent urine drug screens, identification of triggers to use, relapse prevention strategies

be treated as if there were no CD (see Table 2 and specific chapters) and those with significant substance abuse should be referred to appropriate treatment programs. Care providers should be aware that behavioral interventions might not work well until the other psychiatric disorders have been adequately treated and that treatment of co-morbid disorders alone does not always lead to improvements in behavior. Although individual psychotherapy has not proven effective in the treatment of CD, possible beneficial strategies include helping the youth develop empathy, teaching emotion regulation skills, and teaching problem solving skills. Any indication of a possible learning disorder should lead to a referral for further evaluation, since a proper educational environment that addresses learning difficulties may lead to decreases in frustration and decreases in disruptive behavior at school.

MULTIMODAL APPROACHES

Successful treatment approaches for CD are known as multimodal approaches because they provide support and treatment for the family and structure for the youth. The treatment team may include a targeted case manager to assist the family with negotiating the educational and juvenile justice system as well as to help in finding better housing and applying for additional social services. Psychotherapeutic techniques combine parent training, support for regulating the affect in the family, and may involve improving peer relationships. Project Back on Track is an example of an intensive four-week multimodal program for youth offenders. The program consists of parent training, education, group therapy, and empathy building exercises. The youth participate in 32 hr of activities during the four-week program, while the parents have a total of 15 hr of contact with the program. Participation in the program saved society an estimated $1800 per patient during the first year following the program.

PSYCHOPHARMACOLOGIC APPROACHES

There is limited data on the psychopharmacologic treatment of children with conduct disorder outside data for the treatment of co-morbid disorders. Because of the limited data for the psychopharmacologic treatment of CD, we recommend a conservative approach for adding medications that do not treat an obvious co-morbid disorder. Target symptoms should be clearly identified, and baseline rates should be collected from multiple sources, including teachers and parents. Medications that do not demonstrate a clear benefit should not be continued.

Because there is a high rate of co-morbid ADHD associated with CD, and because of the proven efficacy and safety of the stimulants, a stimulant trial should be considered. Even in the absence of obvious inattention and hyperactivity, stimulants may be effective at reducing impulsivity in youth with CD. When a youth is at risk for abusing or selling stimulants, clinicians should consider long-acting stimulants and administering the medication at school where compliance can be closely monitored.

Several open-label clinical trials have demonstrated decreases in aggression with SSRIs, including paroxetine at 20 mg/day and fluoxetine at 20 mg/day. One open-labeled study has suggested that bupropion at 300 mg/ day may be effective in treating youth with co-morbid CD, substance use disorders, and ADHD. Mood stabilizers are sometimes indicated to treat aggression in youth with chronic aggression and disruptive behavior, especially when these symptoms occur in the context of chronic irritability or frequent mood swings. Although lithium at a dose of 300–1200 mg/day or a blood level of 0.8–1.2 mmol/L has the most data supporting its effectiveness at decreasing aggression in youth, there have been two controlled studies that have demonstrated the effectiveness of divalproate at a dose of 750–1500 mg/day in decreasing aggression in youth with CD. Because of the potential for serious side effects of lithium and divalproate, including weight gain and associated negative outcomes, clinicians should continually monitor the effectiveness of these medications. The neuroleptics, both conventional and atypicals, have demonstrated benefits in a few studies. Most recently, a small (20 patients) double-blind, placebo-controlled study demonstrated the efficacy of risperidone (weight <50 kg, 0.25–1.5 mg/day; >50 kg, 0.5–3 mg/day) in the treatment of youth with CD. Unfortunately, to date, data only support short-term benefits. Because of the potential serious side effects of neuroleptics, e.g., weight gain, insulin resistance, and movement disorders, clinicians should continually monitor the effectiveness of the medication. The alpha-2-noradrenergic agonist clonidine, at a dose of up to 0.1–0.2 mg/day, has some efficacy, particularly when added to a stimulant in youth with co-morbid ADHD. Clinicians should monitor for sedation and hemodynamic side effects when using these medications. Although open trials demonstrated some benefit to the use of carbamazepine, a more recent controlled trial failed to confirm a significant difference when compared to placebo. To date, there are no published studies showing that topiramate is beneficial in the treatment of aggressive youth. Propranolol has decreased aggression in children with mental retardation and brain injury, however, there are no studies demonstrating efficacy in youth with CD.

CONCLUSION

While there is no single treatment proven universally effective for CD, the high cost of untreated CD, both to the youth and to society, warrants thoughtful but intensive treatment. A good treatment plan can only be formulated after a thorough assessment including determining the frequency and circumstances of target behaviors, co-morbid disorders, and other contributing factors such as educational needs, housing needs, and parental psychiatric disorders. The treatment plan should include appropriate interventions such as behavior management techniques, psychopharmacologic treatment, and targeted case management.

SUGGESTED READINGS

1. Bassarath L. Conduct disorder: a biopsychosocial review. Can J Psychiatry 2001; 46: 609–616.
2. Borduin CM. Multisystemic treatment of criminality and violence in adolescents. J Am Acad Child Adolesc Psychiatry 1999; 38:242–249.
3. Burke JD, Loeber R, Birmaher B. Oppositional defiant disorder and conduct disorder: a review of the past 10 years, part II. J Am Acad Child Adolesc Psychiatry 2002; 41: 1275–1293.
4. Lambert EW, Wahler RG, Andrade AR, Bickman L. Looking for the disorder in conduct disorder. J Abnorm Psychol 2001; 110:110–123.
5. Myers WC, Burton PR, Sanders PD, Donat KM, Cheney J, Fitzpatrick TM, Monaco L. Project back-on-track at 1 year: a delinquency treatment program for early-career juvenile offenders. J Am Acad Child Adolesc Psychiatry 2000; 39:1127–1134.
6. Stevens V, Van Oost P, De Bourdeaudhuij I. The effects of an anti-bullying intervention programme on peers' attitudes and behaviour. J Adolesc 2000; 23:21–34.
7. Woolfenden SR, Williams K, Peat JK. Family and parenting interventions for conduct disorder and delinquency: a meta-analysis of randomised controlled trials. Arch Dis Child 2002; 86:251–256.

76
Substance Abuse

Nancy P. Dalos
All Children's Hospital, Clearwater, Florida, U.S.A.

First it gave me wings to fly, then it took away the sky.
—*Anonymous*

INTRODUCTION

Along with other risk taking behaviors that increase in the preadolescent and adolescent years, substance abuse remains a significant source of concern for parents, health-care providers, and other professionals working with children. Significant morbidity and mortality remain associated with illicit drug use, including automobile accidents (30% of teen fatalities are associated with elevated blood alcohol levels, i.e., BAL), drownings, and other accidents. Coma or death due to intoxication and overdosage by use of one or more agents may occur at lower dosages of the ingested drug(s) or alcohol for teens compared to adults. Adolescents often consume larger quantities of alcohol and other substances quickly, seeking a rapid state of intoxication or euphoria. Such patterns of use (binging or chugging) may lead to death or irreversible brain damage.

The clinical potential for adverse outcomes in adolescence has been correlated with the patterns of use (Table 1), age, maturity, and other psychosocial factors. The nature of the specific substance utilized also determines the relative risk to the child's health. In children, individual (school and behavior problems, mental health issues) and family risk factors (i.e., degree of parental involvement, famiiy history of substance abuse) have also been noted to impact the potential for a youngster to move from experimenting to dependency or addiction in their pattern of drug use. Additional concerns related to the early use of illicit substances in preadolescence or early adolescence stem from findings of a clinically increased risk of latter addictions as adults. Studies specific to the regular use of alcohol before the age of 15 show a fourfold increase in risk of later alcohol dependence than in individuals who do not begin use of alcohol until age 21. This information as well as specific material regarding trends in use are followed by the National Institute on Drug Abuse (NIDA), and are well presented in Nelson's *Textbook of Pediatrics*, 17th Edition (1).

Table 1 Stages of Adolescent Substance Abuse

Stage	Learned behavior (compulsive coping)	Drugs of choice	Frequency of use	Clinical changes
I.	Experimentation "Learning the euphoria"	Tobacco, alcohol inhalants, marijuana	Occasional/ weekend	None obvious
II.	Regular use "Deliberately seeks euphoria,or effect of other drugs"	Alcohol, marijuana inhalants,uppers and downers	Every weekend	Change in personality, lying, oppositional, angry. Loss of interest in usual activities/friends
III.	Daily use "obsessed with achieving the high"	Alcohol, marijuana inhalants,uppers/ downers LSD, cocaine, heroin	Daily	Lying, stealing, loss of friends, job, school achievement. Depression, suicidal thoughts
IV.	Dependency/addiction burnout Increased levels of alcohol and other drugs to "feel normal"	Same as Stage III	Constant	Weight loss, cough poor health, memory loss, blackouts, risk-taking behavior, suicide

(Adapted with permission from A Family's Guide for the Prevention of Alcohol, Tobacco and Other Drug Use. Lowe Family Foundation, Inc., 2001.)

DIAGNOSIS AND EVALUATION

In the outpatient setting, a good history is the mainstay in the evaluation, along with identification of clinical signs and symptoms of drug use or abuse. Physical changes that may be noted include weight loss or gain, disheveled appearance, pallor, circles under the eyes, slurred or rapid speech, bloodshot eyes, or dilated pupils. Chronic coughing and a dry or runny nose may also be noted. Neurobehavioral changes are common, and may best be detected by parents and professionals who have established relationships with the child.

The most common patterns of adolescent drug use are outlined in Table 1. These include:

- Stage I Experimentation (initial use)
- Stage II Regular use
- Stage III Daily use
- Stage IV Dependency/addiction/burnout

The most common compounds of experimentation, heavy use, and abuse are tobacco (smokeless tobacco—SLT, cigarettes), alcohol, marijuana, inhalants, hallucinogens (LSD, mushrooms, PCP), "club drugs" (MDMA = [3,4-methylenedioxymethamphetamine] = X-Ecstasy; GHB = (gamma hydroxy butyrate) = Liquid Ecstasy/G/GHBuddy/Easy lay/date rape drug), cocaine (used with heroin = "speedball") and amphetamines (methamphetamine = "speed" or "ice"). The astute clinician who can effectively identify concerns regarding the signs and/or symptoms of adolescent substance use and abuse, including changes in behavior, academic performance, family stressors, change in peer group, changes in physical appearance and clinical signs may assist the family by identifying and confronting the problem, and by guiding them toward effective treatment options. Such caring guidance can be life saving for the child. Several brief questionnaires and screening tools have been developed to aid clinicians in this process; however, these are often limited in value due to frequent "refusal to report" on household surveys. School-based surveys also have significant limitations. It is recommended that referral for substance abuse treatment be made as soon as regular usage (Stage II) is identified.

TREATMENT

Prevention

Many educational programs have been developed to provide guidance to elementary, preadolescent, and adolescent patients. These are commonly presented in the schools. The most effective programs are those such as Families and Communities Together (FACT) developed by the Lowe Family Foundation. Such programs educate both students and parents, and enable a healthy dialogue within the family unit. According to the Partnership for a Drug Free America, parents who talk to their teens regularly about issues related to substance abuse experience a 42% decrease in the likelihood that teenagers will become involved in substance abuse. Teens who are nonusers have been noted to have strong parental relationships andguidance, and are able to discuss these issues with parents without fear. Such teens also have parents who are involved in their daily lives, activities, and monitor their activites closely.

Overdose and Withdrawal

In the Pediatric Emergency Room, Hospital, or ICU setting, consideration of drug intoxication must be raised in any patient exhibiting changes in mental status, including delirium, speech changes, delusions, paranoia, coma, confusion, and CNS stimulation or depression. Many times, the clinician may be confronted with signs of overdosage from one agent coexisting with signs of withdrawal from another. Seizures may be associated with opiate, alcohol, cocaine, and other drug use. Therefore, drug screening should be performed in all patients without prior histories of epilepsy.

The *alcohol overdose syndrome* is particularly important for parents, educators, police, and care providers within the health-care system to detect and correctly address. In any teenager who appears disoriented, lethargic, or comatose, a BAL or breathalizer test correlates well with clinical outcome. The BAL levels of 200 mg/dL are associated with risk of death from respiratory depression and levels of 500 mg/dL can be fatal. Respiratory support and monitoring are essential, and dialysis should be considered for patients with BAL greater than 400 mg/dL. The possibility of concurrent head trauma or other drug ingestions should also be considered. At the time of initial clinical assessment, it is also important to realize that the BAL may continue to rise, if large amounts of alcohol have been consumed but not yet absorbed into the vascular system. Therefore, it is always prudent advice to a parent, caregiver, or friend, to bring an intoxicated patient to the Emergency Room for assessment, and not to advise them to "let the teen to sleep it off." Many adolescent and young adult (college age) deaths occur each year, after individuals who have binged or chugged alcohol develop respiratory depression, coma, and

MENTAL STATUS CHANGES

Delerium, Euphoria
Mumbling Speech
Hallucinations

Delusions, Paranoia
Aggitation
Seizures, Myoclonus

Confusion,
Coma CNS
Depression

Obtain serum chemistries, CBC, urine drug screen
Blood Alcohol Level
Head CT if indicated
Assess Respiratory and Cardiovascular Status

Are Pupils

Dilated

Fluctuating

Constricted

SUSPECT

Combination of Agents

Anticholinergics
Antihistamines
Antipsychotics, Antidepressants
Organic agents/Plants Cocaine,
methamphetamine

Opiates
Sedatives
Alcohol
Cholinergic agents
Mushrooms

ASSOCIATED WITH

Tachycardia, Dry Flushed
Skin (Anticholinergic) or
Diaphoresis (Sympathomimetic
Syndrome), Myoclonus, Seizures,
Urinary Retention, Hyperreflexia

Increased Salivation, Diaphoresis
Respiratory Depression
Hypotension
Weakness, Hyporeflexia
Seizures

MONITOR FOR

Arrythmias
Hypotension
Seizures

Respiratory depression
Hypotension
GI, Renal, Hepatic Dysfunction

OVERDOSAGE WITH OTHER "GATEWAY DRUGS"
USUALLY NOT FATAL

Accute Marijuana Ingestion

Present euphoric, relaxed.
Dysphoria with high dosages (Hashish)
Can Rx with Benzodiazapines

Not fatal unless combined with other
Substances.

Inhalants

Usually produce short-term
effects (15-30 minutes)
History of "huffing"

Produce relaxation, euphoria,
Incoordination, slurred speech,
Diplopia

Poor outcomes when associated
Accidents (drowning), Pulmonary
And renal toxicity (Freon), or
Gasoline Sniffing Encephalopathy

Figure 1 Algorithm for acute intoxication/overdose.

death during sleep. Likewise, treatment with cold showers, coffee, fruit juice, and exercise do not accelerate the rate of metabolism of alcohol by the liver or effect the clinical outcome (Fig. 1).

CHRONIC TREATMENT OF ESTABLISHED DEPENDENCE/ADDICTION

Teens who develop usage patterns of chronic daily use (Stage III) and dependency and addiction (Stage IV) require acknowledgement of the problem and confrontation in a loving supportive manner but with initiation of new guidelines for limitation of behavior, and increased monitoring of the child's activities. A network of teachers, parents, physicians, and counselors must then be established to allow the child to enter into the recovery phase of his/her illness. Treatment options should be supervised by an individual specialized in the treatment of substance abuse and addictions, and may require a period of detoxification followed by further inpatient or intensive outpatient rehabilitative therapy which may last for a period of 3 6 weeks. Following the intensive phase of treatment, maintenance of sobriety is best achieved by participation in an outpatient therapeutic community and involvement in programs such as alcoholics annonymous (AA) or narcotics annonymous (NA). Treatment of addictions does not involve an effort to "cure" the individual, but rather to provide a relapse prevention program aimed at eliminating the compulsion to use illicit substances to deal with life and life's problems, and to help teens develop more effective coping strategies. In Barbara Cole's book, Gifts of Sobriety, the process of recovery is described as that of finding our real self, something that the disease of addiction covers up. Our children need to be encouraged to believe that their true self is the precious gift which can be received when the promises of recovery come true. Through the love and caring of the therapeutic recovery community dreams can be restored, and a special vision of hope can be renewed within the world of the affected child and their family.

REFERENCE

1. Jenkins RR. Substance abuse. In: Nelson Textbook of Pediatrics. 17th ed. Philadelphia, PA: Saunders, 2004.

SUGGESTED READINGS

1. Cole BS. Gifts of Sobriety; When the Promises of Recovery Come True. Hazeldon, 2000.
2. Dryfoos JG. Adolescents at Risk, Prevalence and Prevention. Oxford University Press, 1990.
3. Ketchum K, William FA. Beyond the Influence, Understanding and Defeating Alcoholism. Bantum Books, 2000.
4. Lowe Family Foundation. A Family Guide: Alcohol, Tobacco, Other Drugs and Teenagers.
5. NIDA/National Institute on Drug Abuse/National Institutes of Health/www.drugabuse.gov High School and Youth Trends; Trends in Use. 2000–2002.
6. Popkin MH. Active Parenting of Teens, Parents Guide. Atlanta, GA: Active Parenting Publishers, 1988.

77

Neuroleptic Malignant Syndrome, Serotonin Syndrome, and Malignant Hyperthermia

Ian Butler and Pedro Mancias
The University of Texas Medical School at Houston, Houston, Texas, U.S.A.

INTRODUCTION

Neuroleptic malignant syndrome (NMS) and malignant hyperthermia (MH) have both been recognized since the 1960s and are usually diagnosed by psychiatrists or anesthesiologists. Furthermore, MH was diagnosed in an acute clinical setting of succinylcholine induction associated with halogenated anesthetics for surgical procedures, whereas NMS was apparent over several hours or days (subacute) and included neuropsychiatric manifestations in patients on neuroleptics. Serotonin syndrome (SS) was also recognized in the 1960s but has come into prominence with the increased use of selective serotonin reuptake inhibitors (SSRIs) as antidepressants. However, overlap features were readily recognized and included autonomic nervous system (ANS) instability, variable temperature elevations, and muscular rigidity with increased serum creatine kinase (CK) levels. Recently, with increased understanding of the role of calcium homeostasis in neuronal and muscle excitability, such as excitation–contraction coupling (muscle) and neurotransmitter release (neuronal), investigators have questioned a common pathophysiology for these disorders due to defects in calcium metabolism and homeostasis.

Appending "malignant" to these disorders emphasizes their severity and potentially fatal consequences without prompt recognition and urgent management. Furthermore, physicians evaluating children and adolescents are now likely to encounter such cases in their hospitals (MH) or outpatient clinics (NMS and SS) given the frequency of surgical and anesthetic procedures in children and the increasing use of neuroleptics and other psychotropic agents in children and adolescents.

NEUROLEPTIC MALIGNANT SYNDROME (NMS)

Neuroleptic malignant syndrome was recognized in the French literature in the 1960s following the introduction of neuroleptic medications in the 1950s. NMS has been mostly associated with high potency neuroleptics such as haloperidol and thiothixene. However, "atypical" neuroleptics such as risperidone and olanzapine have been associated with NMS, in addition to various other medications that rapidly alter functions of dopaminergic neurons, such as levodopa withdrawal, tetrabenazine administration, and abrupt withdrawal of baclofen.

DIAGNOSIS AND EVALUATION

Clinical awareness and early recognition of neuroleptic malignant syndrome are critical to management and are more likely to occur and be recognized following initial administration of neuroleptics, however, delayed clinical onset may occur while changing or increasing neuroleptics in clinical practice. Clinical features of NMS include hyperthermia, sympathetic nervous system over activity (hypertension, tachycardia), increased muscle tone with elevated serum CK levels, and altered consciousness or mental status (Table 1).

The differential diagnosis of NMS may be difficult since early behavioral manifestations may be mistaken for exacerbations of the underlying neuropsychiatric disorder, and increasing doses of neuroleptics may be recommended. Furthermore, there are a number of important medical conditions that need to be recognized, many having prominent neuropsychiatric presentations (Table 2). Screening for various psychotropic drugs and porphyrins in urine, and thyroid function and CK levels in blood, can be valuable adjuncts to a careful history and examination.

MANAGEMENT

Management of NMS centers around early recognition and careful withdrawal of the presumed offending agent. This may not be readily achieved depending on the

Table 1 Clinical Features of Neuroleptic Malignant Syndrome

Cardinal features	*Associated features*	
• Hyperthermia	• Akinesia	• Fluctuating BP
• Rigidity	• Tremor	• Tachycardia
• Autonomic instability	• Dystonia	• Diaphoresis
• Altered consciousness	• Dysphagia	• Incontinence
	• Sialorrhea	• Pallor
		• Flushing

Table 2 Differential Diagnosis of Neuroleptic Malignant Syndrome

• Malignant hyperthermia	• Thyrotoxicosis
• Heatstroke	• Acute porphyria
• Serotonin syndrome	• Tetanus
• Lethal catatonia	• Tetany
• Encephalitis	• Akinetic mutism
• Drug intoxication—MDMA, cocaine	• Locked-in-syndrome

neuropsychiatric diagnosis and specific drug(s) administered. Drug toxicity screening (blood and urine) may be necessary in clinical settings of uncertain drug access in children. Meticulous supportive care in an intensive-care unit will be necessary in order to correct fluid and electrolyte imbalances in a febrile patient with an impaired level of consciousness and requiring respirator support and artificial cooling (blanket or mattress). Autonomic instability (cardiac arrhythmias and blood pressure fluctuations) requires careful and continuous monitoring of vital signs. Baseline biochemical studies should include serum electrolytes (particularly potassium levels) and indicators of rhabdomyolysis (serum CK, blood, and urine myoglobin levels) with frequent monitoring of renal and hepatic functions. Adequate hydration and acid–base therapy may be valuable in preventing myoglobin-induced renal failure.

There are no specific pharmacological agents that have been rigorously evaluated clinically, however, intravenous dantrolene sodium 3–5 mg/kg/day divided t.i.d. or q.i.d., has been recommended as specific therapy to maintain calcium homeostasis in muscle cytoplasm. Dopaminergic agents are recommended as a counter to dopamine receptor blocking or dopamine depleting actions of the offending psychotropic agent. Bromocriptine 2.5–5 mg q.i.d. or amantadine 200–400 mg daily or levodopa/carbidopa via nasogastric tube has been recommended as dopamine agonists. Benzodiazepines, by indirectly increasing dopaminergic activity by affecting gamma-aminobutyric acid (GABA) action, may be administered for increased muscle rigidity, agitation, or even catatonia. There are reports of improvement with electroconvulsive treatment (ECT). Initiation and withdrawal of specific pharmacological agents require careful clinical judgment and consultation with intensive-care and psychiatric colleagues.

SEROTONIN SYNDROME (SS)

SS has been increasingly recognized with the widespread use (including children) of SSRIs for depression and a variety of neuropsychiatric conditions of childhood. Enhanced central serotoninergic neurotransmission (toxic effect) has been implicated and there is clinical overlap with other malignant syndromes (NMS and MH). Furthermore, subtle forms of this syndrome may be increasingly recognized as child psychiatrists and child neurologists use multiple psychoactive medications with overlapping actions (serotoninergic) in behavioral management of children (Tourette syndrome, autism, and obsessive-compulsive states). With the widespread use of serotonin agonists (e.g., sumatriptan, rizatriptan, and dihydroergotamine) in the symptomatic treatment of childhood onset migraine, often combined with a tricyclic agent for migraine prophylaxis, pediatric neurologists can anticipate an increased incidence of the serotonin syndrome.

DIAGNOSIS AND CLINICAL FEATURES

SS occurs in the context of administration of serotonin elevating drugs (often multiple serotoninergic agents), particularly the various SSRIs, but also including tricyclic antidepressants (TCAs) and monoamine oxidase inhibitors (MAOIs) that can also elevate nervous system levels of serotonin. Clinical features can be similar to NMS, including altered mental status and behavioral changes, autonomic nervous system dysfunction (diaphoresis, diarrhea, and temperature instability) with muscle rigidity and hyper-reflexia, myoclonus, ataxia, and tremors. Rhabdomyolysis and associated metabolic changes are less frequent.

MANAGEMENT

The management of patients with (malignant) SS is very similar to that for NMS, omitting the use of dopamine agonists and also agents for rigidity (dantrolene sodium), unless rigidity is clinically apparent, despite adequate use of benzodiazepines (for agitation and rigidity). The subsequent use of psychotropic agents for the underlying neuropsychiatric disorder will need to be carefully weighed against potential recurrence of the syndrome.

MALIGNANT HYPERTHERMIA (MH)

Malignant hyperthermia (MH) associated with general anesthesia was also described in the 1960s and was recognized as a lethal form of hypermetabolism occurring during or shortly after an anesthetic procedure in which a halogenated anesthetic agent (such as halothane or enflurane or sevoflurane) was administered and often preceded by induction with succinylcholine (masseter spasm). Variable occurrences with similar anesthetic agents for previous or subsequent surgical procedures were recognized, together with a familial tendency (dominant, rarely recessive). Clinical studies suggested a population frequency of 1:8500 with an increased incidence in childhood and patients with neuromuscular disorders, including central core myopathic disorders (CCD) but also muscular dystrophies and myotonic disorders. The incidence of MH crises during general anesthesia varies from 1:15,000 in children to 1:50,000 in adults. There were early attempts at patient identification by phenotypic features (King, Denborough syndrome) and screening for elevated serum CK levels prior to surgery. Advances in understanding and recognizing this pharmaco-toxic entity have included studies of: porcine stress syndrome linked to chromosome 6; MH linked to human chromosome 19q 11.2–13.2; ryanodine receptor (RYRI) mapped to porcine chromosome 6 and human chromosome 19; heterozygous mutations in RYRI gene in some cases of MH and MH/CCD; and interaction of calcium in muscle excitation–contraction coupling with RYR1 receptor (sarcoplasmic reticulum, SR) and dihydropyridine receptor: DHPR component of voltage gated L-type calcium channels (sarcoplasmic-T-tubules).

DIAGNOSIS AND EVALUATION

Over the past two decades, the clinical and metabolic features of MH have been well recognized and described by anesthesiologists. Since phenotypic features are rarely evident and there is rarely a prior or family history of MH, sustained jaw rigidity (masseter spasm with succinylcholine) apparent during intubation may be the initial manifestation of this potentially severe disorder. Only somewhat later does the temperature rise in the patient and anesthetic soda-lime canister and give warning to the anesthesiologist of an impending hypermetabolic crisis. Progression to the late clinical stages is fortunately uncommon in modern anesthetic practice (Table 3). Diagnostic considerations during these critical minutes may include other disorders

Table 3 Clinical Features of Malignant Hyperthermia

Onset	Clinical signs
Early	Sustained jaw rigidity after succinylcholine Tachypnea Rapid exhaustion of soda-lime Hot soda-lime canister Elevated, irregular pulse rate
Middle	Patient hot to touch, elevated temperature Cyanosis with dark blood in wound Elevated, irregular pulse rate
Late	Generalized muscle rigidity Prolonged bleeding Dark urine with oliguria Elevated, irregular pulse rate Death

(Table 4) associated with a hypermetabolic state, such as acute dysautonomia (hyperadrenergic state), febrile (infectious) conditions, and acute rhabdomyolysis (muscle trauma or ischemia).

From a practical viewpoint, in patients with a classical MH response to typical anesthetic agents, further confirmatory (in vitro contracture test) studies are probably not indicated. With increasing understanding of the role of calcium in excitation–contraction coupling in muscle and contraction sensitivity of isolated human muscle fibers to various concentrations of pharmacological agents, there has developed an in vitro contracture test (IVCT) for human and research studies of MH utilizing halothane, caffeine, ryanodine, and 4-chloro-*m*-cresol. Clinical situations in which IVCT is of value may include identification of other family members requiring future surgery (despite previously uneventful surgeries), evaluation of family members with proven or suspected central core disease (and possibly other myopathies), and evaluation of patients with mild MH reactions (e.g., masseter spasm) during previous anesthesias. Unfortunately at this stage, genetic studies of specific mutations in known (RYRI) and putative (DHPR receptor, sodium channel) genes are not practical given the size of the gene (RYR1 has 5000 amino acids encoded by 106 exons) and apparent genetic heterogeneity.

Table 4 Differential Diagnosis of Malignant Hyperthermia

- Inadequate anesthesia or analgesia
- Inappropriate breathing circuit, fresh gas flow or ventilation
- Infection or sepsis
- Tourniquet ischemia
- Anaphylaxis
- Pheochromocytoma
- Thyroid storm
- Cerebral ischemia
- Other muscle disease

MANAGEMENT

The short-term outcome and evaluation of patients with clinical features of MH will depend on the clinical stage (early, middle, late) at recognition and the current stage of the surgical procedure, as to whether management should be initiated (intravenous dantrolene sodium), changing the anesthetic drug to a nonhalogenated agent, and completion or deferral of surgery. There is now excellent clinical and in vitro evidence of a disturbance in calcium metabolism in muscle cell cytoplasm leading to increased muscle contractions in patients with MH. Dantrolene sodium is now the drug of choice in managing patients with MH syndrome at all clinical stages. Dantrolene sodium inhibits RYR1 function by limiting channel activation by calmodulin and calcium. RYR1 (plant alkaloid ryanodine binds to receptor) is a SR protein with calcium^{2+} activated calcium^{2+} ATP-ase pump properties maintaining appropriate gradients of stored (SR) and cytoplasmic calcium for muscle contraction. Intracellular calcium-induced hypermetabolism in muscle (and liver) can be alleviated (or prevented) by intravenous dantrolene sodium 2.5 mg/kg (dissolved in sterile water) and repeated as necessary, such that more than 10 mg/kg may be required to control an acute MH event. Intravenously administered dantrolene sodium is usually effective in 5–10 min. MH patients require intensive-care monitoring, including serum electrolytes (calcium, sodium, potassium, bicarbonate, and glucose levels), CK levels, acid–base studies (ABGs), electrocardiographic monitoring for arrhythmias, and coagulation studies (disseminated intravascular coagulopathy). Dantrolene sodium administered early in the course of an MH episode may prevent the need for further life-saving treatments. However, cardiac arrhythmias from hypocalcemia, hypercapnia, and hyperkalemia will require specific management, including cardiac consultation and intravenous lidocaine with correction of metabolic disturbances. Active cooling to 38°C may be necessary. Since recrudescence of MH reaction may occur, maintenance dantrolene sodium (1 mg/kg every 6 hr) is recommended for 24 hr with intensive-care monitoring for at least 36 hr. Careful observation for muscle injury with elevated CK and myoglobin levels during this period will be necessary to prevent subsequent renal injury from muscle necrosis.

CONCLUSION

Iatrogenic pharmaco-toxicity is well known to practicing physicians, including physicians evaluating children with various neurological and neuromuscular disorders. Including the term "malignant" in a clinical entity emphasizes the seriousness of the condition and potential lethality. Such is the case with the three disorders considered, neuroleptic malignant syndrome, serotonin syndrome, and malignant hyperthermia disorder. All three disorders are relatively rare and most likely will be recognized in a hospital, operating room, or intensive-care setting. However, the two conditions related to the use of psychotropic agents may initially present to a physician or pediatrician in the outpatient clinic. Although withdrawal of the offending (toxic) agent is imperative, managing the toxic effects on various organs (brain, muscle, heart, liver, kidney) becomes critical and modern management has been effective in significantly reducing the morbidity of these pharmo-toxic states. Since all three conditions have significant clinical overlap, all three may need to be considered in the differential diagnosis in particular patients, e.g., comatose patient in which unknown drugs administered (dopamine receptor antagonists, serotonin agonists) and delayed (possibility unrecognized) MH reactions in the postoperative intensive-care setting. The common etiologic role of disturbed calcium homeostasis in these conditions may explain the overlapping clinical manifestations and the common role of dantrolene sodium on decreasing cytoplasmic calcium levels.

SUGGESTED READINGS

1. Carbone JR. The neuroleptic malignant and serotonin syndromes. Emer Med Clin N Am 2000; 18(2):317–325.
2. Frank JP, Harati Y, Butler IJ, Nelson TE, Scott CI. Central core disease and malignant hyperthermia syndrome. Ann Neurol 1980; 7:11–17.
3. Gurrera RJ. Is neuroleptic malignant syndrome a neurogenic form of malignant hyperthermia? Clin Neuropharmacol 2002; 25(4):183–193.
4. Hopkins PM. Malignant hyperthermia; advances in clinical management and diagnosis. Br J Anaesth 2000; 85:118–128.
5. Jurkat-Rott K, McCarthy T, Lehmann-Horn F. Genetics and pathogenesis of malignant hyperthermia. Muscle Nerve 2000; 23:4–17.
6. Mathew NT, Tietjen GE, Lucker C. Serotonin syndrome complicating migraine pharmacotherapy. Cephalgia 1996; 16(5):323–327.
7. Rosenbaum HK, Miller JD. Malignant hyperthermia and myotonic disorders. Anesthesiol Clin N Am 2002; 20:623–664.
8. Susman VL. Clinical management of neuroleptic malignant syndrome. Psychiatric Quart 2001; 72(4):325–336.
9. Ty EB, Rothner AD. Neuroleptic malignant syndrome in children and adolescents. J Child Neurol 2001; 16:157–163.

78
Pediatric Sleep Disorders

Carolyn Elizabeth Hart
Mecklenburg Neurological Associates, Charlotte, North Carolina, U.S.A.

INTRODUCTION

Sleep disorders in infants, children, and adolescents are commonplace but frequently are overlooked. Approximately 25% of children have some type of sleep disturbance, but unlike adults, often go unrecognized. Problems may come to medical attention only under the guise of some resulting symptom, or if the child's sleep pattern creates a problem for the parents. Recognition of this issue should lead physicians to specifically question pediatric patients and their parents about sleep patterns.

DIAGNOSIS

A quick screening history can be obtained by using the mnemonic BuMPSSS: Bedtime Problems (behavioral, circadian), Movements (periodic limb movements, rocking), Parasomnias (sleep talking, walking, terrors, enuresis), Snoring/Sleepiness/and Secondary to other factors. A suspicious finding can then prompt a more detailed sleep history. Often if a child sleeps better in a specific location, the problem is more likely behavioral than pathologic. Inquiring about associated problems such as allergies, asthma, gastroesophageal reflux, overweight, hypertension, medications, and family/environmental difficulties can frequently be helpful. Relevant family history factors include restless legs syndrome, narcolepsy, idiopathic hypersomnia, and attention deficit hyperactivity disorder (ADHD). Further historical details can be obtained through use of patient questionnaires such as the Children's Sleep Habits Questionnaire and completing a 2-week sleep diary.

Physical examination should include a search for tonsillar hypertrophy, narrowed nasal passages, abnormal vital signs, cardiac, pulmonary, neuromuscular, and musculoskeletal abnormalities.

Polysomnogram (PSG) is warranted if there is unexplained daytime sleepiness or suspected sleep apnea and should be considered for paroxysmal arousals. A multiple sleep latency test (MSLT) and CSF hypocretin 1 level may be warranted if narcolepsy is suspected. EEG, EKG, x-rays of chest/head/neck, hematocrit, chemistries, thyroid function tests, sedimentation rate, urinalysis, and urine toxicology screen should be considered selectively.

NORMAL SLEEP DEVELOPMENT

Before determining if there is a sleep disorder, it is important to understand the normal sleep patterns and durations for age. Newborns demonstrate three sleep stages; active (precursor to REM), quiet, and indeterminate, each with EEG and clinical characteristics. Newborns usually enter sleep through REM and sleep 16–20 hr per day in 2–4 hr cycles. A diurnal cycle (circadian entrainment) occurs by about 2–4 months of age so that infants begin to "sleep through the night" (70–80% by 9 months) with a morning and an afternoon nap. Sleep stages 1–4 and REM can usually be differentiated by 4–6 months of age.

Around one year of age, most children give up the second nap, and the diurnal phase of wakefulness lengthens such that total sleep time (TST) is 12–14 hr per day. REM percentage decreases from about 50% in the newborn to about 30% at one year. Bedtime routines and transitional objects are important. Over the next several years, 90-min REM/NREM cycles develop, and TST decreases to 11–12 hr per day. By age 5, many children give up regular naps. In ages 6–12 years, TST gradually shortens from about 11 to about 9 hr per day, and napping is rare. Sleep efficiency is high and slow wave sleep (SWS) is plentiful.

Although adolescents typically need about 9 hr of sleep per night, most only get about 7. Sleep onset is often delayed by circadian and voluntary factors, and sleep offset is often advanced by early school start times. Many teens run a sleep "debt" during the school week and try to "catch up" on weekends. Slow wave sleep percentage, sleep efficiency, and latency to REM onset all decrease.

SPECIFIC DISORDERS AND TREATMENT

The International Classification of Sleep Disorders-Revised (ICSD-R) consists of dyssomnias (disorders of initiating and maintaining sleep and disorders of excessive daytime sleepiness), parasomnias (disorders of arousal and stage transition), secondary disorders (due to mental, neurological, or other conditions), and proposed sleep disorders. Since the aforementioned list was not intended to serve as a differential diagnostic listing, I personally find the following classification to be more useful in the clinical pediatric setting: (A) disorders of sleep timing, arousals, and state; (B) disorders of breathing; (C) disorders of movement; and (D) disorders secondary to other factors. Many sleep disturbances tend to occur most commonly at particular stages of the sleep cycle (Fig. 1).

Disorders of Sleep Timing, Arousals, and State

1. *Limit-setting disorder.* Since the invention of electric lighting (and associated gadgetry), delaying bedtime has been a temptation for children and adults alike. Consistent behavioral management is the treatment.
2. *Delayed sleep phase syndrome.* In this condition, a child's circadian rhythm leads to delayed, but regular sleep onset and offset, a pattern common in adolescence. Treatments include delaying bedtime progressively to reset the internal clock, bright light therapy, and melatonin (1–3 mg q hs).
3. *NREM disorders.* Arousals that occur commonly in NREM sleep include somnambulism, sleep terrors, and confusional arousals. Treatment consists of education/reassurance, scheduled awakenings, protection from

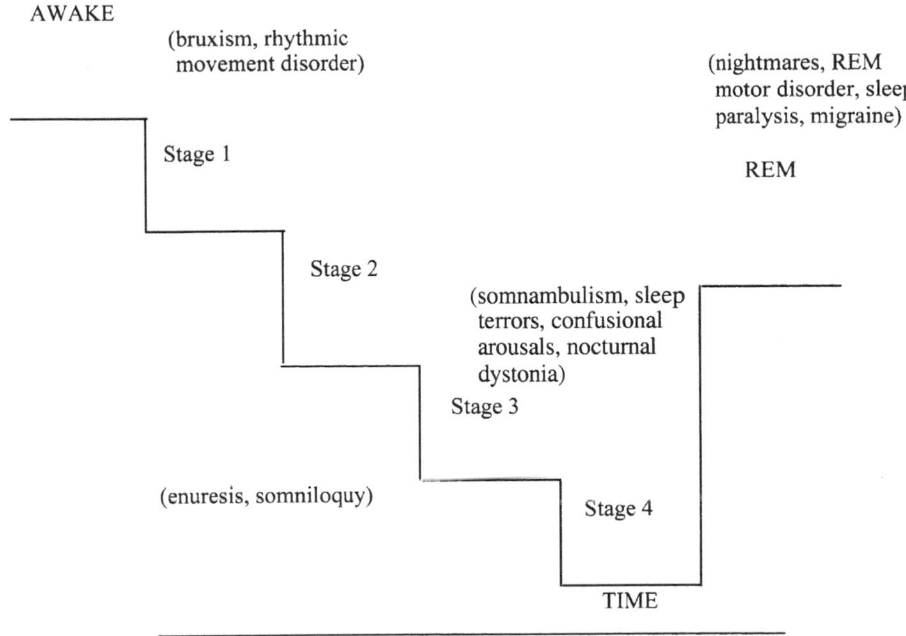

Figure 1 Relationship of parasomnias/arousals to sleep stage.

injury, and relaxation techniques at bedtime. Clonazepam in small doses may be helpful if symptoms are frequent or dangerous (0.01–0.03 mg/kg q hs).

4. *REM disorders*. Arousals associated with REM sleep include nightmares and rarely, sleep paralysis or REM sleep motor disorder.
5. *Nonstate specific*. Somniloquy (sleep talking) and enuresis can occur in any sleep stage. Somniloquy usually does not require treatment. Enuresis is especially common (approximately 25%) among children with ADHD. This problem can be addressed through preventive measures (voiding at bedtime, no caffeine, etc.), moisture alarm, and medications such as imipramine (10–50 mg q hs), DDAVP (desmopressin; 0.2–0.6 mg po or 20–40 mcg IN q hs for children over 6 years of age), and oxybutynin (5 mg q hs for children over 5 years of age).
6. *Narcolepsy*. Narcolepsy can be thought of as a disorder in which sleep and wakefulness are not neatly distinguished and instead intrude on each other. Recent studies have shown an association with low CSF hypocretin 1 levels, probably indicating a deficit in wake-promoting circuits. Symptoms include excessive daytime somnolence, cataplexy, sleep paralysis, and hypnagogic hallucinations. Although symptom onset is often in late childhood or adolescence, manifestations may be only partial and unfortunately, the diagnosis of narcolepsy is commonly delayed for years. PSG and MSLT show rapid sleep onset and shortened latency to REM onset. Treatment involves scheduled naps, education, good sleep habits, stimulants (methylphenidate or amphetamine preparations) or modafinil (100–400 mg q am) to improve diurnal alertness, selective serotonin reuptake inhibitors (e.g., sertraline 25–200 mg/d), tricyclic antidepressants (e.g., amitryptline 25–100 mg q hs), trazodone (25–100 mg q hs), zolpidem (5–10 mg q hs), or zaleplon (5–20 mg q hs) to improve sleep pattern.

Disorders of Breathing

1. *Primary snoring*. Five to ten percent of children snore nightly, and many of these have primary snoring (PS). This is a benign condition that consists of snoring without associated apnea, hypopnea, sleep disturbance, or daytime symptoms. History and physical examination have not proved accurate in distinguishing PS and obstructive sleep apnea/hypopnea (OSA/OH), so PSG may be warranted. Treatment for PS is usually not needed, but it may be a risk factor for later OSA. About one-third of children with ADHD have PS, and about one-third of snoring children have ADHD.
2. *Obstructive sleep apnea/hypopnea*. One to three percent of children have clinically significant OSA. Upper airway and chest wall muscle tone, respiratory rate, tidal volume, and responses to changes in pCO_2 and pO_2 all decrease in sleep. Symptoms include snoring, restlessness, mouth breathing, secondary enuresis, and daytime somnolence (often manifested as ADHD-like symptoms rather than sleepiness). As mentioned above, PSG is warranted if OSA is suspected. Polysomnogram normative values for children are not firmly established, but an Apnea Index of greater than 1 per hour is typically abnormal. Normally end-tidal CO_2 should not be above 50 mmHg for more that 10% of TST. Hypopneas are more common than apneas in children, and children are less likely to arouse due to a respiratory event. Children with OSA often benefit from tonsillectomy or adenoidectomy although some patients experience symptom recurrence after this procedure. Other measures include continuous positive airway pressure (CPAP), nasal steroids, elevation of head of bed and other positional strategies, oral appliances, and other surgical procedures.
3. *Central apnea*. Central apneas are common and usually benign in infants and children. If symptomatic or severe, neuroimaging with attention to posterior fossa and brainstem and treatment with continuous positive airway pressure (CPAP) or may be considered.

Disorders of Movement

1. *Periodic limb movement disorder (PLMD)/restless leg syndrome (RLS)*. The PLMs in sleep are jerky repetitive movements that last 1–5 sec, involve lower more than upper extremities, and recur at 20–40 sec intervals. The PLMD is diagnosed when there is sleep disruption due to PLMs that occur at least 5 times per hour for adults and perhaps 3–4 times per hour for children. The RLS consists of uncomfortable leg sensations, magnified at rest and in the evening and relieved by movement. The PLMD can occur without RLS, but most patients with RLS also have PLMD. Recent studies have shown that PLMD occurs in children, especially among children with ADHD (26%). Treatment options especially in patients with RLS include dopaminergic agents (e.g., pramipexole 0.125–1.5 mg q hs, ropinirole 0.25–5 mg q hs), gabapentin (300–900 mg q hs), clonazepam (0.25–2 mg q hs), and if ferritin is below 50 mcg, ferrous sulfate supplementation (325 mg $FeSO_4$ or 65 mg elemental iron plus 250–500 mg vitamin C to improve absorption).
2. *Rhythmic movement disorder*. Body rocking or head banging occurs in some children, primarily during sleep–wake transitions. There is a familial

component, and the pattern usually disappears by about age 4 without treatment.

Disorders Secondary to Other Factors

Seizures can occur in any sleep stage but may be most common in NREM stage 2. Migraines tend to be REM associated. Depression is associated with decreased SWS, latency to REM onset, and sleep efficiency. Patients with allergies, asthma, GERD, and other systemic illnesses may experience worsening of symptoms at night and suffer consequent sleep disturbance. Hunger, cold, noise, fear, stress, smoke, and strife can all obviously impair sleep onset, quality, and maintenance. Many medications can affect sleep including stimulants, bronchodilators, caffeine, tricyclic antidepressants, benzodiazepines, anticonvulsants, and antihistamines.

Alleviating these myriad causes of sleeplessness, sleep disruption, and sleepiness in children is very rewarding and can have a hugely beneficial impact on public health and well being.

SUGGESTED READINGS

1. American Academy of Pediatrics. Clinical practice guideline: diagnosis and management of childhood obstructive sleep apnea syndrome. Pediatrics 2002; 109:704–712.
2. American Academy of Sleep Medicine. ICSD-International Classification of Sleep Disorders-revised: Diagnostic and Coding Manual. American Academy of Sleep Medicine, 2000.
3. Ferber R, Kryger M. Principles and Practice of Sleep Medicine in the Child. ISBN 0721647618; WB Saunders, 1995.
4. National Sleep Foundation, www.sleepfoundation.org.
5. Owens JA, Spirito A, McGuinn M. The Children's Sleep Habits Questionnaire (CSHQ): psychometric properties of a survey instrument for school-aged children. Sleep 2000; 23(8):1043–1051.
6. Picchietti DL, Walters AS. Moderate to severe periodic limb movement disorder in childhood and adolescence. Sleep 1999; 22(3):297–300.
7. Schechter MS, and the American Academy of Pediatrics, Section on Pulmonology, Subcommittee on Obstructive Sleep Apnea Syndrome. Technical report: diagnosis and management of childhood obstructive sleep syndrome. Pediatrics 2002; 109(4): http://www.pediatrics.org/cgi/content/full/109/4/e69.

79

Sturge–Weber Syndrome

Anne M. Comi
Johns Hopkins University, Baltimore, Maryland, U.S.A.

Bernard L. Maria
Medical University of South Carolina, Charleston, South Carolina, U.S.A.

INTRODUCTION

Sturge–Weber syndrome (SWS) is the third most common neurocutaneous disorder but unlike neurofibromatosis or tuberous sclerosis, it is sporadic. Although clinical and imaging features are heterogeneous, there is typically the presence of a facial port-wine stain, in the ophthalmic distribution of the trigeminal nerve, glaucoma and vascular eye abnormalities, and a parieto-occipital leptomeningeal angioma ipsilateral to the cutaneous and ocular anomalies. Somatic mutation has been proposed as a possible etiology, however the putative gene(s) is unknown.

Children and teenagers with SWS often develop neurologic problems including seizures, migraines, stroke-like episodes, learning difficulties or mental retardation, visual field cuts, and hemiparesis. Children with SWS are also at increased risk for hemiatrophy, visual impairment, ADHD, behavioral and emotional difficulties. Neuro-developmental outcomes in this disorder are highly variable, however. Early diagnosis is required to ensure the appropriate screening and management of associated complications as they arise. Multiple specialists, including a neurologist, ophthalmologist, dermatologist, medical rehabilitation specialist, occupational and physical therapists, speech and language pathologist, psychiatrist and behavioral psychologist, are therefore often involved in the care of individuals with SWS (Fig. 1).

PRESENTATIONS

The diagnosis of SWS can frequently be suspected when an infant is noted to have a facial port-wine stain. The diagnosis of SWS means that the cutaneous port-wine stain is associated with either brain or eye involvement. The risk of an associated underlying leptomeningeal angioma and/or glaucoma is about 8% with a port-wine stain anywhere on the face. Thus, the overwhelming majority of children with a facial port-wine stain do not have SWS. This risk increases to about 25% when the skin angioma is in the V1 ophthalmic distribution on the face. A careful

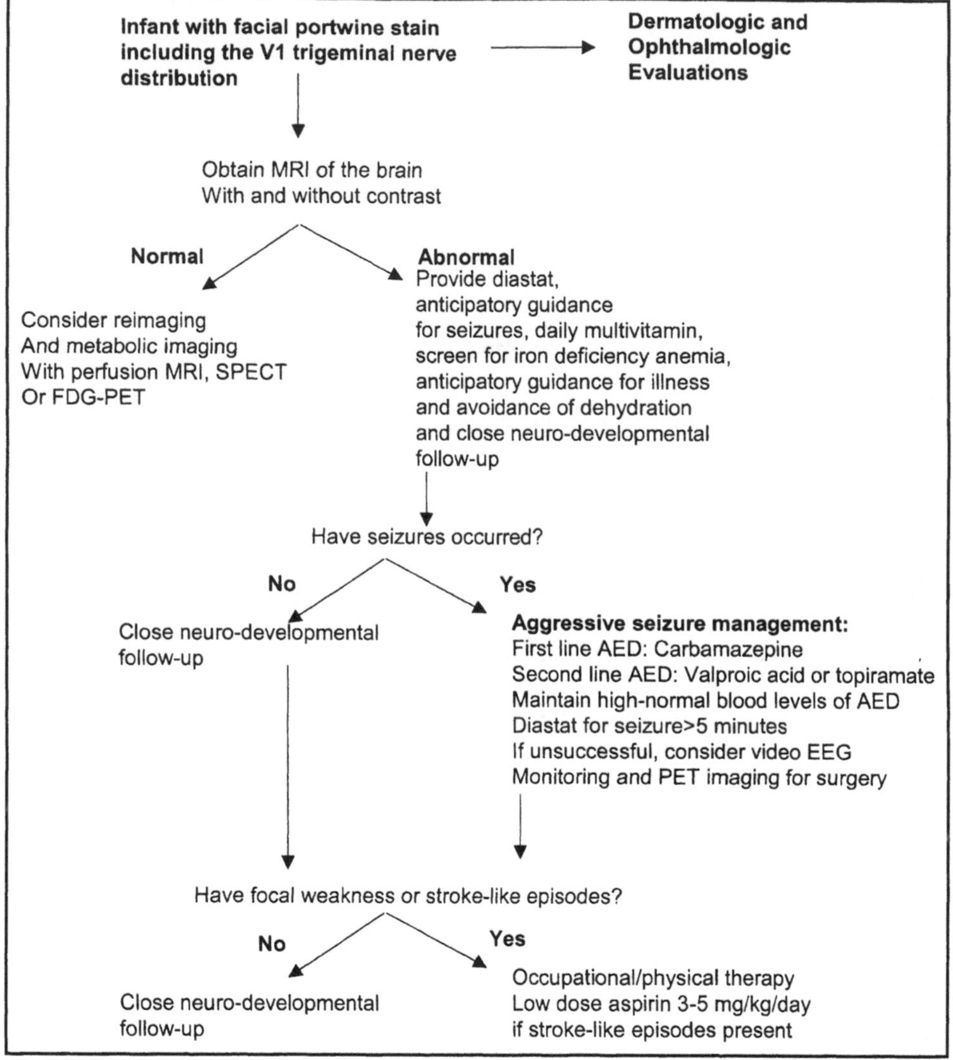

Figure 1 Evaluating an infant with facial cutaneous capillovascular malformation (port-wine stain).

examination of the upper eyelid may reveal cutaneous involvement of just a few millimeters in some cases. The risk of intracranial involvement increases to 33% with bilateral facial port-wine stains. In approximately 85% of children with SWS, the involvement is unilateral with the brain and eye involvement on the same side as the port-wine stain. However, a unilateral port-wine stain can be paired with bilateral leptomeningeal angioma involvement or vice versa.

The most frequent presentation for the neurologic manifestations in SWS is focal and complex partial seizures in an infant with a facial port-wine stain. Onset of seizures is usually in the first two years of life but occasionally can start later in childhood. Other presentations for SWS include a visual field cut presenting as an infant that neglects a hemi-visual space, or the early onset of handedness in a child with a facial port-wine stain. In each case, a through assessment of involvement is needed so that the family can be appropriately counseled and treatment initiated.

DIAGNOSIS AND EVALUATION

Any child with a facial port-wine stain in the V1 distribution, we recommend should have a head CT to image the calcification and an MRI of the brain with and without contrast to detect the angioma (Fig. 1). The typical CT findings are cortical calcifications often in a gyral pattern and atrophy, although these findings may not be present in neonates or infants. The brain MRI demonstrates increased T2 signal in the white matter and focal meningeal enhancement. When possible, we will also ask for postcontrast FLAIR imaging, as this appears to have greater sensitivity for visualizing the angioma. Imaging with technetium-99m hexamethylpropyleneamine oxime single photon emission CT (SPECT) or perfusion MR imaging is useful for assessing the extent and localization of the perfusion defects, and metabolic imaging with FDG-PET or MR spectroscopy may also be helpful in characterizing the extent of brain disease in SWS. Timing of the initial imaging is controversial because if the imaging is done at birth or in the first few months of life it may not be possible to visualize the angioma. If MRI is negative in infancy, one may need to repeat it by the first birthday or with the onset of neurologic symptoms.

Close neurologic and developmental follow-up is essential for children with SWS to diagnose and treat developmental delays, seizures, headaches, hemiparesis, learning difficulties, and behavioral issues as they arise. Most children with SWS will require occupational and physical therapy for their hemiparesis and visual field cut. Developmental and neuropsychological assessments can be very helpful for addressing attentional issues and learning difficulties. Attention-deficit disorder occurs in about 20% of children with SWS, and mental retardation in about 50% of children.

Screening for glaucoma should be done at birth, under anesthesia if necessary, and then at least every 3–4 months in the first year, every six month in the second year and yearly thereafter. Ophthalmologic evaluations can determine the extent of abnormal vessel involvement with the eye. Children with port-wine stains involving both the upper and the lower eyelids are at the greatest risk for glaucoma. Glaucoma in the young child can present with eye enlargement (bupthalmos) or with corneal clouding, and vision loss at any time and these signs and symptoms need immediate evaluation.

Infants with a port-wine stain are also referred for dermatologic assessment. In infancy, the port-wine stain is often pink in color and flat. The port-wine stain generally grows commesurate with growth and often darkens or may become raised with time. It is recommended that port-wine stains be treated in infancy, before hypertrophy and blebbing develop and make treatment more difficult. Presenting the diagnosis of SWS to parents is complex and requires the coordinated input of multiple specialists to address the different organ systems involved in this disorder. It is essential that time is spent answering care-giver questions so that seizures, stroke-like episodes, and other complications are recognized and appropriately managed to minimize brain injury.

THERAPY

In all children with SWS and intracranial involvement, we advise the empiric use of a daily multivitamin. Infants and young children with SWS should be screened for iron deficiency anemia, which is relatively common in young children and if present could exacerbate ischemic brain injury and should be treated.

Seizures

Most infants with SWS will develop complex partial seizures in the first 3 years of life, the majority in the first year. It is essential that parents receive counseling regarding what seizures look like and how to obtain help rapidly for a first seizure. Seizures are managed acutely with benzodiazepines, phosphenytoin and, if necessary phenobarbital. A prolonged hemiparesis, lasting days, weeks, or months is common after a seizure episode, and a permanent hemiparesis frequently develops over time. Although controversial, there is evidence that seizures, particularly if they are frequent or prolonged, may result in increased brain injury resulting from the impairments in blood flow. Therefore, we think that chronic anticonvulsants should be initiated after the first seizure, whether febrile or afebrile, in a child with SWS and brain involvement.

Generally first choice anticonvulsants are carbamazepine, or phenobarbital transitioning to carbamazepine, depending on the age of the child, as most seizures in SWS are complex partial. Oxcarbazepine may also be used. Our second-line choices include topiramate or valproic acid. Rectal or oral diazepam are given to the family for use with seizures lasting longer than 5 min or clusters of seizures. Seizures in SWS, as in other settings, commonly occur during illness. We advise parents to treat fevers and maintain good hydration during illness, even if intravenous fluids are needed. We advise continuing the anticonvulsant for a few years, until the fifth birthday if possible, as older children appear to be less susceptible to permanent neurologic decline that may be exacerbated by seizures in the younger children.

If seizures are not controlled with anticonvulsants, are occurring frequently so as to interfere with development or deterioration in neurologic status is occurring, then children should be considered for surgical resections. Surgery may include focal resections or hemispherectomies. Most candidates for surgery have significant developmental delay and hemiparesis. Timing of surgery should be carefully weighed for risks and benefits; however, in the appropriate situation, surgery can result in cessation of seizures and resumption in development. There is no evidence that surgical resection of the affected cortex is the proper course of action in the absence of intractable epilepsy.

Stroke-like Episodes

Stroke-like episodes can occur in SWS and present as episodes of transient visual field cuts or weakness that can occur independent of seizures or may precede, or follow seizures. It is not entirely clear what these episodes represent; however, thrombosis, hypoxia-seizure, complicated migraine, and/or seizure activity may all have some role in these episodes. Minor head trauma can trigger these events as well. In contrast to status epilepticus, an EEG performed during a stroke-like episode characteristically shows focal cortical slowing.

We recommend prophylactic use of aspirin when stroke-like episodes have occurred. Experience with its use in the prevention of pediatric stroke, and anecdotal evidence in SWS, suggests that low-dose aspirin at 3–5 mg/kg/day is safe and effective; however, no randomized, placebo controlled trial has been done. Children on aspirin therapy should receive varicella immunization and the yearly influenza vaccine because of the association between these illnesses, aspirin use and Reye syndrome in children; however, the international experience with low-dose aspirin use for stroke prophylaxis in children suggests that this therapy is safe. Preventing severe illness with these vaccinations is probably a good idea anyway because episodes of deterioration in SWS often occur in the setting of illness. Occupational and physical therapy is prescribed when weakness is persistent in order to maximize function and prevent contractures.

Headaches

Headaches and migraines are also common in SWS. Acutely, we have used antimigraine medications such as ibuprofen and sumatriptan with good results; however, the safety of triptans has not been studied in SWS. In older children and adults, it seems that seizures can provoke headaches and headaches can precede the onset of seizures or stroke-like episodes. When frequent, valproic acid may provide prophylaxis for both seizures and recurrent headaches. Alternatively, a combination of an anticonvulsant, such as carbamazepine, and a calcium-channel blocker or beta-blocker may be required.

Cognitive and Psychological Issues

Learning disabilities and mental retardation frequently develop in SWS and need to be evaluated and addressed educationally. Attention-deficit disorder is common in SWS and should be addressed with a combination of behavioral and pharmacologic approaches. When behavioral approaches are insufficient, then treatment with either a stimulant or atomoxetine should be initiated and response closely monitored. Depression and anxiety are also common in SWS. Older children and adolescents can demonstrate a decline in function or new behavioral issues, and psychological factors should be evaluated when this occurs. Treatment with a selective serotonin reuptake inhibitor or tricyclic antidepressant may be helpful. However, the safety and efficacy of these approaches have not been studied specifically in SWS.

Treatment of Ophthalmologic and Dermatologic Complications

Treatment of the port-wine stain requires a series of laser treatments. Pulsed-dye laser can improve the appearance of the vascular malformation in about 10 treatments; however, the port-wine stain can recur to some extent as deeper vessels dilate. Some facilities give sedation for these treatments, others utilize only local anesthesia. Without treatment, the port-wines often develop blebbing and hypertrophy of underlying soft-tissue and bone which can lead to significant psychological and functional issues depending on the location and extent of involvement. It is unknown if infancy is the best time for treatment of SWS, given the other systems involved, however, the current practice in SWS is to treat the port-wine stain early. Laser treatments are painful, however, and can occasionally result in scarring, and older children should therefore be included in discussions for timing for treatment.

Glaucoma may occur at any age although two peaks exist in infancy and in early adulthood. The goal of treatment is to reduce intraocular pressure in order to protect vision. Medical and surgical approaches are used and concentrate on either reducing the production of aqueous fluid or promoting its drainage. Medications include beta-agonist eye drops, adrenergic eye drops, and carbonic anhydrase inhibitors. Trabeculectomy and goniotomy are common surgical options.

SUGGESTED READINGS

1. Bodensteiner JB, Roach ES, eds. Sturge–Weber Syndrome. New Jersey: Sturge–Weber Foundation, 1999.
2. Chapieski L, Friedman A, Lachar D. Psychological functioning in children and adolescents with Sturge–Weber syndrome. J Child Neurol 2000; 15(10):660–665.
3. Comi AM. Pathophysiology of Sturge–Weber Syndrome. J Child Neurol 2003; 18(8): 509–516.
4. Kossoff EH, Buck C, Freeman JM. Outcomes of 32 hemispherectomies for Sturge–Weber syndrome worldwide. Neurology 2002; 59(11):1735–1738.
5. Maria BL, Neufeld JA, Rosainz LC, et al. Central nervous system structure and function in Sturge–Weber syndrome: evidence of neurologic and radiologic progression. J Child Neurol 1998; 13(12):606–618.
6. Rothfleisch JE, Kosann MK, Levine VJ, Ashinoff R. Laser treatment of congenital and acquired vascular lesions. Dermatol Clin 2002; 20(1):1–18.

PATIENT RESOURCES

1. Sturge–Weber Foundation. PO Box 418, Mt. Freedom, NJ 07970, U.S.A. Tel.:+1-800-627-5482; fax: +973-895-4846; www.sturge-weber.com
2. Johns Hopkins and Kennedy Krieger Institute, Sturge–Weber Syndrome Center, 123Jefferson Bldg., 600 N Wolfe Street, Baltimore, MD 21287, U.S.A. Tel. :+1-410-614-5807; fax:+1-410-614-2297; http://www.neuro.jhmi.edu/HopkinsSWSCenter/index.htm

80
Neurofibromatosis

Kaleb Yohay
Departments of Neurology and Pediatrics, Johns Hopkins Hospital, Baltimore, Maryland, U.S.A.

INTRODUCTION

Neurofibromatosis types 1 and 2 are separate phakomatoses that have been linked and frequently discussed together for historical reasons. A clear distinction between the two diseases was not made until 1981.

Neurofibromatosis type 1 (NF-1), or von Recklinghausen disease, is a common autosomal dominant disorder with an incidence of 1 in 3000–4000. The gene for NF-1 is located on chromosome 17 (17q11.2) and encodes for neurofibromin. Half of NF-1 cases are sporadic in origin. Mosaicism can occur. Penetrance is essentially 100% but there is significant unpredictable phenotypic variability. Common clinical features of neurofibromatosis are listed in Table 1.

Neurofibromatosis type 2, also known as "central NF," is also an autosomal dominant disorder but is much less common, with an incidence of about 1 in 30,000–40,000 and a symptomatic prevalence of 1 in 210,000. There is wide phenotypic variability. The NF-2 gene is located on chromosome 22 (22q12.2) and encodes for merlin. Like NF-1, about half of NF-2 mutations arise de novo. The clinical hallmark of the disease is bilateral vestibular schwannomas (VS), which occur in about 95% of adults with NF-2. Children with NF-2 more commonly present with tumors other than VS. The average age of onset of symptoms is between 18 and 22 years. CALS are not more common in patients with NF-2 than in the general population and are not part of the diagnostic criteria (Table 1).

The diagnoses of NF-1 and NF-2 are based on clinical features. NIH clinical diagnostic criteria have been developed and are widely used in the diagnosis of NF-1 and 2 (Tables 2 and 3). The NIH criteria for NF-2 may be too restrictive, and alternative criteria with higher sensitivity have been proposed (Table 4). Genetic testing for NF-1 is available but is of limited utility, complicated by the size of the gene and the large number of mutations. The most commonly available test, a premature truncation test, is only about 65–70% sensitive. Testing should be reserved only for clinically equivocal cases. Prenatal testing is limited. The sensitivity of molecular genetic testing for NF-2 is also only about 65%, but linkage analysis in families with more than one affected individuals may be useful for screening unaffected relatives.

Table 1 Comparison of NF-1 and NF-2

	NF-1	NF-2
Incidence	1 in 3000–4000	1 in 30,000–40,000
Typical age of onset	Infancy and early childhood	Adolescence and young adulthood
First manifestations	CALs, frocking	In children: Cataracts and skin schwannomas In adolescents/young adults: Hearing loss, imbalance
Typical tumor types	Neurofibromas, astrocytomas	Schwannomas, meningiomas
OPGS?	Yes	No
Vestibular schwannoma?	No	Yes
Non-tumorous manifestations?	Many	Few
Increased risk of non-CNS cancer?	Yes	No
Chromosomal location	Chromosome 17 (17q11.2)	Chromosome 22 (22q12.2)

NEUROFIBROMATOSIS 1: CLINICAL FEATURES AND TREATMENT

Cutaneous Manifestations

Café-au-lait spots are flat, hyperpigmented macules that usually appear during first year of life but can be present at birth. They typically increase in number and size with age but often fade later in life. About 25% of the normal population have 1–3 CALS, while more than 95% of patients with NF-1 have CALS. Half of children with more than 6 CALS and no other features of NF-1 will later go on to meet criteria for NF-1. Freckling usually is not present at birth and develops during childhood. It most commonly occurs in axillary and/or inguinal areas but can occur in other intertriginous areas.

Neurofibromas are benign tumors of the nerve sheath, composed of a mix of Schwann cells, fibroblasts, and mast cells. There are four types: cutaneous, subcutaneous, nodular plexiform, and diffuse plexiform. Cutaneous neurofibromas are soft fleshy tumors arising from the peripheral nerve sheath, usually appearing in late childhood or young adulthood. They can become cosmetically significant and can cause itching or pain but do not become malignant. Subcutaneous neurofibromas are firm, tender nodules along the course of peripheral nerves that usually appear

Table 2 NIH Diagnostic Criteria for NF-1

NF-1 is present in a person who has two or more of the following signs:
Six or more café-au-lait macules > 5 mm in greatest diameter in prepubertal individuals or > 15 mm in greatest diameter after puberty.
Two or more neurofibromas of any type or one or more plexiform neurofibromas.
Freckling in the axial or inguinal region.
A tumor of the optic pathway.
Two or more Lisch nodules.

Table 3 NIH Diagnostic Criteria for NF-2

NF-2 is present in a person who has either of the following:
1. Bilateral eight nerve masses seen with appropriate imaging techniques (e.g. MRI or CT)
2. A first degree relative with NF-2 and either unilateral eighth nerve mass or two of the following:
   - glioma
   - meningioma
   - schwannoma
   - neurofibroma
   - juvenile posterior subcapsular lenticular opacity

(From Neurofibromatosis Conference statement, National Institutes of Health Consensus Development Conference, Arch Neurol, 1988)

during adolescence or young adulthood. Nodular plexiform neurofibromas cluster along the proximal nerve roots and major nerves and can cause vertebral erosion, cord compression, and scoliosis. Diffuse plexiform neurofibromas involve multiple nerve fascicles and are often highly vascular. They are usually not apparent in infancy though the skin overlying it may be hyperpigmented and/or thickened. They tend to enlarge with age, and can become severely disfiguring.

To date, no effective medical treatment is available for prevention or reduction of cutaneous neurofibromas. Timing and extent of surgical treatment remains variable and controversial. Generally, surgery is reserved for patients with significant discomfort from dermal neurofibromas, or with cosmetically significant lesions. CO_2 laser therapy can also be effective, particularly if a large number of neurofibromas are being treated at one time. Recurrence is typical.

Plexiform neurofibromas are challenging to treat. Because they are often large, irregular in shape, highly vascular, and frequently involve numerous nerves, they are almost impossible to resect completely. Their unpredictable growth patterns also make appropriate treatment choices more difficult. Surgical therapy is generally

Table 4 Proposed Revised Clinical Criteria for NF-2

Definite NF-2	Presumptive or probable NF-2
Bilateral vestibular schwannomas (VS)	Unilateral VS <30 years plus at least one of the following: meningioma, glioma, schwannoma, juvenile posterior subcapsular lenticular opacities
or	or
First degree relative with NF-2 plus 1. Unilateral VS <30 years, or 2. Any two of the following: meningioma, glioma, schwannoma, juvenile posterior subscapsular lenticular opacities	Multiple meningiomas ($\geq$2) plus unilateral VS <30 years or one of the following: glioma, schwannoma, juvenile posterior subcapsular lenticular opacities

(From Gutmann et al. The diagnostic evaluation and multidisciplinary management of neurofibromatosis 1 and neurofibromatosis 2. JAMA 1997; 278:51–570.)

Table 5 Follow up of children with NF-1 and Optic Pathway Gliomas

Time interval following diagnosis of OPG	MRI	Ophthalmologic examination
Diagnosis	X	X
3 Months	X	X
6 Months		X
9 Months	X	X
12 Months		X
15 Months	X	
18 Months		X
24 Months	X	X
36 Months	X	X
Yearly, thereafter	[a]	X

[a]The data are insufficient to make a clear recommendation regarding the intervals for MRI after the first two years after diagnosis. However, assuming there has been no evidence of progression, the intervals between MRI can be gradually lengthened.

(From Listernick et al. Optic pathway gliomas in children with neurofibromatosis 1: Consensus statement from the NF-1 Optic Pathway Glioma Task Force, Ann Neurol. 1997 Feb; 41(2):143-9.)

reserved until the lesion is causing functional limitation or discomfort or is cosmetically significant. More aggressive intervention has been proposed for orbital plexiform neurofibromas but systematic study of outcomes is lacking. Spinal plexiform neurofibromas may also be surgically excised but gross-total resection is often not possible. Regrowth can occur and clinical improvement may be seen in as few as 1–5 patients. Clinical trials for medical therapy of plexiform neurofibromas are underway. Two agents under study include Pirfenidone, an antifibrotic agent that blocks the action of several growth factors, and R115777, a farnesyl transferase inhibitor that interferes with ras functioning.

Lisch nodules are raised, usually pigmented, hamartomas on the iris that are best seen on slit lamp examination. They rarely cause clinically significant symptoms.

Skeletal Manifestations

Osseous lesions present in NF-1 include pseudarthrosis, sphenoid dysplasia, vertebral dysplasias, short stature, and scoliosis. Pseudarthrosis occurs in up to 5% of NF-1 patients. Conversely, 80% of patients with pseudarthrosis have NF-1. Pseudarthrosis results from thinning of long bone cortex, followed by pathologic fracture and impaired healing. Half of cases occur before age 2. Dysplasia of the sphenoid bone can be a disfiguring complication. It can occur with or without an associated plexiform neurofibroma. Short stature is common, with about 13% of patients being 2 standard deviations below the mean for height. Scoliosis can occur as a result of either deformation of the vertebral bodies by nodular plexiform neurofibromas in the vertebral foramina or from vertebral dysplasia. Scoliosis can occur in up to 25% of patients and there is a female preponderance. Cervical or upper thoracic kyphosis is most common. Children with NF-1 and scoliosis should be referred to an orthopedist with experience in treating NF patients. In managing scoliosis, it is important to first differentiate dystrophic from nondystrophic, or more idiopathic disease. Dystrophic scoliosis can be accompanied by vertebral scalloping, spindled ribs, paravertebral soft-tissue masses, foraminal enlargement, a short curve with severe apical rotation, or subluxation or dislocation of a vertebral body. Dystrophic curves are more likely to progress rapidly and, therefore, need early and aggressive surgical management. Nondystrophic scoliosis is managed similarly to idiopathic scoliosis, with observation, bracing, and eventually surgical fusion if indicated.

Neurologic Manifestations

Macrocephaly occurs in 25–50% of children with NF-1. It is uncommonly due to hydrocephalus with aqueductal stenosis. It is usually due to increased brain size, the pathogenesis of which is unclear.

Cognitive deficits are fairly common but tend to be relatively mild. The incidence of mental retardation (FSIQ < 70) is only slightly higher than that of the general population at about 4–8%. However, IQ tends to be 5–10 points lower in comparison to the general population or unaffected siblings, and learning disabilities are quite common, with a prevalence ranging from 30% to 65%. ADHD is also probably more common in the NF-1 population.

Seizures are not a prominent feature of NF-1, but the lifetime risk is approximately twice that of the general population, with a prevalence of approximately 4%. They can begin at any age and can be focal or generalized. Choice of antiepileptic treatment should be based on individual factors in including age, seizure type, and etiology.

Unidentified bright objects (UBOs) are a characteristic radiologic feature of NF-1. They appear as focal areas of T2 bright signal on MRI that do not enhance and cause no mass effect. They most commonly occur in the basal ganglia, cerebellum, brainstem, and subcortical white matter. UBOs may represent areas of increased fluid within myelin in areas of dysplastic glial proliferation and are not thought to be malignant or premalignant. They are not associated with focal neurologic deficits. It has been suggested that the presence of UBOs may correlate with the occurrence of cognitive deficits, though results of studies to date have been mixed.

Malignancy

The reported lifetime risk of malignancy in people with NF-1 ranges from 2% to 10% with an odds ratio of approximately 2–3 times the risk of the general population. The lifetime risk of developing benign or malignant CNS tumors is about 45%. CNS tumors encountered in NF-1 include optic gliomas, astrocytomas, brainstem gliomas, and brain or spinal cord ependymomas. Malignancies outside the CNS include malignant peripheral nerve sheath tumors (MPNSTs), chronic myelogenous leukemia, and pheochromocytoma.

Optic pathway gliomas (OPGs) are the most common CNS tumor in NF-1, occurring in up to 15% of children with the disorder. They are typically histologically low grade and can appear anywhere along the optic pathways. In patients with OPGs, the risk of developing other CNS tumors is increased. Only about 1/3 of optic gliomas are symptomatic, typically presenting with vision loss, proptosis or both. They can also present with accelerated puberty if the tumor originates near the chiasm. Optical pathway gliomas that are destined to become symptomatic or progress typically do so during the first decade of life, so yearly ophthalmologic evaluation for their development should continue until at least 12 years of age.

Most children with NF-1 and OPG can be followed expectantly without intervention, as most of these tumors never progress after diagnosis. Serial MRI and ophthalmologic examinations at predefined intervals (Fig. 5) should be performed in patients with stable disease. The determination of when and how to treat OPGs is complex, controversial, and highly individualized. Surgical resection is usually reserved for patients with anterior optic pathway disease that does not involve the chiasm with no useful residual vision in the affected eye, and in whom there is radiologic or clinical evidence of progression or significant proptosis. If there is useful vision or if the tumor involves the chiasm or posterior visual pathway, radiation therapy (RT) is usually employed. In young children, chemotherapy may be used because of concerns about neurocognitive and endocrinologic side effects of RT.

Malignant peripheral nerve sheath tumors, also called neurofibrosarcomas, result from the malignant transformation of plexiform neurofibromas. These tumors are aggressive and often fatal. The lifetime risk for patients with NF-1 is reported between 5% and 13%. They usually present with pain and rapid growth of a pre-existing nodule within a plexiform neurofibroma. MPNSTs most commonly arise during adulthood but can rarely develop during childhood.

A sudden change in the pattern of growth of plexiform neurofibromas or new onset of pain can be a warning sign of malignant transformation and should be evaluated rapidly. MRI may show areas of necrosis. Biopsy should be considered. Surgical resection is the mainstay of therapy, but adjuvant chemotherapy or radiation may be used, particularly for subtotal resections. Despite therapy, MPNSTs frequently recur and/or metastasize with 5 year survivals around 21% and median survivals of a little over 1 year. A phase II clinical trial examining Gleevec in the treatment of sarcomas in children is currently underway.

General Considerations

Because of the complex and multidisciplinary nature of the disorder, patients with NF-1 are often best served by being followed at an NF center with coordinated multidisciplinary care, including genetics, neurology, neurosurgery, ophthalmology, orthopedics, dermatology, plastic surgery, neuropsychology, and oncology. Patients with NF-1 should undergo biannual physical examinations at least until age 5 and then yearly thereafter. In index cases, other undiagnosed first degree relatives should be examined carefully for stigmata of the disorder. Because of the risk of pheochromocytoma and renal arterial abnormalities, blood pressure should be checked at least twice yearly. Special attention should be paid to early detection of scoliosis, evidence of limb bowing or pseudarthrosis, presence of or change in the cutaneous manifestations, and signs of precocious or delayed puberty. Head circumference should be checked regularly for signs of rapid growth, particularly in the first three years of life. Behavior and development should be followed carefully for signs of learning disability and ADHD. Patients with NF-1 should also undergo yearly neurologic and ophthalmologic evaluation. Screening examinations such as MRI, EEG, and radiographs are not necessary unless specifically indicated by history or examination.

Other manifestations and associations include GI bleeding from gastrointestinal neurofibromas, hemihypertrophy, buphthalmos, congenital glaucoma, vascular abnormalities (including Moymoya and stroke), and neuronal migration defects.

Data on morbidity and mortality in NF-1 are scant. Approximately 1/3 of patients have a serious complication of NF-1. Overall lifespan may be somewhat reduced.

Perhaps the most important role of a clinician working with patients with NF-1 is to provide accurate and up-to-date information on the disorder. Appropriate anticipatory guidance regarding the natural history of the disease, therapeutic options (including available experimental trials), and genetic counseling should be offered to every patient and family.

Neurofibromatosis 2: Clinical Manifestations and Treatment

NF-2 is usually not diagnosed until late adolescence or early adulthood when symptoms referable to the progression of vestibular schwannomas present. Younger children are more likely to present with other CNS tumors, posterior capsular cataracts, or peripheral nerve schwannomas. Unlike NF-1, the pathologic features of NF-2 primarily involve the development of tumors and their complications.

At the time of diagnosis, patients should undergo a thorough evaluation including an ophthalmologic examination, neurologic examination, and audiologic testing. A gadolinium-enhanced MRI of the brain with thin cuts through the internal auditory canals should be performed. Spinal MRI may also be considered. Genetic counseling should be provided.

Any new neurologic signs or symptoms need to be evaluated promptly in patients with NF-2. At a minimum, patients should undergo yearly brain MRI and audiologic evaluation in addition to clinical evaluation. Serial spine MRI need only be performed in patients with large or symptomatic spinal tumors.

Schwannomas are the most prevalent tumor type in NF-2, with vestibular schwannomas occurring in about 98% of affected individuals. Schwannomas can also occur along other cranial nerves (particularly the trigeminal nerve), spinal roots, and peripheral nerves.

Though vestibular schwannomas usually arise from the vestibular portion of the VIIIth cranial nerve, they generally present with auditory symptoms. They are usually slow growing and cause slow deterioration in hearing. Eventually, balance and other cranial nerve functions may become impaired. Brainstem compression and obstructive hydrocephalus can occur. The decision to treat is highly individualized and depends in part on the degree of hearing loss, the size of the tumor, the presence and degree of contralateral symptoms, and the presence of signs or symptoms of other cranial nerve or brainstem dysfunction. Treatment is usually surgical, though RT and radiosurgery are also used. Depending on the type and extent of surgery, hearing loss may be worse postoperatively and may be accompanied by facial or other cranial nerve palsies and headache. Small tumors (<1.5 mm) can often be removed with preservation of hearing. Surgery for larger tumors carries a higher risk of deafness and other cranial nerve dysfunction. For patients who are surgically deafened, one option may include the placement of an auditory brainstem implant (ABI), which is essentially a cochlear implant with a modified proximal electrode. Because of the high risk of eventual deafness, patients and their families should be counseled prior to the onset of complete hearing loss about techniques to facilitate communication such as lip reading and sign language.

Schwannomas arising from other cranial nerves are generally surgically removed if treatment is necessary.

Spinal schwannomas occur in up to 80% of patients with NF-2, though most are small and asymptomatic. They are slow-growing, arise from the dorsal root and are radiologically indistinguishable from spinal neurofibromas. Surgical resection or debulking is performed in patients with severe or progressive symptoms.

Peripheral schwannomas can arise on any peripheral nerve and can cause pain or weakness.

Meningiomas occur in about half of patients with NF-2. Treatment is surgical unless the tumor is inaccessible, in which case, radiation therapy may be considered.

Glial tumors, including ependymomas and astrocytomas, are also more prevalent in patients with NF-2, with estimates of incidence ranging from 6% to 33%. About 80% of gliomas in NF-2 are intramedullary spinal tumors or cauda equina tumors, and 10% arise in the medulla, with ependymomas accounting for most glial tumors in NF-2 and essentially all the spinal tumors. Again, treatment is generally primarily surgical, performed when they become clinically significant.

The prognosis and clinical course in NF-2 are variable and few longitudinal studies have been performed. Lifespan is decreased with a mean actuarial survival of 62 years. Age at diagnosis is the strongest predictor of morbidity and mortality, with earlier onset associated with decreased survival.

SUMMARY

NF-1 and NF-2 are two very different autosomal dominant disorders, with significant potential for central and peripheral nervous system pathology. Familiarity with the disorder, patient education, multidisciplinary access, and vigilance in monitoring patients are essential components of care for these patients who present numerous therapeutic challenges.

SUGGESTED READINGS

1. American Academy of Pediatrics Committee on Genetics. Health supervision for children with neurofibromatosis. Pediatrics 1995; 96:368–372.
2. Baser ME, DG RE, Gutmann DH. Neurofibromatosis 2. Curr Opin Neurol 2003; 16: 27–33.
3. Friedman JM. Neurofibromatosis 1: clinical manifestations and diagnostic criteria. J Child Neurol 2002; 17:548–554.
4. Gutmann DH, Aylsworth A, Carey JC, Korf B, Marks J, Pyeritz RE, Rubenstein A, Viskochil D. The diagnostic evaluation and multidisciplinary management of neurofibromatosis 1 and neurofibromatosis 2. JAMA 1997; 278:51–57.
5. National Institutes of Health Consensus Development Conference Statement: Neurofibromatosis. Bethesda, MD, USA, July 13–15, 1987. Neurofibromatosis 1988; 1:172–178.

PATIENT RESOURCES

1. The National Neurofibromatosis Foundation. www.nf.org (800):323–7939.
2. Neurofibromatosis, Inc. www.nfinc.org (800):942–6825.

81

Tuberous Sclerosis Complex

Raymond S. Kandt
Johnson Neurological Clinic, High Point, North Carolina, U.S.A.

INTRODUCTION

Tuberous sclerosis complex (TSC) is an autosomal dominant disorder caused by a mutation of either the chromosome 9 TSC1 gene or the chromosome 16 TSC2 gene. With a prevalence of about one per 6000, TSC is one of the more common of the neurocutaneous diseases. By comparison, the most common neurocutaneous disorder, neurofibromatosis type 1, has a prevalence of about one per 4000. An inherited or sporadic mutation of either TSC1 or TSC2 results in loss of function or aberrant function of the respective gene product: hamartin (chromosome 9 TSC1) or tuberin (chromosome 16 TSC2). These two genes are thought to act in part as tumor suppressor genes, but also function in various aspects of the regulation of cell growth, migration, and development. In the 1/3 of TSC patients whose families demonstrate autosomal dominant inheritance, the mutation occurs roughly equally in either TSC1 or TSC2. By contrast, TSC2 is more often mutated in the two-thirds of patients who have TSC due to a spontaneous mutation. TSC typically causes problems that affect one or more of four organs: brain, skin, kidneys, and lungs.

DIAGNOSIS AND EVALUATION

The four major impacts of TSC are skin lesions in 95% or more of the patients, seizures in 85% (the most common presenting feature), mental retardation in about 50%, and kidney disease in 60%.

Diagnosis of TSC is dependent upon recognition of the relatively unique hamartomas and hamartias that are characteristic of TSC. These are divided into major and minor diagnostic features (Table 1). A patient is considered to have definite TSC when two major features are present (or one major and two minor features). Additional categories include probable TSC, characterized by one major plus one minor feature, and possible TSC, with one major or two or more minor features.

In the majority of TSC patients, the diagnosis is suspected because of infantile spasms or later onset of seizures, particularly if accompanied by mental retardation. Once TSC is suspected, the diagnosis is confirmed by discovering other

Table 1 Diagnostic and Nondiagnostic Features and Their Prevalence in TSC

Diagnostic features	*Prevalence*
Eleven major features	
Facial angiofibromas/forehead plaque	60–75%
Ungual fibroma, nontraumatic	15–50%
Three or more hypopigmented macules	>90%
Shagreen patch	20%
Multiple nodular retinal hamartomas	50–75%
Cortical tuber/subcortical migration tract	>90%
Subependymal nodule	>80%
Subependymal giant cell astrocytoma	5%
Cardiac rhabdomyomas	60+% children, <20% adults
Pulmonary lymphangioleiomyomatosis	2–5% women (newer studies as high as 40%)
Renal angiomyolipomas	Almost 75% by 10 years
Nine minor features	
Multiple dental pits	50–100% permanent teeth
Hamartomatous rectal polyps (histologic)	
Bone cysts (radiographic diagnosis is sufficient)	
Cerebral white matter radial migration lines (without tuber)	
Gingival fibromas	
Nonrenal hamartoma	Up to 45% hepatic hamartomas
Retinal achromic patch	
"Confetti" skin lesions	<10%
Multiple renal cysts	20% (2% severe cystic disease)

Nondiagnostic features	*Prevalence*
Seizures	85%
Mental retardation	50%
Autism	50%
Renal cell carcinoma	Up to 2%
Aortic or other aneurysms	Rare

manifestations of TSC. The various procedures that allow correct diagnosis and monitoring of TSC are given in Table 2. Attention should also be given to the family history, as this may disclose previously undiagnosed individuals. When typical manifestations are present, the diagnosis is easy. By contrast, because TSC can affect most organ systems (but usually not the spinal cord) and because variability of clinical manifestations among different patients can be striking, diagnosis may be difficult.

Skin Lesions

Among the skin manifestations, 0.5–2 cm or larger hypopigmented macules (also known as ashleaf spots or hypomelanotic macules) are the most common, and are usually present at birth, located on the trunk, extremities, or face. Ultraviolet Wood's light is sometimes necessary to see the macules. The other three common skin manifestations typically occur during the second decade (sometimes earlier) and include facial angiofibromas, shagreen patches, and ungual fibromas. The forehead plaque is often present within the first year.

Table 2 Procedures for Diagnosis and Monitoring of TSC

Phase	Procedures
Suspicion	History and examination
Diagnosis	Confirmation utilizing diagnostic criteria
Completion of baseline evaluations (all can be repeated as necessary)	Skin examination Cranial MRI/CT Renal ultrasound Ophthalmic examination EKG Neurodevelopmental testing
Optional studies for variable manifestations	
Seizures	EEG
Cardiac	Echocardiogram
Family planning	DNA sequencing of TSC1 and TSC2 genes
Enlarging AML	Renal CT
Pulmonary	Chest CT
Follow up	Neurodevelopmental testing at school entrance Renal ultrasound every 1–3 years Cranial MRI/CT every 1–3 years through adolescence Chest CT scan in adult females

Seizures

Although they are the most common neurologic symptom of TSC, seizures are not specific for diagnosis because the seizures of TSC are not unique to TSC nor specific to TSC. Seizures, however, represent one of the major challenges in the medical management. The early onset of infantile spasms in TSC is typically associated with mental retardation. Later onset of seizures is usually manifested with complex partial seizures or a mixed seizure disorder, with or without mental retardation. Although mentally retarded TSC patients always have seizures, a significant minority of TSC patients who have seizures, usually with onset after age 2 years, have normal intelligence.

Mental Retardation

This is the second most common neurologic symptom of TSC, occurring in about 45–50% of patients, and usually associated with infantile spasms. Two-thirds of the retarded are profoundly mentally retarded. When mild, the retardation may not be obvious or diagnosed until school age. Autism is relatively common in TSC, and usually occurs in the mentally retarded patient.

Neuroimaging

There are several possible findings: (1) cortical tubers (>90%); (2) subependymal nodules or SENs (>80%) which appear as periventricular nodular lesions; (3) radial lines extending from the lateral ventricles (migration lines); (4) subependymal giant cell astrocytomas (SEGAs); and (5) dysmorphic ventricles. By CT scan, calcified

SENs are prominent, but the low attenuation of cerebral cortical tubers is difficult to visualize. With MRI, the tubers are easily seen at the gray–white junction of the cerebral and cerebellar cortices as nonenhancing, irregularly bordered areas of high T2 and FLAIR signal. Less commonly, tubers contain calcium or enhance. For diagnosis of TSC, the presence of both tubers and SENs is highly characteristic, particularly if they are joined by migration lines.

Subependymal Giant Cell Astrocytomas

The transformation of SENs in the region of the foramen of Monro into SEGAs is characterized by both enlargement and enhancement (on both CT and MRI). When a SEGA enlarges, it may block CSF circulation and cause elevated intracranial pressure. SEGAs occur in the minority of TSC patients (5%), usually in the second decade but rarely as early as in utero, and rarely enlarge after age 20 years. They are never invasive, but may rarely hemorrhage or worsen seizures.

Renal Disease

Kidney lesions, usually bilateral, occur in about 60% of patients, but are usually not a clinical problem until adulthood. One exception is the children who have a contiguous gene syndrome that affects two adjacent chromosome 16 genes, TSC2 and APKD1 (adult polycystic kidney disease, type 1). These patients may have severe polycystic kidney disease dating from infancy. In other children with TSC, asymptomatic renal lesions, either cysts or angiomyolipomas, can be helpful for diagnosis. Renal ultrasound is the initial screening test, but CT may be necessary to differentiate rapidly enlarging angiomyolipomas, which contain fat, from renal cell carcinomas, which do not.

Other Manifestations

Cardiac rhabdomyomas are usually asymptomatic, but may cause cardiac failure, usually by outflow obstruction. They rarely cause arrhythmias due to involvement of cardiac conduction pathways, e.g., Wolf–Parkinson–White syndrome, and are sometimes detected by EKG when asymptomatic. Cardiac rhabdomyomas generally regress spontaneously during infancy or early childhood. Echocardiogram is helpful for diagnosis of TSC in young children (and even prenatally), but is otherwise unnecessary in asymptomatic or in older persons. Retinal hamartomas, which sometimes look like mulberries, do not affect vision except on the rare occasions that they involve the area of the macula. Pulmonary dysfunction due to lymphangioleiomyomatosis (LAM) occurs either as a rare sporadic disease or in association with TSC. In TSC, LAM affects almost 5% of women older than 20 years. Rarely, LAM in TSC occurs during childhood or in males. Bony changes of TSC are almost always asymptomatic and can include cysts, periosteal new bone, and areas of sclerosis. Hepatic hamartomas (more common in females) are harmless. Cardiogenic cerebral embolization, perhaps from thrombus associated with a rhabdomyoma, is a rare complication.

Genetic Testing

DNA testing is available for the two genes that cause TSC, but the false negative rate is as high as 20%. Most patients who have TSC will fulfill the clinical diagnostic criteria, making DNA testing unnecessary. When the diagnosis is questionable, particularly when prenatal genetic counseling is planned, the DNA test is useful. Prenatal diagnosis is available, but it is most reliable when a causative mutation has been confirmed in a parent.

TREATMENT

Treatments for TSC focus on six aspects: seizure control, education, cosmetic treatments, amelioration of renal disease, CSF shunting or surgical resection of giant cell astrocytomas, and therapy of LAM.

Seizures

Seizures are treated in the same manner as they would be treated in the patient without TSC. ACTH is most commonly used to treat infantile spasms of TSC. Some TSC experts recommend vigabatrin for treatment of infantile spasms in TSC, but others point out the potential hazards including deterioration of visual fields (also difficult to monitor in retarded individuals) and the animal data demonstrating white matter vacuolation. Due to these factors, vigabatrin is unlikely to be approved by the FDA for use in the United States. In addition to standard antiepileptic medications, options for control of seizures include rectal diazepam at home for severe seizures lasting more than 3 min, serial seizures, or status epilepticus. Resection of epileptogenic tubers is limited to selected patients. The ketogenic diet, corpus callosotomy and vagus nerve stimulation have been helpful for many TSC patients.

Education

Early psychological assessment of intellectual function is recommended so that early intervention, resource assistance through the school system, or attendance in a self-contained classroom can be instituted. While education is important for the cognitive disorders of TSC, medications can improve some of the behaviors related to these problems. Useful medications include dextroamphetamine and other psychostimulants for hyperactivity and inattention, fluoxetine for autistic symptoms, clonidine for hyperarousal, and risperidone for aggression.

Cosmetic Treatments

Focused dye laser therapy is effective for treatment of facial angiofibromas that are disfiguring or bleed excessively with minor trauma. Ungual fibromas can be removed surgically if they become symptomatic due to cosmetic concerns, due to excessive accidental trauma or due to discomfort (e.g., poorly fitting shoes).

Renal Lesions

Renal surgery, including tumor enucleation, renal arterial embolization, or partial nephrectomy, is utilized for symptomatic or for large renal angiomyolipomas (e.g., >3.5–4 cm) to help prevent hemorrhage. Treatment with rapamycin to decrease the size of AMLs has entered clinical trials. Rarely, large renal cysts require decompression. Nephrectomy is rarely indicated, particularly since the other kidney may later develop dysfunction. Dialysis or renal transplantation are options in the event of renal failure. The risks of immunosuppression in TSC patients are not increased, and there is no recurrence of TSC lesions in a transplanted kidney. Renal cell carcinoma is treated in the standard manner.

Cerebral Subependymal Giant Cell Astrocytomas

These tumors are low grade. Thus, surgical removal for symptomatic lesions or enlarging lesions is usually successful. Chemotherapy and radiation therapy are not indicated. CSF shunting is performed for hydrocephalus. Because SEGAs rarely enlarge past the age of 20 years, static lesions and those without hydrocephalus are often not treated.

Pulmonary Lymphangioleiomyomatosis (LAM)

Lung transplant or hormonal therapies have been used.

PROGNOSIS

Many patients with TSC are affected by skin lesions only, and often are undiagnosed. TSC skin lesions have no risk for malignant transformation. Prognosis is variable, and is dependent mostly on the presence of one or more neurologic complications or the occurrence of renal or pulmonary complications. Although early seizures are associated with mental retardation, a considerable minority of TSC patients with onset of seizures after age 2 years have normal intelligence. Early onset of infantile spasms in association with mental retardation is associated with a poor prognosis for academic or occupational success. In the past, seizures were associated with mortality, but with the many medical options now available for seizure control, seizures less commonly lead to death. Bronchopneumonia, however, may still be fatal in severely retarded patients with intractable seizures including status epilepticus. Renal lesions are the leading cause of TSC-associated mortality in TSC adults. Placing it in perspective, however, only about 5% of TSC patients develop severe kidney disease. LAM is the second leading TSC-associated cause of death in patients older than 40 years. Less common causes of TSC-associated death include SEGAs, outflow obstruction from rhabdomyomas in infants, and aortic or other aneurysms.

SUGGESTED READINGS

1. Gomez MR, Sampson JR, Whittemore VH. Tuberous Sclerosis Complex. 3rd ed. New York: Oxford University Press, 1999.
2. Kandt RS. Tuberous sclerosis complex and neurofibromatosis type 1: the two most common neurocutaneous diseases. Neurol Clin 2002; 20:941–962.
3. Kwiatkowski DJ. Tuberous sclerosis: from tubers to mTOR. Ann Hum Genet 2003; 67:87–96.
4. Roach ES, Gomez MR, Northrup H. Tuberous sclerosis complex consensus conference: revised clinical diagnostic criteria. J Child Neurol 1998; 13:624–628.

5. Roach ES, DiMario FJ, Kandt RS, et al. Tuberous sclerosis consensus conference: recommendations for diagnostic evaluation. J Child Neurol 1999; 14:401–407.

PATIENT RESOURCE

1. Tuberous Sclerosis Alliance, 801 Roeder Rd, Silver Spring MD 20910, U.S.A., Tel.: +1-800–225–6872; http://www.tsalliance.org

82
Hypomelanosis of Ito

Lori L. Olson and Bernard L. Maria
Medical University of South Carolina, Charleston, South Carolina, U.S.A.

INTRODUCTION

The diagnosis of hypomelanosis of Ito (HI) is appropriate in individuals with hypopigmented skin lesions on the trunk and limbs following the lines of Blaschko. HI was originally named incontinentia pigmenti achromians in 1952 by Ito because the nonrandom streaks, whorls, and patches seen in HI are often described as the "negative pattern" of the hyperpigmented skin lesions in the disorder incontinentia pigmenti. Ito first described the disorder as a cutaneous syndrome, but it now seems clear that 33–94% of individuals have associated neurological, ophthalmological, and other complications. Mental retardation and seizures are characteristically associated with CNS involvement in HI but there is extreme variability in the severity of disease. Recent evidence convincingly suggests that HI is not a discrete disorder as originally believed but instead a nonspecific pigmentary disorder caused by chromosomal mosaicism. HI almost always occurs sporadically, and it seems to be caused by a de novo mutation in early embryogenesis. Although HI is often considered the fourth most common neurocutaneous syndrome, its incidence is very rare, with only 1 in every 600–1000 new patients in a pediatric neurology service.

DIAGNOSIS

The majority of individuals are first diagnosed within the first year of life due to the hypopigmentation of their skin. As in tuberous sclerosis, early diagnosis is enhanced by using a Wood's lamp when evaluating children with new onset seizures; the bilateral or unilateral hypopigmented whorls, streaks, and patches are usually found on the trunk and limbs. These lesions follow the lines of Blashcko, swirling around the trunk and down the arms or legs.

CLINICAL FEATURES

All affected individuals have the hypopigmented skin lesions. A significant number of affected individuals also show CNS involvement, most frequently mental retardation, and seizures. In a study of 76 cases in 1998, Pascual-Castroviejo et al. reported 57% of patients had an IQ below 70 with 40% having an IQ below 50. In addition, 49% suffered from seizures, with generalized tonic–clonic seizures being the most common. Partial, infantile spasms, and myoclonic seizures were also observed. Other significant neurological complications included hypotonia, macrocephaly, microcephaly, speech delay, autistic behaviors, and expressive language disabilities. Skin manifestations include café-au-lait spots, cutis marmorata, angiomatous nevi, nevus of Ota, Mongolian blue spots, hypohidrosis of hypopigmented areas, and morphea. Hair, tooth, and nail abnormalities can also be seen.

Ophthalmologic abnormalities include strabismus, nystagmus, congenital cataracts, and a variety of other nonspecific findings. A number of dental and craniofacial abnormalities can be seen. Some patients have limb asymmetries, scoliosis, pectus anomalies, and foot deformities. Cardiac, kidney, liver, and genital abnormalities, as well as benign and malignant tumors, have also been reported to a lesser extent. However, with such a small number of reported cases and high variability in clinical expression, it is difficult to definitely state the true prevalence of associated problems. There are no reported studies of the natural history of disease in HI.

EVALUATION

Thorough dermatological, neurological, and ophthalmological examinations are extremely important given the heterogeneity and potential severity of HI. Chromosomal analysis of blood, skin fibroblasts, or epidermal keratinocytes or melanocytes is warranted to detect mosaicism or other chromosomal anomalies. For suspected complications, patients may need to be referred to specialists such as an orthopedist, nephrologist, cardiologist, endocrinologist, and dentist. Radiographic examination may be needed to study musculoskeletal abnormalities. Electrocardiograms (EKGs) are required for patients suspected of cardiac abnormalities. It has also been suggested to screen all patients using renal functional and structural tests.

Magnetic resonance imaging (MRIs) and electroencephalograms (EEGs) are justified to characterize structural and neurophysiologic abnormalities upon clinical manifestations. White matter abnormalities are commonly found in MRIs of HI patients. In a 1996 study by Ruggieri et al., MRI findings included increased signal abnormalities in the parietal periventricular and subcortical white matter of both hemispheres in T_2-weighted images. These white matter anomalies are similar to those found in other neurocutaneous syndromes. Electroencephalograms (EEGs) can show focal discharges and slowing, but there has been no consistent finding in HI patients.

GENETICS OF HI

In earlier literature and case reviews, many modes of inheritance were proposed but none have been proven. Recent publications have supported the idea that HI is a phenotype of chromosomal mosaicism. In almost all reported cases, HI occurs sporadically. Using karyotype analysis of blood, skin fibroblasts, epidermal keratinocytes, or melanocytes, many patients have been found to have chromosomal mosaicism. Yet, there is no consistent pattern, as mosaicism has been found in both autosomal and sex chromosomes. Sporadic X:autosome translocations involving

Xp11 have also been found in some girls suffering from HI symptoms. Some authors believe this translocation causes a functional disomy. While some individuals' karyotypes have appeared normal, it is thought there could be mosaicism at the molecular level or minor abnormalities that have gone undetected. Until the genetics of HI are further delineated, physicians should offer families genetic counseling. In addition, when parents of an affected child are considering additional pregnancies, a chromosomal analysis of the affected child and/or the parents is warranted to confirm that the risk of another affected child is extremely low.

DIFFERENTIAL DIAGNOSIS

Hypomelanosis of Ito can be difficult to diagnose but careful examination can differentiate HI from similar disorders. The fourth stage of incontinentia pigmenti (IP) can often be confused with HI because of the presence of linear hypopigmented skin lesions. However, hypopigmentation in HI is not preceded by inflammatory, bullous skin lesions as in IP. A more common neurocutaneous disorder, tuberous sclerosis, is characterized by multiple hypomelanotic, ash leaf-shaped lesions. Nevus depigmatosus is a cutaneous disorder with localized, nonlinear congenital lesions without any of the associated extracutaneous symptoms seen in HI. Vitiligo is a pigment disorder caused by the absence of melanocytes, producing decreased pigmentation in patches of skin. The lesions do not follow the lines of Blaschko and may appear well after birth. The extracutaneous symptoms associated with HI are not commonly seen.

TREATMENT

Treatment for HI is symptomatic. The skin lesions require no special treatment, and individuals do not have to take extra precautions with sun exposure. For individuals without additional neurologic manifestations, an annual follow-up appointment is recommended. The hypopigmented lesions tend to darken with time.

Children with HI and neurologic complications will benefit from special education services. Dentists can frequently treat abnormalities of the teeth. Surgery, corrective glasses, vision therapy, and medication may help some of the ophthalmologic conditions seen in HI.

Patients suffering from seizures may benefit from antiepileptic drugs. Valproate, carbamazepine, and phenytoin are first-line therapies in the treatment of generalized tonic–clonic seizures. First choice drugs for partial seizures include carbamazepine, phenytoin, primidone, phenobartital, and valproate. Treatment of infantile spasms is discussed elsewhere in this book. Almost 30% of patients with HI have refractory epilepsy.

PROGNOSIS

There is extreme variation in the clinical features expressed in patients with HI. There are no published series on natural history of disease so it is difficult to precisely state the prognosis. As many as 70% of affected individuals in reported series have isolated cutaneous abnormalities. However, because of ascertainment bias in clinical series, the true prevalence of brain disease is unknown. A minority suffers from mental retardation and seizures and may depend on another person for self-care. Parents should be reassured that this is rare and that most severe complications are detected early in life.

SUMMARY

HI is a rare neurocutaneous disorder most likely caused by chromosomal mosaicism. HI patients may suffer from numerous clinical manifestations but the expression of the disease is highly variable. There is no systemic treatment for the disorder, except for symptomatic management. Hopefully, further investigation into the genetics of HI will lead to a more tailored approach to treatment.

SUGGESTED READINGS

1. Kuster W, Konig A. Hypomelanosis of Ito: no entity, but a cutaneous sign of mosaicism. Am J Med Gen 1999; 85:346–350.
2. Pascual-Castroviejo I, Roche C, Martinez-Bermejo A, Arcas J, Lopez-Martin V, Tendero A, Esquiroz J, Pascual-Pascual S. Hypomelanosis of Ito: a study of 76 infantile cases. Brain Dev 1998; 20:36–43.
3. Ruggieri M, Pavone L. Hypomelanosis of Ito: clinical syndrome or just phenotype. J Child Neurol 2000; 15:635–644.
4. Ruggieri M, Tigano G, Mazzone D, Tine A, Pavone L. Involvement of the white matter in hypomelanosis of Ito (incontinentia pigmenti achromiens). Neurology 1996; 46:485–492.
5. Ruiz-Maldonado R, Toussaint S, Tamayo L, Laterza A, del Castillo V. Hypomelanosis of Ito: diagnostic criteria and report of 41 cases. Pediatr Dermatol 1992; 9:1–10.

PATIENT RESOURCES

1. H.I.T.S. (UK) (Hypomelanosis of Ito Family Support Network). C/O Terri Grant, Saskatchewan, 99 Great Cambridge Rd, London, Intl N17 7LN, United Kingdom. Tel.: +44-7940-114943; fax: +(44)-208-352-1824; E-mail: tgrant@hitsuk.freeserve.co.uk; Internet: http://www.e-fervour.com/hits.
2. Epilepsy Foundation. 4351 Garden City Drive, Landover, MD 20785, U.S.A. Tel.: +1 301-459-3700; fax: +1 301-577-2684, Tel.: +1 800-332-1000, TDD: +1 800-332-2070, E-mail: postmaster@efa.org, Internet: http://www.epilepsyfoundation.org.

Index

Milton Keynes UK
Ingram Content Group UK Ltd.
UKHW052028071024
449327UK00027B/2477